Oxford Textbook of

Stroke and Cerebrovascular Disease

Oxford Textbook of
Stroke and Cerebrovascular Disease

Edited by

Bo Norrving
Professor in Neurology
Department of Clinical Sciences
Section of Neurology
Lund University
Lund, Sweden

Series Editor
Christopher Kennard

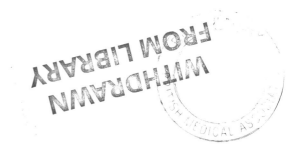
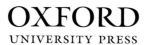
OXFORD
UNIVERSITY PRESS

OXFORD
UNIVERSITY PRESS

Great Clarendon Street, Oxford, OX2 6DP,
United Kingdom

Oxford University press is a department of the University of Oxford.
It furthers the University's objective of excellence in research, scholarship,
and education by publishing worldwide. Oxford is a registered trade mark of
Oxford University press in the UK and in certain other countries

© Oxford University Press 2014

The moral rights of the authors have been asserted

First Edition published in 2014

Impression: 1

Published in the United States of America by Oxford University Press
198 Madison Avenue, New York, NY 10016, United States of America

British Library Cataloguing in Publication Data
Data available

Library of Congress Control Number: 2013952006

ISBN 978–0–19–964120–8

Printed in China by
C&C Offset Printing Co. Ltd

Foreword

Stroke has always been a worldwide problem, but only now is it being recognized as a global, treatable, and preventable condition, largely through scientific advances and the work of stroke leaders such as the contributors to this volume.

Knowledge accrues in pieces but is understood in patterns. The internet has made information available in unprecedented quantities, but of uneven value. Bits and bytes of information are but a few clicks away. However, these pieces have to be put in patterns, in context, and we need to recognize the fact that we still know much less than we need to know, hence the need for a comprehensive, credible, and accessible book.

Bo Norrving and his international cast of authors offer such a volume. In addition to the usual chapters on anatomy, pathophysiology, diagnosis, treatment, and rehabilitation, there are chapters on the increasingly recognized areas of silent infarcts and microbleeds, vascular cognitive impairment and dementia, and the long-term management of stroke. As a former President of the World Stroke Organization, the editor has led efforts to put stroke at the forefront of global health policy by working with the World Health Organization and the United Nations. This enlarged vision of stroke is reflected in a chapter on primary stroke prevention and one on healthcare services, topics that do not usually feature in books on stroke.

May this book enjoy the broad readership that it deserves.

Vladimir Hachinski, CM, MD, FRCPC, DSc,
Dr. honoris causa X5
President, World Federation of Neurology

Preface

Stroke is huge by any measure: often cited data from the Global Burden of Disease project are that there are 6 million deaths due to stroke per year worldwide, 15 million cases of stroke per year, and 30 million persons who have survived a stroke. Other stroke measures are one new stroke every other second, every sixth second stroke kills someone, and one in six will have a stroke during their lifetime. Such numbers have different meanings to different stakeholders. For the patient who has developed a stroke, and for the carers, such data are of little interest (more than possibly telling that 'you are in good company, welcome to the club')—my own stroke is more than enough for me. For health personnel the figures are more alarming: how can we take good care of so many patients, do we have the beds at the stroke unit (and is there a stroke unit at all?), are there rehabilitation and follow-up resources available? Who can do the job, who have the right education and competence? For health administrators, healthcare planners, and politicians the numbers should be alarming: what are the precise numbers in my country or region? What is the trend? What can be done (and what can I do) to help and to prevent stroke? And, will the numbers affect the financial situation in my community?

Fortunately the stroke scene is changing—the Cinderella tale being a good analogy of what has happened. Only a few decades ago (when I started in neurology as my first summer job) stroke had the lowest priority at the emergency department because there was no hurry and nothing could be done acutely. Stroke units were unheard of—at my local hospital there was even a hospital agreement by which patients who were impossible to rehabilitate (definition: age 65 years and above) were outsourced to various other departments (dermatology, renal disease, oncology . . .) so that the burden of stroke to the hospital could be shared. Patients used to stay in bed for 1–2 weeks before any mobilization took place. Heparin treatment was widely used to prevent or treat progressing stroke whereas antiplatelets and statins were unknown at that time. Carotid surgery was performed by thoracic surgeons with rates of serious complication well above 10%. Any ultra-early therapy was regarded as doomed to fail since science told us that brain cells could not survive more than 5–10 minutes of ischaemia. Looking back, I have some difficulties understanding why stroke nevertheless caught my interest and attracted me.

Readers of this preface need not be told in detail what has happened during the last few decades: the introduction of acute neuroimaging and other diagnostic tools, the demonstration of acute thrombolytic therapy as one of medicine's best buys, the glory of organized stroke care (including early mobilization), the development of secondary prevention strategies that have changed the prognosis after stroke drastically, and the demonstration that rehabilitation works—just to mention a few of the groundbreaking changes that have taken place. There has also been an avalanche of knowledge of mechanisms, causes, unusual features, stroke subtypes, and genetics. Advances in science have had a profound impact on clinical practice in stroke.

Another major change is a focus on stroke prevention through joint actions with other non-communicable diseases (NCDs) that share similar risk factors. Stroke is not acting alone in this movement, but is part of the NCD cluster that has rightfully received high governmental attention during the last few years. Stroke shares many risk factors with heart disease, peripheral vascular disease, cancer, dementia, and pulmonary disease—just to mention a few members of the NCD family.

The World Stroke Organization emphasizes three pillars in the Global Agenda for Stroke: prevention, acute care, and long-term management. The latter component has been particularly neglected and warrants much more attention in the future. Few areas in medicine have such broad outreach, involve so many sectors of healthcare, and have such a profound influence on public health as stroke.

For this book I have had the privilege of working together with many of today's most outstanding stroke scientists. I am grateful to all of you for sharing your deep knowledge, and for making yourselves available for the task. I take this opportunity to thank you all most warmly for your contributions to this volume. I also thank the very large number of people in the scientific stroke community, within the World Stroke Organization and regional stroke organizations, who have provided me with inspiration for the present work.

I would also like to thank the staff at Oxford University Press for expert help and support in making this book available. My thanks go to Peter Stevenson who set me the task initially, to Eloise Moir-Ford for keeping track of all manuscript versions and chapter status, to Papitha Ramesh and Nic Williams for copy editing, and to the many other people at Oxford University Press who have been involved with this book. It has been a pleasure working with you.

Finally, my thanks to my wife Lena and my three children (David, Marcus, and Maria) for having been (quite) tolerant of the intrusion of my out-of-usual-business-hours' work into family pleasures and duties.

It is my hope that the book will be read, will be disseminated broadly, and will finally lead to benefits for patients and carers.

Only at the latter stage has a textbook like this one served its ultimate purpose.

Bo Norrving
Lund, Sweden
October 2013

Contents

List of Abbreviations *xi*

List of Contributors *xiii*

1 **Epidemiology of stroke** *1*
Valery Feigin and Rita Krishnamurthi

2 **Risk factors** *9*
Arne Lindgren

3 **Arteries and veins of the brain: anatomical organization** *19*
Laurent Tatu, Fabrice Vuillier, and Thierry Moulin

4 **Pathophysiology of transient ischaemic attack and ischaemic stroke** *35*
Jong S. Kim

5 **Pathophysiology of non-traumatic intracerebral haemorrhage** *51*
Constanza Rossi and Charlotte Cordonnier

6 **Spontaneous intracranial subarachnoid haemorrhage: epidemiology, causes, diagnosis, and complications** *61*
Laurent Thines and Charlotte Cordonnier

7 **Clinical features of transient ischaemic attacks** *79*
David Calvet and Jean-Louis Mas

8 **Clinical features of acute stroke** *85*
José M. Ferro and Ana Catarina Fonseca

9 **Diagnosing transient ischaemic attack and stroke** *94*
Bruce Campbell and Stephen Davis

10 **Management of stroke: general principles** *106*
Mehmet Akif Topcuoğlu and Hakan Ay

11 **Acute phase therapy in ischaemic stroke** *124*
Krassen Nedeltchev and Heinrich P. Mattle

12 **Acute management and treatment of intracerebral haemorrhage** *130*
Marek Sykora, Jennifer Diedler, and Thorsten Steiner

13 **Acute treatment in subarachnoid haemorrhage** *139*
Katja E. Wartenberg

14 **Less common causes of stroke: diagnosis and management** *153*
Turgut Tatlisumak, Jukka Putaala, and Stephanie Debette

15 **Secondary prevention of stroke** *163*
Thalia S. Field and Oscar R. Benavente

16 **Prognosis after stroke** *185*
Vincent Thijs

17 **Silent cerebral infarcts and microbleeds** *194*
Bo Norrving

18 **Complications after stroke** *203*
Hanne Christensen, Elsebeth Glipstrup, Nis Høst, Jens Nørbæk, and Susanne Zielke

19 **Vascular cognitive impairment and dementia** *215*
Didier Leys, Kei Murao, and Florence Pasquier

20 **Brain repair after stroke** *225*
Steven C. Cramer

21 **Rehabilitation after stroke** *234*
Katharina Stibrant Sunnerhagen

22 **The long-term management of stroke** *243*
Reza Bavarsad Shahripour and Geoffrey A. Donnan

23 **Primary prevention of stroke** *255*
Anna M. Cervantes-Arslanian and Sudha Seshadri

24 **Organized stroke care: Germany and Canada** *270*
Silke Wiedmann, Peter U. Heuschmann, and Michael D. Hill

Index *279*

List of Abbreviations

ACA	anterior cerebral artery	DVT	deep vein thrombosis
ACE	angiotensin-converting enzyme	DWI	diffusion-weighted imaging
AChA	anterior choroidal artery	ECG	electrocardiogram
ACoA	anterior communicating artery	eGFR	estimated glomerular filtration rate
ADL	activities of daily living	ESO	European Stroke Organisation
ADL	Alzheimer disease	EVD	extraventricular drain
AF	atrial fibrillation	FDA	Food and Drug Administration
AHA	American Heart Association	FFP	fresh frozen plasma
AICA	anterior inferior cerebellar artery	FHS	Framingham Heart Study
ARB	angiotensin receptor blocker	FLAIR	fluid attenuated inversion recovery
ARER	absolute risk reduction	GABA	gamma-aminobutyric acid
ASA	American Stroke Association	GOS	Glasgow Outcome Scale
AUC	area under the curve	GOS	Glasgow Outcome Scale
AVM	arteriovenous malformation	GRE	gradient echo
BI	Barthel Index	HANAC	hereditary angiopathy with nephropathy, aneurysm, and muscle cramps
CAA	cerebral amyloid angiopathy	HDL	high-density lipoprotein
CADASIL	cerebral autosomal dominant arteriopathy with subcortical infarcts and leucoencephalopathy	HERNS	hereditary endotheliopathy with retinopathy, nephropathy, and stroke
CARASIL	cerebral autosomal recessive arteriopathy with subcortical infarcts and leucoencephalopathy	HR	hazard ratio
CAS	carotid angioplasty and stenting	IA	intra-arterial
CBV	cerebral blood volume	IAT	intra-arterial thrombolysis
CEA	carotid endarterectomy	ICH	intracerebral haemorrhage
CEAD	cervical artery dissection	IDR	incidence density ratio
CEAD	carotid endarterectomy	IHD	ischaemic heart disease
CHS	Cardiovascular Health Study	INR	international normalized ratio
CMB	cerebral microbleed	IST	International Stroke Trial
CNS	central nervous system	ITT	intention-to-treat
CSF	cerebrospinal fluid	LDL	low-density lipoprotein
CT	computed tomography	LP	lumbar puncture
CTV	computed tomography venography	LUTS	lower urinary tract symptoms
CVD	cerebrovascular disease	MAP	mean arterial pressure
CVT	cerebral venous thrombosis	MCA	middle cerebral artery
DALY	disability-adjusted life year	MET S	metabolic syndrome
DAVF	dural arteriovenous fistula	MMSE	Mini Mental State Examination
DCI	delayed cerebral ischaemia	MoCA	Montreal Cognitive Assessment
DNR	do not resuscitate	MRI	magnetic resonance imaging
DOAC	direct oral anticoagulant	mRS	modified Rankin Scale
DSA	digital subtraction angiography	MRV	magnetic resonance venography

MTT	mean transit time	rtPA	recombinant tissue plasminogen activator
NCD	non-communicable disease	SAH	subarachnoid haemorrhage
NG	nasogastric	SCA	superior cerebellar artery
NHS	Nurses' Health Study	SCD	sickle cell disease
NICC	neurocritical care unit	SCI	silent cerebral infarct
NIHSS	National Institutes of Health Stroke Scale	SCM	silent cerebral microbleed
NINDS	National Institute of Neurological Disorders and Stroke	SDB	sleep-disordered breathing
		SD	standard deviation
NMDA	N-methyl-D-aspartate	SES	socioeconomic status
NOAC	novel oral anticoagulant	SIADH	syndrome of inappropriate secretion of antidiuretic hormone
NVAF	non-valvular atrial fibrillation		
OCSP	Oxfordshire Community Stroke Project	SITCH	Surgical Trial in Intracerebral Haemorrhage
OHS	Oxford Handicap Score	SLE	systemic lupus erythematosus
PAR	population attributable risk	SNP	single-nucleotide polymorphism
PbtO$_2$	partial pressure of cerebral tissue oxygen	SWI	susceptibility-weighted imaging
PCA	posterior cerebral artery	TBI	traumatic brain injury
PCC	prothrombin complex concentrate	TCS	Takotsubo cardiomyopathy syndrome
PChA	posterior choroidal arteries	Tmax	time to maximum
PE	pulmonary embolus	TOAST	Trial of Org 10172 in Acute Stroke Treatment
PEG	percutaneous endoscopic gastrostomy	TOF	time-of-flight
PET	positron emission tomography	tPA	tissue plasminogen activator
PFO	patent foramen ovale	TTP	time to peak
PHS	Physicians' Health Study	UK	United Kingdom
PICA	posterior inferior cerebellar artery	US	United States
PoCA	posterior communicating artery	VaD	vascular dementia
PRN	*pro re nata* (as needed)	VCI	vascular cognitive impairment
PSD	post-stroke dementia	WFNS	World Federation of Neurological Surgeons Scale
RCVS	reversible cerebral vasoconstriction syndrome	WHO	World Health Organization
RR	relative risk	WHS	Women's Health Study
RRR	relative risk reduction	WML	white matter lesion

List of Contributors

Hakan Ay Stroke Service, Department of Neurology, A.A. Martinos Center for Biomedical Imaging, Department of Radiology, Massachusetts General Hospital, Harvard Medical School, Boston, MA, USA

Oscar R. Benavente Stroke and Cerebrovascular Health, Vancouver Stroke Program, Brain Research Center, Department of Medicine, Division of Neurology, University of British Columbia, Vancouver, Canada

David Calvet Paris Descartes University, Centre de Psychiatrie et Neurosciences INSERM UMR 894, and Department of Neurology, Centre Hospitalier Sainte-Anne, Paris

Bruce Campbell Department of Neurology, Royal Melbourne Hospital, University of Melbourne, Parkville, Australia

Anna M. Cervantes-Arslanian Boston University Department of Neurology, Boston, MA, USA

Hanne Christensen Department of Neurology, Bispebjerg Hospital, Copenhagen, Denmark

Charlotte Cordonnier Department of Neurology and Stroke Unit, Université Lille Nord de France, Lille, France

Steven C. Cramer Departments of Neurology and Anatomy & Neurobiology, University of California, Irvine, Irvine, CA, USA

Stephen Davis President, World Stroke Organization; Director, Neuroscience and Continuing Care Service; Director, Melbourne Brain Centre at RMH; Director of Neurology, The Royal Melbourne Hospital, Melbourne, Australia

Stephanie Debette Université de Versailles Saint-Quentin-en-Yvelines, France; and Inserm U740, Université Paris, Paris, France; and Department of Neurology, Lariboisière University Hospital, DHU Neurovasc Sorbonne Paris-Cité, Paris, France; and Department of Neurology, Boston University School of Medicine, The Framingham Heart Study, Boston, MA, USA

Jennifer Diedler Department of Neurology, University of Heidelberg, Heidelberg, Germany

Geoffrey A. Donnan Florey Institute of Neuroscience and Mental Health, University of Melbourne, Parkville, Australia

Valery Feigin National Institute for Stroke and Applied Neurosciences, Faculty of Health & Environmental Sciences AUT University, Auckland, New Zealand

José M. Ferro Department of Neurosciences, Hospital de Santa Maria, University of Lisbon, Lisbon, Portugal

Thalia S. Field Vancouver Stroke Program, Brain Research Center, Department of Medicine, Division of Neurology, University of British Columbia, Vancouver, Canada

Ana Catarina Fonseca Department of Neurology, Hospital de Santa Maria, Lisboa, Portugal

Elsebeth Glipstrup Mental Health Services, Bispebjerg Hospital, Copenhagen, Denmark

Nis Høst Department of Cardiology, Bispebjerg Hospital, Copenhagen, Denmark

Peter U. Heuschmann Institute of Clinical Epidemiology and Biometry, University of Würzburg, Würzburg, Germany

Michael D. Hill Calgary Stroke Program, Department of Clinical Neurosciences, Hotchkiss Brain Institute, University of Calgary, Calgary, Canada

Jong S. Kim University of Ulsan, College of Medicine, Seoul, South Korea; and Stroke Center, Asan Medical Center, Seoul, South Korea

Rita Krishnamurthi National Institute for Stroke and Applied Neurosciences, Faculty of Health & Environmental Sciences, AUT University, Auckland, New Zealand

Didier Leys Université Lille Nord de France, Lille, France

Arne Lindgren Department of Neurology Lund, Skåne University Hospital, Lund, Sweden

Jean-Louis Mas Paris Descartes University, Centre de Psychiatrie et Neurosciences INSERM UMR 894 and Department of Neurology, Centre Hospitalier Sainte-Anne, Paris, France

Heinrich P. Mattle Department of Neurology, Inselspital, Bern, Switzerland

Thierry Moulin Service de Neurologie 2,Centre Hospitalier Universitaire, Université de Franche-Comté, Besançon, France

Kei Murao Université Lille Nord de France, Lille, France

Krassen Nedeltchev Triemli Hospital, Zurich, Switzerland

Jens Nørbæk Mental Health Services, Bispebjerg Hospital, Copenhagen, Denmark

Bo Norrving Department of Clinical Sciences, Section of Neurology, Lund University, Lund, Sweden

Florence Pasquier Université Lille Nord de France, Lille, France

Jukka Putaala Department of Neurology, Helsinki University Central Hospital, Helsinki, Finland

Constanza Rossi Department of Neurology and Stroke Unit, University of Lille Nord de France, Lille, France

Sudha Seshadri Boston University Department of Neurology, Boston, MA, USA

Reza Bavarsad Shahripour Florey Institute of Neuroscience and Mental Health, University of Melbourne, Parkville, Australia

Thorsten Steiner Department of Neurology, University of Heidelberg, Heidelberg, Germany; and Department of Neurology, Klinikum Frankfurt Höchst, Frankfurt, Germany

Katharina Stibrant Sunnerhagen Department of Clinical Neurosciences, University of Gothenburg, Institute of Neuroscience and Physiology, Sweden

Marek Sykora Department of Neurology, University of Heidelberg, Heidelberg, Germany; and Department of Neurology, Comenius University, Bratislava, Slovakia

Laurent Tatu Laboratoire d'Anatomie, UFR Sciences médicales et pharmaceutiques, Université de Franche-Comté, Besançon, France; and Service d'Explorations et pathologies neuro-musculaires, Centre Hospitalier Universitaire, Université de Franche-Comté, Besançon, France

Turgut Tatlisumak Department of Neurology, Helsinki University Central Hospital, Helsinki, Finland

Vincent Thijs Department of Neurology, University Hospitals Leuven, Leuven, Belgium

Laurent Thines Division of Neurosurgery, Department of Neurosciences and Locomotive System, Lille University Hospital, Lille, France

Mehmet Akif Topcuoğlu Hacettepe University Hospitals, Department of Neurology, Ankara, Turkey

Fabrice Vuillier Laboratoire d'Anatomie, UFR Sciences médicales et pharmaceutiques, Université de Franche-Comté, Besançon, France; and Service de Neurologie 2, Centre Hospitalier Universitaire, Université de Franche-Comté, Besançon, France

Silke Wiedmann Institute of Clinical Epidemiology and Biometry, University of Würzburg, Würzburg, Germany

Katja E. Wartenberg Neurocritical Care Unit, Department of Neurology, Martin-Luther-University Halle-Wittenberg, Halle (Saale), Germany

Susanne Zielke Department of Neurology, Bispebjerg Hospital, Copenhagen, Denmark

CHAPTER 1

Epidemiology of stroke

Valery Feigin and Rita Krishnamurthi

Introduction

Stroke is the second most common cause of death worldwide and a frequent cause of adult disability in developed countries (1, 2). Stroke burden on families and society is projected to rise from approximately 38 million disability-adjusted life years (DALYs) lost globally in 1990 to 61 million DALYs in 2020 (3) due to population ageing. Stroke also has a large physical, psychological, and financial impact on patients/families, the healthcare system, and society (4, 5). Lifetime costs per stroke patient range from US$59,800 to US$230,000 (5). The majority (about 75%) of cases of stroke occur in people over the age of 65 years (6, 7), and about one-third of patients die of stroke within a year of onset (8, 9). Over half of survivors remain dependent on others for everyday activities, often with significant adverse effects on caregivers (10). Many factors increase the risk of stroke, and these are generally divided into two categories: modifiable and non-modifiable risk factors. Age, gender, and ethnicity are non-modifiable risk factors for stroke. Modifiable or potentially modifiable risk factors include a number of physiological and environmental factors and include hypertension, elevated total cholesterol, smoking, physical inactivity, alcohol consumption, and atrial fibrillation (11).

Stroke mortality data are available from more than 24 countries (12, 13) showing that, in general, rates have declined for several decades. In some countries, stroke mortality has declined since the early 1950s, but the rate of this decline has recently slowed (14–17). While large national or international stroke mortality data may be used for determining overall burden of fatal strokes and trends in stroke mortality, stroke mortality data are often not accurate (diagnosis classification bias) and have limited value for healthcare planning and organization. The role of changes in incidence and improved survival to downward trend in stroke mortality are not adequately quantified, chiefly due to difficulties in measuring stroke incidence accurately (18, 19); however the results from the World Health Organization (WHO) Monitoring Trends and Determinants in Cardiovascular Disease (MONICA) project suggested that both declining and increasing stroke mortality were principally attributable to changes in case fatality rather than changes in incidence (20).

Importance of population-based studies

Epidemiological studies form the basis of much of the medical research and current knowledge in stroke to inform health professionals about best strategies for stroke care organization,

prevention, and management. The gaps in knowledge in stroke prevention and management are continually filled by randomized control trials, case–control, and cohort studies (see Table 1.1). Some of the most informative studies on stroke burden and optimal healthcare organization have arisen from population-based stroke incidence and outcome studies. It is important that stroke is seen and studied in a population context, as a large proportion of the burden of care for stroke is borne outside the hospital sector (11–13). Further, changes in referral patterns can distort longitudinal trends derived from hospitalized cases. Assessing the need for prevention strategies and services is best achieved via population-based stroke registers to determine incidence and outcome (13).

Data on population trends in stroke incidence reflect the success/failure of prevention strategies, while trends in case fatality and outcome reflect changes in stroke management. Both are needed to plan stroke services given high healthcare costs and limited resources. Accurate and representative population-based data are also crucial to: (i) determine the true incidence, causes and outcome of stroke; (ii) implement evidence-based healthcare planning, across the care spectrum; (iii) evaluate the need for and impact of preventative/management strategies; (iv) address persistent uncertainty about what key factors (socioeconomic and health service) impact stroke recovery; (v) examine the natural course of recovery, in particular for cognitive and behavioural outcomes; (vi) provide information on access and satisfaction with stroke services; and (vii) identify service gaps/unmet needs to ensuring evidence-based policy, resource allocation, prevention planning, management services, and evaluation of service performance.

Assessing the need for prevention strategies and services is most sensitively achieved with the use of population-based registers to determine the incidence and outcome of stroke. However, studying stroke in a population-based fashion is particularly challenging (19), so that such epidemiological studies are relatively rare compared with studies using mortality data, hospital-based stroke registers, or incidence studies in younger age groups only.

In 1987, Malmgren et al. (23) published a list of 12 criteria related to definitions, methods, and mode of data presentation, by which the quality of population-based studies of stroke could be judged. These criteria have been updated by Sudlow et al. (19) in 1997 and most recently by Feigin et al. (Table 1.2) (24, 25).

However, these criteria are so demanding in practice that even the stroke component of the WHO MONICA project is generally regarded as having failed to meet them (18). Even among many registers that are population based, many were limited to people under the age of 75 years, yet only half of all strokes occur in these age groups. Although 'ideal' stroke incidence studies based on both core

Table 1.1 Common epidemiological terms

Term	Definition	Comments
Incidence	The number of new cases of a disease that occur over a specified period of time	The incidence rate is a measure of morbidity (illness) and can be looked at in any population group such as males, persons exposed to a particular chemical toxin, etc.
Attack rate	A measure of how fast a disease is occurring in a population	Attack rates tell us how many new cases of a disease occur over a specific period of time
Prevalence	The proportion of the population affected by a disease at that time	Prevalence is calculated by dividing the number of people who have the disease by the number of people in the community. It provides a snapshot of who has the disease at that point in time and does not take into account the duration of the disease
Mortality	A measure of the proportion of deaths over a specific time period in a given population	Mortality is measured in the entire population at risk from dying from the disease, including both those who have and do not have the disease
Case-fatality	A measure of the proportion of deaths over a specific period of time in individuals with a specified disease	Case-fatality is a measure of the severity of that disease. In contrast to mortality, case-fatality is limited to those who already have the disease
Population attributable risk (PAR)	A measure of the proportion of disease incidence in a total population that can be attributed to a specific exposure	The PAR tells us the extent to which the elimination of a particular exposure would reduce the incidence rate of a particular disease in the whole population
Disability-adjusted life year (DALY)	Years of life lost to premature death and years lived with a disability of a specified severity and duration	DALYs are a means of expressing the overall burden of a disease. Each DALY is 1 lost year of healthy life
Randomized clinical trial (RCT)	A type of study design used to evaluate a particular intervention usually for the treatment or prevention of a disease. The subjects are randomly allocated to either the treatment (e.g. the test drug) or control (e.g. no treatment) group	An RCT can be used to study the effectives of a new drug to treat a condition compared to another drug or no treatment at all. In a 'double-blind' RCT both the subjects in the study and the researcher measuring the outcome are unaware of the allocation of the treatment groups, thus reducing bias
Cohort studies	A population with an exposure and a population without the exposure are followed to compare an outcome of interest between the groups	Typically, the study population must be followed up for a long period of time for the outcome of interest to develop. A well-known example is the Framingham study (21)
Case–control studies	A study design aimed to examine the possible relation of an exposure to a certain disease. A group with the disease (cases) is compared with a group without the disease (controls)	If there is an association of an exposure with a disease, there should be a higher prevalence of the exposure in the cases than in the controls

Adapted from Gordis (22).

and supplementary criteria (24, 25) are the most valuable source of information for developing evidence-based strategies for stroke prevention and health services, to address the problem of accurate and comparable stroke incidence studies in less affluent countries with limited resources where most strokes occur, a WHO stepwise stroke surveillance approach (26) can be recommended (Figure 1.1).

An alternative approach for studying stroke incidence and prevalence in countries with very limited resources could include a combination of a stroke prevalence survey (e.g. door-to-door study) with a study of death certificates (verbal autopsy procedures) in the same community (Figure 1.2), as recently recommended by Feigin (27).

Stroke burden in high-income countries

Historically, information on stroke incidence, prevalence, early case-fatality came predominantly from studies in high-income countries. In addition, long-term trends in stroke incidence in different populations are not well characterized, largely due to difficulties of population-based stroke surveillance (19, 28, 29). However recent studies in mid- to low-income countries

have allowed comparisons in stroke burden and current trends. A recent systematic review of worldwide stroke incidence and early case-fatality (29) found that over the last four decades (1970–2008) there was a statistically significant 42% decrease in stroke incidence rates (1.1% annual reduction) in high-income countries (Figure 1.3A), with the more pronounced reduction in people younger than 75 years and in people with ischaemic stroke. This decrease may be attributable to the effective implementation of preventative measures and management of risk factors in these populations.

However, in low- to middle-income countries stroke incidence rates for the same time period have increased by over 100% and currently exceed those in high-income countries. It was also shown that the risk of stroke is increasing with the age of the population in developed countries (Figure 1.4) (30). The reasons for this difference are unclear, but are a matter of great importance for two main reasons: (i) stroke is a leading cause of disability in adults and (ii) the elderly (the most stroke-prone age group) constitute the fastest-growing segment of the population.

Currently (2000–2008), proportional frequency of ischaemic stroke, intracerebral haemorrhage, and subarachnoid haemorrhage

Table 1.2 Gold standards for an 'ideal' stroke incidence study

Domains	Core criteria	Supplementary criteria
Standard definitions	• World Health Organization definition of stroke • At least 80% CT/MRI verification of the diagnosis of ischaemic stroke, intracerebral haemorrhage, and subarachnoid haemorrhage[a] • First-ever-in-a-lifetime stroke	• Classification of ischaemic stroke into subtypes (e.g. large artery disease, cardioembolic, small artery disease, other)[a] • Recurrent stroke[a]
Standard methods	• Complete, population-based case ascertainment, based on multiple overlapping sources of information (hospitals, outpatient clinics, general practitioners, death certificates)[b] • Prospective study design • Large, well-defined and stable population, allowing at least 100,000 person-years of observation[b] • Follow-up of patients' vital status for at least 1 month[a] • Reliable method for estimating denominator (not more than 5 years old census data)[b]	• Ascertainment of patients with TIA, recurrent strokes and those referred for brain, carotid or cerebral vascular imaging[a] • 'Hot pursuit' of cases • Direct assessment of under-ascertainment[a] by regular checking of general practitioners' databases and hospital admissions for acute vascular problems and cerebrovascular imaging studies and/or interventions
Standard data presentation	• Complete calendar years of data; not more than 5 years of data averaged together[b] • Men and women presented separately • Mid-decade age bands (e.g. 55–64 years) used in publications, including oldest age group (≥85 years)[b] • 95% confidence interval around rates	• Unpublished 5-year age bands available for comparison with other studies

[a] New criteria.
[b] Updated, modified from Sudlow and Warlow (19).
Reprinted from Feigin and Carter (25) with permission.

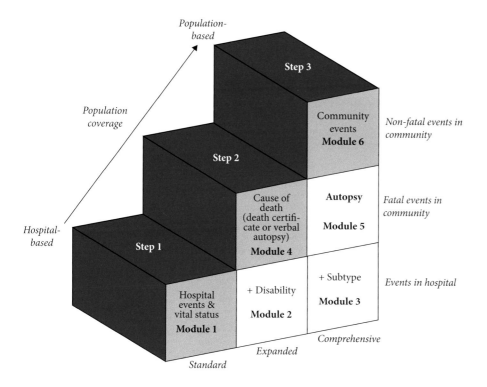

Fig. 1.1 STEP-wise approach to stroke surveillance. (Adapted from Truelsen et al. (24) with permission.)

in high-income countries were estimated as 82%, 11%, and 3%, respectively (29). Early (1-month) case fatality in high-income countries has decreased over the last four decades from 35.9% to 19.8%, potentially due to improved management of acute strokes, and possibly a shift towards less severe strokes. Overall, case-fatality within 1 month of stroke onset in high-income countries is currently about 23% and is higher for intracerebral haemorrhage (42%) and subarachnoid haemorrhage (32%) than for ischaemic stroke (16%) (30).

A recent systematic review of population-based stroke incidence and prevalence studies showed the age-standardized prevalence of stroke in people aged 65 years and older ranges worldwide from 46–72 per 1000 population (Figure 1.5) (30). Stroke makes a significant contribution to disability burden in low- and middle-income

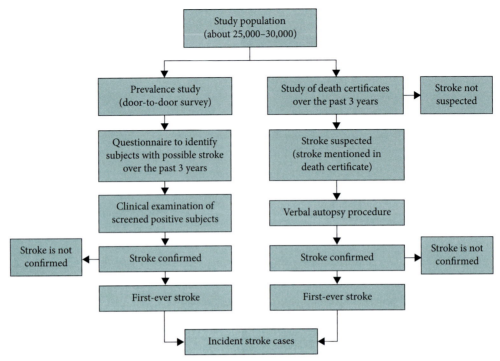

Fig. 1.2 An alternative approach for studying stroke epidemiology in resource-poor countries. (Reprinted from Feigin (25) with permission.)

countries (31), and the recent 2010 Global Burden of Disease Project ranked stroke as the fifth highest cause of DALYs worldwide in 2010 (an increase of 19% from 1990) (32). In terms of global variation, stroke burden was shown to be higher in China, Africa, and South America, and lower national income was associated with higher relative mortality and burden of stroke (33).

Stroke burden in low- to middle-income countries

One of the major challenges in stroke epidemiology is the lack of good-quality epidemiological studies in developing countries (34). According to WHO estimates, death from stroke in developing (low- and middle-income) countries in 2001 accounted for 85.5% of stroke deaths worldwide (35), and the number of DALYs, which comprises years of life lost and years lived with disability (35), in these countries was almost seven times that in developed (high-income) countries (4, 27).

Recent meta-analysis of population-based stroke incidence studies (29) showed that unlike high-income countries, the incidence of stroke in low- to middle-income countries has increased by 100% over the last four decades (1970–2008) (Figure 1.3B). Stroke incidence rates in low- to middle-income countries increased with increasing age in a similar manner to high-income countries (Figure 1.6).

Although ischaemic stroke is the dominating stroke pathological type all over the world, the proportional frequency of intracerebral haemorrhage in low- to middle-income countries tends to be noticeably greater than that in high-income countries (Figure 1.7) (29).

There is evidence from recent studies that the risk factors for stroke in middle- to low-income countries are similar to that in high-income countries, including high blood pressure, smoking, and obesity, although the relative significance of stroke risk factors in high- and low- to middle-income countries may be different (see Chapter 2). The increase in stroke incidence in low- to middle-income counties may be attributed to the poor management of these risk factors. While early case fatality is similar to that of high-income countries, the decrease in early case fatality is not as high as that in high-income countries.

Gender and ethnic differences in stroke burden

There are notable gender and ethnic differences in stroke incidence and outcomes both in high- and mid- to low-income countries. Both socioeconomic and ethnic differences in the risk of stroke have been seen in many countries (36–39). For example, higher risks have been observed among Maori and Pacific people in New Zealand (40, 41), and in the black populations in the United States (36) and United Kingdom (37), compared to the white population. Higher stroke attack rates in lower socioeconomic groups are probably related to several factors. As a general rule, lower socioeconomic groups are more frequently exposed to risk factors for cardiovascular disease, including hypertension, smoking, diabetes, and excessive consumption of alcohol (42). In addition, it has been suggested that lower socioeconomic groups have less access to, or make less effective use of, services that are important to the management of these risk factors, such as early detection and control of hypertension (43). Similarly, many of the ethnic differences in stroke risk have been attributed to differences in socioeconomic circumstances and exposure to risk factors (43). However, studies of cardiovascular disease have found that not all of the differences in attack rates among ethnic groups can be explained by differences

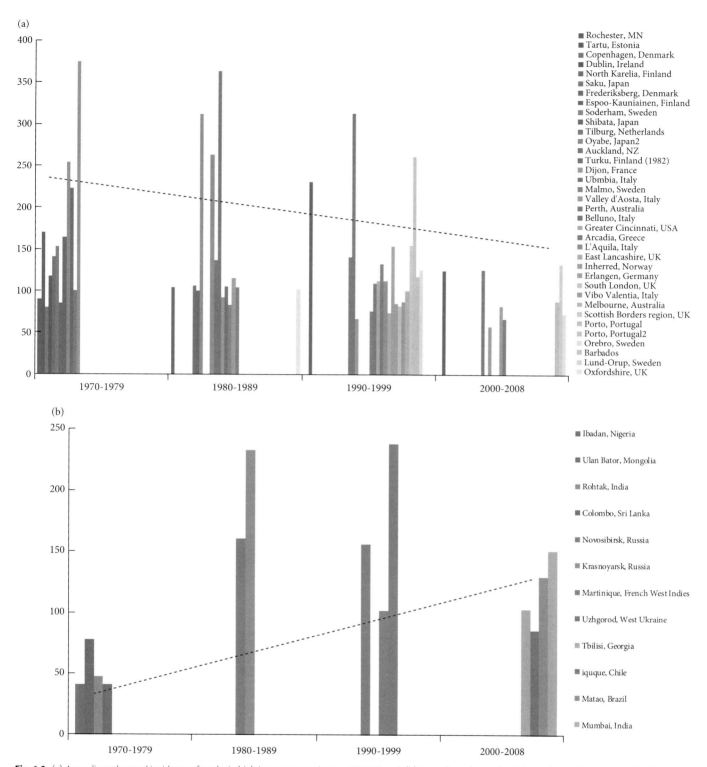

Fig. 1.3 (a) Age-adjusted annual incidence of stroke in high income countries per 100,000/year*. (b) Age-adjusted annual incidence of stroke in low to middle income countries 100,000/year*. (Reprinted from Feigin et al. (13) with permission.)

in conventional cardiovascular risk factors, suggesting genetic and other factors are important (44). Thus, there remains considerable uncertainty regarding the relative importance of stroke risk factor management and control and other factors in the aetiology of these inequalities.

There is also some evidence suggesting ethnic differences in stroke outcomes. In a recent prospective population-based study of 1127 patients with acute stroke in Auckland, New Zealand the risk of dependency, as measured by Frenchay Activities, at 6 months post-stroke was higher in non-Europeans (Asian and Pacific

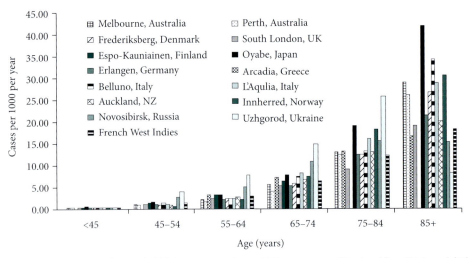

Fig. 1.4 Age-specific stroke incidence rates in selected, primarily high income countries per 1000-person-years. (Reprinted from Feigin et al. (13) with permission.)

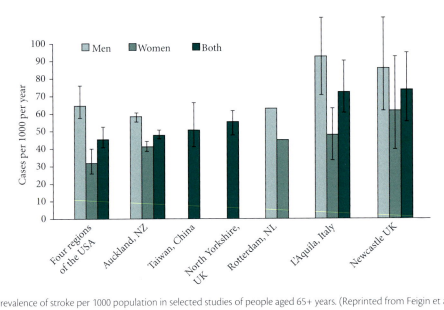

Fig. 1.5 Age-standardized prevalence of stroke per 1000 population in selected studies of people aged 65+ years. (Reprinted from Feigin et al. (26) with permission.)

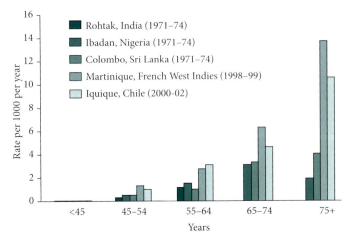

Fig. 1.6 Age-specific annual incidence of first-ever-in-lifetime stroke per 1000 population in selected developing countries. (Reprinted from Feigin (26) with permission.)

people) compared to Europeans (after adjustment for casemix variables) (45). Measures of handicap and quality of life were also worse in non-Europeans. Some ethnic differences particularly in stroke outcomes may be attributable to socioeconomic status and accessibility to healthcare, and/or to a higher prevalence of risk factors in some ethnic groups.

Additionally, there are gender differences in stroke. The lifetime risk of stroke in women (one in five) is greater than in men (one in six) (46). This higher risk is primarily due to the greater life expectancy of women. Worldwide evidence of better outcomes in male stroke survivors is accumulating (47–51), yet reasons for these gender differences in stroke outcomes are also unclear. Recent research shows poorer functional outcomes and quality of life post stroke in women are not due to differences in age, pre-stroke function, and comorbidities (47). As women often have their stroke later in relation to men they are also usually the most important family caregivers (52). Their state of health can affect the health and well-being of other family members and demands placed upon

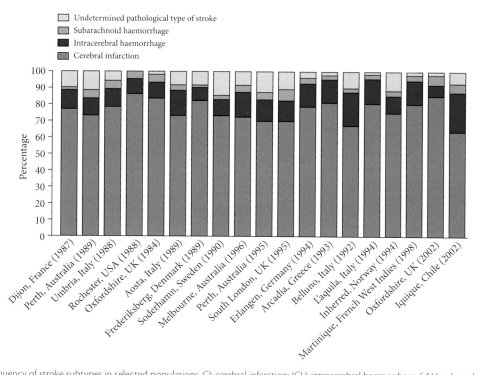

Fig. 1.7 Proportional frequency of stroke subtypes in selected populations. CI: cerebral infarction; ICH: intracerebral haemorrhage; SAH: subarachnoid haemorrhage; UND: undetermined pathological type of stroke. (Modified from Feigin (13) with permission.)

them in providing care to men and others within their social network can also increase their risk of stroke (52, 53). A study of stroke incidence in women showed that two-thirds of women with stroke were not partnered compared with one-third of men (52). Due to their greater life expectancy, more elderly women are likely to be living alone, thus there is a greater risk of the need for institutionalized care after stroke. More intensive treatment/rehabilitation may be needed to improve outcomes for women, along with further research to explore underlying biological mechanism of gender differences in outcome (51). Accurate population-based data on gender and ethnic differences in stroke burden and service use will facilitate implementation of evidence-based recommendations to bridge gaps in health services and increase uptake of lifestyle changes in ethnic and sex groups (39).

Suggested public health strategies to reduce the global stroke burden

The global stroke burden, particularly in low- to middle-income countries is likely to reach epidemic proportions if current trends continue. In developing countries, there has been a shift towards urbanization driven by social and economic changes. This has led to changes towards poorer diet and lifestyle choices thus increasing the prevalence of risk factors, including smoking. With increasing life expectancy leading to older populations, the burden of stroke will become a major cause for concern unless urgent action is taken to implement population-based prevention at local government and international levels.

For stroke prevention programmes to be effective, they should be designed with an understanding of the independent relative risk, prevalence, independent population attributable risk, and adaptation of proven measures to modify or control the specific risk factor

(54, 55). Public health strategies to reduce global stroke burden include increasing public stroke awareness, increasing awareness of stroke risk factors, and the importance and effectiveness of prevention. Additionally, local and national government bodies need to take responsibility to improve lifestyle factors, for example, by making fresh fruits and vegetables more affordable. Ways to reduce tobacco use and reduce dietary salt intake must be explored and implemented to reduce stroke risk. There is sufficient evidence for effective strategies for stroke prevention (see Chapter 22); the challenge now is to apply this knowledge effectively to reduce the burden of stroke globally.

References

1. Johnston SC, Mendis S, Mathers CD. Global variation in stroke burden and mortality: estimates from monitoring, surveillance, and modelling. *Lancet Neurol.* 2009;8(4):345–354.
2. Rothwell PM. The high cost of not funding stroke research: a comparison with heart disease and cancer. *Lancet.* 2001;357(9268): 1612–1616.
3. Mackay J, Mensah GA. *The Atlas of Heart Disease and Stroke.* Geneva: World Health Organization; 2004.
4. Strong K, Mathers C, Bonita R. Preventing stroke: saving lives around the world. *Lancet Neurology.* 2007 Feb;6(2):182–187.
5. Caro JJ, Huybrechts KF, Duchesne I. Management patterns and costs of acute ischemic stroke: an international study. *Stroke.* 2000 Mar;31(3):582–590.
6. Bonita R, Anderson CS, Broad JB, Jamrozik KD, Stewart-Wynne EG, Anderson NE. Stroke incidence and case fatality in Australasia. A comparison of the Auckland and Perth population-based stroke registers. *Stroke.* 1994 Mar;25(3):552–557.
7. Bonita R, Broad JB, Beaglehole R. Changes in stroke incidence and case-fatality in Auckland, New Zealand, 1981-91. *Lancet.* 1993;342(8885):1470–1473.

8. Anderson CS, Jamrozik KD, Broadhurst RJ, Stewart-Wynne EG. Predicting survival for 1 year among different subtypes of stroke. Results from the Perth Community Stroke Study. *Stroke*. 1994;25(10): 1935–1944.

9. Bonita R, Ford MA, Stewart AW. Predicting survival after stroke: a three-year follow-up. *Stroke*. 1988;19(6):669–673.

10. Anderson CS, Linto J, Stewart-Wynne EG. A population-based assessment of the impact and burden of caregiving for long-term stroke survivors. *Stroke*. 1995 May;26(5):843–849.

11. Straus SE, Majumdar SR, McAlister FA. New evidence for stroke prevention: scientific review. *JAMA*. 2002 Sep;288(11):1388–1395.

12. Bonita R, Stewart A, Beaglehole R. International trends in stroke mortality: 1970-1985. *Stroke*. 1990 Jul;21(7):989–992.

13. Thom TJ. Stroke mortality trends. An international perspective. *Ann Epidemiol*. 1993 Sep;3(5):509–518.

14. Bonita R, Beaglehole R. *Primary prevention of cardiovascular disease in older New Zealanders: a report to the National Health Committee*. Wellington, New Zealand: National Advisory Committee on Health and Disability; 1998.

15. Australia NHFo. *Heart Facts: 1995*. Canberra, Australia: National Heart Foundation; 1997.

16. Stroke: a looming epidemic? *Australian Family Physician*. 1997;26: 1137–1143.

17. Gillum RF, Sempos CT. The end of the long-term decline in stroke mortality in the United States? *Stroke*. 1997 Aug;28(8):1527–1529.

18. Bonita R, Beaglehole R. Monitoring stroke. An international challenge. *Stroke*. 1995 Apr;26(4):541–542.

19. Sudlow CLM, Warlow CP. Comparing stroke incidence worldwide: what makes studies comparable? *Stroke*. 1996 Mar;27(3):550–558.

20. Sarti C, Stegmayr B, Tolonen H, Mahonen M, Tuomilehto J, Asplund K. Are changes in mortality from stroke caused by changes in stroke event rates or case fatality? Results from the WHO MONICA Project. *Stroke*. 2003;34(8):1833–1840.

21. Wolf PA, D'Agostino RB, Belanger AJ, Kannel WB. Probability of stroke: a risk profile from the Framingham Study. *Stroke*. 1991 Mar;22(3):312–318.

22. Gordis L. *Epidemiology* (4th edn). Oxford: Elsevier Limited; 2009.

23. Malmgren R, Bamford J, Warlow C, Sandercock P, Slattery J. Projecting the number of patients with first ever strokes and patients newly handicapped by stroke in England and Wales. *BMJ*. 1989;298(6674):656–660.

24. Feigin V, Hoorn SV. How to study stroke incidence. *Lancet*. 2004;363(9425):1920.

25. Feigin VL, Carter K. Stroke incidence studies one step closer to the elusive gold standard? *Stroke*. 2004;35(9):2045–2047.

26. Truelsen T, Bonita R, Jamrozik K. Surveillance of stroke: a global perspective. *Int J Epidemiol*. 2001;30(Suppl):S11–S6.

27. Feigin VL. Stroke in developing countries: can the epidemic be stopped and outcomes improved? *Lancet Neurol*. 2007 Feb;6(2):94–97.

28. Anderson CS, Carter KN, Hackett ML, Feigin V, Barber PA, Broad JB, et al. Trends in stroke incidence in Auckland, New Zealand, during 1981 to 2003. *Stroke*. 2005;36(10):2087–2093.

29. Feigin VL, Lawes CM, Bennett DA, Barker-Collo SL, Parag V. Worldwide stroke incidence and early case fatality reported in 56 population-based studies: a systematic review. *Lancet Neurol*. 2009;8(4):355–369.

30. Feigin VL, Lawes CM, Bennett DA, Anderson CS. Stroke epidemiology: a review of population-based studies of incidence, prevalence, and case-fatality in the late 20th century. *Lancet Neurol*. 2003;2(1):43–53.

31. Sousa RM, Ferri CP, Acosta D, Albanese E, Guerra M, Huang Y, et al. Contribution of chronic diseases to disability in elderly people in countries with low and middle incomes: a 10/66 Dementia Research Group population-based survey. *Lancet*. 2009 Nov 28;374(9704):1821–1830.

32. Murray CJL, Vos T, Lozano R, Naghavi M, Flaxman AD, Michaud C, et al. Disability-adjusted life years (DALYs) for 291 diseases and injuries in 21 regions, 1990–2010: a systematic analysis for the Global Burden of Disease Study 2010. *Lancet*. 2012 Dec;380(9859):2197–223.

33. Kim AS, Johnston SC. Global variation in the relative burden of stroke and ischemic heart disease. *Circulation*. 2011 Jul;124(3):314–323.

34. Feigin VL. Stroke epidemiology in the developing world. *Lancet*. 2005;365(9478):2160–2161.

35. Mathers CD, Lopez AD, Murray CJL. *The burden of disease and mortality by condition: data, methods, and results for 2001. In Lopez AD, Mathers CD, Ezzati M, Jamison DT, Murray CJL (eds) Global Burden of Disease and Risk Factors (pp. 45–240)*. New York: Oxford University Press; 2006.

36. Sacco RL, Boden-Albala B, Gan R, Chen X, Kargman DE, Shea S, et al. Stroke incidence among white, black, and Hispanic residents of an urban community: the Northern Manhattan Stroke Study. *Am J Epidemiol*. 1998;147(3):259–268.

37. Stewart JA, Dundas R, Howard RS, Rudd AG, Wolfe CD. Ethnic differences in incidence of stroke: prospective study with stroke register. *BMJ*. 1999;318(7189):967–971.

38. van Rossum CT, van de MH, Breteler MM, Grobbee DE, Mackenbach JP. Socioeconomic differences in stroke among Dutch elderly women: the Rotterdam Study. *Stroke*. 1999 02;30(2):357–362.

39. Feigin VL, Rodgers A. Ethnic disparities in risk factors for stroke: what are the implications? *Stroke*. 2004;35(7):1568–1569.

40. Bonita R, Broad JB, Beaglehole R. Ethnic variations in stroke incidence and case fatality: the Auckland Stroke study. *Stroke*. 1997;28:758–761.

41. Feigin V, Carter K, Hackett M, Barber PA, McNaughton H, Dyall L, et al. Ethnic disparities in incidence of stroke subtypes: Auckland Regional Community Stroke Study, 2002–2003. *Lancet Neurol*. 2006;5(2):130–139.

42. Kaplan GA, Keil JE. Socioeconomic factors and cardiovascular disease: a review of the literature. *Circulation*. 1993 Oct;88(4:Pt 1):1973–1998.

43. Casper M, Wing S, Strogatz D, Davis CE, Tyroler HA. Antihypertensive treatment and US trends in stroke mortality, 1962 to 1980. *Am J Public Health*. 1992 Dec;82(12):1600–1606.

44. Anand SS, Yusuf S, Vuksan V, Devanesen S, Teo KK, Montague PA, et al. Differences in risk factors, atherosclerosis, and cardiovascular disease between ethnic groups in Canada: the Study of Health Assessment and Risk in Ethnic groups (SHARE). *Lancet*. 2000;356(9226):279–284.

45. Rose SB, Lawton BA, Elley CR, Dowell AC, Fenton AJ. The 'Women's Lifestyle Study', 2-year randomized controlled trial of physical activity counselling in primary health care: rationale and study design. *BMC Public Health*. 2007;7:166.

46. Seshadri S, Beiser A, Kelly-Hayes M, Kase CS, Au R, Kannel WB, et al. The lifetime risk of stroke: estimates from the Framingham Study. *Stroke*. 2006;37(2):345–350.

47. Reeves MJ, Bushnell CD, Howard G, Gargano JW, Duncan PW, Lynch G, et al. Sex differences in stroke: epidemiology, clinical presentation, medical care, and outcomes. *Lancet Neurology*. 2008 Oct;7(10):915–926.

48. Kapral MK, Fang J, Hill MD, Silver F, Richards J, Jaigobin C, et al. Sex differences in stroke care and outcomes: results from the Registry of the Canadian Stroke Network. *Stroke*. 2005 Apr;36(4):809–814.

49. Appelros P, Stegmayr B, Terent A. Sex differences in stroke epidemiology: a systematic review. *Stroke*. 2009 Apr;40(4): 1082–1090.

50. Feigin VL. [Climatologic aspect of the epidemiology of acute cerebral circulatory disorders (review)]. *Zhurnal Nevropatologii i Psikhiatrii Imeni S S Korsakova*. 1984;84(9):1406–1412.

51. The New Zealand Adult Nutrition Survey. *Methodology Report for the 2008/09 New Zealand Adult Nutrition Survey*. Wellington: University of Otago and Ministry of Health 2011.

52. Dyall L, Carter K, Bonita R, Anderson C, Feigin V, Kerse N, et al. Incidence of stroke in women in Auckland, New Zealand. Ethnic trends over two decades: 1981–2003. *N Z Med J*. 2006;119(1245):U2309.

53. Kerr AJ, Broad J, Wells S, Riddell T, Jackson R. Should the first priority in cardiovascular risk management be those with prior cardiovascular disease? *Heart*. 2009 Feb;95(2):125–129.

54. Chen L, Rogers SL, Colagiuri S, Cadilhac DA, Mathew TH, Boyden AN, et al. How do the Australian guidelines for lipid-lowering drugs perform in practice? Cardiovascular disease risk in the AusDiab Study, 1999-2000. *Med J Aust*. 2008 Sep;189(6):319–322.

55. Whisnant JP. Modeling of risk factors for ischemic stroke. The Willis Lecture. *Stroke*. 1997 09;28(9):1840–1844.

CHAPTER 2

Risk factors

Arne Lindgren

Introduction

It is of great importance to identify the risk factors for stroke and to what extent these different risk factors contribute to the general as well as the individual risk burden for stroke. The term risk factor has been used since the 1960s (1). A risk factor has been defined as a factor (trait) associated with a pathological medical condition. However, such an association is not sufficient to establish a factor to be a risk factor. A specific trait may be seen in individuals after disease onset but its occurrence does not prove that this caused the disease. For example, if hypertension is often seen in stroke patients, does this necessarily mean that hypertension is the cause of stroke, or could possibly hypertension be the result of the stroke instead? Because of this, prospective cohort studies are often needed to identify risk factors. If a factor observed before stroke onset can be related to stroke occurring later in life, this indicates that this factor may indeed be a risk factor. However, some factors may be analysed also after stroke onset without this caveat, especially factors that are not influenced by the disease onset, e.g. gender and variations in the human genome. An additional proof that a trait is actually a risk factor for stroke is if treatment of the trait leads to a reduced incidence of stroke. The amount of influence a specific risk factor has on risk is often measured as relative risk, odds ratio (OR), hazard ratio, and population attributable risk (PAR) (Table 2.1).

PAR is the portion of risk for a disease caused by a specific factor. The numerical value of the PAR indicates how much of the disease that would be avoided if the risk factor could be completely eliminated. Therefore it is related to absolute risk for a specific factor.

Interestingly, even though ischaemic heart disease (IHD), stroke, and peripheral artery disease are all arterial diseases, the importance of risk factors influencing these conditions seem to vary. Thus hypertension is most important for stroke whereas lipid alterations seem to be more important for myocardial infarction (Figure 2.1) (4).

Risk factors for ischaemic arterial cerebrovascular disease

Non-modifiable factors

Birth weight

Low birth weight is reported to be associated with increased stroke risk in adult life (5). Even after adjustment for childhood socioeconomic factors the risk of vascular disease in adulthood may remain (6). A relation between low birth weight and higher blood pressure (BP) in adults has been observed (7). The relation between low birth weight and stroke may be more pronounced for haemorrhagic

stroke (8). It could be suggested that the birth weight is, from a population perspective, a modifiable risk factor if taking the nutritional situation of the mother during pregnancy into account.

Gender

Male gender increases the risk for ischaemic stroke (9, 10). The risk of stroke for men is about 1.3 times as high as for women at a given age except in the highest ages (Figure 2.2). However, this gender difference is less evident when taking the number of risk factors in each individual into account (11). Early menopause has been associated with increased stroke risk (12) and after menopause several vascular risk factors become more prevalent in women (10). The difference in risk between the genders seems to disappear in high age over 80–85 years of age (9). The gender risk is different for subarachnoid haemorrhage where the risk is higher for women (13).

Age

Stroke incidence increases markedly with age (Figure 2.2) (9, 14, 15). This steep increase in stroke incidence by age is observed in both men and women. In the OXVASC study, the rate of stroke increased from 1.76 per 1000 individuals per year for individuals aged 55–64 years to 16.47 for those aged 85 or more (14). The increased incidence with age is seen for ischaemic stroke (16) as

Table 2.1 Different terms used for describing influence of risk. For details, see (2, 3)

Term	Definition
Absolute risk	Risk in absolute number, e.g. if the risk is 1/100 for stroke if the person has a trait and 1/200 if the person does not have the trait
Relative risk	Relative comparison between two situations, e.g. if the risk is 1/100 for the person with the trait and 1/200 for the person without the train—then the relative risk is 2
Odds ratio	Used in, e.g. retrospective case–control studies to estimate relative risk. Calculated as the odds of having a disease if having the trait divided by the odds of not having the disease if having the trait
Hazard ratio	Used for comparing survival in two different groups during a specific studied time period. The observed number divided by expected number in group 1 is compared (divided) by the observed number divided by expected number in group 2
Population attributable risk	Proportion of risk for a disease caused by a specific factor. Indicates how much of the disease that could be avoided if the risk factor was not present

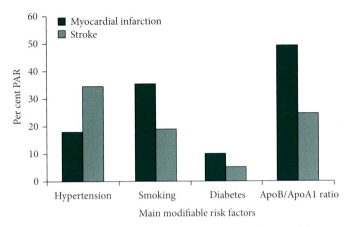

Fig. 2.1 Degree of influence of some risk factors for stroke and myocardial infarction. (Endres M, Heuschmann PU, Laufs U, Hakim AM. Primary prevention of stroke: Blood pressure, lipids, and heart failure. Eur Heart J. 2011;32:545–552)

well as for intracerebral haemorrhage (ICH) (17) and also to some extent for subarachnoid haemorrhage (18). The risk of stroke more than doubles with each decade of increased age after 55 years of age at least up to age 84 (16, 19, 20). Also after age 84, the stroke risk continues to increase (19).

Ethnicity

There are considerable variations in stroke incidence between different ethnic groups. People of African origin have a higher risk of all stroke types compared with Caucasians. This risk is at least 1.2 times higher and even higher for ICH (21). It is possible that this can in part be explained by poorer management of treatable risk factors. The proportion of ICH is higher (about 28%) among Chinese than among Caucasians (22). This increased proportion may remain also after emigration to Western countries; in one study 24% of reported strokes were of haemorrhagic type (23). It has also been reported that in ischaemic stroke, the prevalence of intracranial artery stenosis is more frequent in East Asians (24, 25) and African Americans (26) than in Caucasians.

Familiar/genetic causes (specific or polygenetic)

Even after accounting for all established risk factors there seems to be an increased risk of stroke among some families. This and other observations have led to the conclusion that some inherited factors

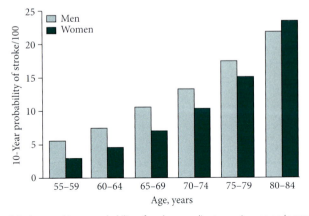

Fig. 2.2 Average 10-year probability of stroke according to age in men and women per 100 (%). (Wolf PA, Belanger AJ, D'Agostino RB. Quantifying stroke risk factors and potentials for risk reduction. Cerebrovasc Dis. 1993;3(Suppl 1):7–14.)

may contribute to the risk of stroke. The heritability of ischaemic stroke when using genome-wide association study data has been calculated as 37.9% overall, ranging from 40.3% for large vessel disease to 32.6% for cardioembolic and 16.1% for small vessel disease (27).

Several rare stroke syndromes have been associated with monogenetic variations, e.g. CADASIL (cerebral autosomal dominant arteriopathy with subcortical infarcts and leucoencephalopathy; *NOTCH3* gene) (28), CARASIL (cerebral autosomal recessive arteriopathy with subcortical infarcts and leucoencephalopathy; *HTRA* gene), MELAS (mitochondrial myopathy, encephalopathy, lactic acidosis and stroke-like episodes; mitochondrial disease), HERNS (hereditary endotheliopathy with retinopathy, nephropathy, and stroke; *TREX1* gene), homocystinuria, Fabry disease (alpha galactosidase gene), Ehlers–Danlos syndrome type IV, Marfan syndrome, pseudoxanthoma elasticum, HANAC (hereditary angiopathy, nephropathy, aneurysm, and muscle cramps syndrome; *COL4A1* mutation), and other syndromes (29). Typically these syndromes include stroke or stroke-like episodes as only one of several different clinical manifestations of the syndrome in question. It should be emphasized that in some cases stroke is the presenting symptom before other symptoms that indicate the specific syndrome are seen. For details, please see Chapter 14.

Sickle cell disease (SCD) increases the risk of stroke in childhood with a prevalence of cerebral infarct of 11% at the age of 20 years (30). SCD children with increased transcranial Doppler ultrasound velocities of the middle cerebral arteries have a particularly high risk. At ages 20–30 years these patients also have a risk of cerebral haemorrhage (30). Cerebral infarcts have also been reported in other related genetic haemoglobin variations though at a lower rate compared with SCD (30). Additional details on SCD are provided in Chapter 14.

The common stroke phenotypes have been more difficult to relate to specific genetic variations. However, there are now reports emerging that certain common genotypes, especially single-nucleotide polymorphism (SNP) variations, are associated with increased risk of intermediate phenotypes that subsequently increase the risk of stroke. Such intermediate phenotypes that may be genetically influenced include hypertension, diabetes mellitus, and heart disease. One example is atrial fibrillation (AF) that has been shown to be related to genetic variations and specific types of ischaemic stroke. AF has in genome-wide association studies been related to SNPs in the *PITX* gene, the *ZHFX3* gene, and the *KCNN3* gene (31).

There are also reports of genetic variations that seem to be more directly related to common subtypes of ischaemic stroke. Typically these reports have included large international collaborations such as the International Stroke Genetics Consortium. SNP variations in the chromosome 9p21 region have been related to ischaemic stroke (32), and these associations seem more evident for the large vessel type of stroke (33). Recently, a new SNP in *HDAC9* on chromosome 7p21.1 was associated with large vessel ischaemic stroke (34). Very recently another study reported a locus on chromosome 6p21.1 related to the ischaemic stroke subtype large artery atherosclerosis (35). The Metastroke collaboration was able to confirm several of these findings (36). Also for ICH there have been reports on genetic associations. The *APOE* ε2 and ε4 alleles are mostly related to lobar ICH and likely amyloid angiopathy whereas ε4 is also, although not with the same high degree of significance, related to deep ICH (37).

Other diseases and measurable traits

Hypertension

Hypertension is the most important treatable risk factor for stroke (4). History of hypertension increases the OR to 2.6 for stroke and has a PAR of 35% (38). The individual relative risk for stroke in hypertensives may be higher—up to 8 in a group of individuals with a mean age of 47 years to develop a stroke during a 10-year follow-up period (39). Hypertension is commonly detected among stroke patients under 55 years of age (40, 41). Hypertension remains to be a stroke risk factor in the elderly and also at ages over 60 is it useful to treat hypertension to prevent stroke (42). At even higher ages the importance of hypertension as a stroke risk factor is somewhat more difficult to assess because the prevalence of hypertension is so high in these age groups (43). However, hypertension treatment seems to reduce stroke risk also in the very elderly, indicating that it is also important to control BP among these individuals (44).

Both systolic (Figure 2.3) (45) and diastolic (46) BP is of importance for stroke risk. Not only hypertension but also BP within the normal range may be a risk factor for stroke. There is no threshold for BP—also rather normal BP levels carry an increased risk of stroke (47) and a considerable proportion of strokes occur among people with high–normal BP or 'mild' hypertension (45).

A systolic BP increase of 20 mmHg or a diastolic BP increase of 10 mmHg more than doubles the risk of stroke death (47).

Not only may the BP measured at a certain time be related to stroke risk, it has been suggested that BP variability and episodic hypertension may increase the stroke risk (48). This may have implications for how BP will be measured and evaluated in the future and also influence which antihypertensive drugs are preferred.

Stroke/transient ischaemic attack

A previous stroke is a powerful risk factor of a new stroke. The risk of a new stroke varies considerably depending on the pathogenetic mechanism of the first stroke and on the simultaneous presence of other risk factors. A risk of about 9% during an average follow-up of 2.5 years, i.e. about 3.6% per year, was reported in the PROFESS trial which included patients with a mean age of 66 years (49).

Also, transient ischaemic attack (TIA) indicates an increased the risk for a subsequent stroke both in the short term and long term. In one study, the risk of stroke within 90 days of a TIA was on average 10.5% but depended on the characteristics of the TIA with higher risk among those with a TIA with weakness or speech impairment, diabetes mellitus, age over 60 years, or longer TIA duration (50).

Silent cerebral infarcts/white matter disease

Presence of silent cerebral infarcts increases the stroke risk by at least two to three times independently of other vascular risk factors (51, 52). Both periventricular and subcortical white matter hyperintensities also increase the risk of subsequent stroke, independently of the presence of silent brain infarcts (52).

Atrial fibrillation

AF is a powerful risk factor for stroke. The abnormal contractions of the atrium of the heart lead to non-laminar blood flow in the left atrium. The blood flow in the left atrial appendage also becomes disturbed and the general opinion is that the blood clots in AF usually develop in the left atrial appendage. Fragments of or the whole clot then detach from the left atrial appendage and embolize to the cerebral arteries or other parts of the arterial system.

The risk for stroke depends on whether other factors are present simultaneously with the AF. The often used $CHADS_2$ score (one point for each of: congestive heart failure, hypertension, age >75, diabetes; and 2 points for stroke or TIA) is a useful method to estimate stroke risk in patients with AF. With none of the factors mentioned in $CHADS_2$, the yearly risk of stroke in patients is on average 1.9%, with one factor present the risk is about 2.8%, and with all factors present the yearly risk is on average 18.2% (53, 54). The more recently developed CHA_2DS_2-VASc may be even more precise in determining stroke risk in AF patients (Table 2.2).

Other cardiac conditions including patent foramen ovale

There are many heart conditions that have been suggested to be associated with increased stroke risk (see Table 2.3). Some of these conditions are well established, e.g. AF (see 'Atrial fibrillation' section above), mitral valve stenosis, acute anterior transmural myocardial infarct, atrial myxoma, mechanical heart valve prosthesis in the mitral or aortic position, whereas other are considered more equivocal regarding stroke risk. The latter include patent foramen ovale (PFO), atrial septal aneurysm, mitral annulus calcifications, and others (55).

A PFO is a remaining connection between the right and left atrium of the heart. If the connection is larger and not having overlapping structures functioning as a valve the condition is instead an atrial septal defect. In both cases there is a theoretical possibility that a venous thrombus travelling as an embolus in the venous system to the heart may pass directly from the right atrium on the venous side of the heart directly to the left atrium on the arterial side of the heart and then continue to travel out into the arterial system. Another possibility that has been proposed is that a thrombus may form *in situ* in the channel that often constitutes the PFO and then detach as an embolus. The relation between PFO and the risk of ischaemic stroke has been debated. PFO is often present in the general population at a rate of about 20–25%. Therefore there is a possibility that the PFO is just a coincident finding in the stroke patient. However, some reports have indicated that among young patients with cryptogenic ischaemic stroke, PFO may be seen more

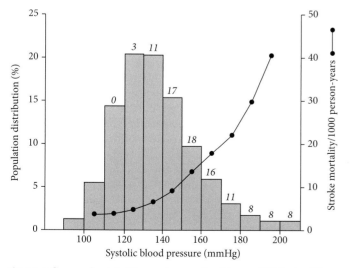

Fig. 2.3 Influence of systolic BP on stroke mortality. (Marmot MG, Poulter NR. Primary prevention of stroke. *Lancet.* 1992;339:344–347.)

Table 2.2 CHA$_2$DS$_2$VASc score and risk of stroke in patients with AF.

Risk factor-based approach expressed as a point based scoring system, with the acronym CHA$_2$DS$_2$–VASc
(Note: maximum score is 9 since age may contribute 0, 1, or 2 points)

Risk factor	Score
Congestive heart failure/LV dysfunction	1
Hypertension	1
Age ≥ 75	2
Diabetes mellitus	1
Stroke/TIA/thrombo-embolism	2
Vascular disease[a]	1
Age 65–74	1
Sex category (i.e. female sex)	1
Maximum score	9

Adjusted stroke rate according to CHA$_2$DS$_2$– VASc score

CHA$_2$DS$_2$ –VASc score	Patients (n = 7329)	Adjusted stroke rate (%/year)[b]
0	1	0%
1	422	1.3%
2	1230	2.2%
3	1730	3.2%
4	1718	4.0%
5	1159	6.7%
6	679	9.8%
7	294	9.6%
8	82	6.7%
9	14	15.2%

a. Prior myocardial infarction, peripheral artery disease, aortic plaque. Actual rates of stroke in contemporary cohorts may vary from these estimates. b. Based on Lip et al. Stroke. 2010;41:2731–2738. LV = left ventricular. Reproduced from Camm AJ, Kirchhof P, Lip GY, Schotten U, Savelieva I, Ernst S, et al. Guidelines for the management of atrial fibrillation: The task force for the management of atrial fibrillation of the European Society of Cardiology. Eur Heart J. 2010;31:2369–2429, with permission.

often than in the general population (56). It has also been discussed that the size of the PFO and a concomitant atrial septal aneurysm (defined as hypermobile part of the septum between the right and left atrium) may increase the risk of stroke (57).

Lipid changes

Serum lipid levels do not play such an important risk factor role for ischaemic stroke as for IHD (20, 58). Even so, increased cholesterol levels are related to ischaemic stroke risk, although this may differ between different pathogenetic subtypes of ischaemic stroke (58). Cholesterol levels are associated with carotid artery atherosclerosis (59) and it is therefore likely that cerebral infarcts caused by large vessel disease are more clearly related to increased cholesterol levels. Conversely, reports indicate that low cholesterol levels may increase the risk of ICH (60, 61) and observations have related intense lowering of cholesterol levels in stroke patients to a slightly

increased risk of ICH (62). The situation regarding triglyceride levels and risk of stroke is unclear (20).

Coagulation disorders

Antiphospholipid antibodies including anticardiolipin antibodies and lupus anticoagulant have been associated with ischaemic stroke. Even though the situation is complex with different assays and cut-off levels used, there is probably an increased stroke risk for patients with high levels of these antibodies (63). Several other coagulation disorders are associated with increased risk of venous thrombosis, but it is much less clear how these affect the arterial situation (63). It is possible that in some situations a coagulation disorder causing a venous thrombosis may give rise to paradoxical embolism through a PFO.

Homocysteine

Increased homocysteine levels have been observed in stroke patients (64). Even so, the importance of increased homocysteine levels for stroke risk has been debated. Two reasons for this are: (i) that the situation is complicated by the relation between homocysteine levels and other vascular risk factors, e.g. age and decreased renal function, both of which in their turn influence stroke risk; and (ii) that studies have been unable to clearly demonstrate that homocysteine lowering therapy decreases stroke risk (65).

Diabetes mellitus

Diabetes mellitus has a deteriorating effect on arterial blood vessels and is a risk factor for ischaemic stroke. The relative risk of ischaemic stroke for diabetic individuals has been estimated to be between 1.3 and 6 (20, 66). Diabetes also increases the risk of stroke recurrence (66). Lacunar infarcts may be more common in diabetic patients (67) although this has not always been reported (68). The effect of diabetes may in part be mediated by other risk factors such as hypertension and lipid alterations and it is also possible that these and other risk factors such as smoking potentiate each other.

Migraine

The relation between migraine and stroke is complex (69). Migraine and ischaemic stroke often occur in the same patients. Migraine-like symptoms may indicate another underlying disease that may cause a stroke, e.g. arteriovenous malformation, arterial dissection, CADASIL, MELAS, encephalitis, or even atherosclerosis. It is also of interest that migraine has been related to increased prevalence of white matter hyperintensities on magnetic resonance imaging. However, also in patients without migraine caused by another disease, there seems to be an increased risk of stroke, and the risk is higher for patients with migraine with aura compared with patients with migraine without aura. The risk of stroke in migraineurs may be higher in women than in men (70). The increased risk among individuals with migraine with aura has been reported to represent a relative risk of 2.27 (71). However, the individual risk in younger patients who report migraine with aura, e.g. under 45 years of age, is still low due to the low overall stroke incidence in younger ages. Migraine as a risk factor for stroke seems to interact with other risk factors such as smoking and use of oral contraceptives. The cerebral infarct supposed to be caused by migraine with aura has symptoms similar to those experienced in the aura phase. It has been suggested that a pronounced cortical spreading depression may cause local ischaemia so profound that an infarct develops. Other theories have included that the increased prevalence of PFO among

Table 2.3 Cardiac changes with possible relation to thromboembolic risk

Major potential sources	Minor potential sources
Atrial fibrillation	Patent foramen ovale
Recent (<3 months) myocardial infarct	Atrial septal aneurysm
Thrombus left atrium or ventricle	Mitral valve prolapse
Dilating cardiomyopathy (EF ≤35 %)	Severe mitral annulus calcification
Mitral stenosis	Calcific aortic stenosis
Myxoma	Spontaneous echo contrast in left atrium on echocardiography
Mechanical prosthetic valve	Other (e.g. hypokinetic left ventricular segment, bioprosthetic valve, mitral valve strands)
Infective endocarditis	
Marantic endocarditis	
Protruding aortic plaque	

Major potential source: causal relation probable. Minor potential source: sometimes over represented in stroke studies but no certain causal relation. EF = ejection fraction. Modified from reference (55).

patients with migraine with aura is a possible mechanism for the increased risk of stroke in these patients. However, this has been questioned and it is possible that this is only an epiphenomen, i.e. that migraine with aura and PFO coexist in the same patients without any additional combined mutual influence on stroke risk. For a detailed, up-to date overview about migraine and stroke, please see reference (69).

Infection

Inflammation measured as, e.g. C-reactive protein or fibrinogen levels, seem to increase the risk of stroke (72). Acute or chronic infections that precede stroke onset and cause an increased stroke risk may at least in part be mediated by inflammation (73). Chronic infections suggested to be related to stroke include agents such as *Chlamydia pneumoniae*, *Helicobacter pylori*, *Cytomegalovirus*, herpes simplex virus (HSV)-1, and HSV-2 even though the effect is perhaps more mediated by a 'total burden' of infections rather than a single agent (72). Periodontitis has also been related to stroke risk (74). It seems clear that Chagas disease causes increased risk of stroke (75). Acute infection, e.g. respiratory or urinary tract infection, may precede stroke onset and indicate increased stroke risk (73).

Obstructive sleep apnoea

Even though obstructive sleep apnoea (OSA) may increase BP and be related to obesity, there seems to be an independent stroke risk related to OSA *per se* (76). Suggested possible mechanisms include hypercoagubility, atherosclerosis, decreased cerebral blood flow, and paradoxical embolization (76). Interestingly, wake-up stroke has recently been linked to OSA (77).

Renal disease

Renal dysfunction increases the risk of stroke in individuals with known atherothrombotic disease (78). Microalbuminuria has been independently associated with stroke risk (79).

Arterial diseases

Carotid artery stenosis or occlusion is a well-known risk factor for stroke. There is a risk in individuals with asymptomatic carotid artery stenosis (80, 81) but the risk is considerably higher in patients with a symptomatic high-degree stenosis (81–83).

Aortic plaques are independent risk factors for stroke and severe aortic arch plaques have been reported to confer a risk of cerebral infarct of 10% or more in 1 year (84). Patients with asymptomatic or symptomatic peripheral arterial disease have an increased risk of stroke (85, 86). In addition, carotid artery disease is more frequently seen in patients with peripheral artery disease (85).

Several diseases with microangiopathy of the brain (87, 88) and sometimes simultaneous vascular involvement of other organs (some with, some without clinical symptoms from other organs than the brain) are related to stroke risk, e.g. CADASIL (28, 89), CARASIL (90), HERNS (91), HANAC (92), HSA (hereditary systemic angiopathy) (93), Fabry disease (94), polyarteritis nodosa (95), and other syndromes.

Other diseases

Several factors that are more uncommon in the general population are also related to stroke risk. These factors include inflammatory disease, e.g. inflammatory bowel disease, haematological disorders, cancer, and different medical or surgical procedures. Please see separate chapters in this book regarding these conditions.

Lifestyle risk factors

Several lifestyle risk factors have been related to stroke risk. A comprehensive review on this topic with both tables of relative risk and information on PAR has been given by Chiuve et al. (96). The Royal College of Physicians has provided tables of evidence that include aspects on life style factors (<http://www.rcplondon.ac.uk/sites/default/files/documents/stroke_evidence_tables_2008.pdf>, accessed 29 Oct 2013). It is of special interest that some factors have been reported as acute triggers of stroke onset (97). The following sections give a more detailed description of lifestyle and stroke risk.

Smoking

Cigarette smoking approximately doubles the risk for ischaemic stroke (38, 98–100). The situation for ICH is less clear but here smoking may also indicate an increased risk (96). There is an even more pronounced relation between cigarette smoking and risk for subarachnoid haemorrhage (101). Also, passive smoking carries a risk for stroke (98). Smoking potentiates the effect of other risk factors (20). Cigarette smoking is associated with an increased risk of atherosclerosis as well as with the risk of thrombus formation. Individuals who stop smoking reduce their risk of stroke (96, 100) by up to 50% (100).

Alcohol

Excessive alcohol consumption increases the risk of stroke. Moreover, individuals who do not use any alcohol may have a slightly increased risk (96), and a J-shaped curve for stroke risk regarding alcohol consumption has been suggested (20). It is possible that temporary heavy alcohol consumption increases the risk of immediate stroke (97).

Drug abuse

Drug abuse can cause stroke due to several pathogenetic mechanisms. Intravenous injection of a drug may be accompanied by other agents such as air or talcum powder with subsequent embolization.

Drugs or other agents administered simultaneously may cause vasculitis due to toxic or hypersensitivity reaction. Infectious agents may be injected due to non-sterile conditions and cause, e.g. infective endocarditis with subsequent cerebral embolization. The use of drugs may also unmask other pre-existing lesions such as arterial aneurysms, arteriovenous malformations, and tumours. Drugs increasing sympathetic activity such as amphetamine can cause acute BP elevation with subsequent ICH (102). Cocaine is a potent vasoconstrictor agent. Cocaine abuse has been related to both cerebral infarct and ICH (102). There are case reports of stroke related to cannabis use but a clear causative risk still remains unsettled (103). It should be mentioned that sympathomimetics and other vasoactive drugs including cannabis, cocaine, and amphetamine—as well as conventional medications with vasoactive effects—have also been associated with the reversible cerebral vasoconstriction syndrome (104).

Obesity

A body mass index (BMI) of 25 kg/m² or more in men and 30 kg/m² or more in women increases the risk of ischaemic stroke, whereas the risk for ICH does not necessarily increase by BMI increase (96). As an example, a BMI of 30.0–31.9 kg/m² in women and of 25.0–29.9 kg/m² in men carry a relative risk of 1.44 and 1.43 for ischaemic stroke, respectively. Waist:hip ratio has also been related to increased stroke risk, even after adjustment for BMI (105).

Physical activity

Physical activity decreases the risk of stroke compared with no physical activity (106). Daily exercise of at least 30 minutes decreases the relative risk of stroke to between 0.69 and 0.74 (96). Physical activity of at least 30 minutes three to five times per week has been recommended (107).

Diet

There are many components in diet and it is unclear how these influence stroke risk. Excessive salt intake is related to higher BP (108). Several diets have been related to lower stroke risk. The Alternate Healthy Eating Index (AHEI)-based diet score is based on intake of trans fat, ratio of polyunsaturated to saturated fat, ratio of chicken and fish to red meat, fruits, vegetables, soy, nuts, cereal fibre, and multivitamin use and has been related to lower risk of stroke in women (96). Fruit and vegetables may have a protective effect against both ischaemic and haemorrhagic stroke: one meta-analysis reported that individuals eating three to five servings per day had a relative risk of stroke of 0.89 compared with those consuming less fruit and vegetables (109). Fish consumption may also decrease the risk of stroke (110).

Hormone therapy (especially oral contraceptives and hormone replacement therapy)

Oral contraceptive use may confer a slightly elevated risk of ischaemic stroke (111). The results have been debated and questions such as influence on stroke risk by oestrogen dose are not clearly understood (20). However, it seems that oral contraceptive use increases the ischaemic stroke risk in females with simultaneous other stroke risk factors such as smoking, hypertension, diabetes mellitus, older age, and hypercholesterolemia (20, 112). The situation regarding risk of ICH is less clear.

Hormone replacement therapy has been related to increased risk of stroke with a relative risk of 1.29 (113). It is possible that transdermal oestrogen hormone replacement therapy carries a lower risk of stroke compared to oral oestrogens and further studies are ongoing (10).

Other drugs with hormone-like actions such as tamoxifen have also been reported to increase stroke risk (114). One review linked tamoxifen to thromboembolic events but not significantly to stroke risk (115). The stroke risk may be limited to the active tamoxifen treatment period and then decrease in the post-treatment period (116).

Stress

Self-perceived psychological stress has been associated with increased stroke risk (117) and individuals experiencing major life events have a dose–response relationship with stroke risk (118). These studies mostly refer to an increased risk in the longer perspective, but it is possible that psychological stress may be a trigger for stroke onset (97). Both negative emotions and anger seem to be more common during the last 2 hours before stroke onset than during the preceding day or year (119).

Socioeconomic factors

Both comparisons within countries and between countries indicate that low socioeconomic status is associated with increased stroke risk (120). In addition, the deficit after stroke tends to be more severe as well as the mortality ratio in stroke patients with lower socioeconomic status. Even though lower socioeconomic status is related to higher frequency of other stroke risk factors such as hypertension and physical activity, this may not be the only explanation why these individuals have an increased risk. The impact of socioeconomic status may vary by age, e.g. in one study there was a clearer association for men 40–59 years old compared to older men (121).

Interaction between different risk factors

Many individuals have more than one stroke risk factor and it is then difficult to assess how important each risk factor is. This important area is complex and it is often difficult to use different suggested score systems to evaluate how much different risk factors potentiate each other (see Chapter 23 regarding these issues). When considering secondary prevention it is also very important to consider the interaction between different risk factors.

Risk factors for intracerebral haemorrhage

Some risk factors for ICH have been discussed previously in this chapter. Hypertension and higher age are risk factors for ICH (17, 60, 123). Other risk factors include African American rather than Caucasian ethnicity and lower cholesterol or low-density lipoprotein-cholesterol levels (21, 60, 61). Frequent alcohol use and diabetes mellitus have been related to ICH (123, 124). Results regarding the influence of triglyceride levels have been equivocal (60, 123). Genetic factors and cerebral amyloid angiopathy are also of importance (see earlier in this chapter). The risk factors for ICH seem to have varying impact depending on whether the ICH is lobar or deep (124). The risk of ICH increases in patients using antiplatelet or anticoagulant medications. Cerebral microbleeds are more often seen in ICH patients than in ischaemic stroke/TIA patients (125). Please see Chapter 5 regarding further discussion on risk factors for ICH.

Risk factors for subarachnoid haemorrhage

Risk factors for subarachnoid haemorrhage are somewhat different than for ischaemic stroke. However, smoking and hypertension are also important independent risk factors for subarachnoid haemorrhage (101, 126, 127). Female gender and increased age are also risk factors (13, 18). Other suggested risk factors include alcohol consumption as well as genetic factors, and many rare causes have also been suggested (13, 127, 128). Oral contraceptive use has been proposed to be a potential risk factor (13) but a large meta-analysis could not confirm this (127).

Risk factors for cerebral venous thrombosis

The risk factors for cerebral venous thrombosis (CVT) vary considerably depending on age and gender. In the large International Study on Cerebral Vein and Dural Sinus Thrombosis, general risk factors observed included: genetic (22%) or acquired (16%) thrombophilia, haematological conditions including polycythaemia, thrombocythaemia, and anaemia (12%), and infection (12%) (129). The spectrum in females younger than 50 years with CVT was somewhat different with a prevalence of oral contraceptive use (54%), pregnancy (6%), and puerperium (14%) (129).

References

1. Kannel WB, Dawber TR, Kagan A, Revotskie N, Stokes J, 3rd. Factors of risk in the development of coronary heart disease—six year follow-up experience. The Framingham study. *Ann Intern Med.* 1961;55:33–50.
2. Altman DG. *Practical Statistics for Medical Research.* London: Chapman & Hall; 1991.
3. Uter W, Pfahlberg A. The application of methods to quantify attributable risk in medical practice. *Stat Methods Med Res.* 2001;10:231–237.
4. Endres M, Heuschmann PU, Laufs U, Hakim AM. Primary prevention of stroke: blood pressure, lipids, and heart failure. *Eur Heart J.* 2011;32:545–552.
5. Osmond C, Kajantie E, Forsen TJ, Eriksson JG, Barker DJ. Infant growth and stroke in adult life: the Helsinki birth cohort study. *Stroke.* 2007;38:264–270.
6. Johnson RC, Schoeni RF. Early-life origins of adult disease: national longitudinal population-based study of the united states. *Am J Public Health.* 2011;101:2317–2324.
7. Davies AA, Smith GD, May MT, Ben-Shlomo Y. Association between birth weight and blood pressure is robust, amplifies with age, and may be underestimated. *Hypertension.* 2006;48:431–436.
8. Hypponen E, Leon DA, Kenward MG, Lithell H. Prenatal growth and risk of occlusive and haemorrhagic stroke in Swedish men and women born 1915-29: historical cohort study. *BMJ.* 2001;323:1033–1034.
9. Wolf PA, Belanger AJ, D'Agostino RB. Quantifying stroke risk factors and potentials for risk reduction. *Cerebrovasc Dis.* 1993;3(Suppl 1):7–14.
10. Lisabeth L, Bushnell C. Stroke risk in women: the role of menopause and hormone therapy. *Lancet Neurol.* 2012;11:82–91.
11. Berry JD, Dyer A, Cai X, Garside DB, Ning H, Thomas A, et al. Lifetime risks of cardiovascular disease. *N Engl J Med.* 2012;366:321–329.
12. Lisabeth LD, Beiser AS, Brown DL, Murabito JM, Kelly-Hayes M, Wolf PA. Age at natural menopause and risk of ischemic stroke: the Framingham heart study. *Stroke.* 2009;40:1044–1049.
13. Longstreth WT, Jr, Koepsell TD, Yerby MS, van Belle G. Risk factors for subarachnoid hemorrhage. *Stroke.* 1985;16:377–385.
14. Rothwell PM, Coull AJ, Giles MF, Howard SC, Silver LE, Bull LM, et al. Change in stroke incidence, mortality, case-fatality, severity, and risk factors in Oxfordshire, UK from 1981 to 2004 (Oxford vascular study). *Lancet.* 2004;363:1925–1933.
15. Hallstrom B, Jonsson AC, Nerbrand C, Norrving B, Lindgren A. Stroke incidence and survival in the beginning of the 21st century in southern Sweden: comparisons with the late 20th century and projections into the future. *Stroke.* 2008;39:10–15.
16. Seshadri S, Wolf PA. Lifetime risk of stroke and dementia: current concepts, and estimates from the Framingham study. *Lancet Neurol.* 2007;6:1106–1114.
17. Rothwell PM, Coull AJ, Silver LE, Fairhead JF, Giles MF, Lovelock CE, et al. Population-based study of event-rate, incidence, case fatality, and mortality for all acute vascular events in all arterial territories (Oxford vascular study). *Lancet.* 2005;366:1773–1783.
18. de Rooij NK, Linn FH, van der Plas JA, Algra A, Rinkel GJ. Incidence of subarachnoid haemorrhage: a systematic review with emphasis on region, age, gender and time trends. *J Neurol Neurosurg Psychiatry.* 2007;78:1365–1372.
19. Johansson B, Norrving B, Lindgren A. Increased stroke incidence in Lund-Orup, Sweden, between 1983 to 1985 and 1993 to 1995. *Stroke.* 2000;31:481–486.
20. Goldstein LB, Bushnell CD, Adams RJ, Appel LJ, Braun LT, Chaturvedi S, et al. Guidelines for the primary prevention of stroke: a guideline for healthcare professionals from the American heart association/American stroke association. *Stroke.* 2011;42:517–584.
21. Kleindorfer D, Broderick J, Khoury J, Flaherty M, Woo D, Alwell K, et al. The unchanging incidence and case-fatality of stroke in the 1990s: a population-based study. *Stroke.* 2006;37:2473–2478.
22. Zhang LF, Yang J, Hong Z, Yuan GG, Zhou BF, Zhao LC, et al. Proportion of different subtypes of stroke in China. *Stroke.* 2003;34:2091–2096.
23. Fang J, Foo SH, Fung C, Wylie-Rosett J, Alderman MH. Stroke risk among Chinese immigrants in New York City. *J Immigr Minor Health.* 2006;8:387–393.
24. Feldmann E, Daneault N, Kwan E, Ho KJ, Pessin MS, Langenberg P, et al. Chinese-white differences in the distribution of occlusive cerebrovascular disease. *Neurology.* 1990;40:1541–1545.
25. Suh DC, Lee SH, Kim KR, Park ST, Lim SM, Kim SJ, et al. Pattern of atherosclerotic carotid stenosis in Korean patients with stroke: different involvement of intracranial versus extracranial vessels. *AJNR Am J Neuroradiol.* 2003;24:239–244.
26. Sacco RL, Kargman DE, Gu Q, Zamanillo MC. Race-ethnicity and determinants of intracranial atherosclerotic cerebral infarction. The northern Manhattan stroke study. *Stroke.* 1995;26:14–20.
27. Bevan S, Traylor M, Adib-Samii P, Malik R, Paul NL, Jackson C, et al. Genetic heritability of ischemic stroke and the contribution of previously reported candidate gene and genomewide associations. *Stroke.* 2012;43:3161–3167.
28. Chabriat H, Vahedi K, Iba-Zizen MT, Joutel A, Nibbio A, Nagy TG, et al. Clinical spectrum of cadasil: a study of 7 families. Cerebral autosomal dominant arteriopathy with subcortical infarcts and leukoencephalopathy. *Lancet.* 1995;346:934–939.
29. Cole JW, Gutwald J. Other monogenetic stroke disorders. In Sharma P, Meschia J (eds) *Stroke Genetics* (pp. 147–170). London: Springer; 2013.
30. Ohene-Frempong K, Weiner SJ, Sleeper LA, Miller ST, Embury S, Moohr JW, et al. Cerebrovascular accidents in sickle cell disease: rates and risk factors. *Blood.* 1998;91:288–294.
31. Lemmens R, Hermans S, Nuyens D, Thijs V. Genetics of atrial fibrillation and possible implications for ischemic stroke. *Stroke Res Treat.* 2011;2011:208694
32. Smith J, Melander O, Lövkvist H, Hedblad B, Engström G, Nilsson P, et al. Common genetic variants on chromosome 9p21 confers risk of ischemic stroke: a large-scale genetic association study. *Circ Cardiovasc Genet.* 2009;2:159–164.
33. Gschwendtner A, Bevan S, Cole JW, Plourde A, Matarin M, Ross-Adams H, et al. Sequence variants on chromosome 9p21.3 confer risk for atherosclerotic stroke. *Ann Neurol.* 2009;65:531–539.
34. International Stroke Genetics Consortium (ISGC); Wellcome Trust Case Control Consortium 2 (WTCCC2), Bellenguez C, Bevan S, Gschwendtner A, Spencer CC, et al. Genome-wide association study identifies a variant in HDAC9 associated with large vessel ischemic stroke. *Nat Genet.* 2012;44:328–333.
35. Holliday EG, Maguire JM, Evans TJ, Koblar SA, Jannes J, Sturm JW, et al. Common variants at 6p21.1 are associated with large artery atherosclerotic stroke. *Nat Genet.* 2012;44:1147–1151.
36. Traylor M, Farrall M, Holliday EG, Sudlow C, Hopewell JC, Cheng YC, et al. Genetic risk factors for ischaemic stroke and its subtypes (the

metastroke collaboration): a meta-analysis of genome-wide association studies. *Lancet Neurol*. 2012;11:951–962.

37. Biffi A, Sonni A, Anderson CD, Kissela B, Jagiella JM, Schmidt H, *et al*. Variants at APOE influence risk of deep and lobar intracerebral hemorrhage. *Ann Neurol*. 2010;68:934–943.

38. Hankey GJ. Stroke: fresh insights into causes, prevention, and treatment. *Lancet Neurol*. 2011;10:2–3.

39. Qureshi AI, Suri MF, Kirmani JF, Divani AA, Mohammad Y. Is prehypertension a risk factor for cardiovascular diseases? *Stroke*. 2005;36:1859–1863.

40. Putaala J, Yesilot N, Waje-Andreassen U, Pitkaniemi J, Vassilopoulou S, Nardi K, *et al*. Demographic and geographic vascular risk factor differences in European young adults with ischemic stroke: the 15 cities young stroke study. *Stroke*. 2012;43:2624–2630.

41. Rolfs A, Fazekas F, Grittner U, Dichgans M, Martus P, Holzhausen M, *et al*. Acute cerebrovascular disease in the young: the stroke in young Fabry patients study. *Stroke*. 2013;44:340–349.

42. Staessen JA, Gasowski J, Wang JG, Thijs L, Den Hond E, Boissel JP, *et al*. Risks of untreated and treated isolated systolic hypertension in the elderly: meta-analysis of outcome trials. *Lancet*. 2000;355:865–872.

43. Whisnant JP, Wiebers DO, O'Fallon WM, Sicks JD, Frye RL. A population-based model of risk factors for ischemic stroke: Rochester, Minnesota. *Neurology*. 1996;47:1420–1428.

44. Beckett NS, Peters R, Fletcher AE, Staessen JA, Liu L, Dumitrascu D, *et al*. Treatment of hypertension in patients 80 years of age or older. *N Engl J Med*. 2008;358:1887–1898.

45. Marmot MG, Poulter NR. Primary prevention of stroke. *Lancet*. 1992;339:344–347.

46. MacMahon S, Peto R, Cutler J, Collins R, Sorlie P, Neaton J, *et al*. Blood pressure, stroke, and coronary heart disease. Part 1, prolonged differences in blood pressure: prospective observational studies corrected for the regression dilution bias. *Lancet*. 1990;335:765–774.

47. Lewington S, Clarke R, Qizilbash N, Peto R, Collins R. Age-specific relevance of usual blood pressure to vascular mortality: a meta-analysis of individual data for one million adults in 61 prospective studies. *Lancet*. 2002;360:1903–1913.

48. Rothwell PM, Algra A, Amarenco P. Medical treatment in acute and long-term secondary prevention after transient ischaemic attack and ischaemic stroke. *Lancet*. 2011;377:1681–1692.

49. Sacco RL, Diener HC, Yusuf S, Cotton D, Ounpuu S, Lawton WA, *et al*. Aspirin and extended-release dipyridamole versus clopidogrel for recurrent stroke. *N Engl J Med*. 2008;359:1238–1251.

50. Johnston SC, Gress DR, Browner WS, Sidney S. Short-term prognosis after emergency department diagnosis of tia. *JAMA*. 2000;284:2901–2906.

51. Vermeer SE, Longstreth WT, Jr, Koudstaal PJ. Silent brain infarcts: a systematic review. *Lancet Neurol*. 2007;6:611–619.

52. Vermeer SE, Hollander M, van Dijk EJ, Hofman A, Koudstaal PJ, Breteler MM. Silent brain infarcts and white matter lesions increase stroke risk in the general population: the Rotterdam scan study. *Stroke*. 2003;34:1126–1129.

53. Gage BF, Waterman AD, Shannon W, Boechler M, Rich MW, Radford MJ. Validation of clinical classification schemes for predicting stroke: results from the national registry of atrial fibrillation. *JAMA*. 2001;285:2864–2870.

54. Camm AJ, Kirchhof P, Lip GY, Schotten U, Savelieva I, Ernst S, *et al*. Guidelines for the management of atrial fibrillation: the task force for the management of atrial fibrillation of the European Society of Cardiology (ESC). *Eur Heart J*. 2010;31:2369–2429.

55. Hart RG. Cardiogenic embolism to the brain. *Lancet*. 1992;339:589–594.

56. Overell JR, Bone I, Lees KR. Interatrial septal abnormalities and stroke: a meta-analysis of case-control studies. *Neurology*. 2000;55:1172–1179.

57. Mas JL, Arquizan C, Lamy C, Zuber M, Cabanes L, Derumeaux G, et al. Recurrent cerebrovascular events associated with patent foramen ovale, atrial septal aneurysm, or both. *N Engl J Med*. 2001;345:1740–1746.

58. Amarenco P, Steg PG. The paradox of cholesterol and stroke. *Lancet*. 2007;370:1803–1804.

59. Wilson PW, Hoeg JM, D'Agostino RB, Silbershatz H, Belanger AM, Poehlmann H, *et al*. Cumulative effects of high cholesterol levels, high blood pressure, and cigarette smoking on carotid stenosis. *N Engl J Med*. 1997;337:516–522.

60. Sturgeon JD, Folsom AR, Longstreth WT, Jr, Shahar E, Rosamond WD, Cushman M. Risk factors for intracerebral hemorrhage in a pooled prospective study. *Stroke*. 2007;38:2718–2725.

61. Iso H, Jacobs DR, Jr, Wentworth D, Neaton JD, Cohen JD. Serum cholesterol levels and six-year mortality from stroke in 350,977 men screened for the multiple risk factor intervention trial. *N Engl J Med*. 1989;320:904–910.

62. Amarenco P, Bogousslavsky J, Callahan A, 3rd, Goldstein LB, Hennerici M, Rudolph AE, *et al*. High-dose atorvastatin after stroke or transient ischemic attack. *N Engl J Med*. 2006;355:549–559.

63. de Lau LM, Leebeek FW, de Maat MP, Koudstaal PJ, Dippel DW. A review of hereditary and acquired coagulation disorders in the aetiology of ischaemic stroke. *Int J Stroke*. 2010;5:385–394.

64. Homocysteine studies collaboration. Homocysteine and risk of ischemic heart disease and stroke: a meta-analysis. *JAMA*. 2002;288:2015–2022.

65. Clarke R, Halsey J, Lewington S, Lonn E, Armitage J, Manson JE, *et al*. Effects of lowering homocysteine levels with b vitamins on cardiovascular disease, cancer, and cause-specific mortality: meta-analysis of 8 randomized trials involving 37 485 individuals. *Arch Intern Med*. 2010;170:1622–1631.

66. Idris I, Thomson GA, Sharma JC. Diabetes mellitus and stroke. *Int J Clin Pract*. 2006;60:48–56.

67. Arauz A, Murillo L, Cantu C, Barinagarrementeria F, Higuera J. Prospective study of single and multiple lacunar infarcts using magnetic resonance imaging: risk factors, recurrence, and outcome in 175 consecutive cases. *Stroke*. 2003;34:2453–2458.

68. Jackson CA, Hutchison A, Dennis MS, Wardlaw JM, Lindgren A, Norrving B, *et al*. Differing risk factor profiles of ischemic stroke subtypes: evidence for a distinct lacunar arteriopathy? *Stroke*. 2010;41:624–629.

69. Kurth T, Chabriat H, Bousser MG. Migraine and stroke: a complex association with clinical implications. *Lancet Neurol*. 2012;11:92–100.

70. Spector JT, Kahn SR, Jones MR, Jayakumar M, Dalal D, Nazarian S. Migraine headache and ischemic stroke risk: an updated meta-analysis. *Am J Med*. 2010;123:612–624.

71. Etminan M, Takkouche B, Isorna FC, Samii A. Risk of ischaemic stroke in people with migraine: systematic review and meta-analysis of observational studies. *BMJ*. 2005;330:63.

72. Elkind MS. Inflammatory mechanisms of stroke. *Stroke*. 2010;41:S3–8.

73. McColl BW, Allan SM, Rothwell NJ. Systemic infection, inflammation and acute ischemic stroke. *Neuroscience*. 2009;158:1049–1061.

74. Grau AJ, Becher H, Ziegler CM, Lichy C, Buggle F, Kaiser C, *et al*. Periodontal disease as a risk factor for ischemic stroke. *Stroke*. 2004;35:496–501.

75. Carod-Artal FJ, Gascon J. Chagas disease and stroke. *Lancet Neurol*. 2010;9:533–542.

76. Yaggi HK, Concato J, Kernan WN, Lichtman JH, Brass LM, Mohsenin V. Obstructive sleep apnea as a risk factor for stroke and death. *N Engl J Med*. 2005;353:2034–2041.

77. Hsieh SW, Lai CL, Liu CK, Hsieh CF, Hsu CY. Obstructive sleep apnea linked to wake-up strokes. *J Neurol*. 2012:259:1433–1439.

78. Koren-Morag N, Goldbourt U, Tanne D. Renal dysfunction and risk of ischemic stroke or tia in patients with cardiovascular disease. *Neurology*. 2006;67:224–228.

79. Lee M, Saver JL, Chang KH, Liao HW, Chang SC, Ovbiagele B. Impact of microalbuminuria on incident stroke: a meta-analysis. *Stroke*. 2010;41:2625–2631.

80. Risk of stroke in the distribution of an asymptomatic carotid artery. The European Carotid Surgery Trialists Collaborative Group. *Lancet.* 1995;345:209–212.

81. Rothwell PM. Carotid artery disease and the risk of ischaemic stroke and coronary vascular events. *Cerebrovasc Dis.* 2000;10 Suppl 5:21–33.

82. MRC European carotid surgery trial: interim results for symptomatic patients with severe (70-99%) or with mild (0-29%) carotid stenosis. European Carotid Surgery Trialists' Collaborative Group. *Lancet.* 1991;337:1235–1243.

83. North American Symptomatic Carotid Endarterectomy Trial Collaborators. Beneficial effect of carotid endarterectomy in symptomatic patients with high-grade carotid stenosis. North American symptomatic carotid endarterectomy trial collaborators. *N Engl J Med.* 1991;325:445–453.

84. Kronzon I, Tunick PA. Aortic atherosclerotic disease and stroke. *Circulation.* 2006;114:63–75.

85. Banerjee A, Fowkes FG, Rothwell PM. Associations between peripheral artery disease and ischemic stroke: implications for primary and secondary prevention. *Stroke.* 2010;41:2102–2107.

86. Criqui MH, Denenberg JO, Langer RD, Fronek A. The epidemiology of peripheral arterial disease: importance of identifying the population at risk. *Vasc Med.* 1997;2:221–226.

87. Ringelstein EB, Kleffner I, Dittrich R, Kuhlenbaumer G, Ritter MA. Hereditary and non-hereditary microangiopathies in the young. An up-date. *J Neurol Sci.* 299:81–85.

88. Yamamoto Y, Craggs L, Baumann M, Kalimo H, Kalaria RN. Review: molecular genetics and pathology of hereditary small vessel diseases of the brain. *Neuropathol Appl Neurobiol.* 37:94–113.

89. Chabriat H, Joutel A, Dichgans M, Tournier-Lasserve E, Bousser MG. Cadasil. *Lancet Neurol.* 2009;8:643–653.

90. Fukutake T. Cerebral autosomal recessive arteriopathy with subcortical infarcts and leukoencephalopathy (carasil): from discovery to gene identification. *J Stroke Cerebrovasc Dis.* 20:85–93.

91. Jen J, Cohen AH, Yue Q, Stout JT, Vinters HV, Nelson S, *et al.* Hereditary endotheliopathy with retinopathy, nephropathy, and stroke (herns). *Neurology.* 1997;49:1322–1330.

92. Alamowitch S, Plaisier E, Favrole P, Prost C, Chen Z, Van Agtmael T, *et al.* Cerebrovascular disease related to col4a1 mutations in hanac syndrome. *Neurology.* 2009;73:1873–1882.

93. Winkler DT, Lyrer P, Probst A, Devys D, Haufschild T, Haller S, *et al.* Hereditary systemic angiopathy (HSA) with cerebral calcifications, retinopathy, progressive nephropathy, and hepatopathy. *J Neurol.* 2008;255:77–88.

94. Brady RO, Schiffmann R. Clinical features of and recent advances in therapy for fabry disease. *JAMA.* 2000;284:2771–2775.

95. Reichart MD, Bogousslavsky J, Janzer RC. Early lacunar strokes complicating polyarteritis nodosa: thrombotic microangiopathy. *Neurology.* 2000;54:883–889.

96. Chiuve SE, Rexrode KM, Spiegelman D, Logroscino G, Manson JE, Rimm EB. Primary prevention of stroke by healthy lifestyle. *Circulation.* 2008;118:947–954.

97. Guiraud V, Amor MB, Mas JL, Touze E. Triggers of ischemic stroke: a systematic review. *Stroke.* 2010;41:2669–2677.

98. Bonita R, Duncan J, Truelsen T, Jackson RT, Beaglehole R. Passive smoking as well as active smoking increases the risk of acute stroke. *Tob Control.* 1999;8:156–160.

99. Shah RS, Cole JW. Smoking and stroke: the more you smoke the more you stroke. *Expert Rev Cardiovasc Ther.* 2010;8:917–932.

100. Shinton R, Beevers G. Meta-analysis of relation between cigarette smoking and stroke. *BMJ.* 1989;298:789–794.

101. Feigin V, Parag V, Lawes CM, Rodgers A, Suh I, Woodward M, *et al.* Smoking and elevated blood pressure are the most important risk factors for subarachnoid hemorrhage in the Asia-Pacific region: an overview of 26 cohorts involving 306,620 participants. *Stroke.* 2005;36:1360–1365.

102. Westover AN, McBride S, Haley RW. Stroke in young adults who abuse amphetamines or cocaine: a population-based study of hospitalized patients. *Arch Gen Psychiatry.* 2007;64:495–502.

103. Singh NN, Pan Y, Muengtaweeponsa S, Geller TJ, Cruz-Flores S. Cannabis-related stroke: case series and review of literature. *J Stroke Cerebrovasc Dis.* 2012;21:555–560.

104. Ducros A. Reversible cerebral vasoconstriction syndrome. *Lancet Neurol.* 2012;11:906–917.

105. Suk SH, Sacco RL, Boden-Albala B, Cheun JF, Pittman JG, Elkind MS, *et al.* Abdominal obesity and risk of ischemic stroke: the northern Manhattan stroke study. *Stroke.* 2003;34:1586–1592.

106. Wendel-Vos GC, Schuit AJ, Feskens EJ, Boshuizen HC, Verschuren WM, Saris WH, *et al.* Physical activity and stroke. A meta-analysis of observational data. *Int J Epidemiol.* 2004;33:787–798.

107. Galimanis A, Mono ML, Arnold M, Nedeltchev K, Mattle HP. Lifestyle and stroke risk: a review. *Curr Opin Neurol.* 2009;22:60–68.

108. He FJ, Li J, MacGregor GA. Effect of longer-term modest salt reduction on blood pressure. *Cochrane Database Syst Rev.* 2013;4:CD004937.

109. He FJ, Nowson CA, MacGregor GA. Fruit and vegetable consumption and stroke: meta-analysis of cohort studies. *Lancet.* 2006;367:320–326.

110. He K, Song Y, Daviglus ML, Liu K, Van Horn L, Dyer AR, *et al.* Fish consumption and incidence of stroke: a meta-analysis of cohort studies. *Stroke.* 2004;35:1538–1542.

111. Gillum LA, Mamidipudi SK, Johnston SC. Ischemic stroke risk with oral contraceptives: a meta-analysis. *JAMA.* 2000;284:72–78.

112. Kemmeren JM, Tanis BC, van den Bosch MA, Bollen EL, Helmerhorst FM, van der Graaf Y, *et al.* Risk of arterial thrombosis in relation to oral contraceptives (ratio) study: oral contraceptives and the risk of ischemic stroke. *Stroke.* 2002;33:1202–1208.

113. Magliano DJ, Rogers SL, Abramson MJ, Tonkin AM. Hormone therapy and cardiovascular disease: a systematic review and meta-analysis. *BJOG.* 2006;113:5–14.

114. Braithwaite RS, Chlebowski RT, Lau J, George S, Hess R, Col NF. Meta-analysis of vascular and neoplastic events associated with tamoxifen. *J Gen Intern Med.* 2003;18:937–947.

115. Nelson HD, Fu R, Griffin JC, Nygren P, Smith ME, Humphrey L. Systematic review: comparative effectiveness of medications to reduce risk for primary breast cancer. *Ann Intern Med.* 2009;151:703–715, W–226-235.

116. Rosell J, Nordenskjold B, Bengtsson NO, Fornander T, Hatschek T, Lindman H, *et al.* Time dependent effects of adjuvant tamoxifen therapy on cerebrovascular disease: results from a randomised trial. *Br J Cancer.* 2011;104:899–902.

117. Jood K, Redfors P, Rosengren A, Blomstrand C, Jern C. Self-perceived psychological stress and ischemic stroke: a case-control study. *BMC Med.* 2009;7:53.

118. Kornerup H, Osler M, Boysen G, Barefoot J, Schnohr P, Prescott E. Major life events increase the risk of stroke but not of myocardial infarction: results from the Copenhagen city heart study. *Eur J Cardiovasc Prev Rehabil.* 2010;17:113–118.

119. Koton S, Tanne D, Bornstein NM, Green MS. Triggering risk factors for ischemic stroke: a case-crossover study. *Neurology.* 2004;63:2006–2010.

120. Addo J, Ayerbe L, Mohan KM, Crichton S, Sheldenkar A, Chen R, *et al.* Socioeconomic status and stroke: an updated review. *Stroke.* 2012;43:1186–1191.

121. Grimaud O, Bejot Y, Heritage Z, Vallee J, Durier J, Cadot E, *et al.* Incidence of stroke and socioeconomic neighborhood characteristics: an ecological analysis of Dijon stroke registry. *Stroke.* 2011;42:1201–1206.

122. Graham I, Atar D, Borch-Johnsen K, Boysen G, Burell G, Cifkova R, *et al.* European guidelines on cardiovascular disease prevention in

clinical practice: Executive summary: fourth joint task force of the European Society of Cardiology and other societies on cardiovascular disease prevention in clinical practice (constituted by representatives of nine societies and by invited experts). *Eur Heart J*. 2007;28:2375–2414.

123. Zia E, Pessah-Rasmussen H, Khan FA, Norrving B, Janzon L, Berglund G, *et al*. Risk factors for primary intracerebral hemorrhage: a population-based nested case-control study. *Cerebrovasc Dis*. 2006;21:18–25.

124. Woo D, Sauerbeck LR, Kissela BM, Khoury JC, Szaflarski JP, Gebel J, *et al*. Genetic and environmental risk factors for intracerebral hemorrhage: preliminary results of a population-based study. *Stroke*. 2002;33:1190–1195.

125. Lovelock CE, Cordonnier C, Naka H, Al-Shahi Salman R, Sudlow CL, Sorimachi T, *et al*. Antithrombotic drug use, cerebral microbleeds, and intracerebral hemorrhage: a systematic review of published and unpublished studies. *Stroke*. 2010;41:1222–1228.

126. Qureshi AI, Suri MF, Yahia AM, Suarez JI, Guterman LR, Hopkins LN, *et al*. Risk factors for subarachnoid hemorrhage. *Neurosurgery*. 2001;49:607–612; Comments 612–613.

127. Feigin VL, Rinkel GJ, Lawes CM, Algra A, Bennett DA, van Gijn J, *et al*. Risk factors for subarachnoid hemorrhage: an updated systematic review of epidemiological studies. *Stroke*. 2005;36: 2773–2780.

128. van Gijn J, Kerr RS, Rinkel GJ. Subarachnoid haemorrhage. *Lancet*. 2007;369:306–318.

129. Ferro JM, Canhao P, Stam J, Bousser MG, Barinagarrementeria F. Prognosis of cerebral vein and dural sinus thrombosis: results of the international study on cerebral vein and dural sinus thrombosis (ISCVT). *Stroke*. 2004;35:664–670.

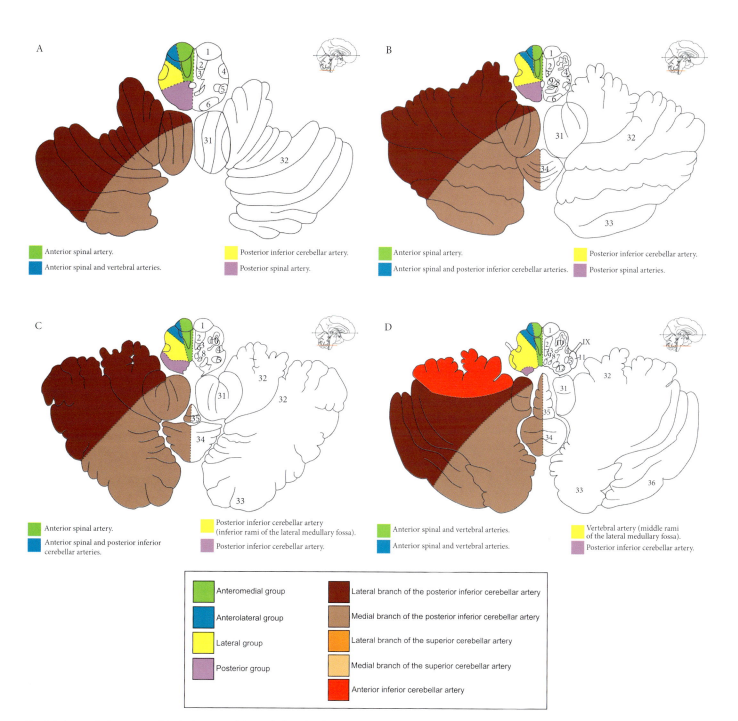

A

Anterior spinal artery.

Anterior spinal and vertebral arteries.

Posterior inferior cerebellar artery.

Posterior spinal artery.

B

Anterior spinal artery.

Anterior spinal and posterior inferior cerebellar arteries.

Posterior inferior cerebellar artery.

Posterior spinal arteries.

C

Anterior spinal artery.

Anterior spinal and posterior inferior cerebellar arteries.

Posterior inferior cerebellar artery
(inferior rami of the lateral medullary fossa).

Posterior inferior cerebellar artery.

D

Anterior spinal and vertebral arteries.

Anterior spinal and vertebral arteries.

Vertebral artery (middle rami
of the lateral medullary fossa).

Posterior inferior cerebellar artery.

Anteromedial group	Lateral branch of the posterior inferior cerebellar artery
Anterolateral group	Medial branch of the posterior inferior cerebellar artery
Lateral group	Lateral branch of the superior cerebellar artery
Posterior group	Medial branch of the superior cerebellar artery
	Anterior inferior cerebellar artery

Fig. 3.1 Anatomical structures of the brainstem and the cerebellum (A–L) and cerebral hemispheres (M–X).

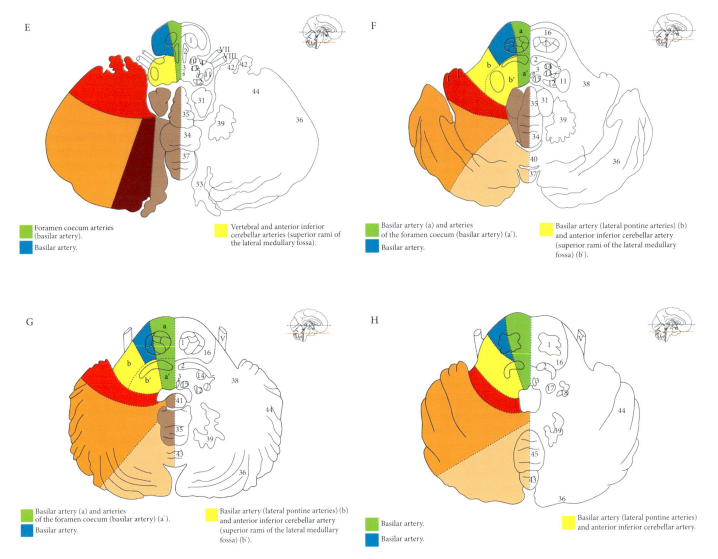

E

Foramen coecum arteries (basilar artery).

Basilar artery.

Vertebral and anterior inferior cerebellar arteries (superior rami of the lateral medullary fossa).

F

Basilar artery (a) and arteries of the foramen coecum (basilar artery) (a´).

Basilar artery.

Basilar artery (lateral pontine arteries) (b) and anterior inferior cerebellar artery (superior rami of the lateral medullary fossa) (b´).

G

Basilar artery (a) and arteries of the foramen coecum (basilar artery) (a´).

Basilar artery.

Basilar artery (lateral pontine arteries) (b) and anterior inferior cerebellar artery (superior rami of the lateral medullary fossa) (b´).

H

Basilar artery.

Basilar artery.

Basilar artery (lateral pontine arteries) and anterior inferior cerebellar artery.

Fig. 3.1 Continued

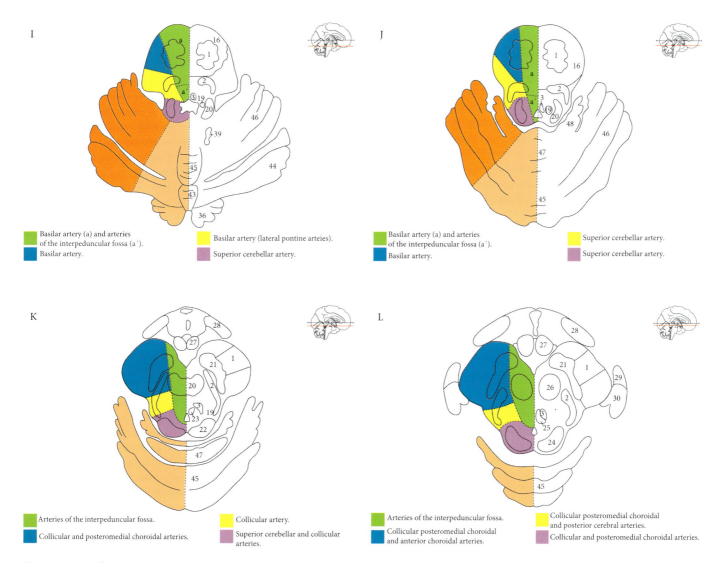

I

16
1
a
2
a′
3 19
20
46
39
45
44
43
36

■ Basilar artery (a) and arteries of the interpeduncular fossa (a′).
■ Basilar artery.
■ Basilar artery (lateral pontine arteies).
■ Superior cerebellar artery.

J

1
16
a
2
3
a′
9 20
48
46
47
45

■ Basilar artery (a) and arteries of the interpeduncular fossa (a′).
■ Basilar artery.
■ Superior cerebellar artery.
■ Superior cerebellar artery.

K

28
27
21 1
20 2
19
23
22
47
45

■ Arteries of the interpeduncular fossa.
■ Collicular and posteromedial choroidal arteries.
■ Collicular artery.
■ Superior cerebellar and collicular arteries.

L

28
27
21 1
29
26
2
30
25
24
45

■ Arteries of the interpeduncular fossa.
■ Collicular posteromedial choroidal and anterior choroidal arteries.
■ Collicular posteromedial choroidal and posterior cerebral arteries.
■ Collicular and posteromedial choroidal arteries.

Fig. 3.1 Continued

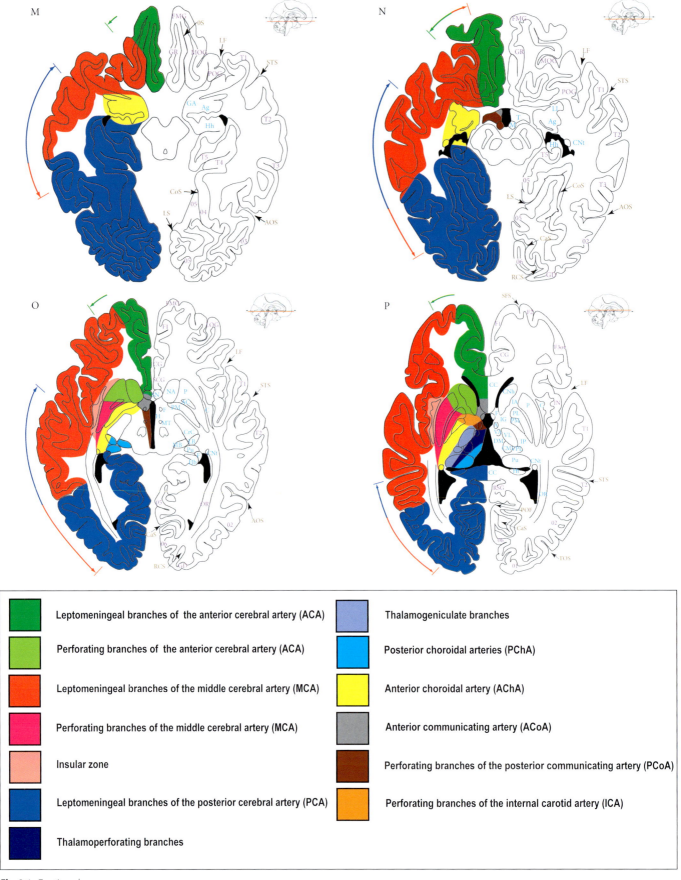

Leptomeningeal branches of the anterior cerebral artery (ACA)

Perforating branches of the anterior cerebral artery (ACA)

Leptomeningeal branches of the middle cerebral artery (MCA)

Perforating branches of the middle cerebral artery (MCA)

Insular zone

Leptomeningeal branches of the posterior cerebral artery (PCA)

Thalamoperforating branches

Thalamogeniculate branches

Posterior choroidal arteries (PChA)

Anterior choroidal artery (AChA)

Anterior communicating artery (ACoA)

Perforating branches of the posterior communicating artery (PCoA)

Perforating branches of the internal carotid artery (ICA)

Fig. 3.1 Continued

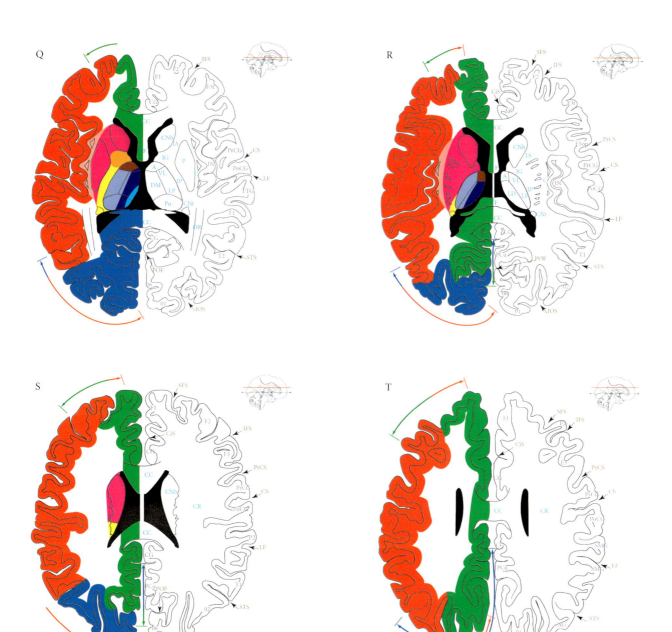

Fig. 3.1 Continued

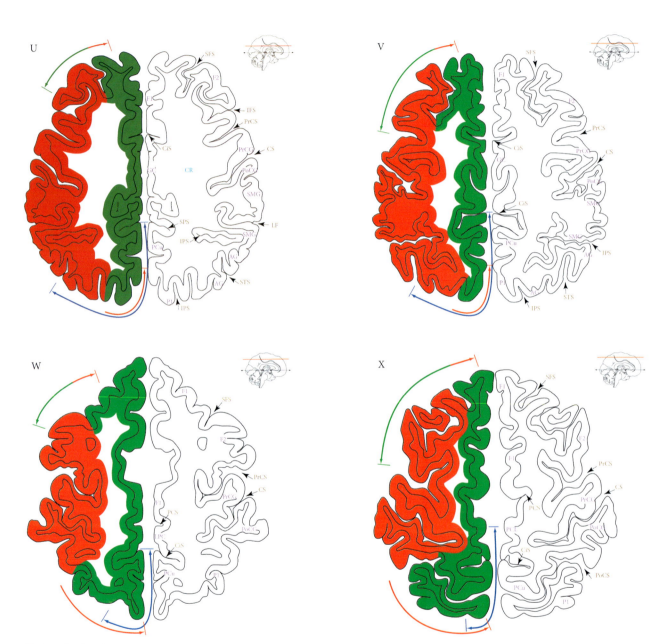

Fig. 3.1 Continued

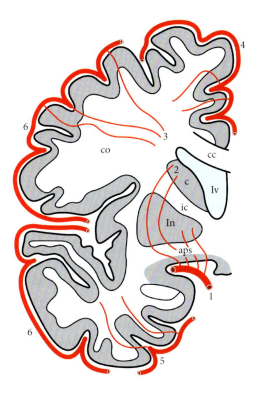

1. Middle cerebral artery
2. Perforating arteries (deep perforating arteries)
3. Medullary arteries (superficial perforating arteries)
4. Leptomeningeal branches of the anterior cerebral artery
5. Leptomeningeal branches of the posterior cerebral artery
6. Leptomeningeal branches of the middle cerebral artery.

Fig. 3.2 Schematic coronal section of the brain showing the general arrangement of the hemispheric arteries (cc: corpus callosum, co: centrum ovale, c: caudate nucleus, lv: lateral ventricule, ic: internal capsule, ln: lentiform nucleus, aps: anterior perforated substance).

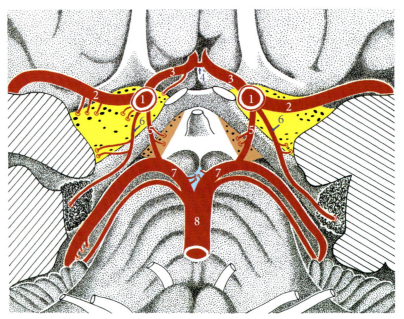

1. Internal carotid artery
2. Middle cerebral artery
3. Anterior cerebral artery
4. Anterior communicating artery
5. Posterior communicating artery
6. Anterior choroidal artery
7. Posterior cerebral artery
8. Basilar artery.

Fig. 3.3 Arterial circle of Willis and perforating branches of the cerebral arteries (yellow: anterior perforated substance receiving ACA, ICA, MCA, AChA perforators; blue: posterior perforated substance receiving PCA perforators; orange: lateral perforated substance receiving PCoA perforators).

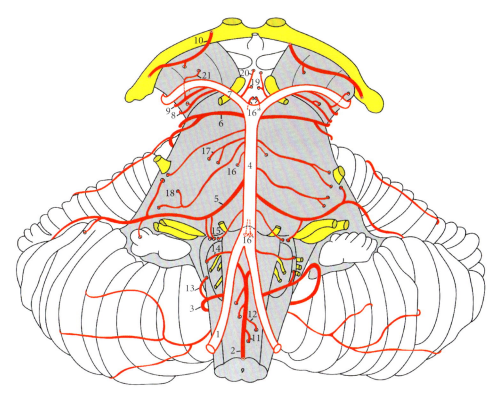

1. Vertebral artery
2. Anterior spinal artery
3. Posterior inferior cerebellar artery
4. Basilar artery
5. Anterior inferior cerebellar artery
6. Superior cerebellar artery
7. Posterior cerebral artery
8. Collicular artery
9. Posteromedial choroidal artery
10. Anterior choroidal artery
11. Anteromedial group of medullary arteries

12. Anterolateral group of medullary arteries
13. Lateral group of medullary arteries. Inferior rami arising from the posterior inferior cerebellar artery
14. Lateral group of medullary arteries. Middle rami arising from the vertebral artery
15. Lateral group of medullary arteries. Superior rami arising from the anterior inferior cerebellar artery and basilar artery
16. Anteromedial group of pontine arteries (16′ arteries penetrating the foramen coecum; 16′ arteries penetrating the interpeduncular fossa)
17. Anterolateral group of pontine arteries
18. Lateral group of pontine arteries
19. Anteromedial group of mesencephalic arteries
20. Anterolateral group of mesencephalic arteries
21. Lateral group of mesencephalic arteries.

Fig. 3.4 Anterior view showing the general arrangement of the brainstem and cerebellar arteries.

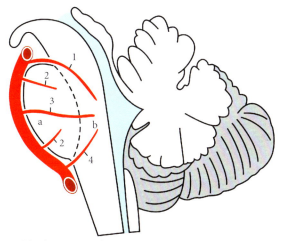

1. Descending arteries supplying the upper part of the pontine tegmentum
2. Pontine arteries supplying ventral part of the pons
3. Pontine arteries supplying the middle part of the pontine tegmentum
4. Ascending arteries penetrating the foramen coecum and supplying the lower part of the pontine tegmentum.

Fig. 3.5 Sagittal section of the pons showing the paths of arterial branches arising from the basilar artery for pons vascularization: (A) ventral part of the pons, (B) pontine tegmentum.

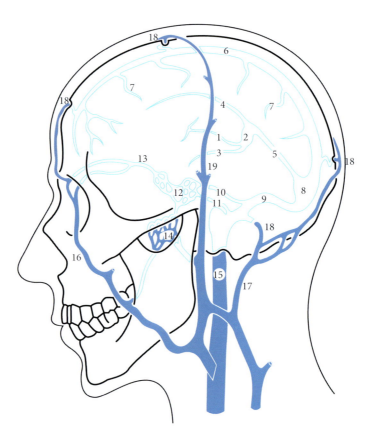

1. Superior sagittal sinus
2. Torcular herophilii
3. Lateral sinus
4. Sigmoid sinus
5. Occipital sinus
6. Jugular foramen
7. Cavernous sinus
8. Superior petrosal sinus
9. Inferior petrosal sinus
10. Intercavernous sinus
11. Sphenoparietal sinus
12. Straight sinus.

Fig. 3.6 Dural sinuses at the base of the skull.

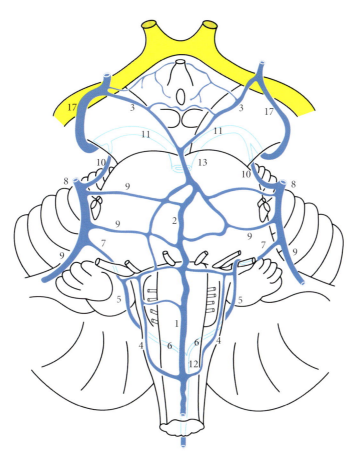

1. Internal cerebral vein
2. Great cerebral vein
3. Basal vein
4. Inferior sagittal sinus
5. Straight sinus
6. Superior sagittal sinus
7. Cortical vein
8. Torcular herophilii
9. Lateral sinus
10. Superior petrosal sinus
11. Inferior petrosal sinus
12. Cavernous sinus
13. Ophthalmic vein
14. Pterygoid plexus
15. Internal jugular vein
16. Facial vein
17. Occipital vein
18. Emissary vein.

Fig. 3.7 Brain venous circulation.

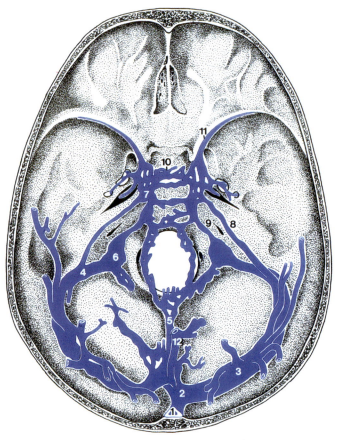

1. Antero-median medullary vein
2. Antero-median pontine vein
3. Interpeduncular vein
4. Retro-olivary vein
5. Lateral medullary vein
6. Inferior cerebellar peduncle vein
7. Lateral pontine vein

8. Superior petrosal vein
9. Anterior cerebellar vein
10. Lateral mesencephalic vein
11. Basal vein
12. Postero-median medullary vein
13. Great cerebral vein.

Fig. 3.8 Posterior fossa veins.

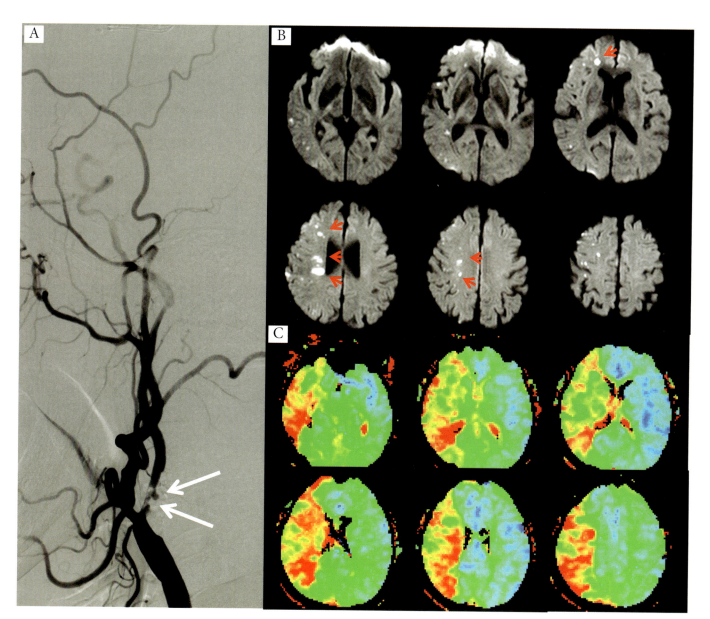

Fig. 4.1 Artery-to-artery embolism and hypoperfusion in a patient with ulcerative internal carotid artery disease. A 64-year-old hypertensive, diabetic man developed dysarthria and left hemiparesis. (A) Angiography showed severe, ulcerative atherosclerotic stenosis in the right carotid bulb area (long arrows). (B) DWI showed multiple scattered embolic infarcts in the right cortical areas, some of them located in the borderzone areas (short arrows). (C) Perfusion-weighted MRI using regional mean transit time showed hypoperfused areas in the right MCA territory.

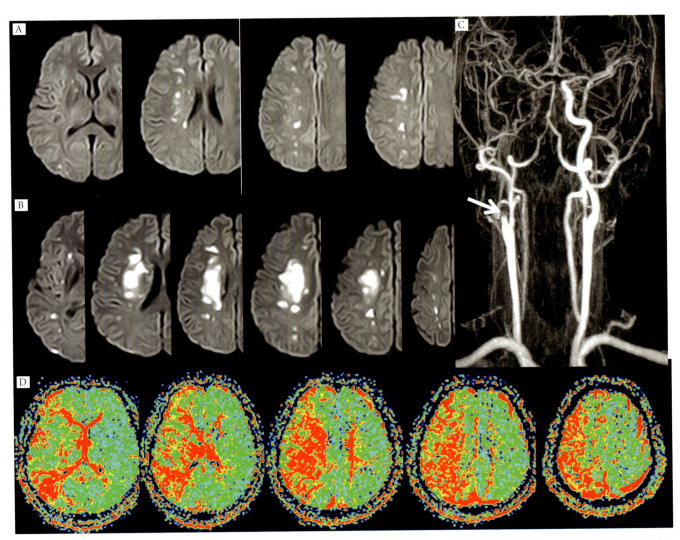

Fig. 4.7 Haemodynamic infarction. A 50-year-old man with uncontrolled diabetes mellitus developed mild left hemiparesis (MRC grade IV). (A) Initial DWI showed scattered infarcts in the right border zone area. Two days later, the limb weakness progressed to grade II. (B) Repeat DWI showed extended lesions. (C) MRA showed right internal carotid artery occlusion (long arrow). (D) Perfusion-weighted MRI (MTT map) showed decreased perfusion in the right MCA territory.

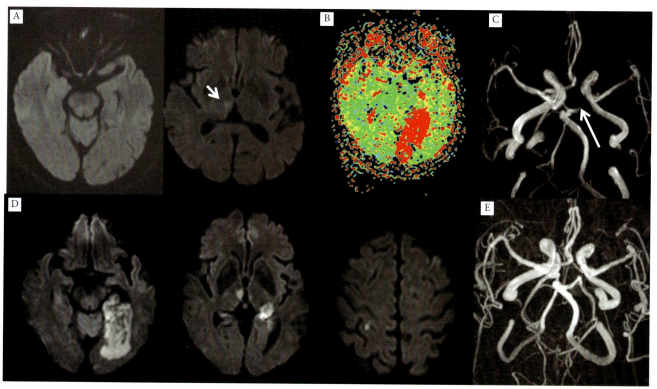

Fig. 4.8 Cardiogenic infarction. A 71-year-old woman with atrial fibrillation suddenly developed confusion. (A) Initial DWI showed right medial thalamic infarction (short arrow) without definite lesion on the occipital area. (B) Perfusion-weighted MRI (MTT map) showed decreased perfusion in the left occipital area. (C) MRA showed occlusion of the left posterior cerebral artery (long arrow). (D) Follow-up DWI 4 days later showed haemorrhagic infarction in the left occipital area, and an infarct in the right thalamus. A small infarct is also shown in the right cortical area of MCA territory. (E) MRA showed complete recanalization of the posterior cerebral artery.

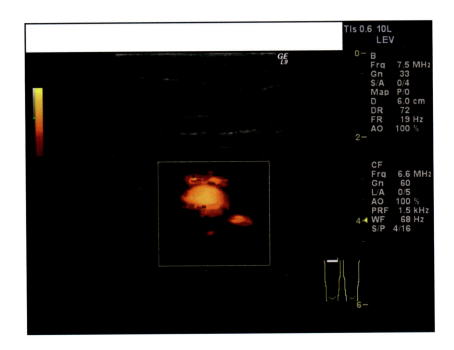

Fig. 18.5 Doppler ultrasound of DVT.

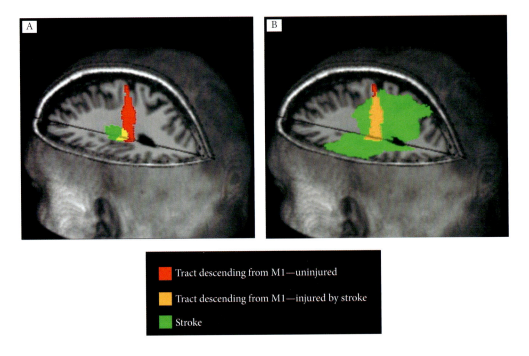

■ Tract descending from M1—uninjured

■ Tract descending from M1—injured by stroke

■ Stroke

Fig. 20.1 Extent of injury to a specific motor tract predicts gains in arm motor function from a course of robotic therapy in subjects with chronic stroke (87). Two examples of stroke injury to the corticospinal tract descending from primary motor cortex are provided. The subject in (A) had only 37.5% of this tract injured by stroke and had a gain of 11 points on the Fugl–Meyer scale, while the subject in (B) had 93.4% of this tract injured by stroke and had a gain of only 1 point. In this study, tract-specific injury was stronger than infarct volume or baseline clinical status at predicting gains. Such findings might be incorporated into clinical trials, for example, as an entry criterion, for identifying subjects with sufficient biological substrate to improve from therapy.

CHAPTER 3

Arteries and veins of the brain: anatomical organization

Laurent Tatu, Fabrice Vuillier, and Thierry Moulin

Brain arterial circulation

We provide an overview of the anatomy of the cerebral arteries including a brain map of the areas supplied by these arteries in the brainstem, cerebellum, and cerebral hemispheres (Figure 3.1; Tables 3.1–3.4). Arterial territories are depicted in such a way that can be directly applied to neuroimaging slices in clinical practice. The map is presented on a series of 24 templates, based on a bicommissural plane. The brainstem and cerebellar sections are 4 mm thick, whereas those of the cerebral hemispheres are 8 mm thick. The anatomical structures listed in Tables 3.1 and 3.3 are shown on the right-hand side of Figure 3.1 sections and the arterial territories captioned in Tables 3.2 and 3.4 appear on the left. This brain map has been previously published and a more detailed description can be found elsewhere (1–3). Certain unresolved issues concerning cerebral arterial blood flow and its clinical or imaging-related consequences are more specifically addressed.

Arterial supply of the cerebral hemispheres

Arterial supply of the cerebral hemispheres is divided into two systems: the perforating arteries and the leptomeningeal arteries (Figure 3.2). The perforating arteries, also called deep perforating arteries, arise from the arterial circle of Willis or its immediate branches. They perforate the brain parenchyma as direct penetrators via the perforated substances. The leptomeningeal arteries, also known as pial arteries, consist of the terminal branches of the anterior (ACA), middle (MCA), and posterior cerebral arteries (PCA) and the anterior choroidal artery, forming an anastomotic network on the surface of the hemispheres. They yield branches that penetrate the cortex, subjacent white matter, and U fibres. The deepest ones form the medullary (or superficial perforating) arteries.

Perforating branches of the cerebral arteries

The perforating branches of the cerebral arteries enter the brain via the anterior, posterior, and lateral perforated substances (Figure 3.3). The perforating arteries arising from the internal carotid artery (ICA), ACA, MCA, anterior communicating artery (ACoA), and anterior choroidal artery (AChA) pass through the anterior perforated substance.

Perforating arteries arising from the PCA enter the brain through the posterior perforated substance forming the interpeduncular arteries. These are classed as three rami: only the superior rami (thalamoperforating arteries) participate in blood supply of the hemispheres. The inferior and middle rami supply the brainstem. The PCA also gives rise to the thalamogeniculate branches and the posterior choroidal arteries (PChA) to supply blood to the thalamus and geniculate bodies.

The posterior communicating artery (PoCA) gives rise to perforating branches, notably the premamillary artery, which passes through the lateral perforated substance.

Perforating branches of the internal carotid artery

The perforating branches of the ICA arise from its supraclinoid portion near the origin of the AChA, and pass through the anterior perforated substance to enter the brain. These branches supply the genu of the internal capsule, the adjacent part of the globus pallidus and the contiguous posterior limb of the internal capsule (4, 5) (Figure 3.1P, Q).

Perforating branches of the anterior choroidal artery

The perforating branches of the AChA enter the anterior perforated substance. They supply the lower part of the two posterior thirds and the retro-lenticular part of the internal capsule, the adjacent optic radiations and acoustic radiations, the medial globus pallidus, and the tail of the caudate nucleus (4, 6–11) (Figure 3.1O–S).

Anterior communicating artery

The ACoA gives off perforating branches that divide into three groups: the hypothalamic arteries, the subcallosal artery and the median callosal artery. The vascular territory of this artery includes the lamina terminalis, anterior hypothalamus, septum pellucidum, part of the anterior commissure and fornix, the paraterminal gyrus including the septal nuclei and occasionally the subcallosal region, the anterior part of the corpus callosum, and the cingulate gyrus (5,12,13,14) (Figure 3.1N–P).

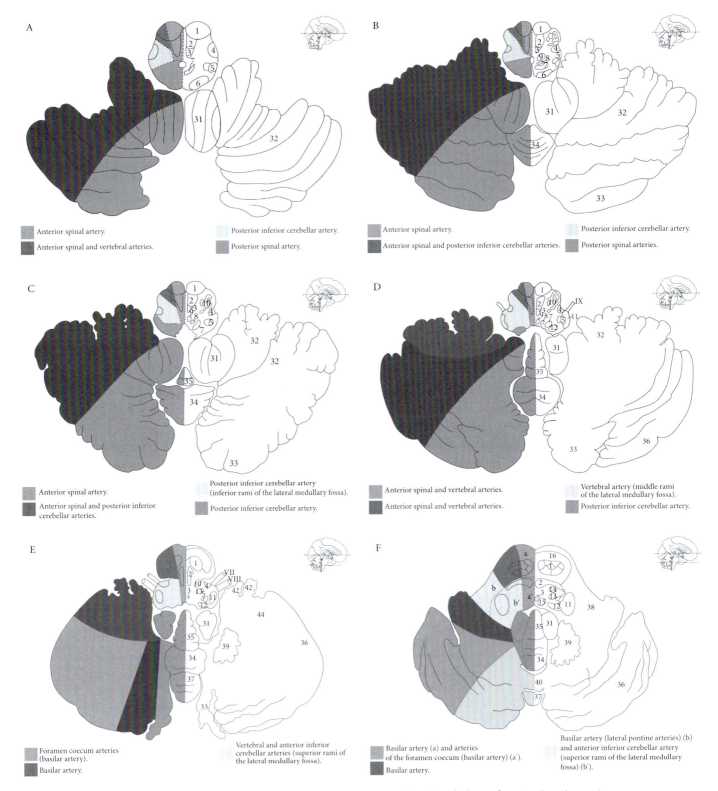

Fig. 3.1 Anatomical structures of the brainstem and the cerebellum (A–L) and cerebral hemispheres (M–X). Also see figure in colour plate section.

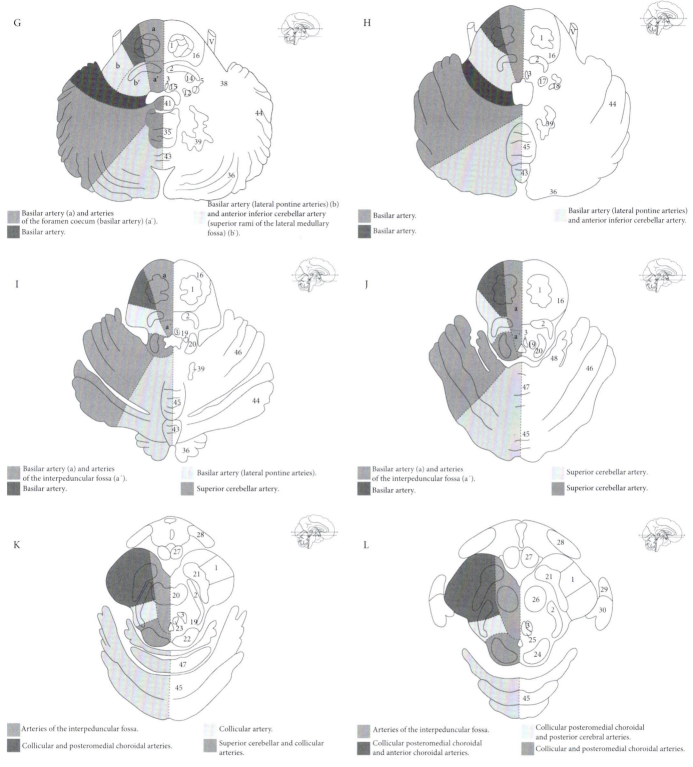

Fig. 3.1 Continued

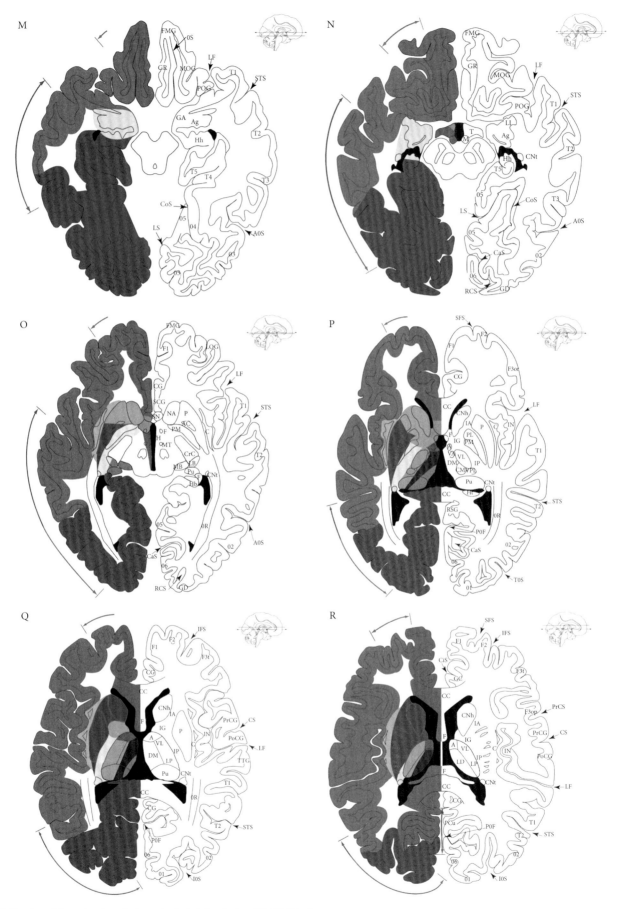

Fig. 3.1 Continued. See color plates for legends of arterial territories of Fig 3.1 M to L

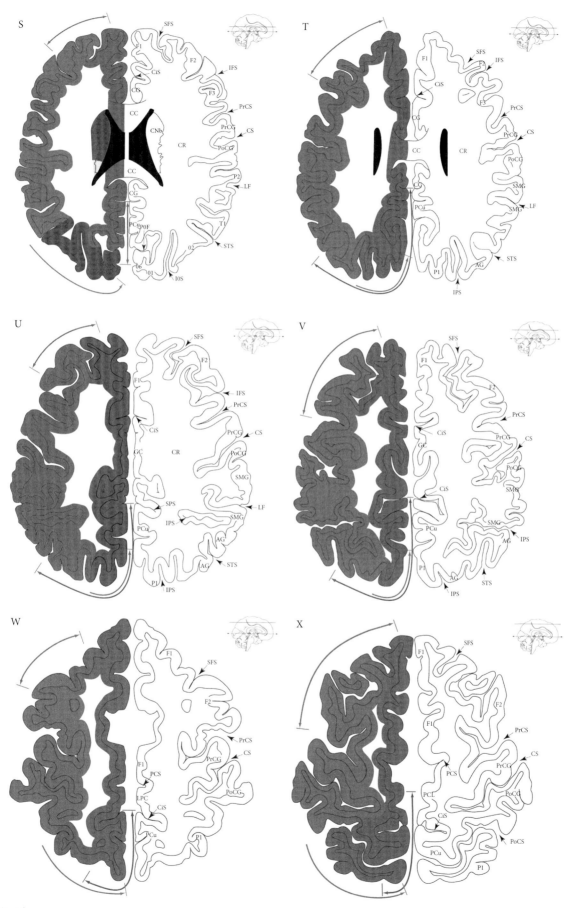

Fig. 3.1 Continued

Table 3.1 Anatomical structures of the brainstem and the cerebellum (Figure 3.1A–L)

1	Corticospinal tract
2	Medial lemniscus
3	Medial longitudinal fasciculus
4	Spinothalamic tract
5	Spinal trigeminal tract and nuclei
6	Gracile and cuneate nuclei
7	Nucleus of the solitary tract
8	Dorsal motor vagal nucleus
9	Hypoglossal nucleus
10	Inferior olivary nucleus
11	Inferior cerebellar peduncle
12	Vestibular nucleus
13	Facial nucleus
14	Superior olivary nucleus
15	Abducens nucleus
16	Pontine nuclei
17	Motor trigeminal nucleus
18	Principal sensory trigeminal nucleus
19	Nucleus coeruleus
20	Superior cerebellar peduncle
21	Sustantia nigra
22	Inferior colliculus
23	Trochlear nucleus
24	Superior colliculus
25	Oculomotor nucleus
26	Red nucleus
27	Mamillary body
28	Optic tract
29	Lateral geniculate body
30	Medial geniculate body
31	Tonsil
32	Biventer lobule
33	Inferior semilunar lobule
34	Pyramid of vermis
35	Uvula
36	Superior semilunar lobule
37	Tuber of vermis
38	Middle cerebellar peduncle
39	Dentate nucleus
40	Folium of vermis
41	Nodulus
42	Flocculus
43	Declive
44	Simple lobule
45	Culmen
46	Quadrangular lobule
47	Central lobule
48	Ala of the central lobule
V	Trigeminal nerve
VII	Facial nerve
VIII	Vestibulocochlear nerve
IX	Glossopharyngeal nerve

Table 3.2 Brainstem and cerebellar territories

Brainstem territories
Anteromedial group (AM)
Anterolateral group (AL)
Lateral group (L)
Posterior group (P)
Cerebellar territories
Lateral branch of the posterior inferior cerebellar artery (l-PICA)
Medial branch of the posterior inferior cerebellar artery (m-PICA)
Lateral branch of the superior cerebellar artery (l-SCA)
Medial branch of the superior cerebellar artery (m-SCA)
Anterior inferior cerebellar artery (AICA)

Perforating branches of the anterior cerebral artery

The perforating branches of the ACA are divided into two groups. The direct ACA perforators usually originate from the proximal pre-communicating segment and the recurrent artery of Heubner, arising from the proximal post-communicating segment. These arteries supply the anterior and inferior parts of the head of the caudate nucleus, the anterior and inferior portions of the anterior limb of the internal capsule, the adjacent part of the putamen and globus pallidus, the caudal rectus gyrus, the subcallosal gyrus, and the medial part of the anterior commissure (5, 6, 15–18) (Figure 3.1O, P).

Perforating branches of the middle cerebral artery

The perforating branches of the MCA, known as the lenticulostriate arteries, usually arise from the basal segment of the artery. They are usually classified in two groups: medial and lateral. These perforating branches supply the superior part of the head and the body of the caudate nucleus, the lateral segment of the globus pallidus, the

Table 3.3 Anatomical structures of cerebral hemispheres (Figure 3.1M–X)

Gyri (purple)	
CG	Cingulate gyrus
F1	Superior frontal gyrus
F2	Middle frontal gyrus
F3	Inferior frontal gyrus
F3op	Inferior frontal gyrus pars opercularis
F3or	Inferior frontal gyrus pars orbitalis
F3t	Inferior frontal gyrus pars triangularis
FMG	Frontomarginal gyrus
GR	Gyrus rectus
LOG	Lateral orbital gyrus
MOG	Medial orbital gyrus
PCu	Precuneus
POG	Posterior orbital gyrus
SCG	Subcallosal gyrus
IN	Insula
PCL	Paracentral lobule
PoCG	Postcentral gyrus
PrCG	Precentral gyrus
AG	Angular gyrus
P1	Superior parietal gyrus
P2	Inferior parietal gyrus
SMG	Supramarginalis gyrus
T1	Superior temporal gyrus
T2	Middle temporal gyrus
T3	Inferior temporal gyrus
T4	Fusiform gyrus
T5	Parahippocampal gyrus
TTG	Transverse temporal gyrus
O1	Superior occipital gyrus
O2	Middle occipital gyrus
O3	Inferior occipital gyrus
O4	Fusiform gyrus
O5	Lingual gyrus
O6	Cuneus
GD	Gyrus descendens (Ecker)
RSG	Retrosplenial gyrus
Sulci (brown)	
AOS	Anterior occipital sulcus
CaS	Calcarine sulcus
CiS	Cingulate sulcus
CoS	Collateral sulcus
CS	Central sulcus
IFS	Inferior frontal sulcus
IOS	Intra-occipital sulcus
IPS	Intraparietal sulcus
LF	Lateral fissure
LS	Lingual sulcus
OS	Olfactory sulcus
PCS	Paracentral sulcus
PoCS	Postcentral sulcus
POF	Parieto-occipital fissure
PrCS	Precentral sulcus
RCS	Retrocalcarine sulcus
SFS	Superior frontal sulcus
SPS	Subparietal sulcus
STS	Superior temporal sulcus (parallel sulcus)
TOS	Transverse occipital sulcus
Internal structures (blue)	
CNb	Caudate nucleus, body
CNh	Caudate nucleus, head
CNt	Caudate nucleus, tail
IA	Internal capsule, anterior limb
IG	Internal capsule, genu
IP	Internal capsule, posterior limb
NA	Nucleus accumbens
P	Putamen
PL	Globus pallidus, pars lateralis
PM	Globus pallidus, pars medialis
SN	Septal nuclei
A	Anterior thalamic nucleus
CM	Centromedian thalamic nucleus
DM	Dorsomedial thalamic nucleus
LD	Lateral dorsal thalamic nucleus
LP	Lateral posterior thalamic nucleus
Pu	Pulvinar
VA	Ventral anterior thalamic nucleus
VL	Ventral lateral thalamic nucleus
VPL	Ventral posterolateral thalamic nucleus
C	Claustrum
CR	Corona radiata
IN	Insula
LI	Limen insulae
CC	Corpus callosum
F	Fornix

(continued)

Table 3.3 Continued

Hb	Hippocampus, body
Hh	Hippocampus, head
Ht	Hippocampus, tail
AC	Anterior commissure
Ag	Amygdala
CrC	Crus cerebri
GA	Gyrus ambiens
H	Hypothalamus
LB	Lateral geniculate body
M	Mamillary body
MB	Medial geniculate body
MT	Mamillo-thalamic tract
OR	Optic radiations
T	Tuber

Table 3.4 Arterial territories of cerebral hemispheres

Leptomeningeal branches of the anterior cerebral artery (ACA)
Perforating branches of the anterior cerebral artery (ACA)
Leptomeningeal branches of the middle cerebral artery (MCA)
Perforating branches of the middle cerebral artery (MCA)
Insular zone
Leptomeningeal branches of the posterior cerebral artery (PCA)
Thalamoperforating branches
Thalamogeniculate branches
Posterior choroidal arteries (PChA)
Anterior choroidal artery (AChA)
Anterior communicating artery (ACoA)
Perforating branches of the posterior communicating artery (PCoA)
Perforating branches of the internal carotid artery (ICA)

putamen, the dorsal half of the internal capsule, and the lateral half of the anterior commissure (15, 19–21) (Figure 3.1O–S).

Posterior communicating artery

Seven to ten branches arise from the PCoA. The largest branch is termed the premamillary artery. The PCoA perforators supply the posterior portion of the optic chiasm and optic tract, as well as the posterior part of the hypothalamus and mamillary body (11, 22, 23). The thalamic territory of the PCoA includes the anterior nucleus and the polar part of the ventralis anterior nucleus and the reticularis nucleus (11, 19, 24) (Figure 3.1N–R).

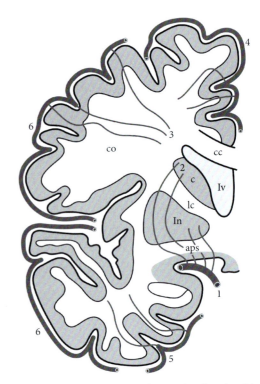

1. Middle cerebral artery
2. Perforating arteries (deep perforating arteries)
3. Medullary arteries (superficial perforating arteries)
4. Leptomeningeal branches of the anterior cerebral artery
5. Leptomeningeal branches of the posterior cerebral artery
6. Leptomeningeal branches of the middle cerebral artery.

Fig. 3.2 Schematic coronal section of the brain showing the general arrangement of the hemispheric arteries (cc: corpus callosum, co: centrum ovale, c: caudate nucleus, lv: lateral ventricule, ic: internal capsule, ln: lentiform nucleus, aps: anterior perforated substance). Also see figure in colour plate section.

Thalamoperforating branches

The thalamoperforating arteries, also called paramedian thalamic arteries, arise from the pre-communicant segment of the PCA and form the superior rami of the interpeduncular arteries. They supply the thalamus, especially the medial nuclei, the intralaminar nuclei, part of the dorsomedial nucleus, the posteromedial portion of the lateral nuclei, and the ventromedial pulvinar (11, 19, 25) (Figure 3.1P–R).

Thalamogeniculate branches

The thalamogeniculate arteries, also named inferolateral thalamic arteries, usually arise from the PCA segment next to the geniculate bodies. They supply a major part of the lateral side of the caudal thalamus including the rostrolateral part of the pulvinar, the posterior part of the lateral nuclei and lateral dorsal nucleus, and the ventroposterior and ventrolateral nuclei (11, 19, 26) (Figure 3.1P–R).

Posterior choroidal arteries

The posterior choroidal group usually includes one or two medial and one to six lateral posterior choroidal arteries. The medial PChA usually arises from the proximal perimesencephalic

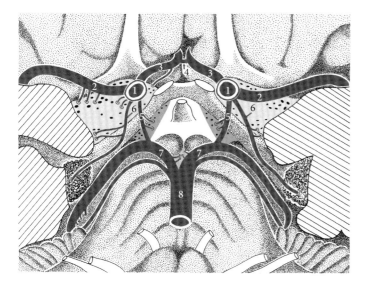

1. Internal carotid artery
2. Middle cerebral artery
3. Anterior cerebral artery
4. Anterior communicating artery
5. Posterior communicating artery
6. Anterior choroidal artery
7. Posterior cerebral artery
8. Basilar artery.

Fig. 3.3 Arterial circle of Willis and perforating branches of the cerebral arteries (yellow: anterior perforated substance receiving ACA, ICA, MCA, AChA perforators; blue: posterior perforated substance receiving PCA perforators; orange: lateral perforated substance receiving PCoA perforators). Also see figure in colour plate section.

segments of the PCA. The lateral PChA arises from the distal perimesencephalic segments of the PCA or from a branch of the PCA. The medial PChA supplies the medial geniculate body, as well as the posterior part of the medial nucleus and of the pulvinar. The lateral PChA supplies part of the lateral geniculate body, part of the dorsomedial nucleus, and part of the pulvinar (10, 11, 19, 26) (Figure 3.1O).

Leptomeningeal branches of the cerebral arteries

Due to the numerous variations in the branching patterns of the leptomeningeal arteries, there is no need to differentiate between the arterial territories of each cortical branch of the anterior, middle, and posterior cerebral arteries and of the AChA. Using the results of the study by Van der Zwann et al. on cortical boundaries, it is more useful to explain in detail the variability of the cortical territories of the three main cerebral arteries and to define the minimal and maximal cortical supply areas (27).

Leptomeningeal branches of the anterior cerebral artery

The distal segment of the ACA, the pericallosal artery, gives rise to the cortical and the callosal branches. The callosal branches supply the rostrum, genu and body of the corpus callosum. These branches join together posterior to the splenial branches of the PCA. In the most frequent arrangement, the ACA supplies the cortical area of the medial surface of the hemisphere extending to the superior frontal sulcus and the parieto-occipital sulcus. On the orbitofrontal surface, the arterial territory includes the medial orbital gyri. The

maximum cortical ACA territory reaches as far as the inferior frontal sulcus and the minimum area includes only the anterior part of the frontal lobe.

Leptomeningeal branches of the middle cerebral artery

The MCA begins its division into cortical arteries at the base of the Sylvian fissure and extends over the surface of the hemisphere to form the cortical segment. The MCA most frequently distributes to the area on the lateral surface of the hemisphere that extends to the superior frontal sulcus, the intraparietal sulcus, and the inferior temporal gyrus. On the orbitofrontal surface, the arterial territory includes the lateral orbital gyri. The maximum area supplied by the MCA covers the whole lateral surface of the hemisphere, reaching the interhemispheric fissure, whereas the minimum area is confined to the territory between the inferior frontal and the superior temporal sulci.

Leptomeningeal branches of the posterior cerebral artery

As the PCA approaches the dorsal surface of the midbrain, it gives rise to cortical branches. These branches include the hippocampal arteries and the splenial artery, which anastomose with the distal part of the pericallosal artery to supply the splenium of the corpus callosum. The most frequent cortical distribution of the PCA includes the inferomedial surfaces of the temporal and the occipital lobe extending to the parieto-occipital fissure. The maximum cortical supply area can extend as far as the superior temporal sulcus and the upper part of the precentral sulcus, and the minimum area extends only as far as the medial face of the occipital lobe, limited by the parieto-occipital fissure.

Leptomeningeal branches of the anterior choroidal artery

The superficial territory includes part of the uncus, part of the head of the hippocampus, part of the amygdaloid nucleus, and the lateral part of the lateral geniculate body (Figure 3.1M, N).

Arterial supply of the brainstem

Arterial trunks supplying the brainstem include the vertebral artery, basilar artery, anterior and posterior spinal arteries, posterior inferior cerebellar artery (PICA), anterior inferior cerebellar artery (AICA), superior cerebellar artery (SCA), PCA, collicular artery, and AChA (Figure 3.4).

According to their point of penetration into the parenchyma, the collaterals of these arteries are divided, over the entire length of the brainstem, into four groups: anteromedial, anterolateral, lateral, and posterior arteries. This classification was first proposed by Lazorthes, who divided the brainstem arteries into anterior, lateral, and posterior groups (28). For the anterior group, an accurate subdivision into anteromedial and anterolateral arteries was then established by Duvernoy (29).

Each of these four arterial groups supplies the corresponding arterial territories in the brainstem. The arterial territories, well described by Duvernoy, have a variable extension at different levels of the brainstem (29, 30). For example, the posterior group does

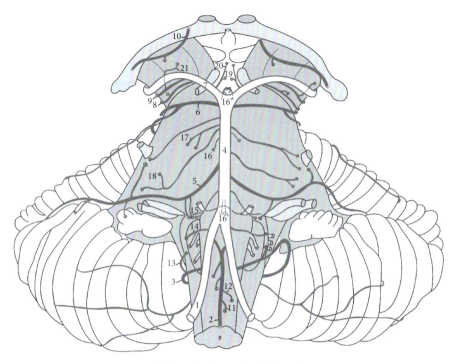

1. Vertebral artery
2. Anterior spinal artery
3. Posterior inferior cerebellar artery
4. Basilar artery
5. Anterior inferior cerebellar artery
6. Superior cerebellar artery
7. Posterior cerebral artery
8. Collicular artery
9. Posteromedial choroidal artery
10. Anterior choroidal artery
11. Anteromedial group of medullary arteries

12. Anterolateral group of medullary arteries
13. Lateral group of medullary arteries. Inferior rami arising from the posterior inferior cerebellar artery
14. Lateral group of medullary arteries. Middle rami arising from the vertebral artery
15. Lateral group of medullary arteries. Superior rami arising from the anterior inferior cerebellar artery and basilar artery
16. Anteromedial group of pontine arteries (16′ arteries penetrating the foramen coecum; 16′ arteries penetrating the interpeduncular fossa)
17. Anterolateral group of pontine arteries
18. Lateral group of pontine arteries
19. Anteromedial group of mesencephalic arteries
20. Anterolateral group of mesencephalic arteries
21. Lateral group of mesencephalic arteries.

Fig. 3.4 Anterior view showing the general arrangement of the brainstem and cerebellar arteries. Also see figure in colour plate section.

not exist in the lower pons. Consequently, the nuclei and tracts that extend into the brainstem may be supplied by several arterial groups.

Arterial groups supplying the medulla

The arterial supply of the medulla comes from the PICA, which gives rise to the inferior rami of the lateral medullary fossa, the vertebral arteries that form the middle rami of the lateral medullary fossa, and the anterior and posterior spinal arteries.

The anteromedial territory is supplied by the anterior spinal artery (Figure 3.1A–C) or the anterior spinal and vertebral arteries (Figure 3.1D).

The anterolateral territory is supplied by the anterior spinal and vertebral arteries (Figure 3.1A), the anterior spinal artery and the PICA (Figure 3.1B, C) or the anterior spinal and vertebral arteries (Figure 3.1D).

The lateral territory is supplied by the PICA (Figure 3.1A–C) or the vertebral artery (Figure 3.1D).

The posterior territory is supplied by the posterior spinal artery (Figure 3.1A, B) or the PICA (Figure 3.1C, D).

Arterial groups supplying the pons

Different arterial trunks supply blood to the pons, including the vertebral arteries, the AICA, which gives off the superior rami of the lateral medullary fossa, the SCA, and the basilar artery.

Basilar artery branches destined for the anteromedial territory enter the ventral part of the pons (medial and lateral pontine arteries), the foramen coecum (foramen coecum arteries), and the interpeduncular fossa (inferior rami of the interpeduncular arteries) (Figure 3.5).

The anteromedial territory is thus supplied by the foramen coecum arteries (Figure 3.1E, part a′ of Figure 3.1F, G), the pontine arteries (Figure 3.1H, part a of Figure 3.1F, G, I, J) or the interpeduncular fossa arteries (part a′ of Figure 3.1I, J).

The anterolateral territory is supplied by the pontine arteries (Figure 3.1E–J).

The lateral territory is supplied by the vertebral artery and the AICA (Figure 3.1E), the pontine arteries (Figure 3.1I, part b of Figure 3.1F, G), the AICA (part b′ of Figure 3.1F, G), the pontine arteries and the AICA (Figure 3.1H) or the SCA (Figure 3.1J).

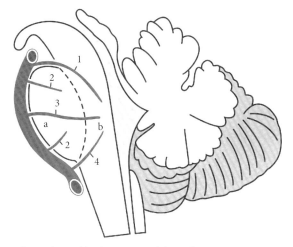

1. Descending arteries supplying the upper part of the pontine tegmentum
2. Pontine arteries supplying ventral part of the pons
3. Pontine arteries supplying the middle part of the pontine tegmentum
4. Ascending arteries penetrating the foramen coecum and supplying the lower part of the pontine tegmentum.

Fig. 3.5 Sagittal section of the pons showing the paths of arterial branches arising from the basilar artery for pons vascularization: (A) ventral part of the pons, (B) pontine tegmentum. Also see figure in colour plate section.

The posterior territory only exists in the upper part of the pons and is supplied by the medial and lateral branches of the SCA (Figure 3.1I, J).

Arterial groups supplying the midbrain

Five arterial trunks supply the arterial midbrain groups. From bottom to top, these are the SCA, the collicular artery, the posteromedial choroidal artery, the PCA forming the middle rami of the interpeduncular arteries, and the AChA.

The anteromedial territory is supplied by the PCA (Figure 3.1K, L).

The anterolateral territory is supplied by the collicular and posteromedial choroidal arteries (Figure 3.1K) or the collicular and posteromedial arteries and the AChA (Figure 3.1L).

The lateral territory is supplied by the collicular artery (Figure 3.1K) or the collicular, posteromedial, and choroidal arteries, and the PCA (Figure 3.1L).

The posterior territory is supplied by the SCA and the collicular arteries (Figure 3.1K) or the collicular and posteromedial choroidal arteries (Figure 3.1L).

Arterial supply of the cerebellum

The cerebellum is supplied by three pairs of long cerebellar arteries, namely the PICA, the AICA, and the SCA (Figure 3.3). The branches of these long cerebellar arteries develop a pial anastomotic network on the surface of the cerebellum. They supply the cerebellar cortex and the central nuclei of the cerebellum. The three long cerebellar arteries also participate in blood supply to the lateral or posterior arterial territories of the brainstem.

The topographic anatomy of the cerebellar arteries has been well studied (31, 32). The territories receiving arterial supply have

been identified in the anatomo-pathological work by Amarenco et al. and the injection studies by Marinkovic et al. (33–36).

The PICA is the most variable of the cerebellar arteries and originates in the vertebral artery. It gives off medial and lateral branches and supplies the inferior vermis as well as the inferior and posterior surfaces of the cerebellar hemispheres (Figure 3.1A–G). The PICA also forms part of the lateral and posterior arterial groups of the medulla, either via its common stem or its medial branch (Figure 3.1A–D).

The AICA usually arises from the bottom third of the basilar artery and supplies the anterior surface of the simple, superior and inferior semilunar lobules as well as the flocculus and the middle cerebellar peduncle (Figure 3.1F, G). In most cases, it gives rise to the internal auditory artery. The AICA participates in supplying the middle cerebellar peduncle and often the lower part of the pontine tegmentum (Figure 3.1F–H).

The SCA divides into medial and lateral branches and supplies the superior half of the cerebellar hemisphere and vermis as well as the dentate nucleus (Figure 3.1E–L). These two branches can arise independently from the basilar artery. The SCA territory often includes the upper part of the pontine tegmentum (Figure 3.1I–L).

Arterial debated topics

A number of points relating to cerebral blood supply remain under debate or are subject to variations. With regard to the arterial supply of the hemispheres, the origin of the leptomeningeal and deep cerebral arteries can vary. Perforating branches may arise from the leptomeningeal arteries and the large perforating arteries may be the origin of some leptomeningeal branches (18). The perforating branches of the MCA can vary and in many cases they emerge from the cortical or early branches of the MCA, the cortical arteries arising from the main trunk of the MCA proximal to its bifurcation or trifurcation (37).

The vascular organization of the centrum ovale is still under debate. It includes transcortical arterioles with exclusive territory as well as terminal ramifications of some perforating branches. The lack of specific anatomical studies on the origin of blood supply to the centrum ovale means that its supply is not taken into account on the brain maps. The arterial supply of the insular zone including the external capsule-claustrum-extreme capsule area is also complex. This area probably has a triple blood supply: a double cortical supply and lateral rami of the lateral striate arteries. Further anatomical studies are required to shed light on these grey areas.

Blood supply to the thalamus is also subject to variations both in terms of the origin of the pedicles, like the thalamoperforating arteries, and the participation of certain arteries in the supply of blood. Anatomical studies have clarified some of these points (38).

In the posterior circulation, the vascular organization of the brainstem is well established. However, the variability of the arteries supplying the cortex and the deep cerebellar nuclei still needs to be clarified. It may be of interest to quantify this variability using the model applied to the arterial territories of the cerebral cortex. In addition, certain variations in the cerebellar territories are not uncommon such as an anterior inferior cerebellar artery replacing a hypoplastic posterior inferior cerebellar artery and taking over most of the anterior and inferior parts of the cerebellar hemisphere. There are also many individual variations in the relative significance of cerebellar artery supply to the brainstem. These aspects require further anatomical research.

Venous circulation of the brain

Cerebral venous blood flow is subject to a number of variations and is not an exact replica of the arterial system. The concept of venous territories is of little value, as few significant correlations exist between the site of venous occlusion and the topography of the corresponding infarction. We therefore present the cerebral veins and their main variations in a more descriptive manner and as they may appear on a magnetic resonance angiogram, without referring to a map of venous territories.

The cerebral venous system is usually divided in four major groups: dural sinuses, deep cerebral veins, cortical cerebral veins, and posterior fossa veins. The dural sinuses collect all the venous blood from the brain that eventually enters the internal jugular veins to join the general venous circulation.

Dural venous sinuses

Dural venous sinuses are venous channels enclosed between two layers of dura mater. They drain blood from the brain, meninges, and skull. They communicate with the meningeal and diploic veins and with the extracranial venous system through emissary veins (Figures 3.6 and 3.7). They can be categorized as medial unpaired sinuses, symmetrical paired sinuses, and cavernous sinuses.

Most of them converge to form the posterior confluence of sinuses (the torcular herophili), opposite the internal occipital protuberance. Others drain to the cavernous sinuses (19, 28, 39–42).

Medial and unpaired sinuses

Superior sagittal sinus

The superior sagittal sinus is contained within the dura mater at the site of attachment of the falx cerebri to the cranial vault. It runs backwards, increasing gradually in size, from the foramen caecum to the torcular herophili. It communicates with the nasal veins via the emissary vein of the foramen caecum. One frequent variation is the termination of the superior sagittal sinus in one of the transverse sinuses.

The superior sagittal sinus communicates, via its lateral expansions, with the arachnoid granulations and constitutes one of the main sites of cerebrospinal fluid resorption. The anterior portion is sometimes replaced by two frontal parasagittal veins. It receives venous blood from the superior, medial and lateral surfaces of the cerebral hemispheres.

Inferior sagittal sinus

The inferior sagittal sinus lies within the free margin of the falx cerebri. It begins near the junction of the anterior and middle third of the falx by the union of veins from the falx and a variable number of corpus callosum and cingulum veins. It extends backwards, increasing in size until it enters the straight sinus.

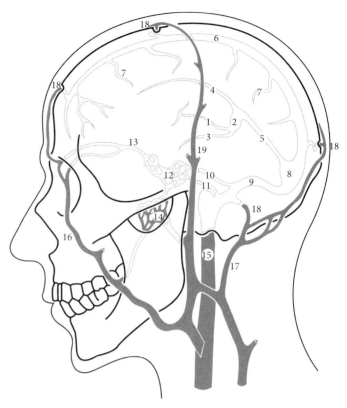

1. Superior sagittal sinus	7. Cavernous sinus
2. Torcular herophilii	8. Superior petrosal sinus
3. Lateral sinus	9. Inferior petrosal sinus
4. Sigmoid sinus	10. Intercavernous sinus
5. Occipital sinus	11. Sphenoparietal sinus
6. Jugular foramen	12. Straight sinus.

Fig. 3.6 Dural sinuses at the base of the skull. Also see figure in colour plate section.

Straight sinus

The straight sinus originates behind the splenium of the corpus callosum and is formed chiefly by the union of the inferior sagittal sinus and the great cerebral vein. It runs its course along the line of junction of the falx cerebri and the tentorium cerebelli, draining into the the torcular herophili. Some segments of the straight sinus can be doubled or tripled. Venous patterns at the junctions of the inferior sagittal sinus, great cerebral vein and straight sinus are also variable.

Occipital sinus

The occipital sinus is a small venous channel situated near the attachment of the falx cerebri. It passes upwards from the margin of the foramen magnum and drains into the torcular herophili. It communicates with the internal vertebral venous plexus and the marginal sinus that surrounds the foramen magnum.

Paired sinuses

Lateral sinus

The lateral sinus extends bilaterally from the internal occipital protuberance to the jugular foramen and divides into two segments. The first horizontal segment, known as the tranverse sinus, runs its course on the occipital bone, along the border of the tentorium cerebelli. The second S-shaped segment, called the sigmoid sinus, bends inwards at

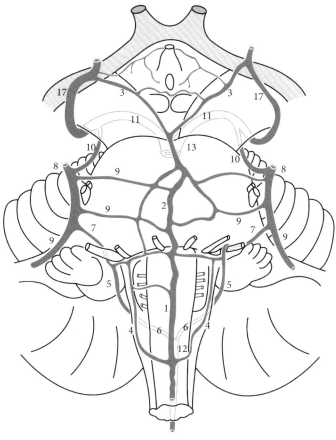

1. Internal cerebral vein
2. Great cerebral vein
3. Basal vein
4. Inferior sagittal sinus
5. Straight sinus
6. Superior sagittal sinus
7. Cortical vein
8. Torcular herophilii
9. Lateral sinus
10. Superior petrosal sinus
11. Inferior petrosal sinus
12. Cavernous sinus
13. Ophthalmic vein
14. Pterygoid plexus
15. Internal jugular vein
16. Facial vein
17. Occipital vein
18. Emissary vein.

Fig. 3.7 Brain venous circulation. Also see figure in colour plate section.

the petrous part of the temporal bone, and descends along the petro-mastoid fissure towards the jugular foramen. The lateral sinuses are frequently asymmetrical, the right lateral sinus more often draining the superior sagittal sinus. The transverse sinus receives the veins from the lateral and inferior parts of the temporal and occipital lobes as well as the cerebellar veins. The sigmoid sinus receives the superior petrous sinuses and the veins from the brainstem.

Superior petrosal sinus

The superior petrosal sinus runs along the superior surface of the petrous part of temporal bone in the attached margin of the tentorium cerebelli, and extends from the initial part of the sigmoid sinus to the posterior part of the cavernous sinuses. It can receive veins from the brainstem.

Inferior petrosal sinus

The inferior petrosal sinus runs along the petrobasilar suture from the postero-inferior part of the cavernous sinus to the jugular foramen. It can also receive veins from the brainstem.

Sphenoparietal sinus

The sphenoparietal sinus corresponds to the combination of two venous structures: a portion of the anterior branch of the middle meningeal vein and a dural sinus located under the lesser sphenoid wing. It runs into the cavernous sinus. There are conflicting views regarding the drainage site of the superficial middle cerebral vein. It is often regarded as terminating in the sphenoparietal sinus or as being an independent vein terminating in isolation in the cavernous sinus.

Cavernous sinus

The cavernous sinus is formed of two parts located on both sides of the hypophyseal fossa and is connected to the intercavernous sinuses, which lie in the diaphragma sellae. It extends to the superior orbital fissure at the front, to the foramen lacerum at the back and laterally to the foramen ovale. The cavernous sinus is a venous confluence of blood from the meninges, the orbital cavity, the brain, and the extracranial blood, particularly via its connection with the facial vein. It constitutes a rigid space in which the internal carotid artery beats surrounded by the sympathetic plexus, veins, and the abducens nerve. The oculomotor, trochlear, and ophthalmic nerves pass along the lateral wall of the cavernous sinus.

At the front, the cavernous sinus drains the superior and inferior ophthalmic veins, the spheno-parietal sinus, and communicates with the pterygoïd plexus via veins in the foramen rotundum. The cavernous sinus joins the pterygoïd plexus laterally, through the veins of the foramen ovale. At the back, the cavernous sinus is connected to the basilar plexus, to the transverse sinus via the superior petrosal sinus, and to the internal jugular vein via the inferior petrosal sinus.

Deep cerebral veins

Less variable than the cortical veins, the deep cerebral veins drain the deep white matter, the periventricular regions, and the diencephalic structures. They comprise the internal cerebral veins, basal veins, great cerebral vein and their collaterals (Figure 3.7 and 3.8) (19, 28, 43–48).

Internal cerebral veins

These paired veins originate in the interventricular foramen by union of the anterior septal and thalamostriate veins. They pass along the roof of the third ventricle between the two layers of the tela choroidea of the third ventricle. They join to form the great cerebral vein under the splenium of the corpus callosum next to the pineal body. The internal cerebral veins drain the superior choroidal, septal, and thalamic veins.

Great cerebral vein

The great cerebral vein (of Galen) is a vessel forming under the splenium of the corpus callosum by the union of the two internal cerebral veins. The great cerebral vein passes behind the splenium of the corpus callosum, terminating at the anterior junction of the falx cerebri and tentorium cerebelli. The inferior sagittal sinus joins the great cerebral vein to form the straight sinus. In addition to the internal cerebral veins, the great cerebral vein receives numerous other veins, in particular the basal veins, superior cerebellar veins, pineal veins, collicular veins, superior thalamic veins, internal occipital veins, and the posterior pericallosal veins.

Basal veins

The basal veins (of Rosenthal) are paired vessels originating on the surface of the anterior perforated space by the union of the anterior cerebral, deep middle cerebral and inferior striate veins. The basal veins circumvent the cerebral peduncle and flow into the great cerebral vein. They form an anastomotic network between the superficial and deep venous systems.

The principal veins flowing into the basal vein are the chiasmatic, hypothalamic, interpeduncular, and the veins of the temporal lobe.

Cortical cerebral veins

The cortical cerebral veins drain the cerebral cortex and the sub-cortical white matter, in particular the U fibres, via the superficial transcerebral venous system. The cortical venous system is extremely variable and specific nomenclatures of cortical veins are of no practical value. The topographical groupings of these veins, proposed by various authors, would appear to be more appropriate (19, 28, 39). The classification most adapted to neurovascular practice is that of Lasjaunias and Berenstein grouping these cortical veins into three systems: dorsomedial, ventrolateral, and anterior (49):

- The dorsomedial system drains the high convexity and midline cortical veins mainly into the superior sagittal sinus, the inferior sagittal sinus, the straight sinus or the great cerebral vein.

- The ventrolateral system drains the temporo-occipital cortical veins into the lateral sinus.

- The anterior system drains the anterior temporal and the anterior inferior frontal lobes into the cavernous sinus and the pterygoïd venous plexus.

There are numerous and variable anastomoses in the cortical venous network. Two large calibre anastomotic and more constant veins are usually described:

- The superior anastomotic vein (of Trolard) is a large vein joining the superior sagittal sinus with the superficial middle cerebral vein, crossing the cortical surface of the frontal and parietal lobes.

- The inferior anastomotic vein (of Labbé) is described as one or two anastomotic veins between the veins of the lateral fissure and the transverse sinus, draining the posterior portion of the temporal lobe (50, 51).

Posterior fossa vein

Brainstem veins

The brainstem veins extend the venous drainage system of the spinal cord (Figure 3.8). They are arranged in three large venous groups called anterior, lateral, and posterior veins (19, 28, 47, 52, 53).

The anterior veins are organized around an anteromedian axis formed by the anteromedian medullary vein. It follows its course in the anteromedian medullary sulcus following the anterior spinal vein and being followed by the anteromedian pontine vein. The latter communicates with the two interpeduncular veins that join the basal veins.

The lateral veins are usually represented on each side by the lateral medullary and the retro-olivary veins. The lateral medullary vein follows a course slightly dorsal to the retro-olivary sulcus. It receives the inferior cerebellar peduncle vein and flows into the

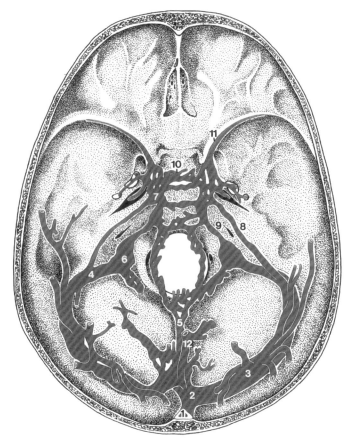

1. Antero-median medullary vein
2. Antero-median pontine vein
3. Interpeduncular vein
4. Retro-olivary vein
5. Lateral medullary vein
6. Inferior cerebellar peduncle vein
7. Lateral pontine vein
8. Superior petrosal vein
9. Anterior cerebellar vein
10. Lateral mesencephalic vein
11. Basal vein
12. Postero-median medullary vein
13. Great cerebral vein.

Fig. 3.8 Posterior fossa veins. Also see figure in colour plate section.

lateral pontine vein. The retro-olivary vein runs parallel to the lateral medullary vein but is anterior to it and is smaller in diameter.

An important structure for lateral drainage called the superior petrosal vein (of Dandy) is situated at the ponto-mesencephalic level. It is formed by the union of the anterior cerebellar vein that emerges from the horizontal fissure of the cerebellum and receives the lateral pontine vein, transverse pontine veins, and the lateral mesencephalic vein arriving from the basal vein. The superior petrosal vein flows into the superior petrosal sinus.

The dorsal veins are organized around the posteromedian medullary vein, an upward prolongation of the posteromedian spinal vein. It divides into two inferior cerebellar peduncle veins that pass along the fourth ventricle and flow into the lateral medullary veins. The posterior and lateral systems are widely anastomosed by veins surrounding the lateral sides of the medulla oblongata.

At the mesencephalic level, dorsal drainage is carried out by the basal and the lateral mesencephalic veins.

Cerebellar veins

The veins that drain the cerebellum are mainly located on its surface. The arrangement of these veins is well known and is of particular interest to neurosurgeons. They can be grouped into three broad categories: superior, inferior and anterior (19, 28, 47, 53).

The superior group mainly drains the upper part of the vermis and the superior hemispheric veins. The mesencephalic and pineal veins also participate in draining the upper part of the cerebellum. All these veins flow into the great cerebral vein.

The veins in the inferior group drain the inferior part of the cerebellum. The inferior vermian veins usually consist of two large veins which terminate in the dural sinuses near the torcular. The inferior hemispheric veins flow into the transverse sinus.

The anterior cerebellar veins drain venous blood form the middle part of the hemispheres and the lateral recess of the fourth ventricle. They flow into the superior petrosal vein that joins the superior petrosal sinus.

References

1. Tatu L, Moulin T, Duvernoy H, Bogousslavsky J. Arterial territories of human brain: brainstem and cerebellum. *Neurology*. 1996;47(5):1125–1135.
2. Tatu L, Moulin T, Duvernoy H, Bogousslavsky J. Arterial territories of the human brain: cerebral hemispheres. *Neurology*. 1998;50(6):1699–708.
3. Tatu L, Moulin T, Duvernoy H, Bogousslavsky J. Arterial territories of human brain. In Bogousslavsky J, Caplan L (eds) *Stroke Syndromes* (2nd edn, pp. 375–404). Cambridge: Cambridge University Press; 2001.
4. Alexander L. The vascular supply of the strio-pallidum. *Assoc Res Nerv Ment Dis*. 1942;21:77–132.
5. Dunker RO, Harris AB. Surgical anatomy of the proximal anterior cerebral artery. *J Neurosurg*. 1976;44(3):359–367.
6. Beevor C. The cerebral arterial supply. *Brain*. 1908;30:403–425.
7. Herman LH, Fernando OU, Gurdjian ES. The anterior choroidal artery: an anatomical study of its area of distribution. *Anat Rec*. 1966;154(1):95–101.
8. Abbie A. The clinical significance of the anterior choroidal artery. *Brain*. 1933;56:233–246.
9. Furlani J. The anterior choroidal artery and its blood supply to the internal capsule. *Acta Anat*. 1973;85(1):108–112.
10. Alicherif A, Raybaud C, Riss M, Poncet M, Khalil R, Salamon G. Arterial vascularization of the retrochiasmatic optic tract in man: recent data. *Rev Neurol*. 1977;133(5):339–352.
11. Plets CJ, De Reuck J, Vander Eecken H, Van den Bergh R. The vascularization of the human thalamus. *Acta Neurol Belg*. 1970;70(6):687–770.
12. Vincentelli F, Lehman G, Caruso G, Grisoli F, Rabehanta P, Gouaze A. Extracerebral course of the perforating branches of the anterior communicating artery: microsurgical anatomical study. *Surg Neurol*. 1991;35(2):98–104.
13. Wolfram-Gabel R, Maillot C, Koritke JG. Arterial vascularization of the corpus callosum in man. *Arch Anat Histol Embryol*. 1989;72:43–55.
14. Duvernoy H, Koritké G, Monnier G. Sur la vascularisation de la lame terminale humaine. *Z Zellforsch*. 1969;102(1):49–77.
15. DeReuck J. Arterial vascularisation and angioarchitecture of the nucleus caudatus in human. *Eur Neurol*. 1971;5(6):130–136.
16. Ostrowski AZ, Webster JE, Gurdjian ES. The proximal anterior cerebral artery: an anatomic study. *Arch Neurol*. 1960;3:661–664.
17. Marinkovic S, Milisavljevic M, Kovacević M. Anatomical bases for surgical approach to the initial segment of the anterior cerebral artery. Microanatomy of Heubner's artery and perforating branches of the anterior cerebral artery. *Surg Radiol Anat*. 1986;8(1):7–18.
18. Marinkovic S, Gibo H, Milisavljević M. The surgical anatomy of the relationships between the perforating and the leptomeningeal arteries. *Neurosurgery*. 1996;39(1):72–83.
19. Stephens R, Stilwell D. *Arteries and Veins of the Human Brain*. Springfield, IL: Charles C. Thomas; 1969.
20. Herman LH, Ostrowski AZ, Gurdjian ES. Perforating branches of the middle cerebral artery. An anatomical study. *Arch Neurol*. 1963;8:32–34.
21. Umansky FS, Juarez SM, Dujovny M, Ausman JI, Diaz FG, Gomes F *et al*. Microsurgical anatomy of the proximal segments of the middle cerebral artery. *J Neurosurg*. 1984;61(3):458–467.
22. Vincentelli F, Caruso G, Grisoli F, Rabehanta P, Andriamamonjy C, Gouaze A. Microsurgical anatomy of the cisternal course of the perforating branches of the posterior communicating artery. *Neurosurgery*. 1990;26(5):824–831.
23. Pedroza A, Dujovny M, Artero JC, Umansky F, Berman SK, Diaz FG, *et al*. Microanatomy of the posterior communicating artery. *Neurosurgery*. 1987;20(2):228–235.
24. Percheron G. Arteries of the human thalamus. I. Artery and polar thalamic territory of the posterior communicating artery. *Rev Neurol*. 1976;132(5):297–307.
25. Percheron G. Arteries of the human thalamus. II. Arteries and paramedian thalamic territory of the communicating basilar artery. *Rev Neurol*. 1976;132(5):309–324.
26. Percheron G. Arteries of the thalamus in man. Choroidal arteries. III. Absence of the constituted thalamic territory of the anterior choroidal artery. IV. Arteries and thalamic territories of the choroidal and postero-median thalamic arterial system. V. Arteries and thalamic territories of the choroidal and postero-lateral thalamic arterial system. *Rev Neurol*. 1977;133(10):547–558.
27. van der Zwan A, Hillen B, Tulleken CA, Dujovny M, Dragovic L. Variability of the territories of the major cerebral arteries. *J Neurosurg*. 1992;77(6):927–940.
28. Lazorthes G. *Vascularisation et circulation de l'encéphale humain*. Paris: Masson; 1972.
29. Duvernoy H. *Human Brain Stem Vessels*. Berlin: Springer-Verlag; 1978 (2nd edn 1999).
30. Duvernoy H. *The Human Brainstem and Cerebellum. Surface, Structure, Vascularization and Three Dimensional Sectional Anatomy with MRI*. Wien: Springer-Verlag; 1995.
31. Rhoton AL. The cerebellar arteries. *Neurosurg*. 2000;47(3 Suppl):S29–68.
32. Rodriguez-Hernandez A, Rhoton AL, Lawton MT. Segmental anatomy of cerebellar arteries: a proposed nomenclature. Laboratory investigation. *J Neurosurg*. 2011;115(2):387–397.
33. Amarenco P, Hauw JJ, Hénin D, Duyckaerts C, Roullet E, Laplane D, *et al*. Cerebellar infarction in the area of the posterior cerebellar artery. Clinicopathology of 28 cases. *Rev Neurol*. 1989;145(4);277–286.
34. Amarenco P, Hauw JJ. Cerebellar infarction in the territory of the superior cerebellar artery: a clinicopathologic study of 33 cases. *Neurology*. 1990;40(9):1383–1390.
35. Amarenco P, Hauw JJ. Cerebellar infarction in the territory of the anterior and inferior cerebellar artery. A clinicopathological study of 20 cases. *Brain*. 1990;113:139–155.
36. Marinkovic S, Kovacevic M, Gibo H, Milisavljević M, Bumbasirević L. The anatomical basis for the cerebellar infarcts. *Surg Neurol*. 1995;44(5):450–460.
37. Vuillier F, Medeiros E, Moulin T, Cattin F, Bonneville JF, Tatu L. Main anatomical features of the M1 segment of the middle cerebral artery: a 3D time-of-flight magnetic resonance angiography at 3 T study. *Surg Radiol Anat*. 2008;30(6):509–514.
38. Cosson A, Tatu L, Vuillier F, Parratte B, Diop M, Monnier G. Arterial vascularization of the human thalamus: extra-parenchymal arterial groups. *Surg Radiol Anat*. 2003;25(5-6):408–415.
39. Hacker H. Superficial supratentorial veins and dural sinus. In Newton T, Potts D (eds) *Radiology of the Skull and Brain* (pp. 1851–1902). St. Louis, MO: The CV Mosby Company; 1974.
40. Browder J, Kaplan HA, Krieger AJ. Anatomical features of the straight sinus and its tributaries. *J Neurosurg*. 1976;44(1):55–61.
41. Bisaria KK. Anatomic variations of venous sinuses in the region of the torcular Herophili. *J Neurosurg*. 1985;62(1):90–95.
42. San Millán Ruíz D, Fasel JH, Rüfenacht DA, Gailloud P. The sphenoparietal sinus of breschet: does it exist? An anatomic study. *Am J Neuroradiol*. 2004;25(1);112–1120.

43. Kilic T, OzdumanK, Cavdar S, Ozek MM, Pamir MN. The galenic venous system: surgical anatomy and its angiographic and magnetic resonance venographic correlations. *Eur J Radiol*. 2005;56(2): 212–219.

44. Chaynes P. Microsurgical anatomy of the great cerebral vein of Galen and its tributaries. *J Neurosurg*. 2003;99(6):1028–1038.

45. Stein R, Rosenbaum A. Normal deep cerebral venous system. In Newton T, Potts D (eds) *Radiology of the Skull and Brain* (pp. 1903–2110). St. Louis, MO: The CV Mosby Company; 1974.

46. Ono M, Rhoton AL, Peace D, Rodriguez RJ. Microsurgical anatomy of the deep venous system of the brain. *Neurosurgery*. 1984;15(5): 621–657.

47. Huang Y, Wolf B. The basal cerebral vein and its tributaries. In Newton T, Potts D (eds) *Radiology of the Skull and Brain* (pp. 2111–2154). St. Louis, MO: The CV Mosby Company; 1974.

48. Tubbs RS, Loukas M, Louis RG Jr, Shoja MM, Askew CS, Phantana-Angkool A, *et al*. Surgical anatomy and landmarks for the basal vein of rosenthal. *J Neurosurg*. 2007;106(5):900–902.

49. Lasjaunias P, Berenstein A. *Surgical Neuroangiography. 3. Functional Vascular Anatomy of Brain, Spinal Cord and Spine*. Berlin: Springer-Verlag; 1990.

50. Guppy KH, Origitano TC, Reichman OH, Segal. Venous drainage of the inferolateral temporal lobe in relationship to transtemporal/transtentorial approaches to the cranial base. *Neurosurgery*. 1997;41(3):615–619, discussion 619–620.

51. Avci E, Dagtekin A, Akture E, Uluc K, Baskaya MK. Microsurgical anatomy of the vein of Labbé. *Surg Radiol Anat*. 2011;33(7):569–573.

52. Duvernoy H. *The Superficial Veins of the Human Brain; Veins of the Brain Stem and of the Base of the Brain*. Berlin: Springer-Verlag; 1975.

53. Matsushima T, Rhoton AL Jr, de Oliveira E, Peace D. Microsurgical anatomy of the veins of the posterior fossa. *J Neurosurg*. 1983;59(1):63–105.

CHAPTER 4

Pathophysiology of transient ischaemic attack and ischaemic stroke

Jong S. Kim

Introduction

Stroke is a heterogeneous disorder associated with diverse pathogenic mechanisms. Understanding these mechanisms is important in determining treatment and prevention strategies in individual patients. Identifying the stroke mechanism requires history taking, neurological examinations, and appropriate laboratory/diagnostic tests.

Careful history taking may provide some insights into stroke mechanism. For example, maximal neurological deficits at stroke onset in a patient with a history of atrial fibrillation suggest a cardiogenic embolic infarction. Recurrent transient ischaemic attacks (TIA) or strokes with the same hemispheric symptoms are suggestive of ipsilateral large artery disease (LAD). Short-lasting stereotactic TIAs evoked by fatigue or dehydration may be signs of haemodynamically significant arterial steno/occlusive lesions. Examination of peripheral pulse and auscultation of cardiac murmurs or carotid bruits further help us delineate stroke mechanisms.

Chest X-ray, electrocardiography, Holter monitoring, transthoracic and transoesophageal echocardiography, and laboratory tests, including serum lipid, glucose and homocysteine concentrations, and coagulation profiles, are usually performed. However, stroke cannot be diagnosed nor its mechanism identified with certainty without neuroimaging evaluation. Neuroimaging commonly used in stroke patients includes computed tomography (CT), magnetic resonance imaging (MRI), conventional angiography, magnetic resonance angiography (MRA), CT angiography (CTA), and Doppler ultrasonography. Diffusion-weighted MRI (DWI), gradient echo MRI (GRE), and perfusion-weighted MRI (PWI), are nowadays increasingly used in the assessment of pathophysiology and management of stroke patients. High-resolution vessel wall MRI (HRMRI) may detect diffuse atherosclerotic plaques not detectable by conventional MRA (1, 2). These neuroimaging techniques are discussed in detail in Chapter 8.

Mechanisms of transient ischaemic attack and stroke

Large artery disease

LAD is the major cause of cerebral infarction in developed countries. Its main pathology consists of thrombosis superimposed on atherosclerosis, although other diseases such as dissection, vasculitis, and moyamoya disease are occasionally encountered.

The process of atherosclerosis is complex. Fibrous plaques in the aorta or internal carotid arteries (ICAs) are observed in many subjects younger than 40 years of age. Recurrent mechanical or toxic injuries to the intima associated with turbulent flow, as well as vascular risk factors such as hypertension, diabetes, hypercholesterolaemia, and cigarette smoking, initiate and promote the process of atherosclerosis. Circulating lipids, especially low-density lipoproteins, enter the vascular wall and inflammatory processes are initiated. Cholesterol containing macrophages and smooth muscle cells proliferate, finally resulting in atheroma formation (3–5).

Atherosclerosis is prone to occur in bifurcation areas, where blood turbulence is expected to occur. These areas include the carotid bulb, siphon, proximal middle cerebral artery (MCA), proximal vertebral artery, mid-basilar artery, and proximal posterior cerebral artery (PCA). Although extracranial atherosclerosis (ECAS), especially ICA bulb disease, is the most common form of LAD in Caucasians, ICAS is more frequent than ECAS in Asian, black, and Hispanic populations (6). Male sex, hyperlipidaemia, and coronary heart disease are more closely associated with ECAS, whereas female sex, advanced hypertension, metabolic syndrome, and insulin resistance are more closely associated with ICAS (7, 8). These differences, however, only partly explain the ethnic differences in the location of cerebral atherosclerosis.

Detailed stroke mechanisms in LAD patients include artery-to-artery embolism, hypoperfusion, branch occlusion, *in situ* atherothrombotic occlusion, and their combinations.

Artery-to-artery embolism

Although ICA stenosis is frequently observed in elderly persons, it is often asymptomatic. Certain characteristics of atherosclerotic plaques have been found to generate embolisms. Examination of carotid endarterectomy specimens revealed that plaque ulceration was significantly more common in symptomatic than asymptomatic patients (9). Plaque erosion or ulceration is a complex process related to shear stress and intra-arterial pressure changes (10). Intraplaque inflammation and subsequent cytokine activation lead to the recruitment of macrophages, lymphocytes, and mast cells. These cells activate metalloproteinases, which degrade the plaque wall and induce ulceration (11–13). Intraplaque haemorrhage also

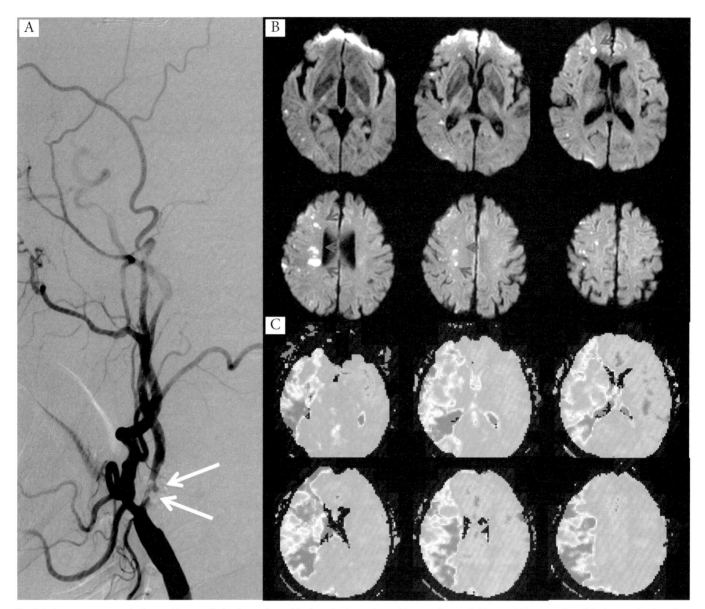

Fig. 4.1 Artery-to-artery embolism and hypoperfusion in a patient with ulcerative internal carotid artery disease. A 64-year-old hypertensive, diabetic man developed dysarthria and left hemiparesis. (A) Angiography showed severe, ulcerative atherosclerotic stenosis in the right carotid bulb area (long arrows). (B) DWI showed multiple scattered embolic infarcts in the right cortical areas, some of them located in the borderzone areas (short arrows). (C) Perfusion-weighted MRI using regional mean transit time showed hypoperfused areas in the right MCA territory. Also see figure in colour plate section.

contributes to plaque destabilization (14). Systemic infection may also play a role in this process; *Chlamydia pneumoniae* is often found in carotid plaques (15). These unstable plaques result in a procoagulation environment, with abnormal expression of tissue factor and plasminogen activator inhibitor. Local turbulence of blood flow and rupture of a plaque into the bloodstream promote thrombus formation (16, 17). These thrombi are prone to be broken up by forceful blood flow and migrate through the bloodstream to occlude distant arteries, resulting in clinical symptoms. Cholesterol debris can also migrate in this way (cholesterol embolism).

Ulcerative plaques can be identified *in vivo* by CTA and MRA, and more clearly by conventional angiography (Figure 4.1). On duplex scans, vulnerable plaques appear as echolucent and heterogeneous, with occasional evidence of intraplaque haemorrhage

(18). Although not widely used in clinical practice, HRMRI may detect characteristics of vulnerable plaques, including fibrous cap rupture, large necrotic core, and juxtaluminal haemorrhage or thrombus (19, 20). Microembolic signals detected by transcranial Doppler represent an embolus passing through the insonated artery, and are helpful in predicting future embolic stroke (21).

Artery-to-artery embolism is the predominant stroke mechanism in patients with ECAS, as well as being one of the important stroke mechanisms in patients with ICAS (i.e. proximal MCA to distal MCA) (22). Although autopsy studies of patients with ICAS producing embolism are rare, pathologies similar to ICA disease have been observed, including plaque rupture, intramural haemorrhage and ulceration (23).

DWI is useful in assessing the embolic mechanism of stroke, in that it can reliably detect small, scattered, cortical infarcts in the territory of the diseased artery. In many patients, DWI-identified lesions are also located in borderzone areas, suggesting that embolism often develops in combination with hypoperfusion (Figure 4.1). Underlying perfusion deficits may contribute to the development of embolic infarction by inducing abnormal clotting or by the impaired clearance of emboli (24). Cortical embolisms in patients with ICAS are often associated with subcortical, perforator territory infarctions, suggesting that a combined mechanism (embolism and branch occlusion) is common (25) (Figure 4.2).

Recent DWI studies in patients with MCA territory infarction found that territorial cortical or superficial infarcts were associated with embolic mechanisms, whereas deep perforator infarcts and internal borderzone infarcts were more common in patients with intrinsic atherosclerotic MCA disease (26, 27). In patients with significant ICA disease, DWI lesion patterns may differ according to the degree of stenosis and perfusion impairment; lesions occurring in haemodynamic risk zones were significantly more common in patients with high degree stenosis/occlusion, along with diffusion–perfusion mismatch (28).

In patients with ICA disease, plaque vulnerability may be more important than the degree of stenosis in predicting embolic strokes (29). Nevertheless, the degree of stenosis is generally severe in patients who experience embolic strokes. In ICAS patients, severe stenosis is more often associated with artery-to-artery embolism than with branch occlusion (22). Therefore, in both conditions, embolism is prone to occur in patients with the presence of perfusion deficits in the territory of a severely stenosed vessel.

Although less frequent than in anterior circulation stroke, artery-to-artery embolism does occur in the posterior fossa. Significant atherothrombosis in the proximal vertebral artery often induces embolization, occluding arteries such as the PCA, superior cerebellar artery, posterior inferior cerebellar artery, and the upper portion of the basilar artery (30). Stenoses in the distal vertebral

and basilar arteries may also produce embolism, although they produce strokes by way of branch occlusion as well (8, 31, 32). As in the anterior circulation, embolisms seem to occur more frequently in the setting of posterior fossa hypoperfusion, related to bilateral vertebral artery disease or hypoplasia.

Finally, embolisms may develop from the large arteries proximal to the ICA, including the common carotid artery, subclavian arteries, ascending aorta and aortic arch. Transoesophageal echocardiography is required to detect plaques in the aorta. Since aortic plaques develop more frequently in the distal aortic arch than in the ascending aorta, embolic stroke tends to occur in the left rather than the right hemisphere (33). Although case–control studies showed that thick (≥4 mm) atherosclerotic plaques are an independent risk factor for recurrent strokes (34), this was not confirmed in recent population-based studies (35, 36).

In situ thrombotic occlusion

Excessive thrombus formation in areas of atherosclerotic plaque can ultimately result in total occlusion of the vessel. In patients with ECAS, the clinical consequences of arterial occlusion are not so grave because of the ample collateral circulations in the circle of Willis. Therefore, total arterial occlusion may remain asymptomatic or produce minor haemodynamic TIAs or strokes. In rare patients with insufficient collaterals or those with previous contralateral ICA occlusion, ICA occlusion may result in devastating infarcts involving whole ICA (MCA and ACA, plus PCA in the presence of fetal circulation) territories (37).

In contrast to ECAS, *in situ* thrombotic occlusion in patients with ICAS more often produces significant cerebral infarction as the collateral circulation is generally less efficient in these patients. The resultant infarcts are usually larger than those caused by branch occlusion. However, unlike cardiogenic embolism, *in situ* thrombotic occlusion rarely produces sudden, whole territory infarction because of the relatively well-developed collateral circulation in patients with a chronic atherosclerotic process (38). In patients with MCA steno-occlusion, the initial lesions are usually restricted

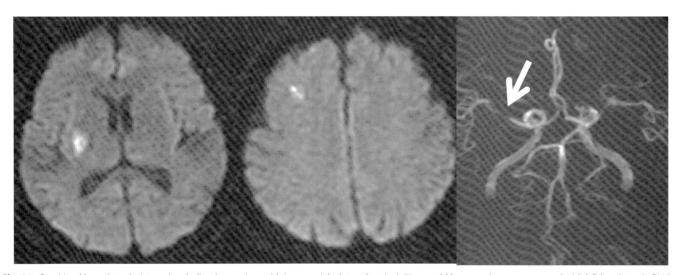

Fig. 4.2 Combined branch occlusion and embolism in a patient with intracranial atherosclerosis. A 72-year-old hypertensive man presented with left hemiparesis. DWI showed a solitary infarct in the right putamen/internal capsule, and another small cortical infarct. MR angiography showed right MCA stenosis (arrow) that probably induced branch (perforator) occlusion and embolism. (From Kang DW, Kim KS. Application of magnetic resonance imaging. In Kim JS, Caplan LR, Wong KSL (eds) *Intracranial Atherosclerosis* (pp. 135–146). Oxford: Wiley-Blackwell; 2008, with permission.)

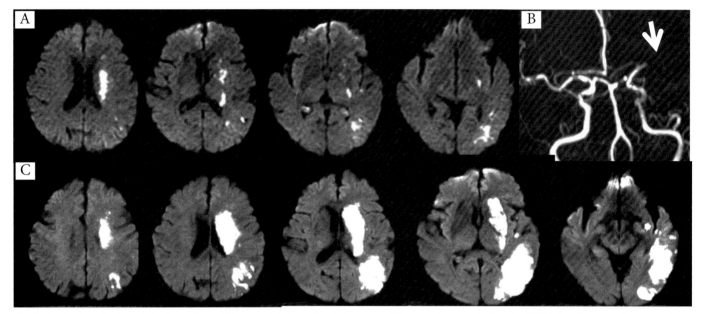

Fig. 4.3 *In situ* thrombotic occlusion in a patient with intracranial atherosclerosis. A 64-year-old hypertensive man developed mild right hemiparesis and sensory aphasia. (A) DWI at the time of admission showed acute infarcts in the left lenticulocapsular and borderzone areas between MCA and posterior cerebral artery. (B) MRA showed thrombotic occlusion of the left MCA. The patient's neurological symptoms progressively worsened to have severe right hemiparesis and global aphasia. (C) Follow up MRI 4 days later showed increased lesion size. (From Wong KSL, Caplan LR, Kim JS. Stroke mechanisms. In, Kim JS, Caplan LR, Wong KSL ed. Intracranial Atherosclerosis, pp 57–68, with permission.)

to the striatocapsular and/or borderzone area. As the occlusion continues, the initial infarct frequently grows, accompanied by progressive neurological worsening (Figure 4.3). Thus, the ultimate infarct size varies according to the status of the collateral circulation, the speed of arterial occlusion and haemodynamic stability after the occurrence of stroke. With sufficient collaterals, total thrombotic intracranial occlusion may result in only minor stroke/TIA or even remain asymptomatic.

Branch occlusion

Branch or perforator occlusion is a stroke mechanism unique to patients with ICAS. Atherosclerotic plaques in the intracranial artery can occlude the orifice of the perforators, causing infarcts limited to the subcortical area (39). Pathological features of this condition have been described (40, 41), with the pathologic substrates occluding the branching vessel being microdissection, plaque haemorrhage, and platelet-fibrin materials. Branch occlusion is an important, but to date neglected mechanism of LAD (42). It is more often observed in posterior than in anterior circulation stroke and is one of the major mechanisms of brainstem stroke (31, 32, 43, 44). Branch occlusion is currently more easily recognized by imaging methodologies such as MRA and CTA, being regarded as an important cause of so-called 'lacunar' infarcts (45–48) (Figure 4.4, left image of panel 1, A of panel 2).

The infarcts associated with branch occlusion do not differ fundamentally from 'lacunar infarcts' caused by lipohyalinotic small artery disease (SAD), although their pathological nature is different. The subcortical infarcts caused by branch occlusion tend to extend to the basal surface, whereas a lacune caused by lipohyalinosis usually produces an island of ischaemic tissues within the parenchyma. Although both conditions equally produce lacunar syndromes clinically, the former is more often associated with

atherosclerosis in other vascular beds (49), larger lesion volume, and an unstable and adverse clinical course than the latter (32, 33, 50).

Compared with arterial lesions producing embolism or haemodynamic impairment, branch occlusion is related to milder atherosclerosis (25). One problem in diagnosing branch occlusion is the sensitivity and specificity of existing imaging techniques in detecting mild vascular lesions; they may not be detected by TCD, and may only be equivocally detected by MRA or CTA. Moreover, because the imaging diagnosis is based on findings of luminal narrowing, atherosclerotic thickening of the vessel walls in the absence of focal narrowing cannot be detected with these methods. Nowadays, HRMRI is increasingly utilized to identify branch occlusion associated with diffuse ICAS (2, 51) (Figure 4.5; Figure 4.4, C of panel 2) which makes us suspect that branch occlusion may be much more common than previously thought (42).

Hypoperfusion

With continued atherosclerotic process, the plaque grows inwardly, and narrowing of the vessel leads to turbulent blood flow and finally hypoperfusion distal to the site of stenosis. Generally, the degree of hypoperfusion depends on the severity of vascular stenosis/occlusion, and there is a close correlation between the recurrence of ischaemic stroke and the severity of occlusive disease (52, 53). However, the occurrence of ischaemic events is also influenced by the status of collateral flow, from arteries at the circle of Willis, external carotid artery system, and cervicothyroid arteries, etc.

In patients with severe vascular stenosis/occlusion and insufficient collaterals, haemodynamic TIAs can occur. Typically, symptoms such as hemiparesis, aphasia, monocular blindness, limb shaking (in anterior circulation disease) or dizziness, diplopia, and visual disturbances (in posterior circulation disease) occur briefly

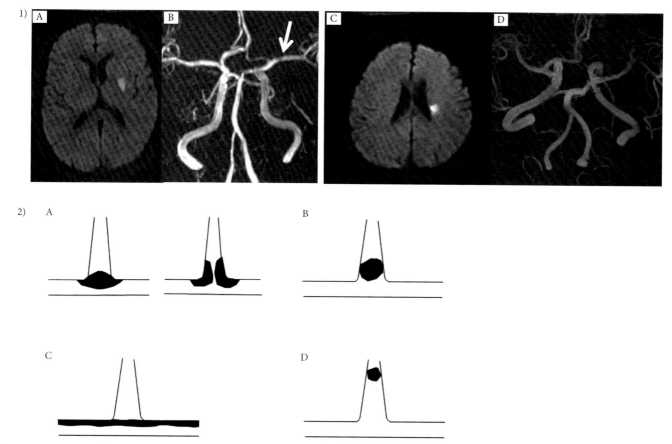

Fig. 4.4 Various causes of small subcortical infarction. Panel 1: (A) Subcortical infarction caused by branch occlusion associated with focal intracranial atherosclerosis (arrow, B). (C) Subcortical infarction presumably caused by lipohyalinotic small artery disease (D). Panel 2: (A) Branch occlusion causing subcortical infarction. Left: obliteration of perforators by focal intracranial atherosclerosis. Right: junctional atherothrombosis. (B) Atherosclerotic proximal small vessel disease. (C) Intracranial disease with diffuse wall involvement. (D) Lipohyalinotic distal small artery disease. 2A=branch occlusion identified by current vascular imaging techniques. 2A, 2B=Caplan's definition of branch atheromatous disease. 2A, 2C=branch occlusion identified by imaging techniques including high-resolution MRI. 2A, 2B, 2C=atherosclerotic causes of single subcortical infarction.

and stereotypically in patients who are dehydrated, fatigued, or at the time when they suddenly stand up. Revascularization therapies, such as angioplasty/stenting or bypass surgery, may rapidly relieve these symptoms (Figure 4.6). When stroke develops, the symptoms may fluctuate widely according to the degree of hydration, blood pressure, and the position of the patient's head. Volume therapy or increasing patient's blood pressure is occasionally helpful in reversing patients' neurological deficits. With persistent perfusion defect, the symptoms may worsen gradually (Figure 4.7).

In the anterior circulation, infarcts caused by haemodynamic impairment usually develop in superficial (anterior cerebral artery–MCA, MCA–PCA) and/or internal (areas between superficial MCA pial penetrators and lenticulostriate arteries) borderzone areas, the latter being more specifically associated with haemodynamic impairment than the former (Figure 4.7). Hypoperfusion as a pathogenic mechanism can therefore be recognized by DWI lesion patterns, the degree of vascular stenosis, the status of collateral vessels, perfusion imaging findings, and appropriate clinical histories. In the posterior circulation, haemodynamic TIAs and strokes occur following severe steno-occlusive lesions occurring in both vertebral arteries or the basilar artery. Here, DWI patterns of haemodynamic infarction have not been clearly established due in part to the many normal variations that influence perfusion status,

such as dominance of the posterior communicating artery or hypoplastic vertebral artery.

Although hypoperfusion is an important stroke mechanism, strokes caused by haemodynamic failure alone are uncommon in clinical practice. More often, hypoperfusion plays an additive role in the development of stroke, together with other major stroke mechanisms.

In patients with abrupt vascular occlusion, with whatever the cause, the core area supplied by this vessel is rapidly damaged, while the surrounding, hypoperfused areas can still survive for a certain period of time. This so-called 'penumbra area' will eventually develop into an ischaemic lesion unless the hypoperfusion status is rapidly reversed. In patients with persistent steno/occlusive vascular lesions, the infarcted area gradually expands over time to include the hypoperfused region unless appropriate therapy is initiated. As discussed earlier, the co-occurrence of hypoperfusion and embolism in patients with severe steno-occlusive vascular diseases is common, due in part to both mechanisms being related to complicated atherosclerotic plaques protruding into the lumen, and in part to ineffective wash out of emboli in hypoperfused areas (24) (Figure 4.1).

The role of hypoperfusion remains less clear in patients with small subcortical infarction. As already discussed, small subcortical infarcts are caused by either a lipohyalinotic SAD or by

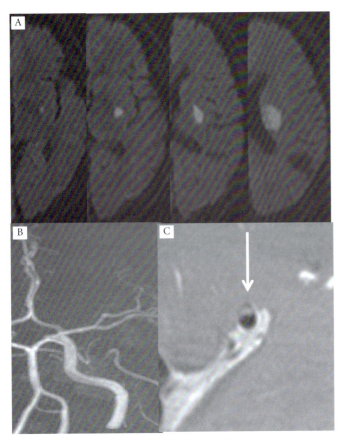

Fig. 4.5 High-resolution vessel wall MRI. A 61-year-old hypertensive woman presented with right hemipareisis. (A) DWI showed a vertically extended infarct in the left putamen/internal capsule. (B) MRA did not show any abnormality in MCA. (C) High-resolution vessel wall MRI identified atherosclerotic plaques in the superior wall of the left MCA trunk (arrow).

branch occlusion associated with parental artery disease (39, 41, 51, 54). Patients with small subcortical infarctions often experience neurological progression (55), often associated with subacute lesion volume increase (32, 56). Presumably, lesion volume expansion may occur in hypoperfused area in these patients. It remains unclear, however, whether hypoperfused areas are larger in patients with neurological progression or those having parental artery disease (32, 56).

Small artery disease

A single subcortical infarction, traditionally called a 'lacunar infarction' usually results from SAD (57). Its pathological hallmarks include irregular cavities, less than 15–20 mm in size, located deep in the cerebral hemisphere, brainstem, and the cerebellum. Penetrating arteries associated with these lesions are associated with disorganized vessel walls, fibrinoid material deposition, and, occasionally, haemorrhagic extravasation through arterial walls, a finding first called 'segmental arterial disorganization' and then lipohyalinosis by Fisher (41, 57–63). More benign and common vascular changes include the deposition of collagen replacing smooth muscles cells, with preserved lumen size and overall vascular architecture. Although these simple vascular changes do not produce arterial occlusions, they are associated with reduced vascular distensibility and are probably related to white matter ischaemic changes commonly seen in elderly patients and those with vascular risk factors (64).

These vascular changes occur at arteries or arterioles 40–400 μm in diameter, and frequently affect the lenticulostriate branches of the MCA (Figure 4.4, right image of panel 1, D of panel 2), the thalamoperforating arteries from the posterior cerebral artery and the perforators of the basilar arteries. The resultant subcortical infarcts produce 'lacunar syndromes', including pure motor stroke, pure sensory stroke, sensorimotor, dysarthria clumsy hands, and ataxic hemiparesis without cortical symptoms.

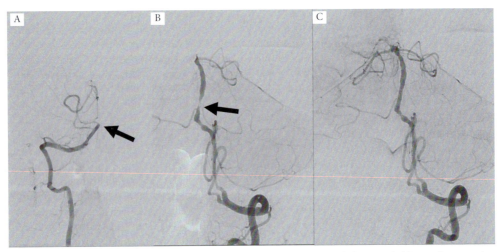

Fig. 4.6 Posterior fossa TIAs associated with haemodynamic failure. A 45-year-old man with hypertension, diabetes, and a history of coronary heart disease developed recurrent attacks of dizziness, diplopia, and gait instability that lasted for a few minutes. MRI showed no abnormal findings. (A) Angiogram shows occlusion of the right vertebral artery just above the posterior inferior cerebellar artery (arrow) and (B) severe stenosis of the basilar artery just above the anterior inferior cerebellar artery (arrow). (C) Angioplasty and stenting was performed and the stenosis was improved. The patient no longer developed such symptoms during 12 months after the procedure. (From Capaln LR, Amarenco P, Kim JS. Posterior circulation disorders. In, Kim JS, Caplan LR, Wong KSL ed. Intracranial Atherosclerosis, pp 83–99, with permission.)

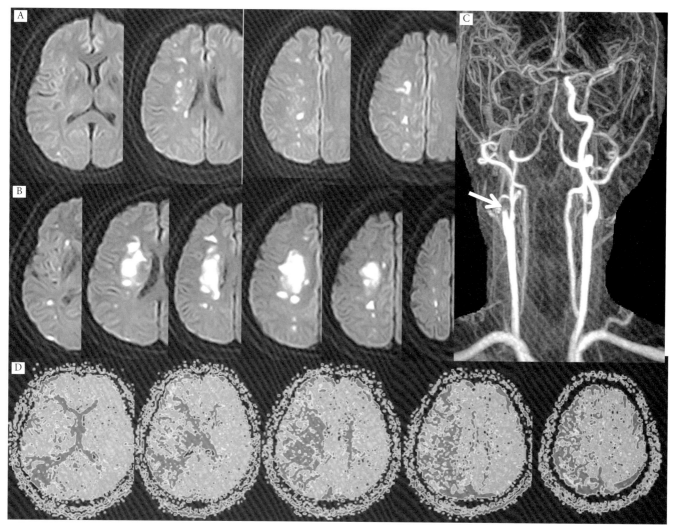

Fig. 4.7 Haemodynamic infarction. A 50-year-old man with uncontrolled diabetes mellitus developed mild left hemiparesis (MRC grade IV). (A) Initial DWI showed scattered infarcts in the right border zone area. Two days later, the limb weakness progressed to grade II. (B) Repeat DWI showed extended lesions. (C) MRA showed right internal carotid artery occlusion (long arrow). (D) Perfusion-weighted MRI (MTT map) showed decreased perfusion in the right MCA territory. Also see figure in colour plate section.

However, lacunar infarctions are not always caused by non-atherosclerotic lesions. In the proximal part of the small artery, the atherosclerotic process is observed although not associated with a profound lipid core or plaque rupture as shown in LAD (Figure 4.4, B of panel 2). In addition, as discussed earlier, single subcortical infarction may be caused by branch occlusion associated with atherothrombotic lesion in the parental, intracranial artery (Figure 4.4, left image of panel 1, A of panel 2). These atherosclerotic causes of subcortical infarction have been collectively described as 'atheromatous branch occlusion (BAD)' by Caplan (39) (Figure 4.4, A and B of panel 2).

The concept of BAD has provided insights into the atherosclerotic causes of lacunar infarction. Using current imaging modalities, however, proximal atherosclerotic SAD cannot be distinguished from distal lipohyalinotic SAD. Because arteriosclerotic SAD usually produces relatively extensive lesions along the diseased artery (39), the size and extension of subcortical infarctions has been used to differentiate arteriosclerotic from lipohyalinotic SAD (65). However, as DWI-detected lesion volumes frequently increase over time (32, 56), lesion size may differ depending on the timing of imaging (65). Moreover, infarcts located distant from parental vessels may also be associated with parental artery disease (51). Thus, BAD may not be reliably defined by MRI criteria alone. To avoid confusion, we may better reserve BAD as a pathological term rather than use it in clinical practice (42). The concept of lipohyalinotic and atherogenic causes of small subcortical infarction is summarized in Figure 4.4.

Finally, subcortical lacunar infarcts, especially large lesions, may be caused by embolism from diseased heart or carotid artery (66, 67). However, more recent studies using DWI showed that the embolic aetiology is actually rare in patients with strictly subcortical infarcts (48).

Cardiac embolism

Embolism from a diseased heart is the cause of approximately 20–25% of ischaemic strokes (68–70) with the proportion depending on the extensiveness of cardiac workup, such as Holter monitoring or transthoracic/transoesophageal echocardiography. A thrombus arising in the heart most frequently travels to the MCA territory, and DWI studies have shown that the most frequent pattern of cardiogenic embolic infarctions was territorial and cortical (25). However, cardiac embolism may affect any part of the brain, including the subcortical and brainstem regions (66, 67).

Infarcts associated with cardioembolism are typically larger than those associated with LAD, partly because the clots are larger and partly because of the insufficiently developed collateral circulation in the absence of chronic atherosclerosis (71). The onset is usually abrupt, with a gradual progression or fluctuation of symptoms being less common than with LAD. However, approximately 5% of embolic strokes may show a non-sudden or fluctuating onset (72). DWI detection of multiple acute infarcts in multiple vascular territories suggests an embolism from the heart rather than LAD (73) (Figure 4.8).

The occluded vessels are visible when angiography is performed soon after stroke. Although the MCA trunk and/or branches are the most frequently affected, larger vessels such as the internal and common carotid arteries may be occluded. Smaller occluded vessels are more difficult to detect with MRA or CTA. Clinical symptoms vary according to the size and location of the occluded vessels. Generally, cardiogenic embolic infarcts tend to produce more severe clinical symptoms than those associated with other aetiologies. Accordingly, patients' mortality is relatively high (69, 74). However, small cortical infarcts may produce minor symptoms: weakness limited to a part of distal limbs (75) or dysarthria only (76). Signs of peripheral artery occlusion, such as a reddish discoloration of the skin in distal limbs, are suggestive of embolic stroke.

In cardioembolic infarcts, the embolic materials are generally evanescent. Previous studies have shown that embolic occlusion of vessels was detected in more than 75% of patients when patients were evaluated by angiography within 8 hours of stroke onset (77), but in only 40% when angiography was delayed for up to 72 hours (78). Follow-up angiograms occasionally show recanalization of occluded vessels or migration of emboli from proximal to distal arteries. These characteristics help us differentiate embolic from atherosclerotic *in situ* occlusion (79). Due in part to large lesion size and in part to frequent recanalization (and reperfusion), haemorrhagic transformation of an infarct is relatively common (Figure 4.8). Haemorrhagic transformation may be associated with development of headache or neurological worsening, and is one of the main concerns in initiating anticoagulation therapy.

In addition, GRE may provide information on the aetiology of vascular occlusion, by revealing the so-called 'GRE susceptibility vessel sign' (GRE SVS) (80–82) (Figure 4.9). The characteristics of an intraluminal clot differ according to the origin of the thrombus. White thrombi formed in areas of high shear stress are composed predominantly of platelet aggregates, whereas red thrombi formed in low-pressure areas such as cardiac chambers are rich in fibrin and trapped red blood cells (83, 84). Therefore, it is expected that thrombus showing a GRE SVS sign contains a large quantity of red blood cells. One study, in which DWI, GRE, and MRA were used to assess ischaemic stroke patients within 24 hours of stroke onset (85), found that GRE SVS was more frequently observed in patients

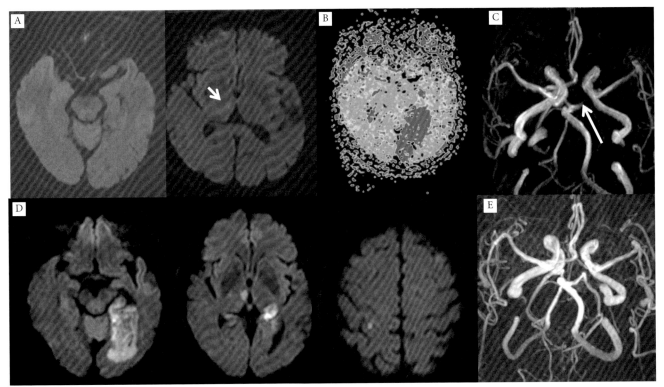

Fig. 4.8 Cardiogenic infarction. A 71-year-old woman with atrial fibrillation suddenly developed confusion. (A) Initial DWI showed right medial thalamic infarction (short arrow) without definite lesion on the occipital area. (B) Perfusion-weighted MRI (MTT map) showed decreased perfusion in the left occipital area. (C) MRA showed occlusion of the left posterior cerebral artery (long arrow). (D) Follow-up DWI 4 days later showed haemorrhagic infarction in the left occipital area, and an infarct in the right thalamus. A small infarct is also shown in the right cortical area of MCA territory. (E) MRA showed complete recanalization of the posterior cerebral artery. Also see figure in colour plate section.

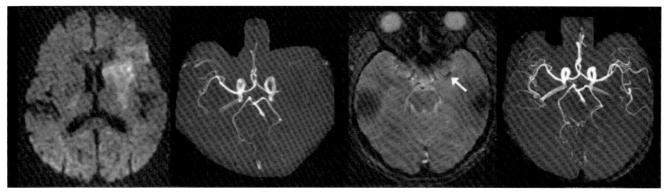

Fig. 4.9 GRE susceptibility vessel sign. A 61-year-old woman with atrial fibrillation presented with right hemiparesis and aphasia. There were acute left MCA infarcts on DWI, a left MCA occlusion on MRA, and susceptibility vessel sign (SVS) in the occluded vessel on GRE (arrow) on acute scans (1 hour after onset). The patient was treated with intravenous tPA. Follow-up MRA (last image) showed complete recanalization of the left MCA. (From Kang DW, Kim KS. Application of magnetic resonance imaging. In, Kim JS, Caplan LR, Wong KSL ed. Intracranial Atherosclerosis, pp 135–146, with permission.)

with cardioembolic stroke (31/40, 78%) than in those with other stroke subtypes (14/55, 25%), illustrating the usefulness of GRE as adjunctive information in evaluating the aetiology of the arterial occlusion.

Table 4.1 summarizes the important heart diseases causing embolism. Due to space limitations, only a few specific aetiologies are briefly discussed here.

Atrial fibrillation

Atrial fibrillation is the most common cause of embolic infarction in developed countries. Because the incidence of atrial fibrillation increases with age, it will likely become an even more important cause of stroke in the future. Paroxysmal atrial fibrillation, which can be detected by Holter monitoring, is equally risky. In patients with atrial fibrillation, the following characteristics are shown to increase the risk of stroke: previous embolic events, advanced age, hypertension, diabetes, and associated cardiac problems such as rheumatic valve disease, left ventricular dysfunction, and enlarged atrium. Based on this information, scales have been developed that can predict the stroke risk and identify the patients who need anticoagulation therapy. One of the best validated schemes is the $CHADS_2$ (86) (Table 4.2). The risk of thromboembolism linearly increases as $CHADS_2$ score increases in both the patients taking warfarin and those who did not (87). More recently, another system called CHA_2DS_2-VASc score was introduced that additionally considered gender factor and put more weight on advanced age (88) (Table 4.2). CHA_2DS_2-VASc seems to improve the predictive value over the $CHADS_2$ schema. A study comparing $CHADS_2$ and CHA_2DS_2-VASc systems in patients with atrial fibrillation showed that the $CHADS_2$ score classified 33% as requiring oral anticoagulation while the CHA_2DS_2-VASc score classified 53% as requiring oral anticoagulation. With CHA_2DS_2-VASc system, many patients, particularly older women, are redistributed from the low- to high-risk categories (89).

It seems clear that these scoring systems help us predict embolism risks and define patients who need anticoagulation among those with atrial fibrillation. However, as many items are also factors predicting prognosis in patients with non-cardiogenic infarction, the scores may not be specifically valuable for patients with cardiogenic stroke. A recent study showed that increased $CHADS_2$ score was associated with increased burden

of concomitant cerebral atherosclerosis (90), and the increased risk of stroke in patients with high $CHADS_2$ scores may be due at least in part to an increased incidence of LAD. Another study showed that prestroke $CHADS_2$ and CHA_2DS_2-VASc scores predict long-term stroke outcomes in non-atrial fibrillation stroke patients as well (91).

Infective endocarditis

Infective endocarditis produces septic emboli, with occluded vessels becoming infected, fragile, and necrotic, sometimes forming mycotic aneurysms. Haemorrhagic complications occur in as many as 20–40% of these patients. Intracerebral and even subarachnoid haemorrhages occur occasionally. Early initiation of appropriate antibiotics is the most effective therapy, whereas anticoagulation should not be given due to an excessive risk of

Table 4.1 Cardiac diseases producing embolic infarction

High risk for ischaemic stroke
Sustained atrial fibrillation
Paroxysmal atrial fibrillation
Sick sinus syndrome
Sustained atrial flutter
Recent (<1 month) myocardial infarction
Rheumatoid mitral or aortic valve disease
Bioprosthetic and mechanical heart valves
Congestive heart failure (with ejection fraction <30%)
Dilated cardiomyopathy
Non-bacterial thrombotic endocarditis
Infective endocarditis
Left atrial myxoma
Low or uncertain risk for ischaemic stroke
Mitral annular calcification
Patent foramen ovale
Atrial septal aneurysm

Table 4.2 CHADS$_2$ and CHA$_2$DS$_2$-VASc score

CHADS$_2$	Points	CHA$_2$DS$_2$-VASc	Points
Congestive heart failure	1	**C**ongestive heart failure/left ventricular dysfunction	1
Hypertension	1	**H**ypertension	1
Age ≥75 years	1	**A**ge ≥75 years	2
Diabetes mellitus	1	**D**iabetes mellitus	1
Stroke/TIA	2	**S**troke/TIA/thromboembolism	2
		Vascular disease (prior myocardial infarction, peripheral artery disease, or aortic plaque)	1
		Age 65–74 years	1
		Sex **c**ategory (i.e. female gender)	1

cerebral haemorrhages. Known cardiac disease, fever, heart murmur, increased ESR, anaemia, leucocytosis, and haemorrhagic infarction are all important items suggestive of infective endocarditis. Blood culture and echocardiography should be performed for a definitive diagnosis.

Patent foramen ovale

The combination of patent foramen ovale (PFO) and right-to-left shunting is a potential source of embolism. Postmortem studies have confirmed that thrombi arising in the venous system, usually in the leg or pelvis, travel to occlude cerebral arteries through a right-to-left cardiac shunt (paradoxical embolism). Therefore, patients with a suspected embolism but without a clear source are generally assessed by transoesophageal echocardiography with shunt tests to detect PFO and right-to-left shunt.

However, the significance of PFO as a cause of stroke remains still unclear; POF is present in 25% of the normal population, and the combination of PFO and right-to-left shunting does not necessarily indicate causality. Moreover, accompanying venous thrombosis is rarely detected (92). A recent meta-analysis showed that the rate of recurrent stroke does not differ between cryptogenic stroke patients with and without PFO (93). Further, although previous studies have suggested a significant association between PFO with a large shunt and atrial septal aneurysm and recurrent stroke (94, 95), more recent studies could not confirm this association (96). Therefore, although many neurologists consider large PFO with a significant amount of shunt as an embolic aetiology of stroke, further studies are needed to elucidate the true role of PFO in patients with stroke.

Uncommon causes or mechanisms of stroke

Uncommon causes of stroke include dissection, moyamoya disease, arteritis, coagulation abnormality, and cerebral autosomal dominant arteriopathy with subcortical infarcts and leucoencephalopathy (CADASIL). Details are described in Chapter 14. The basic stroke mechanisms in patients with these conditions are similar to those previously described, including artery-to-artery embolism,

branch occlusion, hypoperfusion, *in situ* large artery occlusion, and SAD. However, certain stroke mechanisms are more prevalent in a particular disease, depending on the nature and the predilection site of each vascular disease.

Cervicocerebral artery dissections occur in 1–2% of all patients with ischaemic strokes, but are one of the major causes (10–25%) of stroke in younger patients (97). As in atherothrombotic infarction, extracranial dissection usually produces stroke or TIA via artery-to-artery embolism with occasional haemodynamic impairment, whereas branch occlusion is an important stroke mechanism in intracranial dissection. Branch occlusion due to distal vertebral artery dissection is an important mechanism of medullary infarction (31).

Moyamoya disease is characterized by progressive occlusion of the distal ICA or proximal MCA, with the development of fine meshworks of basal collateral vessels. Cerebral hypoperfusion is the predominant stroke mechanism in these patients, and repeated TIAs are observed when patients are dehydrated or hyperventilating (e.g. eating hot noodles or crying). Decreased cerebral perfusion may result in impaired cognition and intelligence in younger patients (98). Less often, cerebral infarction due to embolism or thrombotic occlusion is encountered (99).

Vasculitis may be caused by infectious (e.g. bacterial, tuberculous, spirochetal, fungal, viral) and immunological (e.g. lupus, polyarteritis nodosa, Takayasu disease) disorders. Generally, intracranial arteries adjacent to the brain are involved, with the most frequent stroke mechanisms being *in situ* thrombotic occlusion and branch occlusion. Inflammation surrounding the vessel may produce encephalitis or abscess, which additionally contributes to the clinical symptoms. Takayasu disease is exceptional in that it primarily involves extracranial arteries, such as the aorta, subclavian arteries, and common carotid arteries. Therefore, the main stroke mechanisms in this condition are haemodynamic impairment and artery-to-artery embolism. Subclavian steal syndrome may develop. These inflammatory/immunological conditions may induce hypertension, accelerated atherosclerosis, and cardiac involvement, which can indirectly produce ischaemic strokes.

Coagulation disorders such as factor abnormalities or protein C and S deficiencies more frequently produce venous than arterial strokes. Cancers, especially malignant, advanced ones, may provoke ischaemic stroke via hypercoagulation, non-bacterial thrombotic endocarditis, cancer embolization, and chemotherapy-induced vasculopathy. Patients with cancer-associated stroke frequently have high serum D-dimer and CRP concentrations, with DWI showing multiple scattered lesions in multiple vascular territories (100). Unexplained stroke with these laboratory and imaging characteristics may allow us to suspect the presence of undetected cancers (Figure 4.10).

CADASIL is a hereditary disorder characterized clinically by recurrent migraine, stroke episodes, and vascular dementia. Autopsy findings have shown that the cerebral and leptomeningeal arterioles are involved. The media is thickened and smooth muscle cells are swollen and degenerated, resulting in luminal narrowing and occlusion. Thus, CADASIL is essentially an SAD. However, a recent study suggested that LAD may also occur in these patients (101).

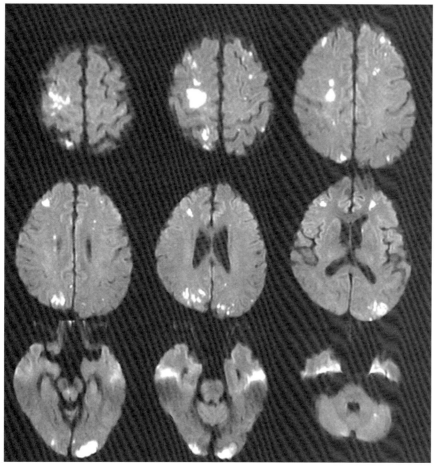

Fig. 4.10 DWI-identified multiple territory infarcts presumably caused by cancer associated hypercoagulopathy. A 64-year-old man without any vascular risk factors developed left hemiparesis. DWI showed multiple scattered infarcts in bilateral anterior and posterior circulations. MRA, electrocardiography, and echocardiography findings were normal. His serum D-dimer and CRP levels were elevated. A further workup revealed that he had lung cancer that metastasized to multiple lymph nodes, bilateral kidneys, and thoracic spines.

Cryptogenic (undetermined) stroke

Cryptogenic stroke or infarct of undetermined origin may be defined when there is an incomplete workup, two or more possible mechanisms, or when the cause is undetermined despite adequate workup. Recent advances in imaging technologies have reduced the proportion of cryptogenic stroke, from 30–40% in the late 1980s (68, 102), to less than 20% more recently (74, 103–105). However, as discussed in the later section 'Classification of stroke based on stroke mechanisms', there are complex issues in defining and classifying stroke mechanisms, and the proportion of patients with cryptogenic infarction should differ according to the classification. It is also influenced by the extensiveness of diagnostic workup, which should be influenced by physicians' enthusiasm, resources for diagnostic workup, and hospital or governmental policies. Thus, the proportion of cryptogenic infarction cannot be directly compared among different stroke centres.

Classification of stroke based on stroke mechanisms

With improved understanding of the pathophysiology of ischaemic stroke, there developed a need to classify stroke. Early registration studies used clinical findings and results of investigations such as CT and cerebral angiogram but without objectively defined criteria on pathophysiology or aetiology (68, 106, 107). The first, and still most widely used classification system using such criteria was the TOAST (Trail of ORG 10172 in acute stroke treatment); the original purpose of TOAST was to better categorize stroke patients who would benefit from danaparoid in the treatment of ischaemic strokes (108). The system was composed of five major subtypes: large artery atherosclerosis (LAA), cardioembolism (CE), small artery occlusion (SAO), stroke of other determined cause (SOC), and stroke of undetermined cause (SUC). SUC was further divided into (i) no cause was found despite an extensive workup or (ii) two or more plausible causes were found. The criteria for each subtype are shown in Table 4.3. The TOAST system is simple, logical, and has been used in epidemiological studies (69) including inter-ethnic comparisons (74), and in the assessment of subtype differences in risk factors (74), stroke recurrence rate (i.e. patients with stroke due to LAA have the highest odds of recurrence) (109), and patients' mortality (i.e. patients with CE have a higher mortality than those of SAO) (69, 74).

One of the limitations of the TOAST system is the high (approximately 40%) proportion of 'SUC'; patients with two or more plausible causes should be classified as SUC, and thorough investigations (such as Holter, echo) may paradoxically increase the rate of SUC. Moreover, there is only moderate inter-rater reliability. For these reasons, another system that modified the original TOAST was introduced (SSS-TOAST, Stop Stroke Study Trial of Org 10172) (110). SSS-TOAST incorporated evidence of research results to identify the most probable TOAST category in the presence of evidence for multiple mechanisms, thereby decreased the proportion of patients with SUC. Based on the weight of evidence, each TOAST subtype was subdivided into three subcategories as 'evident', 'probable', or 'possible' according to predefined specific clinical and imaging criteria. For instance, LAA was categorized as 'evident' only when there is either occlusive or stenotic (≥50% diameter reduction) vascular disease in the clinically relevant extracranial or intracranial arteries, *and* the absence of acute infarction in vascular territories other than the stenotic or occluded artery. An automated version of the SSS-TOAST, the Causative Classification System (CCS), was also developed (111). The CCS is a web-based system that consists of questionnaire-style classification scheme for ischaemic stroke (<http://ccs.martinos.org>), and allows rapid analysis of patient data with excellent intra- and inter-examiner reliability. Therefore, CCS has a potential utility in multicentre/multinational stroke registry or researches (112).

Another system called 'A–S–C–O' was also developed (113). In this phenotype-based classification, every patient is characterized by A–S–C–O: A for atherosclerosis, S for small vessel disease, C for cardiac source, O for other cause. The notable characteristics of this system are that they comprehensibly include all the potential phenotypes of a given patient. According to the level of evidence, each of the four (ASCO) phenotypes is graded 1, 2, or 3; one for 'definitely a potential cause of the index stroke', 2 for 'causality uncertain', 3 for 'unlikely a direct cause of the index stroke (but disease is present)'. When the disease is completely absent, the grade is 0; when grading is not possible due to insufficient workup, the grade is 9. For example, a patient with a 70% ipsilateral symptomatic stenosis, leucoaraiosis, atrial fibrillation, and platelet count of 700,000/mm would be classified as A1–S3–C1–O3. Although this system has a merit in that no information is neglected, formulating too many combinations may give physicians confusion. However, the system may be utilized flexibly according to the need of physicians; patients' treatment can be adapted to the observed phenotypes and the most likely aetiology (e.g. grade 1 in 1 of the 4 A–S–C–O phenotypes), while clinical trials may focus on several of these four phenotypes (e.g. focus on patients A1–A2).

A comparison with these three systems (TOAST, CCS, and ASCO) in a single population showed good-to-excellent agreement of CCS and ASCO with TOAST (114). Each had specific characteristics for subtype assignment; CCS and ASCO assign fewer patients as cause undetermined, and the proportion of subtypes differ according to the grade used (e.g. adapting grade 1 only vs allowing grade 1–3). The three systems can also be used in TIA patients, yielding a similar distribution of underlying aetiologies (115).

Although the classification systems are undoubtedly useful in our clinical practice, they are not without limitations. First, with accumulated research data, especially those from imaging-based studies, some of the criteria used are currently found to be inadequate. For instance, TOAST criteria require the absence of lacunar syndrome for diagnosing LAA, and the small (≤15 mm in diameter) infarct size for defining SAO (Table 4.3). However, it is now well known that patients with LAA occasionally present with lacunar syndrome, and that 15-mm size criteria is not of particular help in defining SAO in patients with subcortical infarction (48).

Second, there is a problem is the classification of infarcts caused by branch occlusion associated with mild (<50%) ICAS (Figure 4.4, left image of panel 1). While LAD has been defined based on significant (>50%) large artery stenosis/occlusion, the presence of cortical symptoms, and appropriate duplex scan findings, infarcts

Table 4.3 TOAST classification

Features	Large artery atherosclerosis	Cardioembolism	Small artery occlusion	Other cause
Clinical				
Cortical or cerebellar dysfunction	+	+	−	±
Lacunar syndrome	−	−	+	±
Imaging				
Cortical, cerebellar, brainstem, or subcortical infarcts >1.5 cm	+	+	−	±
Subcortical or brainstem infarct <1.5 cm	−	−	±	±
Tests				
Stenosis of extracranial internal carotid artery	+	−	−	−
Cardiac source of emboli	−	+	−	−
Other abnormality on tests	−	−	−	+

From Adams et al. (108).

associated with branch occlusion are mostly unassociated with cortical symptoms, undetected by carotid duplex scan, and cannot therefore be classified as LAD in TOAST, SSS-TOAST, and ASCO (42). Therefore some Asian studies modified the TOAST as to categorize ICAS presenting with branch occlusion as LAD (8, 74). A recent study even attempted to classify LAD as branch artery disease, artery-to-artery embolism, and haemodynamic stroke (116), where branch artery disease was defined as an isolated acute infarct in the territory of the penetrating artery, with the parent artery showing evidence of plaque or 'any' degree of stenosis. These trials are an important first step in broadening the concept of LAD. Third, there still remain problems in the categorization of unclear source of embolism such as PFO and aortic atherosclerosis. As discussed earlier, there are lingering controversies regarding the significance of their characteristics as embolic causes of stroke: size of PFO or aortic atheroma or the presence of associated lesions such as atrial septal defect.

Globally speaking, however, an even more important problem in elucidating stroke mechanism and classification is an inadequate aetiological workup due to the lack of resources. Despite the evolution of classification systems based on advanced imaging technologies, countries in many parts of the world, including Africa, south Asia, and South America, simply do not have adequate resources for diagnostic workup, and the stroke subtypes and mechanisms in these countries remain largely unknown. Considerable research is needed worldwide to establish standardized definitions and classifications of strokes that are balanced between eastern and western hemispheres, and can be done with a reasonable amount of cost. At present, each centre should establish its own consensus opinion on standardized aetiological workup and operating definitions. Since stroke mechanisms are often unclear in many patients, establishment of mechanism and subtype classifications should be made by the consensus of teams of physicians who confer regularly after reviewing and discussing all available information on a given patient (70, 74).

References

1. Klein IF, Lavallee PC, Touboul PJ, Schouman-Claeys E, Amarenco P. In vivo middle cerebral artery plaque imaging by high-resolution MRI. *Neurology*. 2006 Jul 25;67(2):327–329.
2. Swartz RH, Bhuta SS, Farb RI, Agid R, Willinsky RA, Terbrugge KG, *et al*. Intracranial arterial wall imaging using high-resolution 3-tesla contrast-enhanced MRI. *Neurology*. 2009 Feb 17;72(7):627–634.
3. Jorgensen L, Packham MA, Rowsell HC, Mustard JF. Deposition of formed elements of blood on the intima and signs of intimal injury in the aorta of rabbit, pig, and man. *Lab Invest*. 1972 Sep;27(3):341–350.
4. Ross R, Glomset J, Kariya B, Harker L. A platelet-dependent serum factor that stimulates the proliferation of arterial smooth muscle cells in vitro. *Proc Natl Acad Sci U S A*. 1974 Apr;71(4):1207–1210.
5. Ross R. Atherosclerosis—an inflammatory disease. *N Engl J Med*. 1999 Jan 14;340(2):115–126.
6. Gorelick PHJ, Huang Y, Wong L. Epidemiology. In Kim JS, Caplan LR, Wong KS (eds) *Intracranial Atherosclerosis* (pp. 33–44). Oxford: Wiley-Blackwell; 2008.
7. Minematsu KBO, Uehara T. Risk factors. In Kim JS, Caplan LR, Wong KS (eds) *Intracranial Atherosclerosis* (pp. 45–54). Oxford: Wiley-Blackwell; 2008.
8. Kim JS, Nah HW, Park SM, Kim SK, Cho KH, Lee J, *et al*. Risk factors and stroke mechanisms in atherosclerotic stroke: intracranial compared with extracranial and anterior compared with posterior circulation disease. *Stroke*. 2012 Dec;43(12):3313–3318.
9. Fisher M, Paganini-Hill A, Martin A, Cosgrove M, Toole JF, Barnett HJ, *et al*. Carotid plaque pathology: thrombosis, ulceration, and stroke pathogenesis. *Stroke*. 2005 Feb;36(2):253–257.
10. Fuster V, Badimon L, Badimon JJ, Chesebro JH. The pathogenesis of coronary artery disease and the acute coronary syndromes (2). *N Engl J Med*. 1992 Jan 30;326(5):310–318.
11. van der Wal AC, Becker AE, van der Loos CM, Das PK. Site of intimal rupture or erosion of thrombosed coronary atherosclerotic plaques is characterized by an inflammatory process irrespective of the dominant plaque morphology.*Circulation*. 1994 Jan;89(1):36–44.
12. DeGraba TJ, Siren AL, Penix L, McCarron RM, Hargraves R, Sood S, *et al*. Increased endothelial expression of intercellular adhesion molecule-1 in symptomatic versus asymptomatic human carotid atherosclerotic plaque. *Stroke*. 1998 Jul;29(7):1405–1410.
13. Jander S, Sitzer M, Schumann R, Schroeter M, Siebler M, Steinmetz H, *et al*. Inflammation in high-grade carotid stenosis: a possible role for macrophages and T cells in plaque destabilization. *Stroke*. 1998 Aug;29(8):1625–1630.
14. Kolodgie FD, Gold HK, Burke AP, Fowler DR, Kruth HS, Weber DK, *et al*. Intraplaque hemorrhage and progression of coronary atheroma. *N Engl J Med*. 2003 Dec 11;349(24):2316–2325.
15. Yamashita K, Ouchi K, Shirai M, Gondo T, Nakazawa T, Ito H. Distribution of Chlamydia pneumoniae infection in the atherosclerotic carotid artery. *Stroke*. 1998 Apr;29(4):773–778.
16. Ogata J, Masuda J, Yutani C, Yamaguchi T. Rupture of atheromatous plaque as a cause of thrombotic occlusion of stenotic internal carotid artery. *Stroke*. 1990 Dec;21(12):1740–1745.
17. Badimon JJ, Lettino M, Toschi V, Fuster V, Berrozpe M, Chesebro JH, *et al*. Local inhibition of tissue factor reduces the thrombogenicity of disrupted human atherosclerotic plaques: effects of tissue factor pathway inhibitor on plaque thrombogenicity under flow conditions. *Circulation*. 1999 Apr 13;99(14):1780–1787.
18. Liapis CD, Kakisis JD, Kostakis AG. Carotid stenosis: factors affecting symptomatology. *Stroke*. 2001 Dec 1;32(12):2782–2786.
19. Saam T, Cai J, Ma L, Cai YQ, Ferguson MS, Polissar NL, *et al*. Comparison of symptomatic and asymptomatic atherosclerotic carotid plaque features with in vivo MR imaging. *Radiology*. 2006 Aug;240(2):464–472.
20. U-King-Im JM, Tang TY, Patterson A, Graves MJ, Howarth S, Li ZY, *et al*. Characterisation of carotid atheroma in symptomatic and asymptomatic patients using high resolution MRI. *J Neurol Neurosurg Psychiatry*. 2008 Aug;79(8):905–912.
21. Molloy J, Markus HS. Asymptomatic embolization predicts stroke and TIA risk in patients with carotid artery stenosis. *Stroke*. 1999 Jul;30(7):1440–1443.
22. Wong KS, Gao S, Chan YL, Hansberg T, Lam WW, Droste DW, *et al*. Mechanisms of acute cerebral infarctions in patients with middle cerebral artery stenosis: a diffusion-weighted imaging and microemboli monitoring study. *Ann Neurol*. 2002 Jul;52(1):74–81.
23. Ogata J, Masuda J, Yutani C, Yamaguchi T. Mechanisms of cerebral artery thrombosis: a histopathological analysis on eight necropsy cases. *J Neurol Neurosurg Psychiatry*. 1994 Jan;57(1):17–21.
24. Caplan LR, Hennerici M. Impaired clearance of emboli (washout) is an important link between hypoperfusion, embolism, and ischemic stroke. *Arch Neurol*. 1998 Nov;55(11):1475–1482
25. Lee DK, Kim JS, Kwon SU, Yoo SH, Kang DW. Lesion patterns and stroke mechanism in atherosclerotic middle cerebral artery disease: early diffusion-weighted imaging study. *Stroke*. 2005 Dec;36(12):2583–2588.
26. Lee PH, Oh SH, Bang OY, Joo IS, Huh K. Isolated middle cerebral artery disease: clinical and neuroradiological features depending on the pathogenesis. *J Neurol Neurosurg Psychiatry*. 2004 May;75(5):727–732.
27. Lee PH, Oh SH, Bang OY, Joo SY, Joo IS, Huh K. Infarct patterns in atherosclerotic middle cerebral artery versus internal carotid artery disease. *Neurology*. 2004 Apr 27;62(8):1291–1296.

28. Szabo K, Kern R, Gass A, Hirsch J, Hennerici M. Acute stroke patterns in patients with internal carotid artery disease: a diffusion-weighted magnetic resonance imaging study. *Stroke*. 2001 Jun;32(6):1323–1329.

29. Bornstein NM, Norris JW. The unstable carotid plaque. *Stroke*. 1989 Aug;20(8):1104–1106.

30. Caplan LR, Amarenco P, Rosengart A, Lafranchise EF, Teal PA, Belkin M, et al. Embolism from vertebral artery origin occlusive disease. *Neurology*. 1992 Aug;42(8):1505–1512.

31. Kim JS. Pure lateral medullary infarction: clinical-radiological correlation of 130 acute, consecutive patients. *Brain*. 2003 Aug;126(Pt 8):1864–1872.

32. Kim JS, Cho KH, Kang DW, Kwon SU, Suh DC. Basilar artery atherosclerotic disease is related to subacute lesion volume increase in pontine base infarction. *Acta Neurol Scand*. 2009 Aug;120(2):88–93.

33. Kwon JY, Kwon SU, Kang DW, Suh DC, Kim JS. Isolated lateral thalamic infarction: the role of posterior cerebral artery disease. *Eur J Neurol*. 2012 Feb;19(2):265–270.

34. Amarenco P, Cohen A, Tzourio C, Bertrand B, Hommel M, Besson G, et al. Atherosclerotic disease of the aortic arch and the risk of ischemic stroke. *N Engl J Med*. 1994 Dec 1;331(22):1474–1479.

35. Meissner I, Khandheria BK, Sheps SG, Schwartz GL, Wiebers DO, Whisnant JP, et al. Atherosclerosis of the aorta: risk factor, risk marker, or innocent bystander? A prospective population-based transesophageal echocardiography study. *J Am Coll Cardiol*. 2004 Sep 1;44(5):1018–1024.

36. Russo C, Jin Z, Rundek T, Homma S, Sacco RL, Di Tullio MR. Atherosclerotic disease of the proximal aorta and the risk of vascular events in a population-based cohort: the Aortic Plaques and Risk of Ischemic Stroke (APRIS) study. *Stroke*. 2009 Jul;40(7):2313–2318.

37. Kwon SU, Lee SH, Kim JS. Sudden coma from acute bilateral internal carotid artery territory infarction. *Neurology*. 2002 Jun 25;58(12):1846–1849.

38. Wong KS CL, Kim JS. Stroke mechanisms. In Kim JS, Caplan LR, Wong KS (eds) *Intracranial Atherosclerosis* (pp. 57–68). Oxford: Wiley-Blackwell; 2008.

39. Caplan LR. Intracranial branch atheromatous disease: a neglected, understudied, and underused concept. *Neurology*. 1989 Sep;39(9):1246–1250.

40. Lhermitte F, Gautier JC, Derouesne C. Nature of occlusions of the middle cerebral artery. *Neurology*. 1970 Jan;20(1):82–88.

41. Fisher CM, Caplan LR. Basilar artery branch occlusion: a cause of pontine infarction. *Neurology*. 1971 Sep;21(9):900–905.

42. Kim JS, Yoon Y. Single subcortical infarction associated with parental arterial disease: important yet neglected sub-type of atherothrombotic stroke. *Int J Stroke*. 2013 Apr;8(3):197–203.

43. Kim JS, Kim J. Pure midbrain infarction: clinical, radiologic, and pathophysiologic findings. *Neurology*. 2005 Apr 12;64(7):1227–1232.

44. Kim JS, Han YS. Medial medullary infarction: clinical, imaging, and outcome study in 86 consecutive patients. *Stroke*. 2009 Oct;40(10):3221–3225.

45. Adachi T, Kobayashi S, Yamaguchi S, Okada K. MRI findings of small subcortical "lacunar-like" infarction resulting from large vessel disease. *J Neurol*. 2000 Apr;247(4):280–285.

46. Bang OY, Heo JH, Kim JY, Park JH, Huh K. Middle cerebral artery stenosis is a major clinical determinant in striatocapsular small, deep infarction. *Arch Neurol*. 2002 Feb;59(2):259–263.

47. Mok VC, Fan YH, Lam WW, Hui AC, Wong KS. Small subcortical infarct and intracranial large artery disease in Chinese. *J Neurol Sci*. 2003 Dec 15;216(1):55–59.

48. Cho AH, Kang DW, Kwon SU, Kim JS. Is 15 mm size criterion for lacunar infarction still valid? A study on strictly subcortical middle cerebral artery territory infarction using diffusion-weighted MRI. *Cerebrovasc Dis*. 2007;23(1):14–19.

49. Nah HW, Kang DW, Kwon SU, Kim JS. Diversity of single small subcortical infarctions according to infarct location and parent artery disease: analysis of indicators for small vessel disease and atherosclerosis. *Stroke*. 2010 Dec;41(12):2822–2827.

50. Bang OY, Joo SY, Lee PH, Joo US, Lee JH, Joo IS, et al. The course of patients with lacunar infarcts and a parent arterial lesion: similarities to large artery vs small artery disease. *Arch Neurol*. 2004 Apr;61(4):514–519.

51. Klein IF, Lavallee PC, Schouman-Claeys E, Amarenco P. High-resolution MRI identifies basilar artery plaques in paramedian pontine infarct. *Neurology*. 2005 Feb 8;64(3):551–552.

52. Chambers BR, Norris JW. Outcome in patients with asymptomatic neck bruits. *N Engl J Med*. 1986 Oct 2;315(14):860–865.

53. Beneficial effect of carotid endarterectomy in symptomatic patients with high-grade carotid stenosis. North American Symptomatic Carotid Endarterectomy Trial Collaborators. *N Engl J Med*. 1991 Aug 15;325(7):445–453.

54. Fisher CM. Bilateral occlusion of basilar artery branches. *J Neurol Neurosurg Psychiatry*. 1977 Dec;40(12):1182–1189.

55. Steinke W, Ley SC. Lacunar stroke is the major cause of progressive motor deficits. *Stroke*. 2002 Jun;33(6):1510–1516.

56. Cho KH, Kang DW, Kwon SU, Kim JS. Lesion volume increase is related to neurologic progression in patients with subcortical infarction. *J Neurol Sci*. 2009 Sep 15;284(1-2):163–167.

57. Fisher CM. Lacunes: small, deep cerebral infarcts. *Neurology*. 1965 Aug;15:774–784.

58. Fisher CM. A lacunar stroke. The dysarthria-clumsy hand syndrome. *Neurology*. 1967 Jun;17(6):614–617.

59. Fisher CM. Lacunar strokes and infarcts: a review. *Neurology*. 1982 Aug;32(8):871–876.

60. Fisher CM. Ataxic hemiparesis. A pathologic study. *Arch Neurol*. 1978 Mar;35(3):126–128.

61. Fisher CM, Curry HB. Pure motor hemiplegia. *Trans Am Neurol Assoc*. 1964;89:94–97.

62. Fisher CM, Cole M. Homolateral ataxia and crural paresis: a vascular syndrome. *J Neurol Neurosurg Psychiatry*. 1965 Feb;28:48–55.

63. Fisher CM. Pure sensory stroke involving face, arm, and leg. *Neurology*. 1965 Jan;15:76–80.

64. Lammie GA. Pathology of small vessel stroke. *Br Med Bull*. 2000;56(2):296–306.

65. Yamamoto Y, Ohara T, Hamanaka M, Hosomi A, Tamura A, Akiguchi I. Characteristics of intracranial branch atheromatous disease and its association with progressive motor deficits. *J Neurol Sci*. 2011 May 15;304(1-2):78–82.

66. Horowitz DR, Tuhrim S, Weinberger JM, Rudolph SH. Mechanisms in lacunar infarction. *Stroke*. 1992 Mar;23(3):325–327.

67. Donnan GA, Bladin PF, Berkovic SF, Longley WA, Saling MM. The stroke syndrome of striatocapsular infarction. *Brain*. 1991 Feb;114 (Pt 1A):51–70.

68. Foulkes MA, Wolf PA, Price TR, Mohr JP, Hier DB. The Stroke Data Bank: design, methods, and baseline characteristics. *Stroke*. 1988 May;19(5):547–554.

69. Kolominsky-Rabas PL, Weber M, Gefeller O, Neundoerfer B, Heuschmann PU. Epidemiology of ischemic stroke subtypes according to TOAST criteria: incidence, recurrence, and long-term survival in ischemic stroke subtypes: a population-based study. *Stroke*. 2001 Dec 1;32(12):2735–2740.

70. Lee BI, Nam HS, Heo JH, Kim DI. Yonsei Stroke Registry. Analysis of 1,000 patients with acute cerebral infarctions. *Cerebrovasc Dis*. 2001;12(3):145–151.

71. Kim HJ, Yun SC, Cho KH, Cho AH, Kwon SU, Kim JS, et al. Differential patterns of evolution in acute middle cerebral artery infarction with perfusion-diffusion mismatch: atherosclerotic vs. cardioembolic occlusion. *J Neurol Sci*. 2008 Oct 15;273(1-2):93–98.

72. Fisher CM, Pearlman A. The nonsudden onset of cerebral embolism. *Neurology*. 1967 Nov;17(11):1025–1032.

73. Grigoliia GN, Chokhonelidze IK, Gvelesiani LG, Sulakvelidze KR, Tutberidze KN. [A possibility of using increased oxygen consumption as a criterion for mechanical respiration weaning in pediatric practice]. *Georgian Med News*. 2007 Jan;142:7–10.

74. Kim JT, Yoo SH, Kwon JH, Kwon SU, Kim JS. Subtyping of ischemic stroke based on vascular imaging: analysis of 1,167 acute, consecutive patients. *J Clin Neurol.* 2006 Dec;2(4):225–230.

75. Kim JS. Predominant involvement of a particular group of fingers due to small, cortical infarction. *Neurology.* 2001 Jun 26;56(12):1677–1682.

76. Kim JS, Kwon SU, Lee TG. Pure dysarthria due to small cortical stroke. *Neurology.* 2003 Apr 8;60(7):1178–1180.

77. del Zoppo GJ, Higashida RT, Furlan AJ, Pessin MS, Rowley HA, Gent M. PROACT: a phase II randomized trial of recombinant pro-urokinase by direct arterial delivery in acute middle cerebral artery stroke. PROACT Investigators. Prolyse in Acute Cerebral Thromboembolism. *Stroke.* 1998 Jan;29(1):4–11.

78. Fieschi C, Bozzao L. Transient embolic occlusion of the middle cerebral and internal carotid arteries in cerebral apoplexy. *J Neurol Neurosurg Psychiatry.* 1969 Jun;32(3):236–240.

79. Cho AH, Kwon SU, Kim JS, Kang DW. Evaluation of early dynamic changes of intracranial arterial occlusion is useful for stroke etiology diagnosis. *J Neurol Sci.* 2011 Aug 25.

80. Chalela JA, Haymore JB, Ezzeddine MA, Davis LA, Warach S. The hypointense MCA sign. *Neurology.* 2002 May 28;58(10):1470.

81. Flacke S, Urbach H, Keller E, Traber F, Hartmann A, Textor J, *et al.* Middle cerebral artery (MCA) susceptibility sign at susceptibility-based perfusion MR imaging: clinical importance and comparison with hyperdense MCA sign at CT. *Radiology.* 2000 May;215(2):476–482.

82. Schellinger PD, Chalela JA, Kang DW, Latour LL, Warach S. Diagnostic and prognostic value of early MR Imaging vessel signs in hyperacute stroke patients imaged <3 hours and treated with recombinant tissue plasminogen activator. *AJNR Am J Neuroradiol.* 2005 Mar;26(3): 618–624.

83. Friedman M, Van den Bovenkamp GJ. The pathogenesis of a coronary thrombus. *Am J Pathol.* 1966 Jan;48(1):19–44.

84. Jorgensen L, Torvik A. Ischaemic cerebrovascular diseases in an autopsy series. I. Prevalence, location and predisposing factors in verified thrombo-embolic occlusions, and their significance in the pathogenesis of cerebral infarction. *J Neurol Sci.* 1966 Sep–Oct;3(5):490–509.

85. Cho KH, Kim JS, Kwon SU, Cho AH, Kang DW. Significance of susceptibility vessel sign on T2*-weighted gradient echo imaging for identification of stroke subtypes. *Stroke.* 2005 Nov;36(11): 2379–2383.

86. Gage BF, Waterman AD, Shannon W, Boechler M, Rich MW, Radford MJ. Validation of clinical classification schemes for predicting stroke: results from the National Registry of Atrial Fibrillation. *JAMA.* 2001 Jun 13;285(22):2864–2870.

87. Go AS, Hylek EM, Chang Y, Phillips KA, Henault LE, Capra AM, *et al.* Anticoagulation therapy for stroke prevention in atrial fibrillation: how well do randomized trials translate into clinical practice? *JAMA.* 2003 Nov 26;290(20):2685–2692.

88. Lip GY, Nieuwlaat R, Pisters R, Lane DA, Crijns HJ. Refining clinical risk stratification for predicting stroke and thromboembolism in atrial fibrillation using a novel risk factor-based approach: the euro heart survey on atrial fibrillation. *Chest.* 2010 Feb;137(2):263–272.

89. Mason PK, Lake DE, DiMarco JP, Ferguson JD, Mangrum JM, Bilchick K, *et al.* Impact of the CHA_2DS_2-VASc score on anticoagulation recommendations for atrial fibrillation. *Am J Med.* 2012 Jun;125(6):603 e1–6.

90. Kim YD, Cha MJ, Kim J, Lee DH, Lee HS, Nam CM, *et al.* Increases in cerebral atherosclerosis according to $CHADS_2$ scores in patients with stroke with nonvalvular atrial fibrillation. *Stroke.* 2011 Apr;42(4):930–934.

91. Ntaios G, Lip GY, Makaritsis K, Papavasileiou V, Vemmou A, Koroboki E, *et al.* $CHADS_2$, CHA_2DS_2-VASc, and long-term stroke outcome in patients without atrial fibrillation. *Neurology.* 2013 Mar 12;80(11):1009–10017.

92. Bogousslavsky J, Garazi S, Jeanrenaud X, Aebischer N, Van Melle G. Stroke recurrence in patients with patent foramen ovale: the Lausanne Study. Lausanne Stroke with Paradoxal Embolism Study Group. *Neurology.* 1996 May;46(5):1301–1305.

93. Almekhlafi MA, Wilton SB, Rabi DM, Ghali WA, Lorenzetti DL, Hill MD. Recurrent cerebral ischemia in medically treated patent foramen ovale: a meta-analysis. *Neurology.* 2009 Jul 14;73(2):89–97.

94. Mas JL, Arquizan C, Lamy C, Zuber M, Cabanes L, Derumeaux G, *et al.* Recurrent cerebrovascular events associated with patent foramen ovale, atrial septal aneurysm, or both. *N Engl J Med.* 2001 Dec 13;345(24):1740–1746.

95. Lamy C, Giannesini C, Zuber M, Arquizan C, Meder JF, Trystram D, *et al.* Clinical and imaging findings in cryptogenic stroke patients with and without patent foramen ovale: the PFO-ASA Study. Atrial Septal Aneurysm. *Stroke.* 2002 Mar;33(3):706–711.

96. Serena J, Marti-Fabregas J, Santamarina E, Rodriguez JJ, Perez-Ayuso MJ, Masjuan J, *et al.* Recurrent stroke and massive right-to-left shunt: results from the prospective Spanish multicenter (CODICIA) study. *Stroke.* 2008 Dec;39(12):3131–3136.

97. Schievink WI. Spontaneous dissection of the carotid and vertebral arteries. *N Engl J Med.* 2001 Mar 22;344(12):898–906.

98. Hogan AM, Kirkham FJ, Isaacs EB, Wade AM, Vargha-Khadem F. Intellectual decline in children with moyamoya and sickle cell anaemia. *Dev Med Child Neurol.* 2005 Dec;47(12):824–829.

99. Horn P, Bueltmann E, Buch CV, Schmiedek P. Arterio-embolic ischemic stroke in children with moyamoya disease. *Childs Nerv Syst.* 2005 Feb;21(2):104–107.

100. Kim SG, Hong JM, Kim HY, Lee J, Chung PW, Park KY, *et al.* Ischemic stroke in cancer patients with and without conventional mechanisms: a multicenter study in Korea. *Stroke.* 2010 Apr;41(4):798–801.

101. Choi EJ, Choi CG, Kim JS. Large cerebral artery involvement in CADASIL. *Neurology.* 2005 Oct 25;65(8):1322–1324.

102. Sacco RL, Ellenberg JH, Mohr JP, Tatemichi TK, Hier DB, Price TR, *et al.* Infarcts of undetermined cause: the NINCDS Stroke Data Bank. *Ann Neurol.* 1989 Apr;25(4):382–390.

103. Madden KP, Karanjia PN, Adams HP, Jr, Clarke WR. Accuracy of initial stroke subtype diagnosis in the TOAST study. Trial of ORG 10172 in Acute Stroke Treatment. *Neurology.* 1995 Nov;45(11):1975–1979.

104. Marti-Vilalta JL, Arboix A. The Barcelona Stroke Registry. *Eur Neurol.* 1999;41(3):135–142.

105. Lee BC, Hwang SH, Jung S, Yu KH, Lee JH, Cho SJ, *et al.* The Hallym Stroke Registry: a web-based stroke data bank with an analysis of 1,654 consecutive patients with acute stroke. *Eur Neurol.* 2005;54(2):81–87.

106. Mohr JP, Caplan LR, Melski JW, Goldstein RJ, Duncan GW, Kistler JP, *et al.* The Harvard Cooperative Stroke Registry: a prospective registry. *Neurology.* 1978 Aug;28(8):754–762.

107. Bamford J, Sandercock P, Dennis M, Burn J, Warlow C. Classification and natural history of clinically identifiable subtypes of cerebral infarction. *Lancet.* 1991 Jun 22;337(8756):1521–1526.

108. Adams HP, Jr, Bendixen BH, Kappelle LJ, Biller J, Love BB, Gordon DL, *et al.* Classification of subtype of acute ischemic stroke. Definitions for use in a multicenter clinical trial. TOAST. Trial of Org 10172 in Acute Stroke Treatment. *Stroke.* 1993 Jan;24(1):35–41.

109. Lovett JK, Coull AJ, Rothwell PM. Early risk of recurrence by subtype of ischemic stroke in population-based incidence studies. *Neurology.* 2004 Feb 24;62(4):569–573.

110. Ay H, Furie KL, Singhal A, Smith WS, Sorensen AG, Koroshetz WJ. An evidence-based causative classification system for acute ischemic stroke. *Ann Neurol.* 2005 Nov;58(5):688–697.

111. Ay H, Benner T, Arsava EM, Furie KL, Singhal AB, Jensen MB, *et al.* A computerized algorithm for etiologic classification of ischemic stroke: the Causative Classification of Stroke System. *Stroke.* 2007 Nov;38(11):2979–2984.

112. Arsava EM, Ballabio E, Benner T, Cole JW, Delgado-Martinez MP, Dichgans M, *et al.* The Causative Classification of Stroke system: an

international reliability and optimization study. *Neurology*. 2010 Oct 5;75(14):1277–1284.

113. Amarenco P, Bogousslavsky J, Caplan LR, Donnan GA, Hennerici MG. New approach to stroke subtyping: the A-S-C-O (phenotypic) classification of stroke. *Cerebrovasc Dis*. 2009;27(5):502–508.

114. Marnane M, Duggan CA, Sheehan OC, Merwick A, Hannon N, Curtin D, *et al*. Stroke subtype classification to mechanism-specific and undetermined categories by TOAST, A-S-C-O, and causative classification system: direct comparison in the North Dublin population stroke study. *Stroke*. 2010 Aug;41(8):1579–1586.

115. Amort M, Fluri F, Weisskopf F, Gensicke H, Bonati LH, Lyrer PA, *et al*. Etiological classifications of transient ischemic attacks: subtype classification by TOAST, CCS and ASCO—a pilot study. *Cerebrovasc Dis*. 2012;33(6):508–516.

116. Gao S, Wang YJ, Xu AD, Li YS, Wang DZ. Chinese ischemic stroke subclassification. *Front Neurol*. 2011;2:6.

CHAPTER 5

Pathophysiology of non-traumatic intracerebral haemorrhage

Constanza Rossi and Charlotte Cordonnier

Introduction

Intracerebral haemorrhage (ICH) is defined as the irruption of blood in the cerebral parenchyma. Terms used in the literature are sometimes confusing. There is no such thing as 'primary' ICH, as much as there is no 'primary' infarct. ICH causes can be differentiated into arterial small and large vessel disease, venous disease, vascular malformation, ICH in the context of other diseases and conditions, and spontaneous. 'Spontaneous' means that no cause has been found with the currently available diagnostic tests, though it is assumed that there is a cause (cryptogenic). 'Spontaneous' also includes that no cause has been found so far, and there is no suspicion about a concept for a cause (idiopathic). 'Spontaneous' haemorrhages may be associated with or without risk factors (like arterial hypertension), and with or without precipitating factors (e.g. oral anticoagulants or antiplatelet agents).

Epidemiology

The epidemiology of ICH is described in Chapter 1; here we will briefly highlight some facts that are specific to ICHs.

During the last decade, spontaneous ICH accounted for approximately 10% of strokes in high-income countries and about 20% of strokes in low- to middle-income countries, with 1-month case fatalities of 30% and 40%, respectively (1). Unfortunately, the 1-month case fatality after ICH has remained stable over the last few decades (2). The incidence of spontaneous ICH is higher in Asian populations (1), and the major risk factors for ICH include male gender, increasing age, arterial hypertension, excessive alcohol consumption, smoking, diabetes mellitus, poor diet, and obesity (waist-to-hip ratio) (3, 4). Despite an apparent stability of incidence (5) over the past decades, the profile of ICH has evolved: there are fewer deep ICHs associated with pre-stroke hypertension, whereas there are more lobar ICHs associated with use of antithrombotic drugs in those aged ≥75 years (possible cerebral amyloid angiopathy (CAA)) (6).

Pathophysiology of ICH

Most data on the pathophysiology of human ICH come from early macroscopic autopsy studies (performed when vascular risk factors such as arterial hypertension were not adequately controlled) and describe neural damage from the hydrostatic pressure of ICH. Most cases of ICH occur when small (50–700 μm) penetrating arteries rupture with subsequent leaking of arterial blood into the brain parenchyma. Part of ICH-induced injury is due to physical disruption of adjacent tissue and the mass effect caused as the ICH forms. ICH volume is often divided into three categories: small when <30 cm^3, medium between 30 and 60 cm^3, and large when >60 cm^3. The fixed shape of the cranium limits its capacity to accommodate the volumetric ICH expansion, and haematoma volumes >150 cm^3 almost inevitably lead to rapid death.

Even if the ICH volume is one of the main prognostic predictors, volume is not the only player in ICH pathophysiology. The intact or partially intact brain tissue around the haematoma may resemble ischaemic brain, and neurons may die by similar mechanisms or may be subject to toxic effects of blood products. Blood–brain barrier disruption and leakage of fluids and proteins contribute to brain oedema, which commonly increases over several days and may further damage the brain (7). Multiple forms of oedema are present after ICH, but its main component is probably vasogenic. There are three phases of oedema formation after ICH: (i) the very early phase (first few hours) which involves hydrostatic pressure and clot retraction with movement of serum from the clot into the surrounding tissue; (ii) the second phase (first few days) in which the coagulation cascade and thrombin production (which also induces inflammatory cell infiltration, mesenchymal cell proliferation, and scar formation) play major roles; (iii) the third phase, related to erythrocyte lysis and haemoglobin toxicity (8), which has been shown to trigger neurotoxic and apoptotic mechanisms in animals (9, 10). Another potential pathogenic mechanism is activation of leucocytes at the injury site within the first few days, attributable to the widespread inflammation seen in animal models of ICH. An inflammatory response in the surrounding brain occurs soon after ICH and peaks several days later (11, 12). Furthermore, inflammation can be associated with the production of matrix metalloproteinases (which can cause a disruption of the blood–brain barrier and secondary brain injury) and the activation in the brain of the complement system.

ICH is a dynamic process and haematoma enlargement occurs in about one-third of patients. This phenomenon contributes to midline shift and accelerates neurological deterioration. The precise mechanisms of haematoma expansion remain unknown, even if accumulating evidence supports a model of ongoing secondary bleeding from ruptured adjacent vessels surrounding the initial bleeding site (13). Most rebleedings occur within the first 24 h (14–16); combinations of various degrees of rebleeding and intraventricular expansion (often causing acute obstructive hydrocephalus) complicate the ICH in up to 70% of all patients within 24 h (17).

Diagnosis

No clinical diagnostic scale

The main difficulty when approaching the epidemiology of ICH is the need to confirm the diagnosis with cerebral imaging (performed as soon as possible after admission), which allows the distinction between ischaemic and haemorrhagic stroke. No clinical scales (such as the Guy's Hospital Score (18) or the Siriraj Hospital Score (19)) can reliably distinguish ischaemic from haemorrhagic strokes.

Radiological investigations have to be performed in the acute phase. Magnetic resonance imaging (MRI) is as reliable as computed tomography (CT) scanning to demonstrate blood in the brain parenchyma (20). When using CT scanning, it is important to remember that after a few weeks, the small ICH will look like a small infarct (21).

Clinical symptoms which are more frequent in ICH

The clinical presentation of the ICH includes non-specific general signs (suggestive of increased intracranial pressure such as headaches, vomiting, and decreased consciousness) and focal symptoms that are related to the location of the ICH. However, none of the clinical signs and symptoms or their combinations have sufficient specificity and sensitivity to differentiate ICH from other types of stroke. About 3% of patients admitted for ICH have experienced a transient neurological deficit and have a normal clinical exam at the admission (C. Cordonnier, unpublished data).

Headaches

In the first 12 h, headaches are present in roughly one-third of patients admitted for ICH. The headaches are more frequent in ICH than in ischaemic stroke (36% vs 16%) (22). However, in the acute phase before imaging, this clinical sign is not reliable enough to distinguish haemorrhagic from ischaemic strokes. The frequency of headaches is similar in supratentorial and infratentorial ICH. The pain is usually diffuse and of progressive appearance, but its characteristics may guide the diagnosis towards certain conditions such as cerebral venous thrombosis, vascular malformations (mainly aneurysms for thunderclap headache), and vasculitis. Usually, the pain is thought to be generated by traction on the meninges or the extracranial vessels, or by irritation of haemosiderin on the trigemino-vascular system (22).

Vomiting

In the posterior fossa, vomiting is a frequent symptom of stroke, either ischaemic or haemorrhagic, due to the dysfunction of vestibular structures or when the floor of the forth ventricle is in contact with the haemorrhage. Vomiting is also frequently present in supratentorial haemorrhages (60% of cases) (23) and is probably due to an increased intracranial pressure or ventricular extension.

Decreased level of consciousness

The prevalence of altered consciousness at admission in ICH patients depends on the setting of recruitment: department of neurology, or neurosurgery, or intensive care unit…In a population-based registry, as well as in a hospital-based cohort that included patients at admission in the emergency department, one ICH patient out of two had a decreased level of consciousness (24). The altered consciousness can occur independently from the location of the ICH:

◆ In supratentorial ICH: it might be due to the intracranial hypertension or to a mass effect on the upper part of the brainstem (both cases more frequent in the presence of a voluminous ICH)

◆ In posterior fossa ICH: (i) in cerebellar ICH, it might be related to a compression of the brainstem or the occurrence of hydrocephalus, while (ii) in the brainstem, the haemorrhage may damage the reticular activating neurons.

The main differential diagnosis encompasses a wide spectrum of diseases (metabolic syndromes, head trauma, hypoxia, intoxication, severe systemic infections, meningitis/encephalitis, brain tumours), and one of the most important to exclude is a decreased level of consciousness due to the presence of non-convulsive epileptic seizures and/or status epilepticus. Electroencephalographic (EEG) monitoring is very helpful in this context and non-convulsive epileptic seizures are frequently underdiagnosed in ICH patients (25).

Seizures

The reported incidence of post-ICH seizures is dependent on study design, diagnostic criteria, duration of follow-up, and population studied, and ranges from 2.7–17% (26). Most of the studies used a clinical definition for the seizures, while a few studies using continuous EEG monitoring reported an incidence of electrical seizures of 42% (25). A recent study found early seizures (ES; i.e. within 7 days after ICH) occurring in 14% of ICH patients, very early in the disease process with half of ES occurring at ICH onset. The only factor associated with ES was a cortical involvement of the ICH, while ES did not influence in-hospital mortality or functional outcome 6 months after ICH onset (27). Lobar location has been described in several studies as a potent predictor of early post-stroke (ischaemic and ICH) seizures due to an increased probability of cortical involvement (28, 29). The pathophysiology of early seizures in ICH is not well known, but a direct irritation caused by the deposits of haemosiderin (and its degradation products containing iron) on the cortex is one possible mechanism by which post-ICH seizures are provoked.

Data in the literature concerning late seizures (LS; i.e. beyond 7 days after ICH) are scarce and mainly come from mixed cohorts. A recent study reported an incidence of 10% in a long-term follow-up investigation with a strong influence of cortical involvement on the occurrence of LS. Furthermore, when evaluating the association with MRI data (cerebral microbleeds, global cortical atrophy, leucoaraiosis), the study found an association between cerebral microbleeds with a cortico-subcortical distribution (i.e. lobar) and the occurrence of LS. The association between lobar brain microbleeds and the risk of LS might suggest a link with the underlying vasculopathy (CAA) (30).

Prognostic scales

The main outcome predictors of ICH are considered to be initial volume and haematoma expansion. Other predictors of poor outcome include age, low Glasgow Coma Scale (GCS) score at admission, location and volume of the haemorrhage, location and amount of intraventricular extension, increased blood pressure levels, and increased blood glucose at admission (26).

Many models have been proposed to predict outcome (including death) (31–33). Among these, the ICH score is the most commonly used (Table 5.1).

The ICH score ranges from 0 (excellent prognosis) to 6 (high probability of death) (31). The aim of the score is to predict the outcome assessed as 30-day mortality and favourable functional outcome throughout the first year after acute ICH (34). Following the first edition of the ICH score, a modified version has been developed (32) by substituting the National Institutes of Health Stroke Scale (NIHSS) with the GCS score. This because: (i) the NIHSS has a wider range than the GCS score, (ii) it measures not only level of consciousness but also neurological deficits, (iii) it has become the standard assessment in all acute stroke patients, and (iv) the NIHSS is a potent predictor of both mortality and good outcome.

Notwithstanding the implementation, this clinical prognostic model has a degree of uncertainty, which might be overcome if other tools are incorporated. For instance, identifying the underlying cause of the ICH might give important clues about the prognosis. In two prospective population-based studies, patients with ICH related to the presence of an arteriovenous malformation (AVM)

Table 5.1 The ICH score (31). ICH volume is calculated using the ABC/2 method

Component	ICH score points
GCS score at admission	
3–4	2
5–12	1
13–15	0
ICH volume in cm³	
≥30	1
<30	0
IVH	
Yes	1
No	0
Infratentorial origin of ICH	
Yes	1
No	0
Age, years	
≥80	1
<80	0
Total ICH score	0–6

GCS: Glasgow Coma Scale; IVH: intraventricular haemorrhage.

had better outcomes than patients with 'spontaneous' ICH, independently of known predictors of outcome (35).

Furthermore, none of the commonly used predictive models have accounted for the impact of 'do not resuscitate' (DNR) orders on mortality after ICH. Early DNR orders are common after ICH (partly due to the high prevalence of decreased level of consciousness) and may lead to a self-fulfilling prophecy (36, 37). Use of ICH predictive models without considering the impact of early DNR orders may lead to inaccurate estimates of mortality risk for individual patients (38).

Causes of ICH

Forget the term 'primary'

ICH encompasses a diverse range of conditions, with different underlying causes (39). Given the large variety of underlying vascular diseases, the concept of *primary* ICH should be replaced by a more systematic stratification into specific diagnostic subtypes (40).

Risk factors differ from causes

The major risk factors for spontaneous ICH are arterial hypertension, excessive alcohol consumption, male sex, increasing age, and smoking. These risk factors may lead to secondary vascular changes, which may eventually cause ICH (39). In recent years, the classical causal role of risk factors for ICH, such as arterial hypertension, has been under revision. In a systematic review of the literature, arterial hypertension was more frequent in patients with deep ICH (odds ratio 2) compared to lobar ICH. However, when methodological limitations were taken into account, the odds ratio was only 1.5 (41). This suggests that arterial hypertension is also very frequent among lobar haemorrhages. The term hypertensive haemorrhage is probably misleading and clinicians should focus on identifying the underlying vascular substrate rather than considering a frequent risk factor as a sole cause.

The main causes of ICH are listed in Table 5.2. In the following sections we will address in detail the two most frequent causes: CAA and arteriolosclerosis.

Most frequent causes

Cerebral amyloid angiopathy (Aβ sporadic form)

Haemorrhages associated with CAA are due to the rupture of amyloid-laden vessels, due to deposition of amyloid protein in the media and adventitia of small to medium-sized cerebral arteries. They typically occur at the border of the grey and white matter of the cerebral hemispheres, and are frequently described as lobar haemorrhages.

Cerebral amyloid angiopathy: the Boston criteria—useful but limited value

The 'Boston criteria' represent an effort to estimate the likelihood of the presence of CAA during life with categories of probable and possible CAA based on the pattern of haemorrhagic lesions on neuroimaging studies. According to these criteria, lobar, cortical, and cortico-subcortical haemorrhages are suggestive of the presence of CAA. The presence of a single haemorrhage in these areas gives rise to the diagnosis of possible CAA, whereas the presence of multiple haemorrhages in these areas is a requirement for probable CAA.

Table 5.2 Commonest causes of apparently 'spontaneous' intracerebral haemorrhage

Causes
Small vessel disease
Small vessel disease (deep ICH)
Cerebral amyloid angiopathy (lobar ICH)
Genetic small vessel disease
Large vessel disease
Haemorrhagic transformation of cerebral infarction
Reversible cerebral vasoconstriction syndrome
Moyamoya disease
Vascular malformations
Cerebral arteriovenous malformation
Intracranial arterial aneurysm
Cerebral cavernous malformation
Dural arteriovenous fistula
Venous disease
Cerebral venous thrombosis
Haemostatic disorders
Haematological diseases
Iatrogenic disorders
ICH in the context of other diseases and conditions
Tumour (primary/metastasis)
Infective endocarditis
Substance abuse
Hypertensive encephalopathy

Adapted from Al-Shahi Salman et al. (39)

Haemorrhages in the basal ganglia, thalamus, or brainstem, regions typically spared by CAA, are exclusion criteria to the diagnosis of CAA. The Boston criteria have been validated with histopathological specimens in only one study that included 39 patients (42). The study had several limitations: (i) only patients with symptomatic lobar ICH and pathological brain specimens were included, therefore it is uncertain whether the results can be extrapolated to other patient categories; (ii) the imaging was based on different radiological modalities (CT or T2-weighted MRI or T2* gradient-recalled echo (GRE)-weighted MRI) with different sensitivities for haemorrhagic lesions.

In the clinical setting, the Boston criteria for 'probable CAA' have excellent specificity (100%; 95% confidence interval (CI) 77–100) and do not misclassify people who have lobar ICH without underlying severe CAA, but their sensitivity and negative predictive value are low (44% (95% CI 28–62) and 39% (95% CI 22–58) respectively). Both standardized use of GRE T2* MRI to identify brain microbleeds and the inclusion of superficial siderosis in the Boston criteria may improve their diagnostic accuracy (43), but false positives and false negatives still exist and the role of other degrees of CAA severity in causing lobar ICH remains to be clarified (44).

Arteriolosclerosis

The consequence of chronic arterial hypertension on vessels that leads to arterial rupture is not fully understood, and the current understanding of the arterial pathology underlying deep haemorrhage is largely based on studies conducted in the 1960s and 1970s by Fisher and colleagues. At that time, prevention and treatment of arterial hypertension were not optimal. In this small case series studied by serial sections, the haemorrhage appeared to arise from structural changes of the small brain vessels, including arteriolosclerosis, lipohyalinosis, and eventual formation of microaneurysms. These lesions were frequently localized on penetrating small arteries and arterioles of the basal ganglia, thalamus, pons, and subcortical white matter (45). Fisher's findings led him to propose that hypertensive changes in the vessel (also known as lipohyalinosis), affecting the small, deep, perforating, intracranial blood vessels, may lead to lacunar infarction in some circumstances and to deep intracerebral haemorrhage in others.

In the absence of prospectively validated diagnostic criteria, clinicians should keep in mind that presence of risk factors is neither necessary nor sufficient to conclude that a deep ICH is due to arteriolosclerosis. Because this vasculopathy has two modalities of expression (haemorrhagic and occlusive), clinicians should try to 'see' the disease: is there leucoaraiosis? Lacunes? Old (often silent) bleeds in the basal ganglia? (Figure 5.1). In the absence of features of arteriolosclerosis, even in an elderly hypertensive patient, clinicians should search for other causes especially small deep AVMs (Figure 5.2).

Cerebral microbleeds

Magnetic resonance imaging of the brain with T2*-weighted GRE sequences has allowed the identification of small foci of chronic blood products, suggesting small, 'silent' haemorrhages called cerebral microbleeds (CMB). CMBs are important biomarkers of underlying vasculopathies: (i) deep perforating vasculopathy is typically associated with CMBs in the basal ganglia, thalamus, brainstem, and cerebellum; while (ii) advanced CAA is associated with a cortico-subcortical (or less commonly cerebellar) distribution (46).

As markers of the severity of underlying haemorrhage-prone vascular pathological changes, CMBs might predict future risk of symptomatic ICH (47). The pathological factors that determine whether a particular bleeding event will result in a microbleed versus a macrobleed are a matter for investigation. The observed bimodal distribution of haemorrhagic volumes raises the possibility of a threshold mechanism, whereby a bleed can either remain small or reach a crucial size that causes it to continue to enlarge fully into the macrobleed range (48).

Intracranial vascular malformations (IVMs)
Cerebral arteriovenous malformations

Brain AVMs are the leading cause of ICH in young adults, even if they account for no more than about one-third of those cases. ICH is the presenting symptom in only half of incident AVM diagnoses (49). The next most frequent manifestation is epilepsy (about one-fifth), while many are asymptomatic at the time of detection. ICH due to a brain arteriovenous malformation (AVM-ICH) appears to have a lower 1-month case fatality than spontaneous ICH (50–53) and have a better long-term outcome (35). The

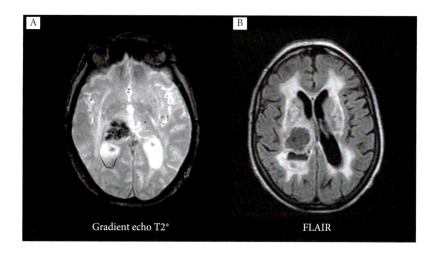

Gradient echo T2*   FLAIR

Fig. 5.1 Brain MRI, axial plane, in a 75-year-old woman treated for arterial hypertension for 10 years. (A) gradient echo T2* showing a right thalamic ICH associated with features of small-vessel disease in its haemorrhagic form and (B) in its occlusive form: severe leucoaraiosis and lacunes on fluid-attenuated inversion recovery (FLAIR) sequence.

annual detection rate of AVM is approximately 1 per 100,000 per year. AVMs are tangles of dilated arteries and veins that form an abnormal communication between the arterial and the venous systems. It is a developmental abnormality, representing persistence of an embryonic pattern of blood vessels, embedded in a normal intervening brain parenchyma. On angiography, they are recognizable by the large feeding arteries which break up into a central nidus of dilated vessels and the rapid shunting of blood to veins that are enlarged and tortuous. There are saccular aneurysms on the feeding arteries or within the nidus itself in about 20% of AVMs: they are a likely source of bleeding. Haemorrhages from AVMs are mostly in the white matter ('lobar'), but they also occur in the deep nuclei of the cerebral hemisphere. When haemorrhage occurs, the blood may reach the surface of the brain, thus

causing a subarachnoid haemorrhage (SAH), but of all haemorrhages secondary to a ruptured AVM only 4% were pure SAH, without a parenchymal component (54). When there is no associated aneurysm on the arterial side, the site of rupture is usually on the venous side of the malformation. Very small vascular malformations may not be seen on angiography. In a series of 72 patients under 45 years with ICH, the proportion of unexplained haemorrhages was as high as 25%, perhaps in part because any AVM could not be seen on angiography (55).

Cerebral cavernous malformations

Cerebral cavernous malformations (or cavernomas) are small (1 mm to several cm in diameter), thin-walled vascular structures, consisting of a mulberry-like conglomerate lined by endothelium

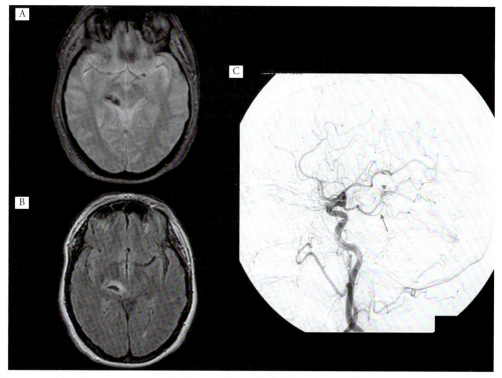

Fig. 5.2 Brain MRI, axial plane: small right thalamo-mesencephalic ICH on gradient echo T2* (A) without any features of small vessel disease in FLAIR sequence (B) in a 62-year-old woman treated for arterial hypertension and diabetes for 5 years. Conventional angiography (C) disclosed a small deep arteriovenous malformation treated by radiosurgery. The nidus is close to the right internal capsule (head of arrow) and is fed by the anterior choroidal artery (arrow).

without muscular or elastic layers, without important arterial feeders, and with no intervening brain tissue. They can be single or multiple and occasionally calcified. Cavernomas may also occur in the skin, orbit, and almost any internal organ. In the brain they are often asymptomatic—their tendency to bleed is close to that of brain AVMs, but the bleeding is often clinically silent. It was only after the advent of imaging modalities such as CT, and especially MRI, that these lesions became regularly recognized during life. A review of more than 14,000 consecutive MRI scans in the late 1980s found them in 0.5% of participants (56). In T2-weighted MRI, they are characterized by a combination of a reticulated core of mixed signal intensity with a surrounding rim of decreased signal intensity, corresponding to deposits of haemosiderin. Smaller lesions appear as areas of decreased signal intensity (black dots) and are even better picked up by T2*-weighted GRE MRI. The lesions are not static but often grow or shrink, and can also appear *de novo* in sporadic cases. Cavernous angiomas are located in the hemispheric white matter or cortex in about one-half of all cases, in the posterior fossa (most often the brainstem) in one-third, and in the basal ganglia or thalamus in one-sixth. Epileptic seizures and transient or permanent focal deficit are common manifestations (56). Estimates of the risk of haemorrhage in patients in whom a cavernoma has been detected vary widely, between 0.25% and 6% per annum. Factors possibly predisposing to a relatively high risk of haemorrhage are a previous haemorrhage, a deep location of the cavernoma (brainstem, cerebellum, basal ganglia, or thalamus), age below 35 years on first presentation, and the presence of multiple lesions, which mostly occur in familial forms (57–60).

Familial forms of the disorder have been detected firstly in Mexican-American families, and later in different European countries and in Asia. Generally, familial variants present multiple cavernous malformations, the number increasing with advancing age. Moreover, given a patient with multiple cavernous malformations, there is a 75% chance that first-degree relatives are affected as well (61). Three CCM genes have been identified: *CCM1/KRIT1* (accounting for 40% of familial cases), *CCM2/MGC4607* (20%), and *CCM3/PDCD10* (20%), genetic linkage analyses mapped three CCM loci on chromosome 7q (*CCM1*), 7p (*CCM2*), and 3q (*CCM3*) (62). *In situ* hybridization studies showed that the three CCM genes have very similar patterns of expression within the central nervous system, suggesting that the three gene products have similar actions (62–64).

Some characteristics of ICH appear to differ between IVM types. In general, ICHs due to cavernous malformations occur at a younger age and tend to be less disabling at onset than those due to cerebral AVM. Furthermore, cavernous malformations tend to cause small ICHs, thereby explaining a mild severity. In this context, ICHs rarely have an extension to other compartments (subarachnoid, subdural, or intraventricular) (65).

Other causes

Cerebral venous thrombosis

Cerebral venous thrombosis (CVT) is a rare type of cerebrovascular disease that accounts for 0.5% of all cases of stroke (66). CVT presents with a wide spectrum of signs and modes of onset, thus mimicking numerous other disorders. The most common symptoms and signs are headache, seizures, focal neurological deficits, altered consciousness, and papilloedema, which can present in isolation or in association with other symptoms.

In about 39% of cases the CVT is associated with an ICH (67). Haemorrhages are most often secondary to engorgement caused by obstruction of cortical veins. Usually, the haemorrhage is preceded by an ischaemic phase, characterized by focal symptoms, headache, seizures, or a global encephalopathy (suggestive of intracranial hypertension), while less frequently the intracerebral bleeding may be the presenting feature of the disease.

The diagnosis can be suspected when the location of the ICH is: parasagittal (mono or bilateral) with thrombosis of the superior sagittal sinus, on the cerebral convexity (when the thrombosis involves a cortical vein), or in the temporal lobes with thrombosis of the lateral sinus (68). Extensive haemorrhages occur in only a minority of patients. The research of CVT should be included in the differential diagnosis of so-called 'primary' intracerebral haemorrhage, and CVT should be suspected especially when: (i) the bleeding is in a lobar location, (ii) the haemorrhage has been preceded by other signs and symptoms (i.e. headache, visual symptoms, ischaemic neurological deficits, seizures), and (iii) the haemorrhage is multiple (mainly in the parasagittal or temporal regions).

Even in the presence of massive ICH there is the indication of full-dose anticoagulants as first-line therapy (66).

Reversible cerebral vasoconstriction syndrome

Reversible cerebral vasoconstriction syndrome (RCVS) is characterized by the association of severe headaches with or without additional neurological symptoms, and constriction of cerebral arteries which resolves spontaneously in 1–3 months (69–71). Although the pathophysiology remains unknown, the prevailing hypothesis is of a transient disturbance in the control of cerebral vascular tone leading to segmental and multifocal arterial constriction and dilatation. This disturbance may be spontaneous, while 25–60% of cases are secondary, mostly to exposure to vasoactive sympathomimetic or serotoninergic substances, and/or to the postpartum state (69, 70). The most common clinical feature is a severe acute headache ('thunderclap' headache) and the major complications are localized cortical SAHs (20–25%) and ischaemic or haemorrhagic strokes (5–10%) eventually leading to permanent sequelae and even death (72, 73). Parenchymal haemorrhages are of variable volume, more frequently single than multiple and lobar than deep, and more often associated with another type of stroke (convexity haemorrhage or infarction, or both) than isolated. They occur early in the course of RCVS and are revealed mostly by a persisting focal deficit concomitant with thunderclap headache. However, parenchymal haemorrhages can also occur in purely cephalalgic cases, and can occur several days after initial normal imaging. Haemorrhagic forms of RCVS seem to be more common in women than in men, and in people with migraine than in those without (71).

Haemorrhagic transformation

Haemorrhagic transformation (HT) occurs in some patients with cerebral infarction (up to 15% in the acute phase of stroke, depending on patient selection and radiological criteria) (74–77). HT may be distinguished from a spontaneous ICH by the lack of homogeneity of the haemorrhagic lesion which lies within an area of infarction (appearing as an area of low density on CT or of hyperintensity in diffusion-weighted imaging (DWI) sequences on MRI) with a typical location confined to a single arterial territory. Sometimes the haemorrhage is so dense that it would have been regarded as a so called 'primary' ICH, had not an earlier CT scan or MRI in the acute phase shown an infarct. Clearly, the main diagnostic problem is represented by the fact that in some patients the first imaging already shows the haemorrhagic transformation and an important diagnostic tool in this case is represented by possible concomitant ischaemic lesions in the same or in other vascular territories. In this view the MRI with DWI sequences in the acute phase of stroke remains the most useful tool to make the differential diagnosis.

There is some evidence suggesting that the major risk factors for HT are the size of the ischaemic lesion and the cardioembolic nature of the stroke (74) together with increasing doses of antithrombotic drugs (78).

Aetiological workup

History

The cause of ICH may occasionally be identified from the history:

◆ A past history of ICH in the same location may suggest a structural lesion (such as an AVM), while if the recurrent lobar haemorrhage is distant from the earlier lesion the underlying condition may be CAA.

◆ A family history of ICH may suggest cavernomas, hereditary haemorrhagic telangiectasia, or a rare genetic familial form of CAA.

◆ Previous epileptic seizures should raise suspicion about an arteriovenous or cavernous malformation, or a tumour.

◆ CAA is often associated with a history of cognitive decline.

◆ If the patient is known to have had cancer, haemorrhage into a brain metastasis should be excluded.

◆ The presence of valvular heart disease should raise the suspicion of septic embolism due to infective endocarditis, although this is a rare cause of ICH.

◆ The use of oral anticoagulants is key information in patients with ICH, because their action has to be neutralized as soon as possible by intravenous prothrombin complex concentrate or fresh frozen plasma and vitamin K.

◆ Recreational drugs should be screened for (cocaine and amphetamines), especially among young ICH patients.

◆ The circumstances preceding ICH may contribute to identifying its cause, e.g. an earlier phase of the illness with a dense neurological deficit (haemorrhagic transformation of an infarct) or puerperium (intracranial venous thrombosis).

Radiological workup

Brain imaging is the cornerstone for ICH diagnosis because haemorrhagic and ischaemic stroke cannot be differentiated on clinical grounds alone.

The location of the haemorrhage may point to some underlying causes. While IVM may lead to all types of ICH, arteriolosclerosis leads to deep ICH and CAA to lobar ICH. Old (and often silent) lobar bleeds or focal haemosiderosis may suggest CAA, at least in an elderly patient.

At admission, after the first brain imaging demonstrating the ICH, it is not always clear whether, how, and when to undertake further radiological investigation. In a survey of current practice in three European countries, younger patient age strongly influenced whether further investigation of ICH was performed, followed by the absence of prestroke hypertension and lobar ICH location, which is in line with existing recommendations. Nevertheless, the types and timing of investigations varied considerably among specialties and countries (79).

1. Brain CT detects symptomatic ICH within minutes of symptom onset but may lack sensitivity if delayed for >1 week after ICH onset (haemorrhage isodense to brain tissue).

   • Hyperacute CT angiography followed by a postcontrast scan may identify a 'spot sign' in up to 40%—one or more hyperintense spots in the haemorrhage—representing a contrast leak. Its presence might suggest a risk of haematoma expansion, poor outcome and mortality even if the translation of its value into clinical practice remains controversial (80–82).

   • While the use of CT angiography (CTA) has been demonstrated in the aetiological workup of SAH, very few data are available regarding predictive values, sensitivity, and specificity of CTA in the setting of an ICH. Most of the studies were performed in selected young patients with a high risk of vascular malformation. These small and biased studies have a very poor external validity. CT-venography is useful to search for a venous thrombosis.

2. MRI with GRE T2* sequences identifies ICH soon after onset and reliably detects chronic posthaemorrhagic iron deposits.

   Conventional sequences may give indirect clues for a diagnosis: old lobar haemorrhages disseminated in the brain in a context of an acute lobar ICH suggesting CAA; leucoaraiosis and lacunes in a context of deep ICH suggesting arteriolosclerosis; acute lesions in DWI suggesting a haemorrhagic transformation of an infarct. The added value of MRI has been described in patients with a spontaneous ICH or isolated IVH (83, 84). The routine use of MRI may be beneficial in all ICH patients, with a meaningful clinical benefit of brain MRI performed even within the first week following symptom onset.

   MR-venography is useful to search for a venous thrombosis. Besides conventional sequences, intracranial MRA associated with dynamic sequences (DSA-MRA) have been evaluated in small studies and might be of interest when IVMs such as AVM or AVF are suspected (85).

3. In patients with ICH, catheter angiography is still the gold standard to detect underlying vascular lesions (arteriovenous malformation, arteriovenous fistula, and arterial aneurysms). This should apply to all patients with ICH, provided they are fit for surgery or interventional neuroradiology, or with no other identified cause. Data regarding the diagnostic accuracy of conventional angiography result from a small, non-randomized, biased cohort of young patients (86, 87). Therefore, the exact prevalence of underlying vascular malformation in deep ICH and/or in hypertensive patients older than 60 years remains unknown.

Initial imaging may also be used as part of prognostic scores predicting clinical outcome after acute ICH. After the ascertainment of the haemorrhagic nature of the stroke, a swift diagnosis of the underlying cause can expedite management to improve

Table 5.3 Diagnostic biological workup suggested at the admission of a patient with a non-traumatic ICH

• Complete blood count including platelets
• Prothrombin time, partial thromboplastin time, INR: if abnormal search for a treatment prior to admission (e.g. oral anticoagulants)
• C-reactive protein and fibrinogen/blood cultures, in case of a suspicion of underlying infectious disease (e.g. endocarditis)
• Liver function
• Renal function
• Illicit drugs (blood and/or urine) in case of suspected angiitis and/or drug addiction

outcome or prevent recurrent ICH. For both MRI and CT, baseline and serial studies can be used to identify patients who may benefit from acute interventions (e.g. anticoagulation for intracranial venous thrombosis or placement of an external ventricular drain for hydrocephalus). The reliable detection of an underlying arterial aneurysm, AVM, or dural arteriovenous fistula may require additional intra-arterial digital subtraction angiography because timely treatment can prevent recurrent ICH.

Alternative non-invasive imaging tools, such as transcranial duplex sonography (TDS), should be explored for early ICH diagnosis and non-invasive follow-up imaging. TDS may represent a potentially useful and reliable method for monitoring early haematoma growth at the patient's bedside during the hyperacute phase (88).

Biological workup

Routine laboratory investigations are important for general medical management of a patient with an ICH, but they rarely uncover its cause.

Haemostatic disorders are frequently a precipitating factor but rarely result in a 'hole' in a vessel. An international normalized ratio (INR) below 5, or platelet count higher than 20,000, should not be considered as a cause but as a precipitating factor of ICH. The clotting system (coagulation factors) can be assessed with the partial thromboplastin time (PTT), the prothrombin time (PT), the thrombin time (TT), or, preferably, the INR (Table 5.3). Abnormalities of primary haemostasis have to do with defects of platelet aggregation or with thrombocytopenia (which rarely result in haemorrhages in the brain). In the acute phase, their monitoring is relevant in case-specific treatments such as platelet infusion or when clotting factors are available.

If infective endocarditis is suspected, the diagnosis may be supported by a high erythrocyte sedimentation rate or C-reactive protein, echocardiography, and blood cultures. In the acute phase, leucocyte count is frequently elevated and may result from the ICH itself, especially when it is large.

In young patients, the abuse of recreational drugs (cocaine, amphetamines, etc.) should be ruled out with a complete screening (blood and/or urine).

Conclusion

The first step in the management of ICH patients is to identify as quickly as possible the underlying vasculopathy that led to bleeding.

Indeed, the cause will determine the short-term and long-term prognosis, helping the clinician to tailor an effective management. Unfortunately, to date, ICHs are still underinvestigated and that fact may contribute to the 40% in-hospital mortality rate.

References

1. Feigin VL, Lawes CM, Bennett DA, Barker-Collo SL, Parag V. Worldwide stroke incidence and early case fatality reported in 56 population-based studies: a systematic review. *Lancet Neurol.* 2009;8(4):355–369.
2. van Asch CJ, Luitse MJ, Rinkel GJ, van der Tweel I, Algra A, Klijn CJ. Incidence, case fatality, and functional outcome of intracerebral haemorrhage over time, according to age, sex, and ethnic origin: a systematic review and meta-analysis. *Lancet Neurol.* 2010 Feb;9(2):167–176.
3. O'Donnell MJ, Xavier D, Liu L, Zhang H, Chin SL, Rao-Melacini P, et al. Risk factors for ischaemic and intracerebral haemorrhagic stroke in 22 countries (the INTERSTROKE study): a case-control study. *Lancet.* 2010 Jul 10;376(9735):112–123.
4. Ariesen MJ, Claus SP, Rinkel GJ, Algra A. Risk factors for intracerebral hemorrhage in the general population: a systematic review. *Stroke.* 2003 Aug;34(8):2060–2065.
5. Bejot Y, Cordonnier C, Durier J, Aboa-Eboule C, Rouaud O, Giroud M. Intracerebral haemorrhage profiles are changing: results from the Dijon population-based study. *Brain.* 2013 Feb;136(Pt 2):658–664.
6. Lovelock CE, Molyneux AJ, Rothwell PM. Change in incidence and aetiology of intracerebral haemorrhage in Oxfordshire, UK, between 1981 and 2006: a population-based study. *Lancet Neurol.* 2007 Jun;6(6):487–493.
7. Sansing LH, Kaznatcheeva EA, Perkins CJ, Komaroff E, Gutman FB, Newman GC. Edema after intracerebral hemorrhage: correlations with coagulation parameters and treatment. *J Neurosurg.* 2003 May;98(5):985–992.
8. Wagner KR, Xi G, Hua Y, Kleinholz M, de Courten-Myers GM, Myers RE, et al. Lobar intracerebral hemorrhage model in pigs: rapid edema development in perihematomal white matter. *Stroke.* 1996 Mar;27(3):490–497.
9. Xi G, Fewel ME, Hua Y, Thompson BG, Jr, Hoff JT, Keep RF. Intracerebral hemorrhage: pathophysiology and therapy. *Neurocrit Care.* 2004;1(1):5–18.
10. Gong C, Boulis N, Qian J, Turner DE, Hoff JT, Keep RF. Intracerebral hemorrhage-induced neuronal death. *Neurosurgery.* 2001 Apr;48(4):875–882; discussion 82–83.
11. Enzmann DR, Britt RH, Lyons BE, Buxton JL, Wilson DA. Natural history of experimental intracerebral hemorrhage: sonography, computed tomography and neuropathology. *AJNR Am J Neuroradiol.* 1981 Nov-Dec;2(6):517–526.
12. Gong C, Hoff JT, Keep RF. Acute inflammatory reaction following experimental intracerebral hemorrhage in rat. *Brain Res.* 2000 Jul 14;871(1):57–65.
13. Brouwers HB, Greenberg SM. Hematoma expansion following acute intracerebral hemorrhage. *Cerebrovasc Dis.* 2013 Feb 28;35(3):195–201.
14. Xi G, Keep RF, Hoff JT. Mechanisms of brain injury after intracerebral haemorrhage. *Lancet Neurol.* 2006 Jan;5(1):53–63.
15. Brott T, Broderick J, Kothari R, Barsan W, Tomsick T, Sauerbeck L, et al. Early hemorrhage growth in patients with intracerebral hemorrhage. *Stroke.* 1997 Jan;28(1):1–5.
16. Kazui S, Minematsu K, Yamamoto H, Sawada T, Yamaguchi T. Predisposing factors to enlargement of spontaneous intracerebral hematoma. *Stroke.* 1997 Dec;28(12):2370–2375.
17. Davis SM, Broderick J, Hennerici M, Brun NC, Diringer MN, Mayer SA, et al. Hematoma growth is a determinant of mortality and poor outcome after intracerebral hemorrhage. *Neurology.* 2006 Apr 25;66(8):1175–1181.
18. Allen CM. Clinical diagnosis of the acute stroke syndrome. *Q J Med.* 1983 Autumn;52(208):515–523.

19. Poungvarin N, Viriyavejakul A, Komontri C. Siriraj stroke score and validation study to distinguish supratentorial intracerebral haemorrhage from infarction. *BMJ*. 1991 Jun 29;302(6792):1565–1567.

20. Kidwell CS, Chalela JA, Saver JL, Starkman S, Hill MD, Demchuk AM, *et al*. Comparison of MRI and CT for detection of acute intracerebral hemorrhage. *JAMA*. 2004 Oct 20;292(15):1823–1830.

21. Keir SL, Wardlaw JM, Warlow CP. Stroke epidemiology studies have underestimated the frequency of intracerebral haemorrhage. A systematic review of imaging in epidemiological studies. *J Neurol*. 2002 Sep;249(9):1226–1231.

22. Kumral E, Bogousslavsky J, Van Melle G, Regli F, Pierre P. Headache at stroke onset: the Lausanne Stroke Registry. *J Neurol Neurosurg Psychiatry*. 1995 Apr;58(4):490–492.

23. Foulkes MA, Wolf PA, Price TR, Mohr JP, Hier DB. The Stroke Data Bank: design, methods, and baseline characteristics. *Stroke*. 1988 May;19(5):547–554.

24. Cordonnier C, Rutgers MP, Dumont F, Pasquini M, Lejeune JP, Garrigue D, *et al*. Intra-cerebral haemorrhages: are there any differences in baseline characteristics and intra-hospital mortality between hospital and population-based registries? *J Neurol*. 2009 Feb;256(2):198–202.

25. Garrett MC, Komotar RJ, Starke RM, Merkow MB, Otten ML, Connolly ES. Predictors of seizure onset after intracerebral hemorrhage and the role of long-term antiepileptic therapy. *J Crit Care*. 2009 Sep;24(3):335–339.

26. Morgenstern LB, Hemphill JC, 3rd, Anderson C, Becker K, Broderick JP, Connolly ES, Jr, *et al*. Guidelines for the management of spontaneous intracerebral hemorrhage: a guideline for healthcare professionals from the American Heart Association/American Stroke Association. *Stroke*. 2010 Sep;41(9):2108–2129.

27. De Herdt V, Dumont F, Henon H, Derambure P, Vonck K, Leys D, *et al*. Early seizures in intracerebral hemorrhage: incidence, associated factors, and outcome. *Neurology*. 2011 Nov 15;77(20):1794–1800.

28. Giroud M, Gras P, Fayolle H, Andre N, Soichot P, Dumas R. Early seizures after acute stroke: a study of 1,640 cases. *Epilepsia*. 1994 Sep–Oct;35(5):959–964.

29. Weisberg LA, Shamsnia M, Elliott D. Seizures caused by nontraumatic parenchymal brain hemorrhages. *Neurology*. 1991 Aug;41(8):1197–1199.

30. Rossi C, De Herdt V, Dequatre-Ponchelle N, Hénon H, Leys D, Cordonnier C. Incidence and predictors of late seizures in intracerebral hemorrhage. *Stroke*. 2013 Jun;44(6):1723–1725.

31. Hemphill JC, 3rd, Bonovich DC, Besmertis L, Manley GT, Johnston SC. The ICH score: a simple, reliable grading scale for intracerebral hemorrhage. *Stroke*. 2001 Apr;32(4):891–897.

32. Cheung RT, Zou LY. Use of the original, modified, or new intracerebral hemorrhage score to predict mortality and morbidity after intracerebral hemorrhage. *Stroke*. 2003 Jul;34(7):1717–1722.

33. Rost NS, Smith EE, Chang Y, Snider RW, Chanderraj R, Schwab K, *et al*. Prediction of functional outcome in patients with primary intracerebral hemorrhage: the FUNC score. *Stroke*. 2008 Aug;39(8):2304–2309.

34. Hemphill JC, 3rd, Farrant M, Neill TA, Jr Prospective validation of the ICH Score for 12-month functional outcome. *Neurology*. 2009 Oct 6;73(14):1088–1094.

35. van Beijnum J, Lovelock CE, Cordonnier C, Rothwell PM, Klijn CJ, Al-Shahi Salman R. Outcome after spontaneous and arteriovenous malformation-related intracerebral haemorrhage: population-based studies. *Brain*. 2009 Feb;132(Pt 2):537–543.

36. Becker KJ, Baxter AB, Cohen WA, Bybee HM, Tirschwell DL, Newell DW, *et al*. Withdrawal of support in intracerebral hemorrhage may lead to self-fulfilling prophecies. *Neurology*. 2001 Mar 27;56(6):766–772.

37. Hemphill JC, 3rd, Newman J, Zhao S, Johnston SC. Hospital usage of early do-not-resuscitate orders and outcome after intracerebral hemorrhage. *Stroke*. 2004 May;35(5):1130–1134.

38. Zahuranec DB, Morgenstern LB, Sanchez BN, Resnicow K, White DB, Hemphill JC, 3rd. Do-not-resuscitate orders and predictive models after intracerebral hemorrhage. *Neurology*. 2010 Aug 17;75(7):626–633.

39. Al-Shahi Salman R, Labovitz DL, Stapf C. Spontaneous intracerebral haemorrhage. *BMJ*. 2009;339:b2586.

40. Steiner T, Petersson J, Al-Shahi Salman R, Christensen H, Cordonnier C, Csiba L, *et al*. European research priorities for intracerebral haemorrhage. *Cerebrovasc Dis*. 2011;32(5):409–419.

41. Jackson CA, Sudlow CL. Is hypertension a more frequent risk factor for deep than for lobar supratentorial intracerebral haemorrhage? *J Neurol Neurosurg Psychiatry*. 2006 Nov;77(11):1244–1252.

42. Knudsen KA, Rosand J, Karluk D, Greenberg SM. Clinical diagnosis of cerebral amyloid angiopathy: validation of the Boston criteria. *Neurology*. 2001 Feb 27;56(4):537–539.

43. Linn J, Halpin A, Demaerel P, Ruhland J, Giese AD, Dichgans M, *et al*. Prevalence of superficial siderosis in patients with cerebral amyloid angiopathy. *Neurology*. 2010 Apr 27;74(17):1346–1350.

44. Samarasekera N, Smith C, Al-Shahi Salman R. The association between cerebral amyloid angiopathy and intracerebral haemorrhage: systematic review and meta-analysis. *J Neurol Neurosurg Psychiatry*. 2012 Mar;83(3):275–281.

45. Fisher CM. Pathological observations in hypertensive cerebral hemorrhage. *J Neuropathol Exp Neurol*. 1971 Jul;30(3):536–550.

46. Greenberg SM, Vernooij MW, Cordonnier C, Viswanathan A, Al-Shahi Salman R, Warach S, *et al*. Cerebral microbleeds: a guide to detection and interpretation. *Lancet Neurol*. 2009 Feb;8(2):165–174.

47. Cordonnier C, Al-Shahi Salman R, Wardlaw J. Spontaneous brain microbleeds: systematic review, subgroup analyses and standards for study design and reporting. *Brain*. 2007 Aug;130(Pt 8):1988–2003.

48. Greenberg SM, Nandigam RN, Delgado P, Betensky RA, Rosand J, Viswanathan A, *et al*. Microbleeds versus macrobleeds: evidence for distinct entities. *Stroke*. 2009 Jul;40(7):2382–2386.

49. Wedderburn CJ, van Beijnum J, Bhattacharya JJ, Counsell CE, Papanastassiou V, Ritchie V, *et al*. Outcome after interventional or conservative management of unruptured brain arteriovenous malformations: a prospective, population-based cohort study. *Lancet Neurol*. 2008 Mar;7(3):223–230.

50. Rosenow F, Hojer C, Meyer-Lohmann C, Hilgers RD, Muhlhofer H, Kleindienst A, *et al*. Spontaneous intracerebral hemorrhage. Prognostic factors in 896 cases. *Acta Neurol Scand*. 1997 Sep;96(3):174–182.

51. Hartmann A, Mast H, Mohr JP, Koennecke HC, Osipov A, Pile-Spellman J, *et al*. Morbidity of intracranial hemorrhage in patients with cerebral arteriovenous malformation. *Stroke*. 1998 May;29(5):931–934.

52. Al-Shahi R, Warlow C. A systematic review of the frequency and prognosis of arteriovenous malformations of the brain in adults. *Brain*. 2001 Oct;124(Pt 10):1900–1926.

53. Choi JH, Mast H, Sciacca RR, Hartmann A, Khaw AV, Mohr JP, *et al*. Clinical outcome after first and recurrent hemorrhage in patients with untreated brain arteriovenous malformation. *Stroke*. 2006 May;37(5):1243–1247.

54. Aoki N. Do intracranial arteriovenous malformations cause subarachnoid haemorrhage? Review of computed tomography features of ruptured arteriovenous malformations in the acute stage. *Acta Neurochir (Wien)*. 1991;112(3–4):92–95.

55. Toffol GJ, Biller J, Adams HP, Jr Nontraumatic intracerebral hemorrhage in young adults. *Arch Neurol*. 1987 May;44(5):483–485.

56. Robinson JR, Awad IA, Little JR. Natural history of the cavernous angioma. *J Neurosurg*. 1991 Nov;75(5):709–714.

57. Kondziolka D, Lunsford LD, Kestle JR. The natural history of cerebral cavernous malformations. *J Neurosurg*. 1995 Nov;83(5):820–824.

58. Porter PJ, Willinsky RA, Harper W, Wallace MC. Cerebral cavernous malformations: natural history and prognosis after clinical deterioration with or without hemorrhage. *J Neurosurg*. 1997 Aug;87(2):190–197.

59. Kupersmith MJ, Kalish H, Epstein F, Yu G, Berenstein A, Woo H, *et al*. Natural history of brainstem cavernous malformations. *Neurosurgery*. 2001 Jan;48(1):47–53; discussion 53–54.

60. Zabramski JM, Wascher TM, Spetzler RF, Johnson B, Golfinos J, Drayer BP, *et al*. The natural history of familial cavernous malformations: results of an ongoing study. *J Neurosurg*. 1994 Mar;80(3):422–432.

61. Labauge P, Laberge S, Brunereau L, Levy C, Tournier-Lasserve E. Hereditary cerebral cavernous angiomas: clinical and genetic features in

57 French families. Societe Francaise de Neurochirurgie. *Lancet.* 1998 Dec 12;352(9144):1892–1897.

62. Labauge P, Denier C, Bergametti F, Tournier-Lasserve E. Genetics of cavernous angiomas. *Lancet Neurol.* 2007 Mar;6(3):237–244.

63. Seker A, Pricola KL, Guclu B, Ozturk AK, Louvi A, Gunel M. CCM2 expression parallels that of CCM1. *Stroke.* 2006 Feb;37(2):518–523.

64. Petit N, Blecon A, Denier C, Tournier-Lasserve E. Patterns of expression of the three cerebral cavernous malformation (CCM) genes during embryonic and postnatal brain development. *Gene Expr Patterns.* 2006 Jun;6(5):495–503.

65. Cordonnier C, Al-Shahi Salman R, Bhattacharya JJ, Counsell CE, Papanastassiou V, Ritchie V, *et al.* Differences between intracranial vascular malformation types in the characteristics of their presenting haemorrhages: prospective, population-based study. *J Neurol Neurosurg Psychiatry.* 2008 Jan;79(1):47–51.

66. Bousser MG, Ferro JM. Cerebral venous thrombosis: an update. *Lancet Neurol.* 2007 Feb;6(2):162–170.

67. Ferro JM, Canhao P, Stam J, Bousser MG, Barinagarrementeria F. Prognosis of cerebral vein and dural sinus thrombosis: results of the International Study on Cerebral Vein and Dural Sinus Thrombosis (ISCVT). *Stroke.* 2004 Mar;35(3):664–670.

68. Stam J. Thrombosis of the cerebral veins and sinuses. *N Engl J Med.* 2005 Apr 28;352(17):1791–1798.

69. Calabrese LH, Dodick DW, Schwedt TJ, Singhal AB. Narrative review: reversible cerebral vasoconstriction syndromes. *Ann Intern Med.* 2007 Jan 2;146(1):34–44.

70. Ducros A, Boukobza M, Porcher R, Sarov M, Valade D, Bousser MG. The clinical and radiological spectrum of reversible cerebral vasoconstriction syndrome. A prospective series of 67 patients. *Brain.* 2007 Dec;130(Pt 12):3091–3101.

71. Ducros A. Reversible cerebral vasoconstriction syndrome. *Lancet Neurol.* 2012 Oct;11(10):906–917.

72. Ducros A, Fiedler U, Porcher R, Boukobza M, Stapf C, Bousser MG. Hemorrhagic manifestations of reversible cerebral vasoconstriction syndrome: frequency, features, and risk factors. *Stroke.* 2010 Nov;41(11):2505–2511.

73. Moskowitz SI, Calabrese LH, Weil RJ. Benign angiopathy of the central nervous system presenting with intracerebral hemorrhage. *Surg Neurol.* 2007 May;67(5):522–527; discussion 7–8.

74. Paciaroni M, Agnelli G, Corea F, Ageno W, Alberti A, Lanari A, *et al.* Early hemorrhagic transformation of brain infarction: rate, predictive factors, and influence on clinical outcome: results of a prospective multicenter study. *Stroke.* 2008 Aug;39(8):2249–2456.

75. Motto C, Aritzu E, Boccardi E, De Grandi C, Piana A, Candelise L. Reliability of hemorrhagic transformation diagnosis in acute ischemic stroke. *Stroke.* 1997 Feb;28(2):302–306.

76. Lindley RI, Wardlaw JM, Sandercock PA, Rimdusid P, Lewis SC, Signorini DF, *et al.* Frequency and risk factors for spontaneous hemorrhagic transformation of cerebral infarction. *J Stroke Cerebrovasc Dis.* 2004 Nov–Dec;13(6):235–246.

77. Lovelock CE, Anslow P, Molyneux AJ, Byrne JV, Kuker W, Pretorius PM, *et al.* Substantial observer variability in the differentiation between primary intracerebral hemorrhage and hemorrhagic transformation of infarction on CT brain imaging. *Stroke.* 2009 Dec;40(12):3763–3767.

78. Larrue V, von Kummer RR, Muller A, Bluhmki E. Risk factors for severe hemorrhagic transformation in ischemic stroke patients treated with recombinant tissue plasminogen activator: a secondary analysis of the European-Australasian Acute Stroke Study (ECASS II). *Stroke.* 2001 Feb;32(2):438–441.

79. Cordonnier C, Klijn CJ, van Beijnum J, Al-Shahi Salman R. Radiological investigation of spontaneous intracerebral hemorrhage: systematic review and trinational survey. *Stroke.* 2010 Apr;41(4):685–690.

80. Wada R, Aviv RI, Fox AJ, Sahlas DJ, Gladstone DJ, Tomlinson G, *et al.* CT angiography "spot sign" predicts hematoma expansion in acute intracerebral hemorrhage. *Stroke.* 2007 Apr;38(4):1257–1262.

81. Demchuk AM, Dowlatshahi D, Rodriguez-Luna D, Molina CA, Blas YS, Dzialowski I, *et al.* Prediction of haematoma growth and outcome in patients with intracerebral haemorrhage using the CT-angiography spot sign (PREDICT): a prospective observational study. *Lancet Neurol.* 2012 Apr;11(4):307–314.

82. Wardlaw JM. Prediction of haematoma expansion with the CTA spot sign: a useful biomarker? *Lancet Neurol.* 2012; 11(4):294–295.

83. Wijman CA, Venkatasubramanian C, Bruins S, Fischbein N, Schwartz N. Utility of early MRI in the diagnosis and management of acute spontaneous intracerebral hemorrhage. *Cerebrovasc Dis.* 2010; 30(5):456–463.

84. Lummel N, Lutz J, Bruckmann H, Linn J. The value of magnetic resonance imaging for the detection of the bleeding source in non-traumatic intracerebral haemorrhages: a comparison with conventional digital subtraction angiography. *Neuroradiology.* 2012 Jul;54(7):673–680.

85. Evans AL, Coley SC, Wilkinson ID, Griffiths PD. First-line investigation of acute intracerebral hemorrhage using dynamic magnetic resonance angiography. *Acta Radiol.* 2005; 46(6):625–630.

86. Halpin SF, Britton JA, Byrne JV, Clifton A, Hart G, Moore A. Prospective evaluation of cerebral angiography and computed tomography in cerebral haematoma. *J Neurol Neurosurg Psychiatry.* 1994; 57(10):1180–1186.

87. Zhu XL, Chan MS, Poon WS. Spontaneous intracranial hemorrhage: which patients need diagnostic cerebral angiography? A prospective study of 206 cases and review of the literature. *Stroke.* 1997; 28(7):1406–1409.

88. Perez ES, Delgado-Mederos R, Rubiera M, Delgado P, Ribo M, Maisterra O, *et al.* Transcranial duplex sonography for monitoring hyperacute intracerebral hemorrhage. *Stroke.* 2009; 40(3):987–990.

CHAPTER 6

Spontaneous intracranial subarachnoid haemorrhage: epidemiology, causes, diagnosis, and complications

Laurent Thines and Charlotte Cordonnier

Introduction

The occurrence of subarachnoid haemorrhage (SAH) is generally related to the rupture of an intracranial aneurysm and its pathophysiological description coincides in many aspects with their natural history. Despite the fact that intracranial aneurysms are relatively common (2–5% of adults are carrying an unruptured intracranial aneurysm), SAH only represents 1–7% of all strokes (1–3). Nevertheless, its occurrence at a young age and its frequent poor prognosis have a severe impact on public health with considerable loss of productive life years in the population similar to that of far more frequent diseases such as ischaemic strokes (1, 4–6). Thus the knowledge of SAH characteristics might help to improve its diagnosis, management, and prevention in order to reduce its individual and social cost.

Definition

Subarachnoid spaces are delimited by an external layer covering the brain surface but not penetrating the sulci, namely the arachnoid, and an internal layer firmly adherent to the brain surface, namely the pia mater (Figure 6.1). These spaces are very narrow over the cortex and enlarge to form cisterns particularly around the brainstem, between both hemispheres (interhemispheric fissure), in the depth of the main cortical sulci as the lateral sulcus (lateral or Sylvian cistern), or around the spinal cord. They are filled with cerebrospinal fluid (CSF) and they communicate with the cerebral ventricles through the foramen of Magendie. Therefore, SAH is defined by the irruption of blood in those subarachnoid spaces, with or without extension to the ventricles or to the brain parenchyma. In this chapter, we have limited the description to spontaneous intracranial SAH because the natural history of traumatic or spinal SAH, despite a similar substratum, is completely different.

Epidemiology

Incidence and prevalence

The overall incidence of SAH in Western countries is about 9 per 100,000 person-years with wide variations between nations

(1, 5, 7–9). The mean age at diagnosis is around 60 years. The incidence of SAH increases with age: the incidence ratio (taking age 45–55 years as the reference category) varies with age and it is 0.10 in those under 25 years and 1.61 over 85 years (7, 8, 10, 11). One of the empirically known features of SAH incidence is its waveform annual distribution. Some studies have found a seasonal peak in winter and spring and a moderate influence of atmospheric pressure changes on daily occurrence of SAH (1, 9). The annual prevalence of SAH itself is not well documented in most countries, but as an example it has been evaluated to represent up to 133,269 admissions in the US between 1996 and 2001 (26,654/year) (12).

Gender, ethnic, and region influence

Females have an increased risk of SAH with sex ratios around 1.2–1.6 depending on the region of origin (1, 7, 8, 10). This is mainly due to the prevalence of intracranial aneurysms in women. Furthermore, women seem more susceptible than men to cardio-neurovascular risk factors usually associated with the risk of SAH (13). Finnish and Japanese women are inversely exposed to the occurrence of SAH, the former being exposed to the greatest risk (7). Nevertheless, incidence is higher in men aged between 25 and 45 years and inversely in women aged between 55 and 85 years (7).

'Non-white' ethnicity is in some studies associated with an increased risk of SAH from 2- to 3.4-fold (13). This has been suggested by studies comparing 'black' versus 'white' Americans or Maori and Pacific people versus 'white' New-Zealanders (1, 14).

Regional differences in SAH prevalence are very important (7). The disease seems to be more diagnosed in some countries as Finland or Japan where the incidence is twice that of others nations (around 20 per 100,000 person-year) whereas the incidence in Central and South-America or China is respectively more than two or four times lower (around 2 to 4 per 100,000 person-year) (15). A higher risk of rupture, prevalence of risk factors (smoking and hypertension in Finland, for example), and genetic factors might explain those differences (7).

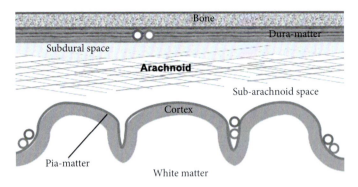

Fig. 6.1 Schematic representation of meningeal spaces.

Time trends

Despite an overall decline in stroke incidence, thanks to a better management of vascular risk factors, the incidence of SAH has only scarcely declined over the last decade (1, 5, 7, 16). This might be explained by the fact that the disease is probably mainly influenced by non-modifiable risk factors such as gender or genetic factors, and that the control of vascular risk factors might be counterbalanced by the aging of the population, which favours the occurrence of SAH.

Risk factors

Acquired risk factors

Epidemiological studies (longitudinal and case–control) have shown with multivariate analyses that smoking, arterial hypertension, and excessive alcohol consumption were independent risk factors for SAH. These risk factors are also regarded as promoting factors for the development of intracranial aneurysms, especially in the setting of multiple ones. The awareness of these modifiable risks factors is the basis of primary and secondary prevention of SAH.

Smoking

Smoking is the main risk factor for SAH, and is present in up to 75% of patient with aneurysmal rupture (14, 17). Smoke products play a negative role through the induction of a deficit in alpha-1 antitrypsin, which is an inhibitor of elastase, leading to the increased degradation of elastic fibres in the arterial wall (18). This is responsible for a decreased resistance of the arterial wall against haemodynamic constraints and to the formation of aneurismal dilatations. The risk of SAH for former smokers is twice the risk of never smoking individuals (relative risk (RR) 1.9; odds ratio (OR) 2.3) (13). Ever smoking or current smoking was associated with a higher risk of SAH (RR 2.2; OR 3.1) compared with never smoking (13, 19). There is therefore some indirect evidence that smoking cessation could reduce the risk of SAH. Smoking has also been associated with the risk of multiple intracranial aneurysms (20).

Arterial hypertension

Arterial hypertension is only the second highest risk factor for SAH, present in 20% of patients with aneurysmal rupture (14). It increases the probability of occurrence of SAH by 2.5-fold (13, 19). Until now, if active prevention of arterial hypertension in the general population has been effective in reducing stroke incidence, little impact on SAH incidence has been observed (21). Hence, blood pressure control will probably not be helpful in reducing SAH frequency, but perhaps it will improve the prognosis of the disease since arterial hypertension is also an independent risk factor of poor outcome after SAH (1).

Alcohol

Alcohol consumption increases the probability of SAH by twofold. The risk only appears for an intake of more than 150 g per week (13, 19). There might be a regional predisposition to the influence of this factor since the Finnish population appeared particularly exposed according to three population-based studies (19).

Others

Use of hormonal treatments (oral contraceptives and hormone replacement therapy) do not significantly affect the risk of SAH. Nevertheless, when analysing specifically the results of studies taking place before 1987, at a time when higher oestrogens levels were used in oral contraceptive pills, a higher risk of SAH was found. Similarly, hormone replacement therapy was in some studies associated with a tendency towards a decreased risk of SAH (up to 40%) without reaching statistical significance (13, 19).

There is also a lack of evidence that hypercholesterolemia and physical activity are risk factors for SAH. On the contrary, some studies demonstrated a protective effect of these two factors on its occurrence (13).

Genetic and familial risk factors

Genetic factors only explain 5–15% of SAH (22, 23). Some gene polymorphisms (i.e. endothelial nitric oxide synthetase, elastin, collagen 1A2) have been associated with a higher risk of development or rupture of intracranial aneurysms (22–25). Gene expression profiles have also been identified in the process of development and rupture of intracranial aneurysms. They modulate the muscle system, cell adhesion processes (downregulation) and the immune/inflammatory response (upregulation) (26). To date, no single gene has been proven to be responsible for intracranial aneurysms formation or rupture and genome-wide linkage studies are suggestive of the involvement of several susceptibility loci that may contain one or more predisposing genes modulated by multiple environmental factors (27, 28).

Familial aneurysms

A family history of intracranial aneurysms or SAH seems to be associated with a higher risk of both diseases but specific genes have not been identified yet (1, 27–31). The risk in first-degree relatives of intracranial aneurysm patients seems to be higher than that of the standard population (1.8 to as high as 6.6 times that of an age-matched control) but not sufficiently to warrant preventive measures such as systematic screening (27, 32). The definition of true familial intracranial aneurysms syndrome is usually restricted to families with at least two first-degree relatives carrying ruptured or unruptured intracranial aneurysm(s) (33). Inheritance patterns are variable: autosomal recessive, autosomal dominant, or autosomal dominant with incomplete penetrance (34). It is associated with a higher risk of unruptured intracranial aneurysms (4.2-fold, incidence 8%) often multiple and rupturing more frequently (overall annual risk 1.2% vs 0.07%) and at a younger age than sporadic cases (1, 35–37). Members of those families are also exposed to a higher susceptibility of other risk factors such as smoking, arterial hypertension or female sex (38).

Connective tissue disorders

Certain genetic syndromes are associated with a higher risk of intracranial aneurysms and SAH: autosomal dominant polycystic kidney disease (polycystin mutation), type IV Ehlers–Danlos syndrome (collagen 3 anomaly), Marfan disease (fibrillin 1 deficit), pseudoxanthoma elasticum (elastic fibres fragmentation), fibromuscular dysplasia (alpha-1 antitrypsin deficit), neurofibromatosis type 1 (39–41). Those diseases are known to be associated with a higher risk of intracranial aneurysms often multiple and rupturing at a younger age than sporadic lesions. In fact, this risk is only significantly increased in clusters of polycystic kidney disease families (2% of all SAH), and the development of intracranial aneurysms seems to be rather rare in other connective tissue diseases (34).

Causes of subarachnoid haemorrhage

Intracranial aneurysms

The rupture of an intracranial aneurysm is the classical and most feared cause of SAH representing 72–85% of cases (5, 42, 43) (Table 6.1). Intracranial aneurysm is an acquired condition that tends to develop preferentially at arterial bifurcations (Figure 6.2). Why certain persons do develop aneurysms and some does not, remains poorly understood. The presence of an underlying arterial wall weakness, though intuitive, has not been established (44). The promotion of the disease relies probably on biomechanical/haemodynamic constraints (i.e. increased wall shear stress at

Table 6.1 Causes and associated location of bleeding (with relative frequencies) of non-traumatic SAH

Frequent neurovascular causes (95%)
Intracranial aneurysm rupture—80% (C-SAH > ICH)
Benign idiopathic haemorrhage—15% (C-SAH)
Rare neurovascular causes (5%)
Cerebral arteriovenous malformation (ICH > c-SAH > C-SAH)
Intracranial dural arteriovenous fistula (subdural > ICH > c-SAH or C-SAH)
Spinal arteriovenous malformation (C-SAH)
Intracranial artery dissection (C-SAH)
Cavernous malformation (ICH > c-SAH > C-SAH)
Moyamoya disease (ICH > c-SAH > C-SAH)
Cerebral vasculitis (c-SAH > ICH > C-SAH)
Cerebral venous thrombosis (ICH > c-SAH > C-SAH)
Cerebral amyloid angiopathy (ICH > c-SAH > C-SAH)
Exceptional medical causes
Pituitary apoplexy
Embolic diseases (cardiac myxoma, choriocarcinoma or endocarditis)
Sickle cell disease
Sympathomimetic drugs abuse
Anticoagulant therapy

c-SAH: convexal SAH; C-SAH: cisternal SAH; ICH: intracerebral haemorrhage.

bifurcations) (45, 46) modulated by an individual genetic susceptibility and amplified by modifiable risk factors as smoking, arterial hypertension, and alcohol consumption. The overall annual risk of rupture on an unruptured intracranial aneurysm is about 1% per year but it is highly variable depending on different parameters: gender, age of the patient or previous history of SAH, location or size of the aneurysm, and associated risk factors. Patient characteristics associated with a higher risk of rupture are age older than 60, female gender, and smoking. Aneurysm characteristics associated with a higher risk of rupture are size greater than 5 mm, posterior circulation location, and symptoms due to the aneurysm other than SAH (2).

Benign idiopathic SAH

Approximately 10–20% of SAH patients will not have a discernible cause of bleeding identified at the end of the workup (5, 10, 42, 47). Among those, one-third (5% of all SAH) will present a specific pattern often referred as benign perimesencephalic (or truncal) haemorrhage (43). This subset of SAH is characterized by mild symptoms at onset, a typical pattern of haemorrhage on computed tomography (CT) (haemorrhage restricted to the cisterns surrounding the brainstem and suprasellar cistern with scant blood allowed in the ventricles or the proximal Sylvian fissure, Figure 6.3), a negative cerebral angiogram, an uneventful clinical course, and an excellent outcome (10, 19, 43, 47). Repeated angiography is not necessary when clinical and radiological presentations are typical and initial CT angiography (CTA)/angiography are negative (47). A venous origin of the bleeding has been suggested to explain its very limited extension (48).

Convexal SAH

Convexal SAH (c-SAH) is characterized by the presence of blood collections in one or several adjacent sulci in the absence of blood at the basal cisterns of the brain or elsewhere (49). It is sometimes referred in the literature as 'focal SAH' or 'focal superficial siderosis'. c-SAH has been described in various settings: vascular malformations (arterio-venous malformations, dural arterio-venous fistulae, cavernomas), arterial dissections, cortical venous thrombosis, vasculitis, reversible cerebral vasoconstriction syndrome (RCVS), posterior reversible encephalopathy syndrome, moyamoya disease and syndrome, infective endocarditis, coagulation disorders, and cerebral amyloid angiopathy (CAA) (50).

While aneurysmal SAH typically present with acute headache, c-SAH are often unexpected findings or associated with transient neurological symptoms. c-SAH are increasingly recognized as a potential diagnostic *in vivo* biomarker of CAA (51). Retrospective data suggest that c-SAH in the context of CAA may be a warning sign of future SAH or ICH (52, 53).

Rare neurovascular causes of SAH

These rare neurovascular causes of SAH account for 5% of all cases (5).

Cerebral arteriovenous malformations

Arteriovenous malformation (AVM) ruptures are rarely disclosed by SAH (9–20% of cases) and usually it is in association with parenchymal (Figure 6.4) or ventricular haemorrhage (54–56). Similarly, SAH represents only 10% of AVM recurrent haemorrhages (57). When pure SAH is encountered in this context, the rupture of a

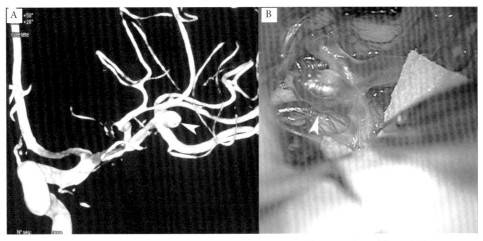

Fig. 6.2 Angiographic ((A) 3D DSA, anterior view) and intraoperative ((B) left Sylvian fissure approach) aspect of a middle cerebral artery aneurysm.

prenidal feeding artery aneurysm should be searched for with CTA or conventional digitalized subtraction angiography (DSA). These aneurysms develop because of increased blood flow on the arterial pathways directed to the AVM (44). Magnetic resonance imaging (MRI) and magnetic resonance angiography (MRA) will show the nidus and conventional DSA will depict its precise angioarchitecture.

Intracranial dural arteriovenous fistulae

Dural arteriovenous fistulae (DAVFs) are constituted by direct arteriovenous shunts into the dural layer. Types II b, III and IV DAVF carry draining pathways involving cortical veins and are associated with a high annual risk of bleeding (8% per year). Haemorrhage is classically subdural but can either be parenchymal or subarachnoid (Figure 6.5) (58). Previous sinus thrombosis, head trauma or intracranial surgery can be the triggering factor for the development of this type of malformation (59). MRA could disclose dilated veins around the shunt area but final diagnosis will be provided with conventional DSA.

Spinal arteriovenous malformations

A history of low cervical pain or stabbing pain between scapulae should evoke the diagnosis of spinal AVM or fistula

(Figure 6.6), particularly if intracranial investigations are negative and SAH concentrates at the posterior fossa or foramen magnum (60, 61). A spinal angiography will be needed to show the malformation.

Cervical or intracranial artery dissections

Cervical artery dissection (CAD) is a classical differential clinical diagnosis of aneurismal SAH that should be considered when a thunderclap headache occurs (frequently after a history of neck trauma or unusual head movements). CADs are rarely associated with intracranial SAH unless the dissection extends to or arises from intracranial arteries (1.5% of cases) (42). In the context of CADs, SAH results from the direct disruption of the arterial wall or the rupture of a pseudoaneurysm (62). Imaging workup will entail, depending on local availability, CTA, DSA, cervical/transcranial Doppler, or MRI/MRA (Figure 6.7).

Others

Cavernous malformation is usually a cause of intracerebral haemorrhage that rarely extents to other brain compartments. It is a very uncommon source of SAH and this could append in this context only with a very superficial pial lesion rupturing

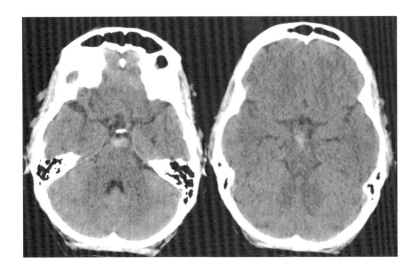

Fig. 6.3 Typical pattern of a benign perimesencephalic haemorrhage on axial CT scan: haemorrhage restricted to the cisterns surrounding the brainstem (interpeduncular cistern) without blood in the ventricles or the proximal Sylvian fissures.

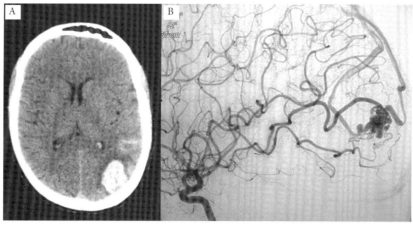

Fig. 6.4 Subarachnoid haemorrhage with parenchymal haematoma ((A) axial brain CT scan) revealing an occipital arteriovenous malformation ((B) lateral view of left internal carotid angiography).

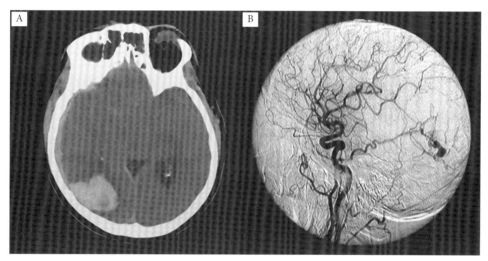

Fig. 6.5 Subdural, parenchymal and subarachnoid haemorrhages ((A) axial CT scan) in relation with the rupture of a right dural arteriovenous fistula with cortico-venous reflux and ectasia ((B) right common carotid artery angiography).

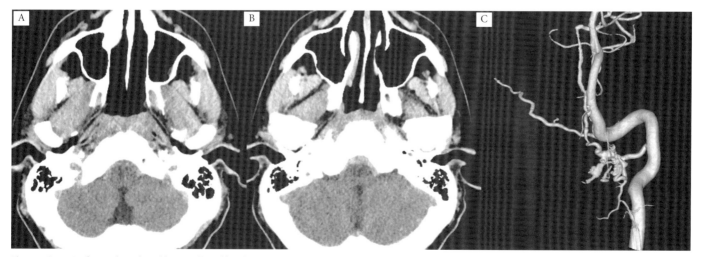

Fig. 6.6 Posterior fossa subarachnoid haemorrhage ((A, B) axial CT scan) revealing a cervical spine dural arteriovenous fistula ((C) 3D DSA of the left vertebral artery).

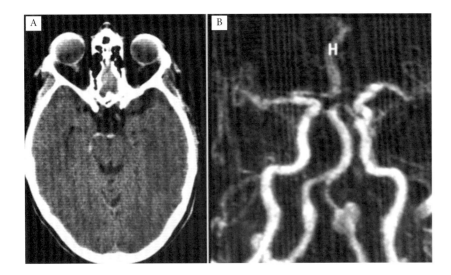

Fig. 6.7 Posterior fossa subarachnoid haemorrhage ((A) axial CT scan) due to a left intracranial (V4 segment) vertebral artery aneurismal dissection ((B) MRA, anterior view).

in the subarachnoid space. Diagnosis is based on MRI disclosing the typical aspect of a nodular lesion with mixed intensity on T2-weighted sequence and surrounded by a haemosiderin halo (63).

Moyamoya disease is a rare cerebrovascular disease consisting of a progressive steno-occlusion of main cerebral arteries in association with the development of neovessels at the base of the brain (lenticulostriate territory) and at the surface of the brain (leptomenigeal collaterals). In children, the disease is usually responsible for ischaemic symptoms but in adults, haemorrhage is the most frequent complication (50%). Although classical, isolated SAH in this context is quite uncommon (Figure 6.8) and could be the consequence of rupture of an associated aneurysm or fragile leptomeningeal neovessels (64).

Cerebral vasculitis is a rare cause of SAH and should be suspected when SAH distribution is very peripheral (Figure 6.9). The diagnosis will be made with angiography showing irregularities of distal cortical arteries (42).

Cerebral venous thrombosis may be diagnosed in a context of a thunderclap headache revealing a focal cortical SAH. Exploring sinuses and cortical veins is therefore mandatory in the setting of an isolated non-aneurismal SAH.

Rare medical causes of SAH

Pituitary apoplexy is a rare aetiology of SAH. It consists of a haemorrhagic necrosis of a pituitary macroadenoma leading to a rapid increase in tumour volume and sometimes its subarachnoid rupture. Neurological symptoms are a sudden retroocular or frontal headache in association with ophthalmological signs as decreased visual acuity, oculomotor nerves palsies, or bitemporal hemianopsia (5). Head CT scan will show a haemorrhage centred in the sella or suprasellar area.

Embolic diseases as cardiac myxoma, choriocarcinoma, or endocarditis could be the source of cerebral arteries infiltration and dilatation until the formation of one or several pseudoaneurysms often referred as 'mycotic aneurysms'. Diagnostic DSA will usually show typical and multiple small distal aneurysms, most of the times located in the middle cerebral artery territory. The main complication of these lesions is their rupture in the parenchyma or subarachnoid spaces (5).

Sickle cell disease might be a direct cause of SAH in children and the pathophysiology in this context is similar to that of moyamoya disease (65).

Sympathomimetic drug abuse, such as cocaine or phenylpropanolamine, might be a cause of SAH. In this case, the haemorrhage

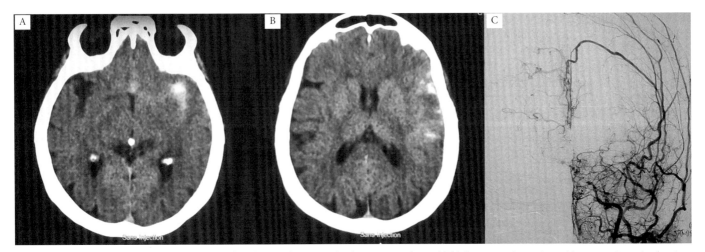

Fig. 6.8 Left Sylvian subarachnoid haemorrhage ((A, B) axial CT scan) associated with moyamoya disease ((C) left common internal carotid artery angiography showing distal ICA occlusion and leptomeningeal collaterals).

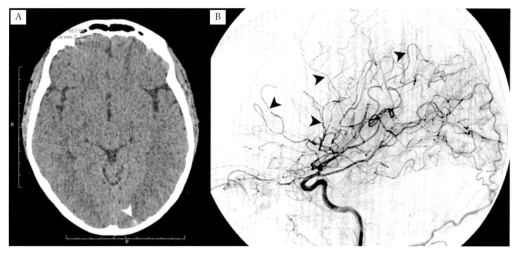

Fig. 6.9 Left convexal parietal subarachnoid haemorrhage. (A) Axial CT scan (white arrow-head) caused by cerebral vasculitis diagnosed on cerebral angiography. (B) Left internal carotid artery angiogram showing multiple irregularities (black arrowheads) of anterior and middle cerebral arteries branches.

usually occurs at a younger age but has the same prognosis as in the usual form. No evidence of associated toxic vasospasm or vasculitis was found on radiological examinations or during autopsy (1, 66, 67).

The use of anticoagulant therapy is found in 5% of patients with non-aneurysmal SAH (43). Nevertheless, anticoagulants alone have been proven to be the cause of SAH in only 2.6% of intracranial haemorrhage (68).

Clinical diagnosis of subarachnoid haemorrhage

Qualification of the headache

The diagnosis of SAH is clinical in essence and will be later confirmed by a non-enhanced head CT scan or a lumbar puncture (LP). The pivotal symptom of SAH is a thunderclap headache. Unfortunately, headaches are not always specific and account for 4–5% of the referrals to the emergency departments among which, SAH represents only 1–2% of the causes (1, 69–71). Therefore it is very important to precisely know how to characterize an aneurismal SAH headache and to be able to differentiate it from the three main differential diagnosis: migraine, tension headache, and RCVS (6, 72, 73). The goal is to appropriately triage patients in order to avoid overinvestigating the disease or, more seriously, misdiagnosing it, which would occur in about 5–12% of patients (43% in emergency departments and 32% at physicians' offices) (1, 6, 72). In the first situation, inappropriate head CT scan then LP will be required. In the second eventuality, no head CT scan (73% of misdiagnosed patients) or LP (7% of misdiagnosed patients) will be performed (6). The average diagnostic delay in the context of SAH is around 3–4 days and during this period, the patient will be exposed to re-rupture (22%) with or without other complications as acute hydrocephalus, intraparenchymal haemorrhage, vasospasm (Figure 6.10), or decreased level of consciousness occurring in 39% of misdiagnosed patients (6, 72). In every instance, when the diagnosis is considered, all efforts have to be made to rule out or to confirm the diagnosis (wide indication of head CT scan), particularly in good clinical and good radiological grade patients (more than half of SAH patients)

which constitute the subgroup at the highest risk of misdiagnosis, and who will instead benefit the most from prompt treatment (8, 10, 69, 72).

Clinical presentation

The following description focuses mainly on aneurismal SAH that combines the more typical features. If the diagnosis is (or should be) easy within the first hours, it is much more difficult to reconstitute the exact clinical sequence when the patient is admitted after a few days. None of the symptoms taken alone is pathognomonic of the disease.

The irruption of blood in the intracranial subarachnoid spaces is accompanied by an acute and severe headache (called 'thunderclap'), which is the pivotal symptom that should lead to consideration of diagnosis (5). The characteristics of the headache are quite specific. In one-third of patients, it is the only symptom (10). The onset is very sudden (like an 'explosion') with a peak intensity reached almost instantaneously (50%) or in a few seconds or minutes (<5 minutes in 93% of cases), which is responsible for the description as a 'thunderclap' headache (10). Usually the patient is also able to remember the exact time or concomitant occupation at the headache onset, which forced him, in most cases, to stop his activity. Indeed, the pain is often severe and classically described by 80% of subject as the 'worst headache ever'. In 20% of cases, a milder headache, called by some authors warning or sentinel headache and corresponding to a minimal bleed, could happen 2–8 weeks before overt SAH (1). Some precipitating circumstances are classically described in half of patients as intense physical exertion (i.e. sport or sexual activity, 6%) or Valsalva-like manoeuvres (i.e. defecation) but in fact fatal SAH attacks usually occur at night (39%) (1, 10, 74). The site of the headache might be in some case restricted to a definite region of the head but it usually becomes rapidly diffuse. The headache lasts several days and in patients presenting late after the beginning of the symptoms, the recurrence of the headache might be a sign of re-rupture that should urge radiological diagnosis and treatment. When a history of chronic cephalalgia is found, it is important to differentiate the current episode with the usual type presented by the patient, particularly in terms of location and intensity.

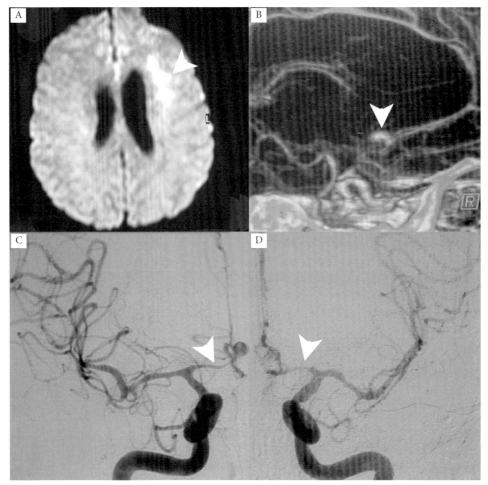

Fig. 6.10 Patient admitted with delayed cerebral ischaemia in the anterior cerebral artery (ACA) territory (A) after the rupture of an anterior communicating aneurysm (B). Cerebral angiography disclosed bilateral severe ACA narrowing due to vasospasm (C, D).

Accompanying symptoms are also present in two-thirds of cases and very suggestive of aneurismal SAH as intense dizziness or syncopal loss of consciousness (25–53%), generalized seizure (7–20%), diplopia, or other focal deficit (1, 10). SAH headache is also frequently followed by the occurrence of meningeal symptoms as nausea/vomiting (77%), neck stiffness (33%), or dorso-lumbar rachialgia (1).

Neurological examination

The clinician will look for meningismus classical symptoms (Kernig or Brudzinsky signs, nuchal or diffuse spinal stiffness, prostration, and pyramidal irritation signs). A focal neurological deficit might be present when SAH is associated with parenchymal haemorrhage or later on when the patient presents several days after SAH onset with symptomatic vasospasm and 'inaugural' delayed cerebral ischaemia.

Ophthalmological symptoms are also classically observed after aneurismal SAH. Diplopia due to third nerve palsy (Figure 6.11) is seen in ruptured postero-carotid or termino-basilar aneurysms (superior cerebellar artery aneurysms). Sixth nerve palsy, which is non-localizing in this context and often bilateral, is due to global intracranial hypertension after SAH. Involvement of lower cranial nerves or a Horner's syndrome should point to dissection of the vertebral artery or the internal carotid artery. Patient could also

complain of a decrease in visual acuity or the feeling of a brown stain in their visual field. These symptoms are usually related to sub-hyaloidal haemorrhages (Terson syndrome) that will be confirmed at fundoscopy (Figure 6.12). They are related to a rapid increase in intracranial pressure during SAH onset. In aneurysmal SAH, 13% of patients present with this syndrome, which is often associated with a more severe presentation and a worst clinical prognosis (higher mortality) (75).

The acute intracranial hypertension resulting from the initial bleed is sometimes responsible for moderate to severe insult on the brainstem structures and particularly on the reticular activating system. This could lead to sudden and transitory loss of consciousness, often revealing the aneurysm rupture, or to a prolonged comatose state observed in cataclysmic SAHs. Thus, emergency symptoms will also be sought as confusion or decreased level of consciousness (from obnubilation to coma) (Glasgow Coma Scale), intracranial hypertension or temporal herniation (bradycardia, homolateral dilated pupil) symptoms, and vegetative or cardiorespiratory dysfunctions.

Two main classifications are used to determine the clinical grade of the patient: Hunt–Hess and World Federation of Neurological Surgeons (WFNS) grading systems (Table 6.2). The clinical status at admission is one of the leading parameters that predict clinical outcome (76).

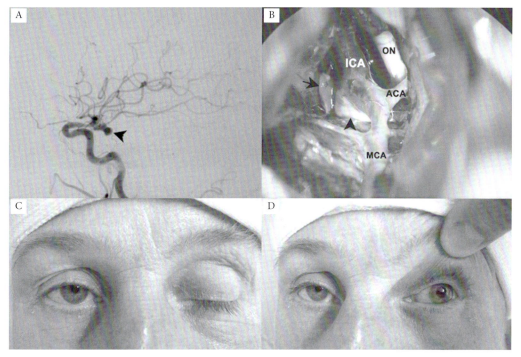

Fig. 6.11 Left posterior carotid ruptured aneurysm revealed by thunderclap headache and left third nerve palsy. (A) Lateral view of left internal carotid angiography (arrow-head = posterior carotid aneurysm). (B) Left pterional approach showing the aneurysm (arrow-head) and the compressed oculomotor nerve before its entry in the cavernous sinus (arrow), ICA: internal carotid artery; ON: optic nerve; ACA: anterior cerebral artery; MCA: middle cerebral artery. (C, D) Left third nerve palsy with ptosis, pupillary dilatation, lateral deviation of the eye.

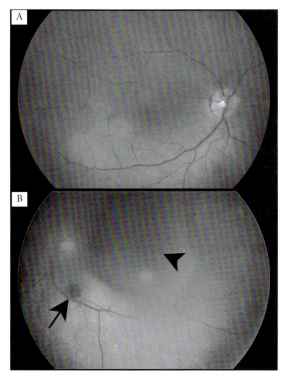

Fig. 6.12 Subarachnoid haemorrhage patient with Terson syndrome. (A) Right eye, normal fundoscopy. (B) Left eye fundoscopy showing a large premacular subhyaloidal haemorrhage (arrowhead) and a small prepapillar haemorrhage (arrow). (By courtesy of Pr Defoort-Dhellemmes and Dr Derlyn, Department of neuro-ophthalmology, Lille University Hospital.)

Table 6.2 Assessment of clinical and radiological grades after SAH

World Federation of Neurological Surgeons (WFNS) grading scale
I—Glasgow Coma Scale score 15
II—Glasgow Coma Scale score 14 or 13 without focal deficit
III—Glasgow Coma Scale score 14 or 13 with focal deficit
IV—Glasgow Coma Scale score 12 to 7 with or without focal deficit
V—Glasgow Coma Scale score 6 to 3 with or without focal deficit
Hunt–Hess grading scale
Grade 0—unruptured aneurysm without symptoms
Grade 1—asymptomatic or minimal headache and slight nuchal rigidity
Grade 2—moderate-to-severe headache, nuchal rigidity, no neurological deficit other than cranial nerve palsy
Grade 3—drowsy, confused, or mild focal deficit
Grade 4—stupor, moderate to severe hemiparesis, possible early decerebrate rigidity and vegetative disturbances
Grade 5—deep coma, decerebrate rigidity, moribund appearance
Fisher grading scale (CT scan)
Grade 1—no SAH
Grade 2—thin SAH <1 mm and clot <3 mm
Grade 3—thick SAH and local or diffused clot >5 × 3 mm
Grade 4—intraventricular haemorrhage, intracerebral haemorrhage

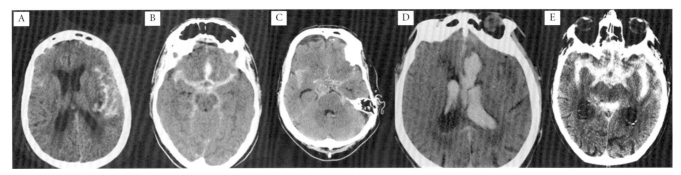

Fig. 6.13 Different patterns of subarachnoid haemorrhage according to the location of the ruptured aneurysm. (A) Left Sylvian fissure haemorrhage from a middle cerebral artery aneurysm. (B) Symmetric and interhemispheric haemorrhage from an anterior communicating aneurysm. (C) Right carotid cistern haemorrhage from a posterior carotid aneurysm. (D) Pericallosal and left frontal medial haemorrhage from a distal anterior cerebral artery aneurysm. (E) Diffuse cisternal symmetric haemorrhage from a basilar termination aneurysm.

Radiological diagnosis of subarachnoid haemorrhage

CT scanner

The diagnosis relies on a clinical expertise immediately followed by a non-enhanced head CT scan showing the typical aspect of SAH: spontaneous hyperdensity located in subarachnoid spaces, basal cisterns, Sylvian or interhemispheric fissures (Figure 6.13). The probability of finding this typical aspect depends on the importance of the initial bleeding and the time elapsed since haemorrhage. Indeed, subarachnoid blood will progressively be resorbed in 1 or 2 weeks depending on the initial amount of blood. Therefore, the sensitivity of CT scan will also decline over time from 98–100% in the first 12 hours, 93% at 24 hours, and 57-85% at 6 days after the bleeding (77–81). There is growing evidence in the literature that a multi-detector CT scan prescribed in less than 6 hours of symptom onset has a sensitivity and specificity of 100% for SAH detection when interpreted by a qualified neuroradiologist and performed in neurologically intact adults with a new acute headache (worst headache ever) peaking in intensity within 1 hour of onset (82, 83). This underlines the imperious need for a prompt clinical diagnosis. In patients presenting late to the emergency department or with delayed diagnosis, attention should be paid to the presence of blood deposits (hyperdensities) at the convexity (to be distinguished from true c-SAH), the posterior areas of the brain as the parieto-occipital sulci or the occipital horns of the lateral ventricles.

In cases of multiple aneurysms (15–30% of cases), the location of blood on the CT scan is very important to determine which aneurysm has bled (Table 6.3) (20). When initial loss of consciousness has been responsible for a head trauma, it is not always easy to differentiate spontaneous from traumatic SAH, especially if the patient is unresponsive. Conversely, patients may have an accident while bicycling or driving at the time of SAH onset and might be quoted as traumatic SAH rather than spontaneous. Other radiological aspects consistent with a trauma will be sought like sub-galeal haematoma, contrecoup contusions, or subdural bleeds along the falx or the cerebellar tentorium. Usually SAH in this context concentrates at the convexity of the brain and rarely in the cisterns or the Sylvian fissure. If any doubt persists, CTA should be performed.

CT scan results are used to establish the radiological grade according to the Fischer grading scale (Table 6.2) depending on the amount and location of blood after the initial bleeding (84). This grading scale is correlated with clinical severity at admission, risk of vasospasm or delayed cerebral ischaemia, and long-term outcome.

CT scan is also useful to detect early complications associated with SAH: mass effect due to intraparenchymal haemorrhage, intraventricular haemorrhage, acute hydrocephalus and global early vasogenic oedema, or ischaemia.

MRI

MRI is not routinely performed for the diagnosis of SAH but some sequences might be useful when blood is distributed along the skull base or when CT scan is negative, particularly in patients with delayed management. Fluid attenuated inversion recovery (FLAIR) images are very sensitive (Figure 6.14A), at the acute stage, for the detection of subarachnoid blood (hyperintense signal), even when the initial bleed was minimal (85). Gradient echo T2* sequences are also effective, at the subacute or chronic stage, for the diagnosis of haemosiderin deposits (hypointense signal) in subarachnoid spaces several days after the bleeding (Figure 6.14). This is very important when the question arises whether an aneurysm has bled or not, and when the clinical history is old, unclear or non-contributive.

Table 6.3 Suspected location of a ruptured aneurysm according to the pattern of SAH

Location of SAH	Location of the ruptured aneurysm
Anterior interhemispheric fissure	Anterior cerebral artery or anterior communicating artery
Pericallosal cistern	Distal anterior cerebral artery
Sylvian fissure	Middle cerebral artery
Pericarotid cistern	Ophthalmic artery, posterior communicating artery, or carotid artery termination
Interpeduncular cistern	Basilar artery termination or superior cerebellar artery
Bulbar or cerebello-bulbar cisterns	Posterior inferior cerebellar artery or vertebrobasilar junction
Diffuse supratentorial	Anterior communicating artery
Diffuse infratentorial	Basilar artery termination

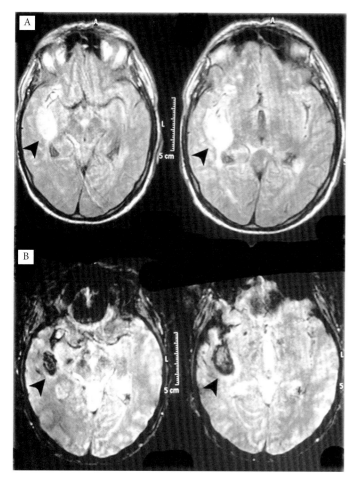

Fig. 6.14 Right Sylvian subarachnoid haemorrhage diagnosed on brain MRI (arrow). (A) FLAIR sequence. (B) Gradient echo T2* sequence (note the presence of blood deposits in the occipital horns).

In patients presenting with a focal neurological deficit and the absence of a parenchymal haematoma, diffusion and/or perfusion sequences will show areas of infarctions or reduced perfusion related to severe vasospasm with delayed cerebral ischaemia.

Lumbar puncture: indication, value, and interpretation

As mentioned earlier, the possibility of diagnosing SAH on LP within the first 6 hours of symptom onset (in neurologically intact adults) after a normal CT scan (interpreted by a qualified neuroradiologist) might be considered very unlikely. According to these results many centres have now changed their practice and do not require LP after a normal CT scan if performed in these conditions and in this time frame (86). In all other situations (i.e. delayed diagnosis, abnormal examination, inexperienced radiologist, low CT scan quality) and if the diagnosis of SAH is suspected despite a negative head CT scan (7% of SAH patients), it is recommended to perform an LP (87). One should note that even in this subgroup of patients the probability of having SAH from a ruptured aneurysm is also very low (1–2%) (5, 77, 88, 89).

When the LP is delayed after SAH onset, CSF samples could be rosy or xanthochromic, which makes the positive diagnosis paradoxically easier. In acute setting, a positive LP is usually defined by successive haemorrhagic CSF samples, not clearing over time and not coagulating in the different tubes (at least three). This presentation of the 'three-tube test' is classical when the LP is done soon after SAH occurrence, but sometimes unreliable. Indeed, it is not always simple to differentiate a true-positive tap from a traumatic one. This led some authors to propose other diagnostic criteria based on the red blood cell count or intensity of xanthochromia (attributable to haemoglobin oxidation products that appear several hours after the headache onset). A CSF tap is usually considered positive when red blood cells count is higher than 5×10^6/L in the third or fourth tube (90), or when visible xanthochromia is identified by direct visual inspection of the centrifuged sample on a background of white paper under full spectrum light (sensitivity 50–93%, specificity 95–97%) (91). The sensitivity of xanthochromia has been reported to be better after 12 hours following the ictus (100%) (92). Although this would argue for delaying the LP, it would also hinder the diagnosis and treatment of real aneurismal SAH patients. Some authors have advocated the use of spectrophotometry for the detection of xanthochromia because of its high sensitivity (100%) but this technique has been found to have a relatively low specificity (29–83% depending of the technique), which might result in an increased number of CTA or conventional DSA rate and a higher detection of incidental (silent) aneurysms. This, in return, would make the management decision-making process more difficult and could lead to treat benign lesions more frequently (69). A normal head CT scan together with a normal LP rule out the diagnosis of SAH and other causes of thunderclap headaches should be searched for (i.e. with MRI).

Diagnosis of the cause of subarachnoid haemorrhage
Cerebral CTA

SAH and ruptured intracranial aneurysms have traditionally been assessed using DSA, and this has remained the gold standard for this purpose. Nevertheless, recent advances in non-invasive imaging technologies have raised the possibility of replacing DSA in order to optimize access to the diagnostic modality, to reduce patient discomfort and the risks associated with this technique: groin haematoma (4%), transitory neurological symptoms (0.7–2%), and possible permanent neurological deficits (0.14–0.5%), particularly in elderly patients for which atherosclerotic arterial changes may limit vascular access and impose a higher risk of embolic events (93–95). Multidetector CT angiography (MDCTA) is now a widely accessible and quickly available alternative. It enables the acquisition of thin overlapping images in a short scanning time thus increasing the spatial resolution of two-dimensional (2D) source images and three-dimensional (3D) reconstructions obtained with the maximum intensity projection technique (MIP) and volume rendering technique (VRT) (Figure 6.15) and allows the recognition of very small structures (voxel dimension obtained with 64-MDCTA: 0.30 mm^3) (96). Interpretation of images should be preferentially done on native images or MIP reconstructions. Because of its qualities, MDCTA is now used worldwide by cerebrovascular teams as the first-line imaging method for the diagnosis and treatment planning of SAH and ruptured intracranial aneurysms. Reported sensitivity for aneurysm detection varies from 84–92% for less than 5 mm and from 96–100% for greater than

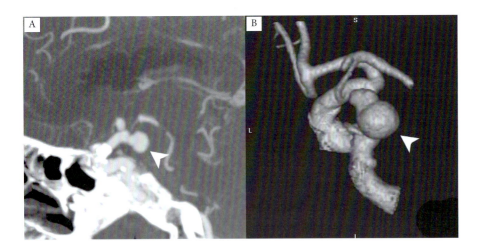

Fig. 6.15 Left posterior carotid aneurysm (arrowhead) diagnosed with cerebral CTA. (A) MIP technique. (B) VRT technique.

5 mm (42, 97–104), and is also dependent on aneurysm location (bony artefacts close to the skull base), image quality, or experience of the neuroradiologist. In the clinical setting, when the diagnostic CT scan is positive for SAH, CTA is immediately performed.

Conventional DSA

DSA is used in many centres as the gold standard for intracranial aneurysm detection (105–107). Adjunction of 3D reconstructions improves the accuracy of the radiological analysis with very high spatial resolution: neck and sac measurement, neck and sac relationships with parental artery and neighbouring branches (Figure 6.16). Three-dimensional DSA is actually perfectly adapted to the planning (neck location, road-mapping, coils placement) and the postoperative control of the endovascular treatment (108–111). This technique is also widely used for the preoperative evaluation and for the postoperative follow-up of clipped aneurysms (112–114). With the advent and improvement of CTA technique, DSA is now commonly performed after SAH diagnosis only when no aneurysm has been evidenced or if CTA was insufficient to clearly depict the angioarchitecture and to allow precise treatment decision

(5, 98, 99, 115). If SAH is typical for an aneurismal origin and the initial DSA is negative, it should be repeated about 7–10 days after the first exam to definitely rule out an underlying aneurysm, which occurs in 1–2% of initially negative cases (1). DSA remains also the most reliable technique for the analysis of other causes of SAH such as cerebral AVM, DAVF, intracranial arterial dissection, and Moyamoya disease.

MRA

Despite technical progress in the technique and its non-invasiveness, MRA has not yet become the gold standard for the management of aneurismal SAH. The anatomical definition of MRA sequences is insufficient for the accurate detection, localization, and depiction of the angioarchitecture of these lesions compared with CTA or DSA (Figure 6.17). The sensitivity of 3D time-of-flight MRA for the detection of intracranial ruptured aneurysms ranges from 55% to 93% depending on the size: the sensitivity is 85–100% and 35–56% respectively for aneurysms larger than 5 mm and smaller than 5 mm (116–122). Many ruptured aneurysms are small which makes MRA usually unsuitable in the setting of aneurismal SAH (123). Nevertheless, the technique is improving and recent studies with 3-Tesla MRI scan found similar results between CTA and MRA (124). One other limitation of the technique is its lack of spatial resolution to represent relationship between the aneurismal neck and neighbouring branches, precluding the use of the technique as the only diagnosis tool in 65% of cases (125, 126). Furthermore, the need for perfect patient compliance, the longer study time, and its sensitivity to motion artefact make the technique difficult in acutely ill SAH patients. On the contrary, when an aneurismal cause of SAH has been excluded, MRI/MRA will be the cornerstone of the diagnosis and management (i.e. intracranial dissection or cerebral venous thrombosis).

Acute complications of subarachnoid haemorrhage

Vegetative disorders and neuroendocrine effects

Medical complications are responsible for 23% of the deaths of SAH patients (127). At the time of aneurysm rupture, a systemic catecholaminergic burst could be responsible for cardiac complications due to left ventricular dysfunction. This neurogenic stress cardiomyopathy

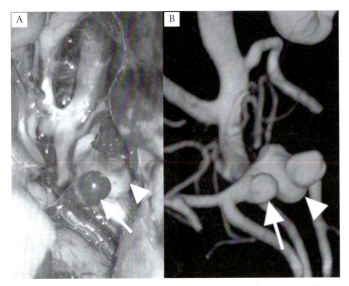

Fig. 6.16 Left ruptured middle cerebral artery aneurysms: (A) diagnosed with cerebral angiography, (B) 3D-DSA.

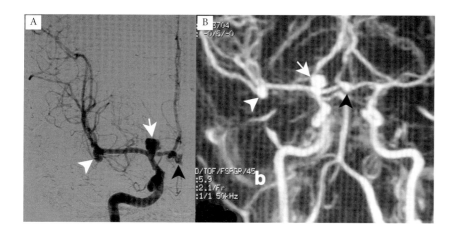

Fig. 6.17 Conventional angiography (A) and MRA (B) showing multiple intracranial aneurysms: middle cerebral artery (white arrowhead), carotid artery termination (white arrow), and anterior communicating artery (black arrowhead).

(128), also referred to in the literature as neurogenic stunned myocardium or Takotsubo syndrome, could associate a decrease in the ejection fraction, aspects of linear myocardial infarction, electrocardiogram abnormalities (ST depression), and troponin elevation. Cardiac arrhythmia occurs in 30% of the cases and is severe in 5%. Neurogenic pulmonary oedema occurs in 23% of the cases and is life threatening in 6% with a maximum incidence between days 3 and 7. It is due to left ventricular dysfunction and to alveolocapillary membrane alterations. Some degree of hepatic dysfunction was noted in 24% of patients with moderate elevation of hepatic enzymes and was severe in only 4% of the cases. Thrombocytopenia and renal failure were encountered in 4% and 7% of cases and were respectively mostly related to sepsis or antibiotic use (127).

Hydroelectrolytic balance disorders can also be encountered and preferentially affect sodium regulation. The reported incidence of hyponatraemia after SAH ranges from 10–30%. It is the consequence of a cerebral salt wasting syndrome or of a syndrome of inappropriate antidiuretic hormone secretion. Hyponatraemia is more common in patients with poor clinical grade, anterior communication artery aneurysms, and hydrocephalus, and may be an independent risk factor for poor outcome (1).

Acute hydrocephalus

Acute hydrocephalus is present at admission in 20–40% of patients (Figure 6.18). It can also appear in the first hours after SAH diagnosis and is often announced by a progressive decrease of consciousness sometimes preceded by a state of agitation or confusion and accompanied by signs of intracranial hypertension (increased headache and blood pressure, then alteration of pupils' responsiveness to light). It is mainly due to CSF blockage on ventricular pathways (53% of SAH patients with intraventricular haemorrhage at admission) or by thick collections of blood in the subarachnoid cisterns and/or occlusion of CSF absorption sites (1, 6). It is often associated with a poor clinical grade at admission (1) and requires, in most cases, the emergent placement of an external ventricular drain to release the intracranial hypertension, which results in patient improvement in more than half of these cases (1). Nevertheless, acute hydrocephalus remains a factor of worst final prognosis in one-third of these patients (8).

Intracerebral and subdural haematoma

The presence of a focal neurological deficit with a SAH clinical presentation could reveal an intraparenchymal bleed (Figure 6.19).

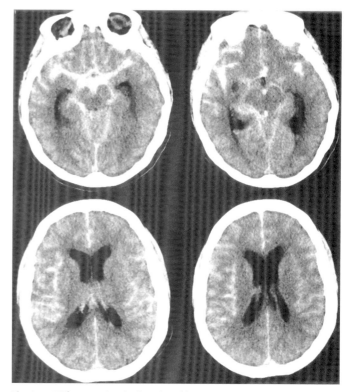

Fig. 6.18 Diffuse aneurismal subarachnoid haemorrhage complicated by acute hydrocephalus.

Intracranial aneurysms might be partially embedded in the brain parenchyma. If the intraparenchymal surface involves the weakest part of the aneurysm wall, the rupture at this site could lead to intracerebral haemorrhage, which is present at admission in 17–30% of patients with aneurysm rupture (5, 6). Pure intracerebral haemorrhage is rare after aneurysm rupture and might be mistaken with other causes of non-aneurysmal haemorrhage. This diagnosis should be considered with haematomas in the vicinity of the interhemispheric fissure (anterior communicating aneurysms), the Sylvian fissure (middle cerebral artery aneurysms), and the anterior perforated substance (carotid termination aneurysms). Acute subdural haematoma is also an infrequent mode of presentation of aneurysm rupture but could be associated with posterior carotid aneurysms.

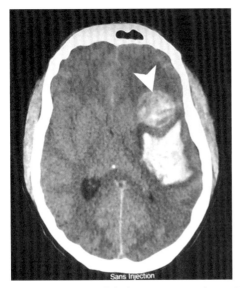

Fig. 6.19 Left compressive temporal lobe haematoma secondary to the rupture of a giant thrombosed middle cerebral aneurysm (arrowhead).

Early rebleeding

Rebleeding usually presents with a new episode of sudden headache and often followed by a degradation of the patient's neurological status or consciousness. The risk of re-rupture is at the highest level the first day after aneurismal SAH onset (4–16%) and occurs in most of the cases during the first 12 hours (5, 129). It is often preceded by increased blood pressure (>150 mmHg) (1, 8, 130, 131). The risk is then about 1–2% per day the following month (30% at 1 month) and 3% the subsequent years (1). It is commonly associated with more severe complications, worst clinical prognosis (1.5-fold increase in any disability, 78% with poor outcome) or survival (global mortality about 60–70%, out-hospital death in 15 to 50% of cases, fourfold increase in in-hospital mortality) and decreased quality of life (1, 6, 8, 129).

Seizure

Generalized seizures usually occur within the first hours after SAH onset in 6–18% of cases. They are more frequent with anterior circulation aneurysms rupture and when parenchymal haemorrhage is associated. Most of seizures occurred at onset and in-hospital seizures were rare (4%) (1, 132).

Global cerebral ischaemia and early death

The sudden eruption of blood in the subarachnoid spaces causes a severe raise in intracranial pressure and decrease in cerebral perfusion pressure, leading sometimes to cerebral circulatory arrest when bleeding has been massive. This initiates a cascade of pathophysiological processes responsible for loss of cerebrovascular autoregulation, acute vasospasm, microvascular platelets activation, blood–brain barrier alteration, and increased permeability leading to acute vasogenic oedema or ischaemia (133). Global cerebral oedema is present in 16% of patients at admission (6). Early focal or diffuse cerebral ischaemia could be the final stage of this evolution resulting in sudden or rapid death that accounts for 3–12% of SAH patients (8, 134).

Secondary complications of subarachnoid haemorrhage

Cranial nerve deficits

Cranial nerve deficits after SAH mainly affect the oculomotor nerves (135, 136). This occurs in about 9% of SAHs. The high incidence of third nerve involvement (80%) is due to its close relationship with posterior carotid aneurysms. At the time of rupture, the nerve is injured either by the blood jet or by direct compression from the aneurysm sac or surrounding clots. The abducens nerve is less frequently affected (37.5%). Its pathophysiological implication is mostly related to raised intracranial pressure following SAH and diffuse suffering of the nerve along its cisternal course. Bilateral sixth nerve palsies are not infrequent in this context. Oculomotor nerve palsies recover usually in 3–6 months and complete recovery is observed more frequently for the abducens than the oculomotor nerve (50% of cases) and more often after surgical clipping than endovascular coiling (137).

Vasospasm and delayed cerebral ischaemia

Vasospasm is a very frequent complication of SAH, angiographically diagnosed in 30–70% of patients and maximal between days 5 and 14 (1). It is related to main and small cerebral arteries' delayed vasoconstriction/thrombosis initiated by the initial insult due to aneurysm rupture followed by the inflammatory response to blood degradation products. Local inflammation is believed to modify the size of large vessels but also to impact microvascular circulation through the overexpression of inflammatory adhesion molecules or endothelial cell activation factors leading to the concentration of inflammatory cells and molecules, vessel wall changes, thrombosis, and eventually delayed cerebral ischaemia (138).

Vasospasm becomes symptomatic in half of the cases depending on the importance of the initial bleed: it is twice as important in Fisher grade 4 than Fisher grade 1 patients. Early vasospasm at angiographic or transcranial Doppler, history of arterial hypertension, poor neurological grade, and elevated admission mean arterial pressure were identified as risk factors for symptomatic vasospasm (84, 139). Delayed cerebral ischaemia occurs in 15–20% of these cases (Figure 6.20), which results in neurological deficit or death and is associated with poor outcome in 42% of patients (1, 8).

Symptomatic vasospasm might be announced by an increased severity of headaches, a new-onset neurological deficit, confusion or decreased level of consciousness, moderate hyperthermia (38.5°C), or elevation of mean arterial pressure, and this in the absence of hydrocephalus or rebleeding documented by an emergent head CT scan. In high-grade patients, every change in clinical state, even minimal, should lead one to consider the diagnosis.

Subacute and chronic hydrocephalus

Subacute or chronic hydrocephalus is encountered in 19–26% of SAH patients (1, 140). Increased intracranial pressure might be evidenced in those patients and the term 'normal pressure hydrocephalus' might be inappropriate in some cases. It is accompanied by signs of progressive and chronic intracranial hypertension, cognitive decline, or walking/gait disturbance. It can develop within a few weeks or later after the bleeding. Most of the time, it is detected during the hospital stay by follow-up head CT scans. When repeated depletive lumbar punctures are ineffective, a definitive

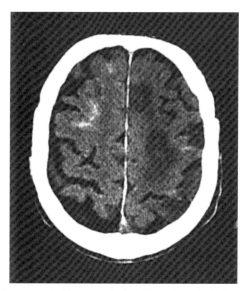

Fig. 6.20 Delayed cerebral ischaemia in the left anterior and middle cerebral artery territories.

shunt (ventriculoperitoneal, ventriculoatrial) is usually inserted. The risk factors for the need of permanent CSF diversion are the presence of acute hydrocephalus, intraventricular haemorrhage, and older age at admission (1, 140).

References

1. Bederson JB, Connolly ES, Jr, Batjer HH, Dacey RG, Dion JE, Diringer MN, *et al.* Guidelines for the management of aneurysmal subarachnoid hemorrhage: a statement for healthcare professionals from a special writing group of the Stroke Council, American Heart Association. *Stroke.* 2009 Mar;40(3):994–1025.

2. Wermer MJ, van dSI, Algra A, Rinkel GJ. Risk of rupture of unruptured intracranial aneurysms in relation to patient and aneurysm characteristics: an updated meta-analysis. *Stroke.* 2007;38(4):1404–1410.

3. Feigin VL, Lawes CM, Bennett DA, Anderson CS. Stroke epidemiology: a review of population-based studies of incidence, prevalence, and case-fatality in the late 20th century. *Lancet Neurol.* 2003 Jan;2(1):43–53.

4. Johnston SC, Selvin S, Gress DR. The burden, trends, and demographics of mortality from subarachnoid hemorrhage. *Neurology.* 1998 May;50(5):1413–1418.

5. van Gijn J, Rinkel GJ. Subarachnoid haemorrhage: diagnosis, causes and management. *Brain.* 2001;124(Pt 2):249–278.

6. Kowalski RG, Claassen J, Kreiter KT, Bates JE, Ostapkovich ND, Connolly ES, *et al.* Initial misdiagnosis and outcome after subarachnoid hemorrhage. *JAMA.* 2004 Feb 18;291(7):866–869.

7. de Rooij NK, Linn FH, van der Plas JA, Algra A, Rinkel GJ. Incidence of subarachnoid haemorrhage: a systematic review with emphasis on region, age, gender and time trends. *J Neurol Neurosurg Psychiatry.* 2007 Dec;78(12):1365–1372.

8. Roos YB, de Haan RJ, Beenen LF, Groen RJ, Albrecht KW, Vermeulen M. Complications and outcome in patients with aneurysmal subarachnoid haemorrhage: a prospective hospital based cohort study in the Netherlands. *J Neurol Neurosurg Psychiatry.* 2000 Mar;68(3):337–341.

9. Epidemiology of aneurysmal subarachnoid hemorrhage in Australia and New Zealand: incidence and case fatality from the Australasian Cooperative Research on Subarachnoid Hemorrhage Study (ACROSS). *Stroke.* 2000 Aug;31(8):1843–1850.

10. Linn FH, Rinkel GJ, Algra A, van Gijn J. Headache characteristics in subarachnoid haemorrhage and benign thunderclap headache. *J Neurol Neurosurg Psychiatry.* 1998 Nov;65(5):791–793.

11. Molyneux A, Kerr R, Stratton I, Sandercock P, Clarke M, Shrimpton J, *et al.* International Subarachnoid Aneurysm Trial (ISAT) of neurosurgical clipping versus endovascular coiling in 2143 patients with ruptured intracranial aneurysms: a randomised trial. *Lancet.* 2002 Oct 26;360(9342):1267–1274.

12. Qureshi AI, Suri MF, Nasar A, Kirmani JF, Divani AA, He W, *et al.* Trends in hospitalization and mortality for subarachnoid hemorrhage and unruptured aneurysms in the United States. *Neurosurgery.* 2005 Jul;57(1):1–8; discussion 1–8.

13. Feigin VL, Rinkel GJ, Lawes CM, Algra A, Bennett DA, van Gijn J, *et al.* Risk factors for subarachnoid hemorrhage: an updated systematic review of epidemiological studies. *Stroke.* 2005 Dec;36(12):2773–2780.

14. Kissela BM, Sauerbeck L, Woo D, Khoury J, Carrozzella J, Pancioli A, *et al.* Subarachnoid hemorrhage: a preventable disease with a heritable component. *Stroke.* 2002 May;33(5):1321–1326.

15. Ingall T, Asplund K, Mahonen M, Bonita R. A multinational comparison of subarachnoid hemorrhage epidemiology in the WHO MONICA stroke study. *Stroke.* 2000 May;31(5):1054–1061.

16. Ingall TJ, Whisnant JP, Wiebers DO, O'Fallon WM. Has there been a decline in subarachnoid hemorrhage mortality? *Stroke.* 1989 Jun;20(6):718–724.

17. Weir BK, Kongable GL, Kassell NF, Schultz JR, Truskowski LL, Sigrest A. Cigarette smoking as a cause of aneurysmal subarachnoid hemorrhage and risk for vasospasm: a report of the Cooperative Aneurysm Study. *J Neurosurg.* 1998;89(3):405–411.

18. Gaetani P, Tartara F, Tancioni F, Klersy C, Forlino A, Baena RR. Activity of alpha 1-antitrypsin and cigarette smoking in subarachnoid haemorrhage from ruptured aneurysm. *J Neurol Sci.* 1996 Sep 15;141(1-2):33–38.

19. Teunissen LL, Rinkel GJ, Algra A, van Gijn J. Risk factors for subarachnoid hemorrhage: a systematic review. *Stroke.* 1996 Mar;27(3):544–549.

20. Qureshi AI, Suarez JI, Parekh PD, Sung G, Geocadin R, Bhardwaj A, *et al.* Risk factors for multiple intracranial aneurysms. *Neurosurgery.* 1998;43(1):22–26.

21. Klag MJ, Whelton PK, Seidler AJ. Decline in US stroke mortality. Demographic trends and antihypertensive treatment. *Stroke.* 1989 Jan;20(1):14–21.

22. Khurana VG, Meissner I, Meyer FB. Update on genetic evidence for rupture-prone compared with rupture-resistant intracranial saccular aneurysms. *Neurosurg Focus.* 2004 Nov 15;17(5):E7.

23. Ruigrok YM, Rinkel GJ, Wijmenga C. Genetics of intracranial aneurysms. *Lancet Neurol.* 2005 Mar;4(3):179–189.

24. Li L, Yang X, Jiang F, Dusting GJ, Wu Z. Transcriptome-wide characterization of gene expression associated with unruptured intracranial aneurysms. *Eur Neurol.* 2009;62(6):330–337.

25. Hofer A, Hermans M, Kubassek N, Sitzer M, Funke H, Stogbauer F, *et al.* Elastin polymorphism haplotype and intracranial aneurysms are not associated in Central Europe. *Stroke.* 2003;34(5):1207–1211.

26. Pera J, Korostynski M, Krzyszkowski T, Czopek J, Slowik A, Dziedzic T, *et al.* Gene expression profiles in human ruptured and unruptured intracranial aneurysms: what is the role of inflammation? *Stroke.* 2010 Feb;41(2):224–231.

27. Wang MC, Rubinstein D, Kindt GW, Breeze RE. Prevalence of intracranial aneurysms in first-degree relatives of patients with aneurysms. *Neurosurg Focus.* 2002;13(3):e2.

28. Foroud T, Sauerbeck L, Brown R, Anderson C, Woo D, Kleindorfer D, *et al.* Genome screen in familial intracranial aneurysm. *BMC Med Genet.* 2009;10:3.

29. Ruigrok YM, Rinkel GJ. Genetics of intracranial aneurysms. *Stroke.* 2008 Mar;39(3):1049–1055.

30. Krischek B, Inoue I. The genetics of intracranial aneurysms. *J Hum Genet.* 2006;51(7):587–594.

31. Verlaan DJ, Dube MP, St-Onge J, Noreau A, Roussel J, Satge N, *et al.* A new locus for autosomal dominant intracranial aneurysm, ANIB4, maps to chromosome 5p15.2-14.3. *J Med Genet.* 2006 Jun;43(6):e31.

32. Raaymakers TW. Aneurysms in relatives of patients with subarachnoid hemorrhage: frequency and risk factors. MARS Study Group. Magnetic

Resonance Angiography in Relatives of patients with Subarachnoid hemorrhage. *Neurology*. 1999;53(5):982–988.

33. Ruigrok YM, Rinkel GJ, Wijmenga C, Van Gijn J. Anticipation and phenotype in familial intracranial aneurysms. *J Neurol Neurosurg Psychiatry*. 2004 Oct;75(10):1436–1442.

34. Wills S, Ronkainen A, van der Voet M, Kuivaniemi H, Helin K, Leinonen E, *et al*. Familial intracranial aneurysms: an analysis of 346 multiplex Finnish families. *Stroke*. 2003 Jun;34(6):1370–1374.

35. Broderick JP, Brown RD, Jr, Sauerbeck L, Hornung R, Huston J, 3rd, Woo D, *et al*. Greater rupture risk for familial as compared to sporadic unruptured intracranial aneurysms. *Stroke*. 2009 Jun;40(6): 1952–1957.

36. Lee JS, Park IS, Park KB, Kang DH, Lee CH, Hwang SH. Familial intracranial aneurysms. *J Korean Neurosurg Soc*. 2008 Sep;44(3):136–140.

37. Brown BM, Soldevilla F. MR angiography and surgery for unruptured familial intracranial aneurysms in persons with a family history of cerebral aneurysms. *AJR Am J Roentgenol*. 1999;173(1):133–138.

38. Connolly ES, Jr, Choudhri TF, Mack WJ, Mocco J, Spinks TJ, Slosberg J, *et al*. Influence of smoking, hypertension, and sex on the phenotypic expression of familial intracranial aneurysms in siblings. *Neurosurgery*. 2001 Jan;48(1):64–68; discussion 8–9.

39. Ring T, Spiegelhalter D. Risk of intracranial aneurysm bleeding in autosomal-dominant polycystic kidney disease. *Kidney Int*. 2007;72(11):1400–1402.

40. Rossetti S, Chauveau D, Kubly V, Slezak JM, Saggar-Malik AK, Pei Y, *et al*. Association of mutation position in polycystic kidney disease 1 (PKD1) gene and development of a vascular phenotype. *Lancet*. 2003;361(9376):2196–2201.

41. Torres VE, Cai Y, Chen X, Wu GQ, Geng L, Cleghorn KA, *et al*. Vascular expression of polycystin-2. *J Am Soc Nephrol*. 2001;12(1):1–9.

42. Agid R, Lee SK, Willinsky RA, Farb RI, terBrugge KG. Acute subarachnoid hemorrhage: using 64-slice multidetector CT angiography to "triage" patients' treatment. *Neuroradiology*. 2006;48(11): 787–794.

43. Flaherty ML, Haverbusch M, Kissela B, Kleindorfer D, Schneider A, Sekar P, *et al*. Perimesencephalic subarachnoid hemorrhage: incidence, risk factors, and outcome. *J Stroke Cerebrovasc Dis*. 2005 Nov-Dec;14(6):267–271.

44. da Costa L, Wallace MC, Ter Brugge KG, O'Kelly C, Willinsky RA, Tymianski M. The natural history and predictive features of hemorrhage from brain arteriovenous malformations. *Stroke*. 2009 Jan;40(1):100–105.

45. Valencia A, Morales H, Rivera R, Bravo E, Galvez M. Blood flow dynamics in patient-specific cerebral aneurysm models: the relationship between wall shear stress and aneurysm area index. *Med Eng Phys*. 2008 Apr;30(3):329–340.

46. Tateshima S, Murayama Y, Villablanca JP, Morino T, Nomura K, Tanishita K, *et al*. In vitro measurement of fluid-induced wall shear stress in unruptured cerebral aneurysms harboring blebs. *Stroke*. 2003;34(1):187–192.

47. Rinkel GJ, Wijdicks EF, Hasan D, Kienstra GE, Franke CL, Hageman LM, *et al*. Outcome in patients with subarachnoid haemorrhage and negative angiography according to pattern of haemorrhage on computed tomography. *Lancet*. 1991 Oct 19;338(8773):964–968.

48. van der Schaaf IC, Velthuis BK, Gouw A, Rinkel GJ. Venous drainage in perimesencephalic hemorrhage. *Stroke*. 2004 Jul;35(7):1614–1618.

49. Beitzke M, Gattringer T, Enzinger C, Wagner G, Niederkorn K, Fazekas F. Clinical presentation, etiology, and long-term prognosis in patients with nontraumatic convexal subarachnoid hemorrhage. *Stroke*. Nov;42(11):3055–3060.

50. Raposo N, Viguier A, Cuvinciuc V, Calviere L, Cognard C, Bonneville F, *et al*. Cortical subarachnoid haemorrhage in the elderly: a recurrent event probably related to cerebral amyloid angiopathy. *Eur J Neurol*. Apr;18(4):597–603.

51. Linn J, Halpin A, Demaerel P, Ruhland J, Giese AD, Dichgans M, *et al*. Prevalence of superficial siderosis in patients with cerebral amyloid angiopathy. *Neurology*. Apr 27;74(17):1346–1350.

52. Linn J, Wollenweber FA, Lummel N, Bochmann K, Pfefferkorn T, Gschwendtner A, *et al*. Superficial siderosis is a warning sign for future intracranial hemorrhage. *J Neurol*. Jan;260(1):176–181.

53. Charidimou A, Baron JC, Werring DJ. Transient focal neurological episodes, cerebral amyloid angiopathy, and intracerebral hemorrhage risk: looking beyond TIAs. *Int J Stroke*. Feb;8(2):105–108.

54. Choi JH, Mast H, Sciacca RR, Hartmann A, Khaw AV, Mohr JP, *et al*. Clinical outcome after first and recurrent hemorrhage in patients with untreated brain arteriovenous malformation. *Stroke*. 2006 May;37(5):1243–1247.

55. Chappell PM, Steinberg GK, Marks MP. Clinically documented hemorrhage in cerebral arteriovenous malformations: MR characteristics. *Radiology*. 1992 Jun;183(3):719–724.

56. Al-Shahi R, Warlow C. A systematic review of the frequency and prognosis of arteriovenous malformations of the brain in adults. *Brain*. 2001 Oct;124(Pt 10):1900–1926.

57. Mast H, Young WL, Koennecke HC, Sciacca RR, Osipov A, Pile-Spellman J, *et al*. Risk of spontaneous haemorrhage after diagnosis of cerebral arteriovenous malformation. *Lancet*. 1997 Oct 11;350(9084):1065–1068.

58. van Dijk JM, terBrugge KG, Willinsky RA, Wallace MC. Clinical course of cranial dural arteriovenous fistulas with long-term persistent cortical venous reflux. *Stroke*. 2002 May;33(5):1233–1236.

59. Sarma D, ter Brugge K. Management of intracranial dural arteriovenous shunts in adults. *Eur J Radiol*. 2003 Jun;46(3):206–220.

60. da Costa L, Dehdashti AR, terBrugge KG. Spinal cord vascular shunts: spinal cord vascular malformations and dural arteriovenous fistulas. *Neurosurg Focus*. 2009 Jan;26(1):E6.

61. Kai Y, Hamada J, Morioka M, Yano S, Mizuno T, Kuratsu J. Arteriovenous fistulas at the cervicomedullary junction presenting with subarachnoid hemorrhage: six case reports with special reference to the angiographic pattern of venous drainage. *AJNR Am J Neuroradiol*. 2005 Sep;26(8):1949–1954.

62. Thines L, Zairi F, Taschner C, Leclerc X, Lucas C, Bourgeois P, *et al*. Subarachnoid hemorrhage from spontaneous dissection of the anterior cerebral artery. *Cerebrovasc Dis*. 2006;22(5-6):452–456.

63. Al-Shahi Salman R, Berg MJ, Morrison L, Awad IA. Hemorrhage from cavernous malformations of the brain: definition and reporting standards. Angioma Alliance Scientific Advisory Board. *Stroke*. 2008 Dec;39(12):3222–3230.

64. Kuroda S, Houkin K. Moyamoya disease: current concepts and future perspectives. *Lancet Neurol*. 2008 Nov;7(11):1056–1066.

65. Carey J, Numaguchi Y, Nadell J. Subarachnoid hemorrhage in sickle cell disease. *Childs Nerv Syst*. 1990 Jan;6(1):47–50.

66. Aggarwal SK, Williams V, Levine SR, Cassin BJ, Garcia JH. Cocaine-associated intracranial hemorrhage: absence of vasculitis in 14 cases. *Neurology*. 1996 Jun;46(6):1741–1743.

67. Levine SR, Brust JC, Futrell N, Ho KL, Blake D, Millikan CH, *et al*. Cerebrovascular complications of the use of the "crack" form of alkaloidal cocaine. *N Engl J Med*. 1990 Sep 13;323(11):699–704.

68. Mattle H, Kohler S, Huber P, Rohner M, Steinsiepe KF. Anticoagulation-related intracranial extracerebral haemorrhage. *J Neurol Neurosurg Psychiatry*. 1989 Jul;52(7):829–837.

69. Perry JJ, Sivilotti ML, Stiell IG, Wells GA, Raymond J, Mortensen M, *et al*. Should spectrophotometry be used to identify xanthochromia in the cerebrospinal fluid of alert patients suspected of having subarachnoid hemorrhage? *Stroke*. 2006 Oct;37(10):2467–2472.

70. Ramirez-Lassepas M, Espinosa CE, Cicero JJ, Johnston KL, Cipolle RJ, Barber DL. Predictors of intracranial pathologic findings in patients who seek emergency care because of headache. *Arch Neurol*. 1997 Dec;54(12):1506–1509.

71. Vermeulen M, van Gijn J. The diagnosis of subarachnoid haemorrhage. *J Neurol Neurosurg Psychiatry*. 1990 May;53(5):365–372.

72. Vermeulen MJ, Schull MJ. Missed diagnosis of subarachnoid hemorrhage in the emergency department. *Stroke*. 2007 Apr;38(4):1216–1221.

73. Ducros A. Reversible cerebral vasoconstriction syndrome. *Lancet Neurol*. Oct;11(10):906–917.

74. Gambhir S, O'Grady G, Koelmeyer T. Clinical lessons and risk factors from 403 fatal cases of subarachnoid haemorrhage. *J Clin Neurosci.* 2009 Jul;16(7):921–924.

75. McCarron MO, Alberts MJ, McCarron P. A systematic review of Terson's syndrome: frequency and prognosis after subarachnoid haemorrhage. *J Neurol Neurosurg Psychiatry.* 2004 Mar;75(3):491–493.

76. Hutchinson PJ, Power DM, Tripathi P, Kirkpatrick PJ. Outcome from poor grade aneurysmal subarachnoid haemorrhage—which poor grade subarachnoid haemorrhage patients benefit from aneurysm clipping? *Br J Neurosurg.* 2000;14(2):105–109.

77. Morgenstern LB, Luna-Gonzales H, Huber JC, Jr, Wong SS, Uthman MO, Gurian JH, *et al.* Worst headache and subarachnoid hemorrhage: prospective, modern computed tomography and spinal fluid analysis. *Ann Emerg Med.* 1998 Sep;32(3 Pt 1):297–304.

78. van der Wee N, Rinkel GJ, Hasan D, van Gijn J. Detection of subarachnoid haemorrhage on early CT: is lumbar puncture still needed after a negative scan? *J Neurol Neurosurg Psychiatry.* 1995 Mar;58(3):357–359.

79. Sidman R, Connolly E, Lemke T. Subarachnoid hemorrhage diagnosis: lumbar puncture is still needed when the computed tomography scan is normal. *Acad Emerg Med.* 1996 Sep;3(9):827–831.

80. Sames TA, Storrow AB, Finkelstein JA, Magoon MR. Sensitivity of new-generation computed tomography in subarachnoid hemorrhage. *Acad Emerg Med.* 1996 Jan;3(1):16–20.

81. van Gijn J, van Dongen KJ. The time course of aneurysmal haemorrhage on computed tomograms. *Neuroradiology.* 1982;23(3):153–156.

82. Cortnum S, Sorensen P, Jorgensen J. Determining the sensitivity of computed tomography scanning in early detection of subarachnoid hemorrhage. *Neurosurgery.* May;66(5):900–902; discussion 903.

83. Perry JJ, Stiell IG, Sivilotti ML, Bullard MJ, Emond M, Symington C, *et al.* Sensitivity of computed tomography performed within six hours of onset of headache for diagnosis of subarachnoid haemorrhage: prospective cohort study. *BMJ.* 343:d4277.

84. Frontera JA, Claassen J, Schmidt JM, Wartenberg KE, Temes R, Connolly ES, Jr, *et al.* Prediction of symptomatic vasospasm after subarachnoid hemorrhage: the modified fisher scale. *Neurosurgery.* 2006;59(1):21–27.

85. Noguchi K, Ogawa T, Seto H, Inugami A, Hadeishi H, Fujita H, *et al.* Subacute and chronic subarachnoid hemorrhage: diagnosis with fluid-attenuated inversion-recovery MR imaging. *Radiology.* 1997 Apr;203(1):257–262.

86. Edlow JA, Fisher J. Diagnosis of subarachnoid hemorrhage: time to change the guidelines? *Stroke.* Aug;43(8):2031–2032.

87. Byyny RL, Mower WR, Shum N, Gabayan GZ, Fang S, Baraff LJ. Sensitivity of noncontrast cranial computed tomography for the emergency department diagnosis of subarachnoid hemorrhage. *Ann Emerg Med.* 2008 Jun;51(6):697–703.

88. Foot C, Staib A. How valuable is a lumbar puncture in the management of patients with suspected subarachnoid haemorrhage? *Emerg Med (Fremantle).* 2001 Sep;13(3):326–332.

89. Wood MJ, Dimeski G, Nowitzke AM. CSF spectrophotometry in the diagnosis and exclusion of spontaneous subarachnoid haemorrhage. *J Clin Neurosci.* 2005 Feb;12(2):142–146.

90. MacDonald A, Mendelow AD. Xanthochromia revisited: a re-evaluation of lumbar puncture and CT scanning in the diagnosis of subarachnoid haemorrhage. *J Neurol Neurosurg Psychiatry.* 1988 Mar;51(3):342–344.

91. Dupont SA, Wijdicks EF, Manno EM, Rabinstein AA. Thunderclap headache and normal computed tomographic results: value of cerebrospinal fluid analysis. *Mayo Clin Proc.* 2008 Dec;83(12):1326–1331.

92. van Gijn J, Vermeulen M, Hasan D. Xanthochromia. *Lancet.* 1989 Oct 28;2(8670):1036.

93. Heiserman JE, Dean BL, Hodak JA, Flom RA, Bird CR, Drayer BP, *et al.* Neurologic complications of cerebral angiography. *AJNR Am J Neuroradiol.* 1994;15(8):1401–1407.

94. Kaufmann TJ, Huston J, III, Mandrekar JN, Schleck CD, Thielen KR, Kallmes DF. Complications of diagnostic cerebral angiography: evaluation of 19,826 consecutive patients. *Radiology.* 2007;243(3):812–819.

95. Willinsky RA, Taylor SM, TerBrugge K, Farb RI, Tomlinson G, Montanera W. Neurologic complications of cerebral angiography: prospective analysis of 2,899 procedures and review of the literature. *Radiology.* 2003 May;227(2):522–528.

96. Thines L, Dehdashti AR, Howard P, Da Costa L, Wallace MC, Willinsky RA, *et al.* Postoperative assessment of clipped aneurysms with 64-slice computerized tomography angiography. *Neurosurgery.* Sep;67(3):844–853; discussion 53–54.

97. Chappell ET, Moure FC, Good MC. Comparison of computed tomographic angiography with digital subtraction angiography in the diagnosis of cerebral aneurysms: a meta-analysis. *Neurosurgery.* 2003;52(3):624–631.

98. Dehdashti AR, Rufenacht DA, Delavelle J, Reverdin A, de Tribolet N. Therapeutic decision and management of aneurysmal subarachnoid haemorrhage based on computed tomographic angiography. *Br J Neurosurg.* 2003 Feb;17(1):46–53.

99. Taschner CA, Thines L, Lernout M, Lejeune JP, Leclerc X. Treatment decision in ruptured intracranial aneurysms: comparison between multi-detector row CT angiography and digital subtraction angiography. *J Neuroradiol.* 2007;34(4):243–249.

100. Tipper G, King-Im JM, Price SJ, Trivedi RA, Cross JJ, Higgins NJ, *et al.* Detection and evaluation of intracranial aneurysms with 16-row multislice CT angiography. *Clin Radiol.* 2005;60(5):565–572.

101. Pechlivanis I, Schmieder K, Scholz M, Konig M, Heuser L, Harders A. 3-Dimensional computed tomographic angiography for use of surgery planning in patients with intracranial aneurysms. *Acta Neurochir (Wien).* 2005;147(10):1045–1053.

102. Teksam M, McKinney A, Casey S, Asis M, Kieffer S, Truwit CL. Multi-section CT angiography for detection of cerebral aneurysms. *AJNR Am J Neuroradiol.* 2004;25(9):1485–1492.

103. Hoh BL, Cheung AC, Rabinov JD, Pryor JC, Carter BS, Ogilvy CS. Results of a prospective protocol of computed tomographic angiography in place of catheter angiography as the only diagnostic and pretreatment planning study for cerebral aneurysms by a combined neurovascular team. *Neurosurgery.* 2004;54(6):1329–1340.

104. Anderson GB, Steinke DE, Petruk KC, Ashforth R, Findlay JM. Computed tomographic angiography versus digital subtraction angiography for the diagnosis and early treatment of ruptured intracranial aneurysms. *Neurosurgery.* 1999;45(6):1315–1320.

105. Tu RK, Cohen WA, Maravilla KR, Bush WH, Patel NH, Eskridge J, *et al.* Digital subtraction rotational angiography for aneurysms of the intracranial anterior circulation: injection method and optimization. *AJNR Am J Neuroradiol.* 1996;17(6):1127–1136.

106. Sugahara T, Korogi Y, Nakashima K, Hamatake S, Honda S, Takahashi M. Comparison of 2D and 3D digital subtraction angiography in evaluation of intracranial aneurysms. *AJNR Am J Neuroradiol.* 2002;23(9):1545–1552.

107. Hochmuth A, Spetzger U, Schumacher M. Comparison of three-dimensional rotational angiography with digital subtraction angiography in the assessment of ruptured cerebral aneurysms. *AJNR Am J Neuroradiol.* 2002;23(7):1199–1205.

108. Missler U, Hundt C, Wiesmann M, Mayer T, Bruckmann H. Three-dimensional reconstructed rotational digital subtraction angiography in planning treatment of intracranial aneurysms. *Eur Radiol.* 2000;10(4):564–568.

109. Kiyosue H, Tanoue S, Okahara M, Hori Y, Nakamura T, Nagatomi H, *et al.* Anatomic features predictive of complete aneurysm occlusion can be determined with three-dimensional digital subtraction angiography. *AJNR Am J Neuroradiol.* 2002;23(7):1206–1213.

110. Anxionnat R, Bracard S, Ducrocq X, Trousset Y, Launay L, Kerrien E, *et al.* Intracranial aneurysms: clinical value of 3D digital subtraction angiography in the therapeutic decision and endovascular treatment. *Radiology.* 2001;218(3):799–808.

111. Abe T, Hirohata M, Tanaka N, Uchiyama Y, Kojima K, Fujimoto K, *et al.* Clinical benefits of rotational 3D angiography in endovascular

treatment of ruptured cerebral aneurysm. *AJNR Am J Neuroradiol.* 2002;23(4):686–688.

112. Tanoue S, Kiyosue H, Kenai H, Nakamura T, Yamashita M, Mori H. Three-dimensional reconstructed images after rotational angiography in the evaluation of intracranial aneurysms: surgical correlation. *Neurosurgery.* 2000;47(4):866–871.

113. Kang HS, Han MH, Kwon BJ, Jung SI, Oh CW, Han DH, *et al.* Postoperative 3D angiography in intracranial aneurysms. *AJNR Am J Neuroradiol.* 2004;25(9):1463–1469.

114. Raabe A, Beck J, Rohde S, Berkefeld J, Seifert V. Three-dimensional rotational angiography guidance for aneurysm surgery. *J Neurosurg.* 2006;105(3):406–411.

115. Hashimoto Y, Kin S, Haraguchi K, Niwa J. Pitfalls in the preoperative evaluation of subarachnoid hemorrhage without digital subtraction angiography: report on 2 cases. *Surg Neurol.* 2007 Sep;68(3):344–348.

116. White PM, Teasdale EM, Wardlaw JM, Easton V. Intracranial aneurysms: CT angiography and MR angiography for detection prospective blinded comparison in a large patient cohort. *Radiology.* 2001;219(3):739–749.

117. Huston J, 3rd, Nichols DA, Luetmer PH, Goodwin JT, Meyer FB, Wiebers DO, *et al.* Blinded prospective evaluation of sensitivity of MR angiography to known intracranial aneurysms: importance of aneurysm size. *AJNR Am J Neuroradiol.* 1994 Oct;15(9):1607–1614.

118. Schuierer G, Huk WJ, Laub G. Magnetic resonance angiography of intracranial aneurysms: comparison with intra-arterial digital subtraction angiography. *Neuroradiology.* 1992;35(1):50–54.

119. Anzalone N, Triulzi F, Scotti G. Acute subarachnoid haemorrhage: 3D time-of-flight MR angiography versus intra-arterial digital angiography. *Neuroradiology.* 1995 May;37(4):257–261.

120. Horikoshi T, Fukamachi A, Nishi H, Fukasawa I. Detection of intracranial aneurysms by three-dimensional time-of-flight magnetic resonance angiography. *Neuroradiology.* 1994 Apr;36(3):203–207.

121. Atlas SW. Magnetic resonance imaging of intracranial aneurysms. *Magn Reson Imaging Clin N Am.* 1998 Nov;6(4):835–848.

122. Wilcock D, Jaspan T, Holland I, Cherryman G, Worthington B. Comparison of magnetic resonance angiography with conventional angiography in the detection of intracranial aneurysms in patients presenting with subarachnoid haemorrhage. *Clin Radiol.* 1996 May;51(5):330–334.

123. Beck J, Rohde S, Berkefeld J, Seifert V, Raabe A. Size and location of ruptured and unruptured intracranial aneurysms measured by 3-dimensional rotational angiography. *Surg Neurol.* 2006;65(1):18–25.

124. Hiratsuka Y, Miki H, Kiriyama I, Kikuchi K, Takahashi S, Matsubara I, *et al.* Diagnosis of unruptured intracranial aneurysms: 3T MR angiography versus 64-channel multi-detector row CT angiography. *Magn Reson Med Sci.* 2008;7(4):169–178.

125. Watanabe Z, Kikuchi Y, Izaki K, Hanyu N, Lim FS, Gotou H, *et al.* The usefulness of 3D MR angiography in surgery for ruptured cerebral aneurysms. *Surg Neurol.* 2001;55(6):359–364.

126. Schwab KE, Gailloud P, Wyse G, Tamargo RJ. Limitations of magnetic resonance imaging and magnetic resonance angiography in the diagnosis of intracranial aneurysms. *Neurosurgery.* 2008 Jul;63(1):29–34; discussion 34–35.

127. Solenski NJ, Haley EC, Jr, Kassell NF, Kongable G, Germanson T, Truskowski L, *et al.* Medical complications of aneurysmal subarachnoid hemorrhage: a report of the multicenter, cooperative aneurysm study. Participants of the Multicenter Cooperative Aneurysm Study. *Crit Care Med.* 1995;23(6):1007–1017.

128. Lee VH, Oh JK, Mulvagh SL, Wijdicks EF. Mechanisms in neurogenic stress cardiomyopathy after aneurysmal subarachnoid hemorrhage. *Neurocrit Care.* 2006;5(3):243–249.

129. Tanno Y, Homma M, Oinuma M, Kodama N, Ymamoto T. Rebleeding from ruptured intracranial aneurysms in North Eastern Province of Japan. A cooperative study. *J Neurol Sci.* 2007;258(1-2):11–16.

130. Ohkuma H, Tsurutani H, Suzuki S. Incidence and significance of early aneurysmal rebleeding before neurosurgical or neurological management. *Stroke.* 2001 May;32(5):1176–1180.

131. Fujii Y, Takeuchi S, Sasaki O, Minakawa T, Koike T, Tanaka R. Ultra-early rebleeding in spontaneous subarachnoid hemorrhage. *J Neurosurg.* 1996 Jan;84(1):35–42.

132. Rhoney DH, Tipps LB, Murry KR, Basham MC, Michael DB, Coplin WM. Anticonvulsant prophylaxis and timing of seizures after aneurysmal subarachnoid hemorrhage. *Neurology.* 2000 Jul 25;55(2):258–265.

133. Sehba FA, Bederson JB. Mechanisms of acute brain injury after subarachnoid hemorrhage. *Neurol Res.* 2006 Jun;28(4):381–398.

134. Huang J, van Gelder JM. The probability of sudden death from rupture of intracranial aneurysms: a meta-analysis. *Neurosurgery.* 2002 Nov;51(5):1101–1105; discussion 5–7.

135. Laun A, Tonn JC. Cranial nerve lesions following subarachnoid hemorrhage and aneurysm of the circle of Willis. *Neurosurg Rev.* 1988;11(2):137–141.

136. Chen PR, min-Hanjani S, Albuquerque FC, McDougall C, Zabramski JM, Spetzler RF. Outcome of oculomotor nerve palsy from posterior communicating artery aneurysms: comparison of clipping and coiling. *Neurosurgery.* 2006;58(6):1040–1046.

137. Guresir E, Schuss P, Setzer M, Platz J, Seifert V, Vatter H. Posterior communicating artery aneurysm-related oculomotor nerve palsy: influence of surgical and endovascular treatment on recovery: single-center series and systematic review. *Neurosurgery.* 2011 Jun;68(6):1527–1533; discussion 33–34.

138. Frijns CJ, Kasius KM, Algra A, Fijnheer R, Rinkel GJ. Endothelial cell activation markers and delayed cerebral ischaemia in patients with subarachnoid haemorrhage. *J Neurol Neurosurg Psychiatry.* 2006 Jul;77(7):863–867.

139. Qureshi AI, Sung GY, Razumovsky AY, Lane K, Straw RN, Ulatowski JA. Early identification of patients at risk for symptomatic vasospasm after aneurysmal subarachnoid hemorrhage. *Crit Care Med.* 2000;28(4):984–990.

140. O'Kelly CJ, Kulkarni AV, Austin PC, Urbach D, Wallace MC. Shunt-dependent hydrocephalus after aneurysmal subarachnoid hemorrhage: incidence, predictors, and revision rates. Clinical article. *J Neurosurg.* 2009 Nov;111(5):1029–1035.

CHAPTER 7

Clinical features of transient ischaemic attacks

David Calvet and Jean-Louis Mas

Introduction

Approximately 20% of ischaemic strokes are preceded by one or several transient ischaemic attacks (TIA) and 10–15% of TIA patients have a stroke within 3 months, with half occurring within 48 hours (1–5). These 'warning' events provide an opportunity for stroke prevention and current guidelines highlight the need for urgent assessment of patients with TIA (6). The diagnosis of TIA, however, can prove difficult because symptoms of TIA are not specific; it relies on obtaining a careful history from the patient and/or a witness of the attack.

An evolving definition

TIA was classically defined as 'a brief episode of focal loss of brain function, thought to be due to ischaemia, that can usually be localized to that portion of the brain supplied by one vascular system (left or right carotid or vertebrobasilar system) and for which no other cause can be found' (7). This definition is simple to use, particularly for epidemiological purposes, but the arbitrary 24-hour time limit doesn't reflect the fact that the majority of TIAs resolve within a few minutes (see 'Duration' section) (8). Moreover, the 24-hour time limit doesn't differentiate transient from permanent ischaemia, since about 40% of patients with classically defined TIAs have signs of acute brain infarction on diffusion-weighted magnetic resonance imaging (MRI) (9, 10).

These limitations led the TIA working group to redefine TIA as 'a brief episode of neurological dysfunction caused by focal brain or retinal ischaemia, with clinical symptoms typically lasting less than 1 hour, and without evidence of acute infarction' (11). The part of the sentence on the duration of the usual symptoms—'typically lasting less than 1 hour'—was removed from the most recent definition of TIA—'a transient episode of neurological dysfunction caused by focal brain or retinal ischaemia, without evidence of acute infarction'—recommended by the American Heart Association and the American Stroke Association (6). By using a tissue rather than a time criterion, the new definition recognizes TIA as a pathophysiological entity, which is similar to an attack of angina in patients with coronary artery disease (12).

However, as the definition requires brain imaging, the diagnosis of TIA versus stroke depends on the availability of imaging facilities and the type of imaging technique used for the diagnosis (MRI vs computed tomography scan). The upcoming World Health Organization International Classification of Diseases (ICD)-11 revision, due by 2015, will use a tissue-based definition with an upper time limit of 24 hours. To date, almost all research publications have used the classical time-based classification.

Symptoms of transient ischaemic attack

Duration

In a hospital-based study (8) which enrolled 1343 patients admitted for a stroke, 382 had a final diagnosis of TIA according to the classic definition (symptoms lasting <24 hours). Among these 382 patients, symptoms lasted less than 30 minutes in 50%, 30–60 minutes in 9.7%, and 60–180 minutes in 15.2% of the patients. In 90% of cases, symptoms disappeared in less than 240 minutes. Among 1115 patients with symptoms lasting 60 minutes or more, only 154 (13.8%) recovered within 24 hours and could thus be considered to have had a TIA. In the OXVASC population-based study (3) about two-thirds of TIA patients had symptoms lasting less than one hour, whereas in the German Stroke data bank TIAs lasted less than one hour in one-third of cases (13).

Various studies have reported an association between symptom duration and presence of lesions on diffusion-weighted imaging (DWI)-MRI (14–17). In a multicentre, patient-level analysis of 808 patients (33% with DWI lesions), the median duration of symptoms was 60 minutes (interquartile range, 15–240 min) in patients with DWI abnormalities compared to 30 minutes (interquartile range, 10–180 min) in those without DWI lesions (p=0.01) (18). In a meta-analysis of 19 studies (1242 patients) (9), the probability to find DWI lesions was 50% higher in patients whose symptoms lasted 60 minutes or more (odds ratio (OR) 1.50; 95% confidence interval (CI) 1.16–1.96).

Clinical features

Symptoms compatible with TIAs are usually classified as 'definite' (probable) or 'possible' depending on the likelihood that the symptoms are related to focal brain ischaemia rather than to other mechanisms (7, 19). In addition, symptoms are classified according to the affected vascular system (carotid vs vertebrobasilar system) (7). This distinction is clinically important, particularly when revascularization procedures are considered. Table 7.1 shows the classification used in the French clinical practice guidelines for immediate management of TIA patients (20).

Table 7.1 Symptoms of probable and possible TIA[a]

Probable TIA	Possible TIA
Symptoms suggesting carotid TIA	VertigoDiplopia
– Amaurosis fugax	Dysarthria
– Speech deficit (aphasia)	Dysphagia
– Unilateral motor and/or sensory symptoms affecting the face and/or limbs; these symptoms usually indicate ischaemia in the carotid territory, but in the absence of other signs it is not possible to tell whether the attack is of carotid or vertebrobasilar origin	Loss of balance
	Isolated sensory symptoms, hemifacial or affecting only part of a limb
Symptoms suggesting vertebrobasilar TIA	Drop attack
– Motor and/or sensory symptoms affecting the face and/or limbs, bilateral or changing sides between attacks	
– Loss of vision in the right and left field of vision (cortical blindness); homonymous hemianopsia may also be seen in carotid TIAs.	

[a] TIA is probable if there is rapid onset, usually <2 min, of one or more of the symptoms listed under 'Probable TIA' (left column). The symptoms in the right column are compatible with a TIA but other diagnoses should be considered first, if one of these symptoms occurs in isolation. The diagnosis becomes 'probable TIA' if these symptoms are combined, successively or concomitantly, with each other or with the symptoms listed under 'Probable TIA'.

TIAs are commonly rapid in onset (no symptoms to maximal symptoms in <5 minutes and usually <2 minutes). Fleeting episodes lasting only a few seconds are not likely to be TIAs.

Definite or probable TIA

Unilateral motor and/or sensory symptoms affecting the face and/or limbs usually indicate ischaemia in the carotid territory, but in the absence of other signs, it is not possible to tell whether the attack is of carotid or vertebrobasilar origin. Motor and/or sensory symptoms suggest vertebrobasilar TIA when they affect the face and/or limbs bilaterally or when they change sides between attacks. The diagnosis of TIA very often remains uncertain when the patient presents with isolated sensory symptoms involving only part of one extremity or one side of the face during a single attack. Aphasia is almost invariably related to carotid system. Very rare exceptions are caused by ischaemia in the distribution of the posterior cerebral artery (cases of amnesic aphasia due to lesions in the left postero-interior temporal lobe and transcortical sensory aphasia explained by lesions involving the thalamus, possibly its dorsomedial and ventrolateral nuclei) (21).

Complete or partial loss of vision in one eye ('amaurosis fugax') indicates carotid-distribution TIA, whereas homonymous hemianopsia indicates vertebrobasilar (mainly)—or carotid-distribution TIA. The distinction between transient monocular blindness and homonymous hemianopsia can be difficult unless the patient alternately covered each eye during the attack. It is common for amaurosis fugax to occur without other symptoms during the episode and to last for only a few minutes (7).

Among 1707 TIA patients included in a large emergency department-based study (2), 46% had unilateral motor deficit, 40% had sensory symptoms, 42% had speech disturbance (dysarthria and/or aphasia), and 13% had loss in vision (homonymous hemianopsia or transient molecular blindness). In a population-based study (3), 52% of 399 patients with definite TIA had unilateral weakness, 17% had speech disturbance (dysarthria and/or aphasia) without unilateral weakness and 31% had symptoms other than unilateral weakness and speech disturbance (3).

Some studies have shown that patients with motor deficit and/or aphasia more often have DWI lesions than patients without these symptoms (Table 7.2) (14, 16, 22). In a meta-analysis of 19 studies (1242 patients) (9), aphasia (OR 2.25; 95% CI 1.57–3.22) and motor weakness (OR 2.20; 95% CI 1.56–3.10) were associated with DWI lesions.

Possible TIA

The group of 'possible' TIA includes symptoms such as loss of balance, vertigo, diplopia, and dysphagia that are mainly suggestive of transient vertebrobasilar territory ischaemia. These symptoms are classified as possible TIA when they occur in isolation, because in this case they are often provoked by other mechanisms than focal brain ischaemia. These symptoms suggest 'probable TIA' when they occur in combination with each other, successively or concomitantly, or in combination with symptoms listed under 'probable TIA' (see Table 7.1).

Although dysarthria has been included among 'possible' TIAs (7), DWI lesions are more common in patients with dysarthria than in those without this symptom (32% vs 21%, adjusted OR 1.73; 95% CI 1.11–2.68) (9). Dysarthria can accompany either carotid or vertebrobasilar TIAs. Because it is either often very difficult to retrospectively distinguish aphasia from dysarthria and because aphasia and dysarthria have very similar predictive value to predict the presence of acute ischaemic lesions on DWI, the term of

Table 7.2 Prevalence of DWI lesions according to TIA symptoms in 98 consecutive patients admitted in a stroke unit (16)

Symptoms of attack	DWI–, n=64	DWI+, n=34	P value
Aphasia	16 (25.0%)	17 (50.0%)	0.01
Motor weakness	30 (46.9%)	25 (73.5%)	0.01
Sensory disturbances	26 (40.6%)	16 (47.1%)	0.5
Visual deficits	7 (10.9%)	2 (5.9%)	0.5
Brainstem symptoms	10 (15.6%)	4 (11.8%)	0.8
Cerebellar symptoms	7 (10.9%)	1 (2.9%)	0.3

speech disturbance is often used (3, 23, 24), particularly in prognostic studies.

In the Oxford Vascular Study, a prospective, population-based study of all stroke and TIA in 91,105 individuals, authors assessed the frequency and characteristics of transient isolated brainstem symptoms (e.g. isolated vertigo, dysarthria, diplopia) before vertebrobasilar ischaemic stroke (25). Of 59 transient isolated brainstem symptoms preceding (median 4 days, interquartile range 1–30) 275 vertebrobasilar strokes, only five (8%) fulfilled the National Institute of Neurological Disorders and Stroke (NINDS) criteria for TIA (probable or definite TIA). The other 54 cases were isolated vertigo (n=23), non-NINDS binocular visual disturbance (n=9), vertigo with other non-focal symptoms (n=10), isolated slurred speech, hemisensory tingling, or diplopia (n=8), and non-focal events (n=4). Only 10 (22%) of the 45 patients with transient isolated brainstem symptoms sought medical attention before the stroke and a vascular cause was suspected by their physician in only one of these cases. This study emphasizes how difficult a diagnosis of TIA can be, particularly in the vertebrobasilar territory.

Non-focal symptoms

Finally, many non-focal symptoms such as impaired consciousness, confusion, dizziness, or fainting do not indicate TIA, except under exceptional circumstances. Patients presenting with these symptoms should first be investigated for mechanisms other than transient brain ischaemia.

Application of an apparently simple definition is far from straightforward in clinical practice, as shown by the poor interobserver agreement in diagnosis of TIA. The kappa index of true agreement between two neurologists has been reported to be only 0.65 for the diagnosis of TIA and 0.31 for determination of the vascular system involved (26). In a subsequent report from the same group (27), the inter-observer agreement for the diagnosis of TIA was improved when symptoms were recorded on a checklist in everyday language rather than in abstract diagnostic terms (kappa value = 0.77). For every item such as vision, muscle strength, or speech, the checklist contained a number of possible symptoms in ordinary language, which could be ticked by the observers. For instance, amaurosis fugax was defined as a complete loss of vision of one eye or of the upper or lower half of the visual field, with the exclusion of blurred, distorted or grey vision (27). Neurologists and non-neurologists often disagree regarding TIA diagnosis (3, 28). In the Oxfordshire community stroke project, among 512 patients referred to neurologists for a suspected TIA, the final diagnosis was TIA in only 195 (38%) patients (28).

Clinical features of TIAs as predictors of early stroke

There is good evidence that some clinical features of a TIA can provide substantial prognostic information. In a large emergency department-based study, five factors (age ≥60 years, symptom duration >10 minutes, motor weakness, speech impairment, and diabetes mellitus) were independently associated with a high risk of recurrent stroke at 3 months. Using these predictive factors, Rothwell et al. (3) developed the ABCD score (Age, Blood pressure, Clinical features: motor weakness and speech disturbance, and Duration of symptoms), which was highly predictive of the 7-day risk of stroke in two independent population-based studies. Subsequent refinements led to the unified $ABCD^2$ score, which incorporates elements from the previous scores (Table 7.3). Although no randomized trial has evaluated the benefit of hospitalization or the utility of the $ABCD^2$ score for triage decisions, a scientific statement from the American Heart Association/American Stroke Association recommended to hospitalize patients with TIA if they present within 72 hours and have an $ABCD^2$ score of 3 or higher (6).

Recently, dual TIA, defined as an earlier transient ischaemic attack within 7 days of the index event, was found to be strongly associated with early stroke risk, independently of other items of the $ABCD^2$ score (24). Dual TIA has been incorporated in the $ABCD^3$ score, but further validation of this score is needed. The ABCD clinical score system should be used cautiously in addition to other predictive factors such as DWI data (29–31).

Transient ischaemic attack mimics

Distinguishing TIA from TIA mimics has major implications for prognosis and management. The diagnosis of TIA remains very challenging in patients with negative neuroimaging, only supported by obtaining a careful history. Differential diagnoses of TIA include neurological or non-neurological disorders (Table 7.4).

Table 7.3 Items of the $ABCD^2$ score and their odds ratios from multivariate model of stroke at 7 days (23)

Items of $ABCD^2$ score, point(s)	Number (%), n=4809	7-day risk of stroke odds ratio (95% CI)
Age >60 years, 1 point	3690 (77%)	1.4 (1.0–2.0)
Blood pressure (BP):	3420 (71%)	1.9 (1.4–2.6)
Systolic BP>140 mmHg or diastolic BP >90 mmHg, 1 point		
Clinical features:	1979 (41%)	3.5 (2.5–4.8)
Focal weakness, 2 points	899 (19%)	1.5 (1.0–2.4)
Speech impairment without focal weakness, 1 point		
Duration:	993 (21%)	1.9 (1.1–3.3)
10–59 min vs <10 min, 1 point	2973 (62%)	2.6 (1.6–4.3)
>60 min vs <10 min, 2 points		
Diabetes mellitus, 1 point	797 (17%)	1.4 (1.1–1.9)

Although TIAs may occasionally manifest as *focal epileptic attacks* (32) and limb shaking TIAs can be seen patients with exhausted cerebrovascular perfusion reserve from large artery stenoses or occlusions, closely linked to orthostatic postures (7), focal epilepsy should be distinguished from TIA. This distinction is usually straightforward because most focal seizures cause 'positive' phenomena. However, focal motor seizures can be mistaken for TIA when the patient emphasizes postictal weakness rather than jerking, or if seizures are of the inhibitory type (33), which may also give rise to aphasic seizures (i.e. speech arrest). Sensory and aphasic seizures may be difficult to distinguish from TIA. Sensory seizures with paraesthesia are typically characterized by rapid march of the symptoms, which usually begin distally and spread up the entire limb of half the body. MRI abnormalities can also be observed in patients with postictal deficit. Epileptic seizures induce abnormalities located at cerebral cortex, hippocampus, amygdale and medial thalamus, that can be detected with DWI and T2-weighted imaging (34). The hippocampus is particularly vulnerable to the effects of seizures. Areas of diminished diffusion after seizures frequently resolve on follow-up. Occasionally, they can evolve into areas with increased apparent diffusion coefficient (ADC) and T2 prolongation consistent with tissue damage, particularly in the hippocampus (34).

Differentiation between TIA and *migraine* can be difficult since TIAs can be accompanied by headache (35), and, conversely, migraine without headache is not unusual. A clue favouring the diagnosis of migraine is the nature of symptoms, which are often positive and frequently involve the visual system (e.g. scintillating scotomas), whereas clinical manifestations of TIA almost invariably represent a decrease or absence of function. Even more important is the mode of spread of symptoms. Symptoms of TIA arise swiftly, affect several body parts simultaneously, and peak in seconds to a few minutes. In migraine, symptoms build-up gradually over 15–30 minutes, with slow march from one part of the body to another and often with serial progression of new symptoms while the initial ones are abating. Nevertheless, these criteria have no absolute value and migraine with aura may be indistinguishable from TIA (36). Migrainous aura can occur without headache, more often but not exclusively in older people with a history of migraine (37). In a report on late-life migraine with aura (38), 29% of episodes lasted less than 5 minutes; 60% of attacks were not associated with headache; and 35% of patients denied a history of recurrent headache (38). Reversible MRI

signal abnormalities such as post gadolinium T1-weighted meningeal enhancement, cortical swelling, or fluid attenuated inversion recovery (FLAIR) cortical hyperintensities have been also reported in patients with familiar hemiplegic migraine and other forms of migraine with prolonged aura (39–42). Occasionally, patients with migraine with prolonged aura may also have DWI hyperintensity involving the cortex and subcortical white matter, with or without corresponding hypointensity on the ADC map which can be confused with an acute infarct (41, 42). These lesions are reversible (40, 41). An association between migraine and the presence of chronic white matter lesions on MRI has also been reported (43, 44).

Intracranial haemorrhage and subdural haematoma are rare but important TIA mimics. Convexal subarachnoid haemorrhage can present with transient repetitive symptoms compatible with migraine auras, epileptic seizures and TIA. Awareness of this entity is important because misdiagnosis as cerebral ischaemic events could lead to incorrect treatment (45). In patients with cerebral amyloid angiopathy, transient repetitive focal neurological deficits can also occur days to weeks before the occurrence of haemorrhage (46, 47). A loss of signal consistent with cortical haemosiderin deposits on T2*-imaging may be a reliable marker for cerebral amyloid angiopathy (47).

Transient global amnesia (TGA) is characterized by isolated, sudden, and reversible loss of anterograde memory. Its prognosis is benign, with a long-term stroke rate similar to that of an age-matched normal population (48). Punctate DWI hyperintense foci have been reported in 41–100% of TGA cases imaged within the first 3 days after the event, depending on the time from TGA onset to MRI and the use of specialized sequences (thinner section and coronal acquisitions) (49–53). The lesions typically measure 1–3 mm in diameter and involve the lateral aspect of the hippocampus, are frequently unilateral and reversible (49).

The main differential diagnoses of amaurosis fugax are listed in Table 7.4. It is critical to determine whether the visual loss involved one eye or both. This distinction can be done when patients alternately covered each eye during the attack.

Patients with metabolic disorders, particularly hypoglycaemia could also present transient episode of neurological dysfunction. Exclusion of an ischaemic origin is sometimes very challenging because of abnormalities in DWI in some cases of hypoglycaemia (54). The differential diagnosis of TIAs also include, Ménière's syndrome, sensory phenomena associated with hyperventilation, and syncope or near-syncope due to hypotension.

Table 7.4 Differential diagnoses

Neurological disorders	Non-neurological disorders	In case of amaurosis fugax
Migraine with aura	Metabolic disorders (particularly hypoglycaemia)	Amaurosis related to malignant hypertension
Focal epileptic seizure		Acute glaucoma
Other	Vertigo of ENT origin (Ménière's disease, benign paroxysmal positional vertigo, vestibular neuritis	Intracranial hypertension
	Syncope	Central retinal vein thrombosis
	Orthostatic hypotension	Retrobulbar optic neuritis
	Hyperventilation syndrome	Detached retina
	Hysteria, simulation	Temporal arteritis
	Psychosomatic disorders	

Diagnostic workup

The first goal of neuroimaging is to confirm or support the ischaemic origin of the symptoms. The American Heart Association and American Stroke Association recommend that 'patients with TIA should preferably undergo neuroimaging evaluation within the 24 hours of symptom onset (6). MRI, including DWI, is the preferred brain diagnostic imaging modality' (6). Neuroimaging may demonstrate signs of recent ischaemia in the corresponding territory (ischaemic stroke according to the new definition). Pooled data from 19 studies showed a rate of DWI positivity of 39% (25–67%) (6). The vast majority (76–100%) of patients with DWI lesions have corresponding T2-weighted signal evidence of permanent injury on follow-up imaging (54, 55). MRI can also show signs of previous cerebral ischaemia and provide indirect evidence for a vascular origin, particularly when previous ischaemic lesions are in the suspected vascular distribution. Brain imaging helps to eliminate some differential diagnoses, particularly intracranial bleeding. MRI also provides prognostic information. Several studies have shown that DWI positivity is associated with an increased risk of early stroke, independently of clinical features included in predictive scores (24, 56) and may help in secondary triage of TIA patients.

The second goal of the workup is to identify the cause of the TIA, in particular those that have urgent therapeutic implications, such as severe carotid stenosis or atrial fibrillation. The aetiological workup should urgently include vessel imaging, cardiac evaluation, and laboratory testing, including C-reactive protein and erythrocyte sedimentation rate (6).

Conclusion

TIA is a great opportunity for stroke prevention but rapid and specialized medical attention is needed because of a short time window. The identification by patient and physicians of the symptoms are the first step of this urgent management. Thus, physicians should inform patients with risk factors for ischaemic stroke about the symptoms of TIA and the necessity of urgent management.

References

1. Rothwell PM, Warlow CP. Timing of TIAs preceding stroke: time window for prevention is very short. *Neurology*. 2005;64(5):817–820.
2. Johnston SC, Gress DR, Browner WS, Sidney S. Short-term prognosis after emergency department diagnosis of TIA. *JAMA*. 2000;284(22): 2901–2906.
3. Rothwell PM, Giles MF, Flossmann E, Lovelock CE, Redgrave JN, Warlow CP, *et al*. A simple score (ABCD) to identify individuals at high early risk of stroke after transient ischaemic attack. *Lancet*. 2005;366(9479):29–36.
4. Giles MF, Rothwell PM. Risk of stroke early after transient ischaemic attack: a systematic review and meta-analysis. *Lancet Neurol*. 2007;6(12):1063–1072.
5. Wu CM, McLaughlin K, Lorenzetti DL, Hill MD, Manns BJ, Ghali WA. Early risk of stroke after transient ischemic attack: a systematic review and meta-analysis. *Arch Intern Med*. 2007;167(22):2417–2422.
6. Easton JD, Saver JL, Albers GW,GW, Alberts MJ, Chaturvedi S, Feldmann E, *et al*. Definition and evaluation of transient ischemic attack: a scientific statement for healthcare professionals from the American Heart Association/American Stroke Association Stroke Council; Council on Cardiovascular Surgery and Anesthesia; Council on Cardiovascular Radiology and Intervention; Council on Cardiovascular Nursing; and the Interdisciplinary Council on Peripheral Vascular Disease. The American Academy of Neurology affirms the value of this statement as an educational tool for neurologists. *Stroke*. 2009;40(6):2276–2293.
7. Special report from the National Institute of Neurological Disorders and Stroke. Classification of cerebrovascular diseases III. *Stroke*. 1990;21(4):637–676.
8. Levy DE. How transient are transient ischemic attacks? *Neurology*. 1988; 38(5):674–677.
9. Redgrave JN, Coutts SB, Schulz UG, Briley D, Rothwell PM. Systematic review of associations between the presence of acute ischemic lesions on diffusion-weighted imaging and clinical predictors of early stroke risk after transient ischemic attack. *Stroke*. 2007;38(5):1482–1488.
10. Oppenheim C, Lamy C, Touze E, Calvet D, Hamon M, Mas JL, *et al*. Do transient ischemic attacks with diffusion-weighted imaging abnormalities correspond to brain infarctions? *AJNR Am J Neuroradiol*. 2006;27(8):1782–1787.
11. Albers GW, Caplan LR, Easton JD, Fayad PB, Mohr JP, Saver JL, *et al*. Transient ischemic attack—proposal for a new definition. *N Engl J Med*. 2002;347(21):1713–1716.
12. European Stroke Organisation (ESO) Executive Committee; ESO Writing Committee. Guidelines for management of ischaemic stroke and transient ischaemic attack. *Cerebrovasc Dis*. 2008;25(5):457–507.
13. Weimar C, Kraywinkel K, Rodl J, Hippe A, Harms L, Kloth A, *et al*. Etiology, duration, and prognosis of transient ischemic attacks: an analysis from the German Stroke Data Bank. *Arch Neurol*. 2002;59(10):1584–1588.
14. Crisostomo RA, Garcia MM, Tong DC. Detection of diffusion-weighted MRI abnormalities in patients with transient ischemic attack: correlation with clinical characteristics. *Stroke*. 2003;34(4):932–937.
15. Prabhakaran S, Chong JY, Sacco RL. Impact of abnormal diffusion-weighted imaging results on short-term outcome following transient ischemic attack. *Arch Neurol*. 2007;64(8):1105–1109.
16. Lamy C, Oppenheim C, Calvet D, Domigo V, Naggaro O, Méder NL, *et al*. Diffusion-weighted MR imaging in transient ischaemic attacks. *Eur Radiol*. 2006;16(5):1090–1095.
17. Kidwell CS, Alger JR, Di Salle F, Starkman S, Villablanca P, Bentson J, *et al*. Diffusion MRI in patients with transient ischemic attacks. *Stroke*. 1999;30(6):1174–1180.
18. Shah Sh, Saver JL, Kidwell CS, Albers G, Rothwell P, Ay H, *et al*. A multicenter pooled, patient-level data analysis of diffusion-weighted MRI in TIA patients. *Stroke*. 2007;38:463–463.
19. Landi G. Clinical diagnosis of transient ischaemic attacks. *Lancet*. 1992;339(8790):402–405.
20. Albucher JF, Martel P, Mas JL. Clinical practice guidelines: diagnosis and immediate management of transient ischemic attacks in adults. *Cerebrovasc Dis*. 2005;20(4):220–225.
21. Servan J, Verstichel P, Catala M, Yakovleff A, Rancurel G. Aphasia and infarction of the posterior cerebral artery territory. *J Neurol*. 1995;242(2):87–92.
22. Cucchiara BL, Messe SR, Taylor RA, Pacelli J, Maus D, Shah Q, *et al*. Is the ABCD score useful for risk stratification of patients with acute transient ischemic attack? *Stroke*. 2006;37(7):1710–1714.
23. Johnston SC, Rothwell PM, Nguyen-Huynh MN, Giles MF, Elkins JS, Bernstein AL, *et al*. Validation and refinement of scores to predict very early stroke risk after transient ischaemic attack. *Lancet*. 2007;369(9558): 283–292.
24. Merwick A, Albers GW, Amarenco P, Arsava EM, Ay H, Calvet D, Coutts SB, *et al*. Addition of brain and carotid imaging to the ABCD2 score improve identification of patients at high early risk after transient ischaemic attack. *Lancet Neurol*. 2010; 9(11):1060–1069.
25. Paul NL, Simoni M, Rothwell PM. Transient isolated brainstem symptoms preceding posterior circulation stroke: a population-based study. *Lancet Neurol*. 2013;12(1):65–71.
26. Kraaijeveld CL, van GJ, Schouten HJ, Staal A. Interobserver agreement for the diagnosis of transient ischemic attacks. *Stroke*. 1984;15(4): 723–725.
27. Koudstaal PJ, van GJ, Staal A, Duivenvoorden HJ, Gerritsma JG, Kraaijeveld CL. Diagnosis of transient ischemic attacks: improvement of interobserver agreement by a check-list in ordinary language. *Stroke*. 1986;17(4):723–728.

28. Dennis MS, Bamford JM, Sandercock PA, Warlow CP. Incidence of transient ischemic attacks in Oxfordshire, England. *Stroke.* 1989;20(3):333–339.

29. Sanders LM, Srikanth VK, Blacker DJ, Jolley DJ, Cooper KA, Phan TG. Performance of the ABCD2 score for stroke risk post TIA: meta-analysis and probability modeling. *Neurology.* 2012;79(10):971–980.

30. Lemmens R, Smet S, Thijs VN. Clinical scores for predicting recurrence after transient ischemic attack or stroke: how good are they? *Stroke.* 2013;44(4):1198–1203.

31. Edlow JA. Risk stratification in TIA patients: "It's the vascular lesion, stupid!". *Neurology.* 2012;79(10):958–959.

32. Ferracci F, Moretto G, Gentile M, Kuo P, Carnevale A. Can seizures be the only manifestation of transient ischemic attacks? A report of four cases. *Neurol Sci.* 2000;21(5):303–306.

33. Lee H, Lerner A. Transient inhibitory seizures mimicking crescendo TIAs. *Neurology.* 1990;40(1):165–166.

34. Milligan TA, Zamani A, Bromfield E. Frequency and patterns of MRI abnormalities due to status epilepticus. *Seizure.* 2009;18(2):104–108.

35. Portenoy RK, Abissi CJ, Lipton RB, Berger AR, Mebler MF, Baglivo J, et al. Headache in cerebrovascular disease. *Stroke.* 1984;15(6):1009–1012.

36. Larsen BH, Sorensen PS, Marquardsen J. Transient ischaemic attacks in young patients: a thromboembolic or migrainous manifestation? A 10 year follow up study of 46 patients. *J Neurol Neurosurg Psychiatry.* 1990;53(12):1029–1033.

37. Ziegler DK, Hassanein RS. Specific headache phenomena: their frequency and coincidence. *Headache.* 1990;30(3):152–156.

38. Fisher CM. Late-life migraine accompaniments—further experience. *Stroke.* 1986;17(5):1033–1042.

39. Gomez-Choco M, Capurro S, Obach V. Migraine with aura associated with reversible sulcal hyperintensity in FLAIR. *Neurology.* 2008;70(24 Pt 2):2416–2418.

40. Gentile S, Rainero I, Daniele D, Binello E, Valfre W, Pinessi L. Reversible MRI abnormalities in a patient with recurrent status migrainosus. *Cephalalgia.* 2009;29(6):687–690.

41. Resnick S, Reyes-Iglesias Y, Carreras R, Villalobos E. Migraine with aura associated with reversible MRI abnormalities. *Neurology.* 2006;66(6):946–947.

42. Bhatia R, Desai S, Tripathi M, Garg A, Padma MV, Prasad K, et al. Sporadic hemiplegic migraine: report of a case with clinical and radiological features. *J Headache Pain.* 2008;9(6):385–388.

43. Rao R, Rosati A, Liberini P, Gipponi S, Venturelli E, Sapia E, et al. Cerebrovascular risk factors and MRI abnormalities in migraine. *Neurol Sci.* 2008;29(Suppl 1):S144–S145.

44. Kruit MC, van Buchem MA, Launer LJ, Terwindt GM, Ferrari MD. Migraine is associated with an increased risk of deep white matter lesions, subclinical posterior circulation infarcts and brain iron accumulation: the population-based MRI CAMERA study. *Cephalalgia.* 2010;30(2):129–136.

45. Izenberg A, Aviv RI, Demaerschalk BM, Dodick DW, Hopyan J, Black SE, et al. Crescendo transient aura attacks: a transient ischemic attack mimic caused by focal subarachnoid hemorrhage. *Stroke.* 2009;40(12):3725–3729.

46. Thanvi B, Robinson T. Sporadic cerebral amyloid angiopathy—an important cause of cerebral haemorrhage in older people. *Age Ageing.* 2006;35(6):565–571.

47. Roch JA, Nighoghossian N, Hermier M, Cakmak S, Picot M, Honnorat J, et al. Transient neurologic symptoms related to cerebral amyloid angiopathy: usefulness of T2*-weighted imaging. *Cerebrovasc Dis.* 2005; 20(5):412–414.

48. Hodges JR, Warlow CP. The aetiology of transient global amnesia. A case-control study of 114 cases with prospective follow-up. *Brain.* 1990;113(Pt 3):639–657.

49. Bartsch T, Deuschl G. Transient global amnesia: functional anatomy and clinical implications. *Lancet Neurol.* 2010;9(2):205–214.

50. Sedlaczek O, Hirsch JG, Grips E, Peters CN, Gass A, Wöhrle J, et al. Detection of delayed focal MR changes in the lateral hippocampus in transient global amnesia. *Neurology.* 2004;62(12):2165–2170.

51. Toledo M, Pujadas F, Grive E, varez-Sabin J, Quintana M, Rovira A. Lack of evidence for arterial ischemia in transient global amnesia. *Stroke.* 2008;39(2):476–479.

52. Yang Y, Kim S, Kim JH. Ischemic evidence of transient global amnesia: location of the lesion in the hippocampus. *J Clin Neurol.* 2008; 4(2):59–66.

53. Weon YC, Kim JH, Lee JS, Kim SY. Optimal diffusion-weighted imaging protocol for lesion detection in transient global amnesia. *AJNR Am J Neuroradiol.* 2008;29(7):1324–1328.

54. Cordonnier C, Oppenheim C, Lamy C, Meder JF, Mas JL. Serial diffusion and perfusion-weighted MR in transient hypoglycemia. *Neurology.* 2005;65(1):175.

55. Inatomi Y, Kimura K, Yonehara T, Fujioka S, Uchino M. DWI abnormalities and clinical characteristics in TIA patients. *Neurology.* 2004;62(3):376–380.

56. Giles MF, Albers GW, Amarenco P, Arsava MM, Asimos A, Ay H, et al. Addition of brain infarction to the ABCD2 Score (ABCD2I): a collaborative analysis of unpublished data on 4574 patients. *Stroke.* 2010; 41(9):1907–1913.

CHAPTER 8

Clinical features of acute stroke

José M. Ferro and Ana Catarina Fonseca

Introduction

Advances in neuroimaging, namely the introduction of magnetic resonance (MRI) with diffusion-weighted imaging (DWI), have allowed us to better study and identify acute ischaemic stroke patterns. Nevertheless, clinical evaluation of patients remains essential. Although MRI DWI is very useful in acute ischaemic stroke, it has a rate of false-negatives that ranges from 0–31% within 24 hours of ischaemic stroke (1). False negatives are higher in vertebrobasilar ischaemic stroke, small lacunar strokes, and low National Institutes of Health Stroke Scale (NIHSS) scores. Therefore, the diagnosis of ischaemic stroke must still be made attending to the clinical findings, without depending solely on DWI MRI.

Early identification of ischaemic stroke subtypes and patterns has several heuristic values. It helps the physician to answer the patient's and their relatives' anxieties concerning the risk of early death, disability, stroke recurrence, and length of stay. It guides the neurologist to choose the most cost-effective ancillary procedures and the therapy with best efficacy and suggests stroke aetiology. It also helps the hospital manager to calculate the average cost of care for stroke subtypes.

The use of thrombolysis in routine clinical practice has influenced stroke subtype presentation. An increased incidence of striatocapsular infarcts has been reported after the introduction of treatment with intravenous recombinant tissue plasminogen activator. This pattern results from a successful recanalization of the main stem of the middle cerebral artery (MCA) (2). In this chapter we will review the clinical-imagiological patterns of acute territorial infarcts and their clinical relevance.

Clinical patterns of acute territorial infarcts

Middle cerebral artery infarcts

The MCA territory is the arterial territory most frequently affected by ischaemic stroke. MCA infarcts can be divided into superficial (involving the cortex and underlying white matter), deep (involving the basal ganglia, the internal capsule and the deep white matter), and combined (3, 4).

MCA infarcts are mainly caused by cardioembolism, internal carotid artery (ICA) thrombosis, dissection, or embolism and rarely in Caucasians but commonly in Asians, by intrinsic MCA disease.

Superficial middle cerebral artery infarcts

Stroke patterns of superficial (pial) MCA infarcts are due to complete pial infarct and infarcts in the distribution of the anterior and posterior division of the MCA. Clinical presentation differs depending on whether the left (dominant for language) or the right (non-dominant) hemisphere is involved. In left hemispheric stroke oral and written language disturbances dominate, in right-sided strokes neglect is almost always present. The MCA generally has 12 pial branches, which cause clinically identifiable syndromes.

Large middle cerebral artery infarcts

Large infarcts cover at least two subterritories of the MCA (deep, superficial, anterior or superior, and posterior or inferior) (Figure 8.1). They have an unfavourable prognosis and produce a severe neurological deficit (gaze deviation, contralateral hemiplegia, global aphasia or neglect with anosognosia, hemianopia) including reduced consciousness. They are caused by cardioembolism, ICA occlusion or dissection (5).

Middle cerebral artery anterior or superior division infarcts

These cause a contralateral hemiparesis with predominant facio-brachial deficit, hemisensory loss, gaze deviation towards the lesion, or decreased visual exploration toward the opposite side. Left-sided infarcts also produce a non-fluent aphasia, ranging from mutism to typical Broca's aphasia and to articulatory, syntactical and naming difficulties. Bucco-facial apraxia is common. In right hemisphere strokes, neglect with anosognosia is sometimes found. Patients may have monotonous speech and be unable to correctly perceive or express the appropriate emotional inflection owing to aprosodia (6).

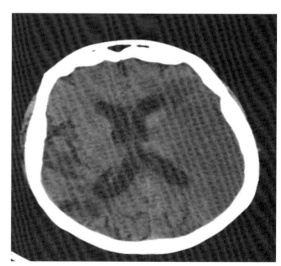

Fig. 8.1 Large left middle cerebral artery acute infarct.

Middle cerebral artery posterior or inferior division infarcts

Hemisensory loss is common and visual field defects (homonymous hemianopia or upper quadrantanopia) are usually present. Motor deficits are absent or mild. In left-sided strokes, fluent aphasia predominates. The most severe form is Wernicke's aphasia with anosognosia and behavioural disturbances including persecutory delusions. In right hemispheric stroke, neglect, anosognosia, and an agitated confusional state usually occur. Constructional apraxia can be present.

Cortical branch syndromes

Infarcts involving the orbitofrontal and prefrontal arteries can produce a frontal syndrome. Left prefrontal infarcts can result in transcortical aphasia, right prefrontal infarcts can produce motor neglect.

Precentral artery territory infarcts result in hemiparesis with predominant proximal arm involvement. In left-sided strokes non fluent aphasia, usually transcortical motor aphasia, apraxia and agraphia are present, in right sided strokes, neglect and motor impersistence can be found.

Central sulcus or rolandic artery territory infarcts produce contralateral motor and sensory defect with faciobrachial predominance, when the occlusion is proximal. In distal occlusion, motor deficit may be restricted to the arm or distal upper extremity. Involvement of the post central gyrus can cause cheiro-oral sensory loss. Central sulcus artery territory infarct typically cause mild Broca's aphasia (left-sided strokes) combined with dysarthria and transient tongue, palatal, and pharyngeal weakness, and faciobrachial weakness. Bilateral central sulcus infarcts cause the cortical form of the anterior opercular syndrome (Foix–Chavany–Marie syndrome), with bilateral voluntary paresis of the facial, masticatory, lingual, and pharyngeal muscles, featuring bilateral lower facial weakness, anarthria or severe dysarthria, and dysphagia (Figure 8.2).

There are three parietal MCA branches: anterior, angular, and posterior (Figure 8.3). Anterior parietal or postcentral sulcus artery infarct causes contralateral sensory loss, mainly in the upper limb (pseudothalamic syndrome) with touch, pain, temperature, and vibration senses impairment. Pain, hyperpathia, and parietal ataxia can also be present. Conduction aphasia, which is a fluent form of aphasia with disproportionate impairment of repetition, anomia,

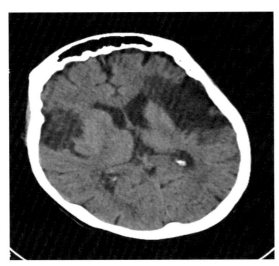

Fig. 8.2 Bilateral central sulcus infarcts.

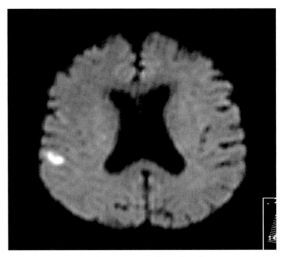

Fig. 8.3 Right middle cerebral artery cortical branch infarct.

agraphia, and apraxia are present in left hemispherical infarcts and neglect in right hemispherical.

Posterior parietal artery territory infarcts are unusual and usually occur in combination with angular gyrus territory artery infarcts. These infarcts cause lower quadrantanopia, cortical sensation dysfunction with astereognosia and impairment of position sense, two-point discrimination, and graphesthesia, with sparing of light touch, vibration, pain, and temperature senses. On the left side fluent aphasia with alexia, Gerstmann syndrome (agraphia, acalculia, digitoagnosia and left–right disorientation), and ideomotor apraxia occur, while on the right, neglect and constructional apraxia result. Upper parietal lobe involvement may show elements of Balint syndrome, including disturbance in manual reaching (optic or visuo-motor ataxia), visual attention, and 'psychic paralysis of gaze'—difficulty in directing the gaze towards targets of interest and easily losing fixation.

The MCA usually has five temporal branches. Temporal MCA infarcts are often combined with lower posterior parietal infarcts. They cause upper quadrantanopia. Vertigo has been reported in superior temporal or insular infarcts. On the left side, Wernicke's aphasia dominates. On the right, limited infarcts can be paucisymptomatic. Extended infarcts cause amusia, neglect, acute agitation, and sometimes delusions symptoms.

Striatocapsular infarcts

Striatocapsular infarcts may mimic a superficial MCA infarct, causing a partial anterior circulation syndrome or present as a lacunar syndrome (pure motor, ataxic hemiparesis, or sensory motor stroke) (Figure 8.4). Hypophonia and abnormal movements due to basal ganglia involvement may be present. Cortical signs are minor or absent. Non-fluent aphasia and neglect can appear. These cortical signs may be due to cortical diaschisis, cortical hypoperfusion or scattered cortical lesions not apparent on CT.

Anterior choroidal artery infarcts

The most frequent presentation of anterior choroidal artery (AChA) infarcts is pure motor deficit followed by motor and sensory dysfunction (7). The classical '3H' syndrome composed by hemiparesis, hemihypesthesia, hemianopia is less common (8). Isolated hemianopia can occur (9). Aphasia and neglect can be

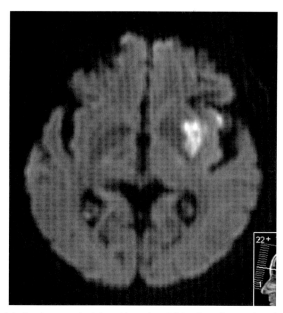

Fig. 8.4 Left striatocapsular infarct. Note the additional small cortical insular infarct.

found following respectively dominant and non-dominant infarcts. Aphasia is most often transcortical motor. Acute bilateral AChA infarct, can cause severe pseudobulbar palsy (7).

AChA territory infarcts are generally caused by cardioembolim or large artery disease with occlusion or artery-to-artery embolism (10) (Figure 8.5).

Thalamic infarcts

Thalamic infarcts can be divided into four main types: (i) tuberothalamic (anterior or polar), in the territory of the tuberothalamic artery, a branch of the posterior communicating artery; (ii) paramedian (thalamoperforate or posterior thalamicsubthalamic), in the territory of the paramedian artery, that originates from the P1 segment of the PCA; (iii) inferolateral (thalamogeniculate),

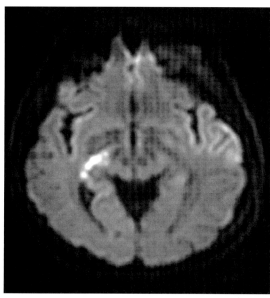

Fig. 8.5 Right anterior choroidal artery infarct.

in the territory of the inferolateral artery, that originates from the P2 segment of the posterior cerebral artery (PCA); (iv) posterior (posterior choroidal artery), that arises from the P2 segment of the PCA (11, 12). Sometimes two territories are involved simultaneously. Bilateral infarcts, in particular tuberothalamic or paramedian, are not infrequent. They may be due to simultaneous emboli or to a common unilateral origin of the arterial branches supplying the anterior and the paramedian thalamus. Bilateral paramedian infarct may be caused by occlusion of Percheron artery. It is a variant arterial supply where the bilateral medial thalamic and rostral midbrain perforators arise from a single trunk from the P1 segment of one PCA.

The four major topographical patterns of bilateral thalamic infarcts are: bilateral paramedian, bilateral inferolateral, combined unilateral paramedian and inferolateral, and combined unilateral tuberothalamic and inferolateral. Infarcts involving the four arterial thalamic territories are exceptional. Occlusion of the PCA in the absence of an ipsilateral posterior communicating artery may explain this uncommon infarct (13).

Inferolateral or thalamogeniculate infarcts usually present as a hemisensory loss with pain or dysaesthesia, plus hemiataxia (14), hemiataxia–hypaesthesia (15), hypaesthesic ataxic hemiparesis and ataxic hemiparesis, and involuntary movements (chorea or dystonia). Tuberothalamic infarcts usually cause drowsiness, apathy, executive deficits, personality changes, amnesia, and aphasia or neglect (depending on the involved side). In paramedian infarcts drowsiness is prominent. Amnesia, abulia, impaired learning, and altered social skills and personality are also apparent. Oculo-motor troubles may be present, namely vertical eye movement disorders (11, 16). In bilateral paramedian thalamic infarcts, the neuropsychological and psychic changes tend to be persist, causing a strategic infarct vascular dementia syndrome (17).

Posterior choroidal artery infarcts result in visual field defects, variable sensory loss, hemiparesis, dystonia, hand tremor, and occasionally amnesia and aphasia. Visual field defects, commonly quadrantanopia or hemianopia are found if the lateral posterior choroidal arteries branches are involved in isolation. Unusual field defects, such as homonymous horizontal sectoranopia or wedge-shaped homonymous hemianopia, may also be found and be due to the dual blood supply to the lateral geniculate body by the lateral posterior choroidal arteries and the anterior choroidal artery (18).

Posterior cerebral artery infarcts

Visual field defects, including hemianopia are the main clinical findings of PCA infarcts. Headache, generally unilateral, is rather frequent and may be severe. PCA infarcts can be superficial (cortical) (19) or combined with lateral thalamic or rostral mesencephalic infarcts (Figure 8.6). The thalamic infarct produces a sensory defect in variable combination with ataxia or involuntary movements. The midbrain lesion is usually limited and causes a transient paresis. More extensive midbrain lesions produce vigilance and oculomotor troubles. Sensory abnormalities in PCA stroke are associated with ventrolateral thalamic infarcts in the thalamogeniculate or lateral posterior choroidal arteries or less frequently to ischaemia to the white matter tracts to the somatosensory motor cortex (20). Hemiparesis in PCA infarcts can be due to infarction of the cerebral peduncle or less frequently to infarction of the anterior segment of the posterior limb of the internal capsule (21).

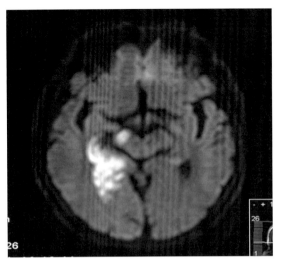

Fig. 8.6 Right posterior cerebral artery territorial infarct. Notice the anterolateral mesencephalic extension.

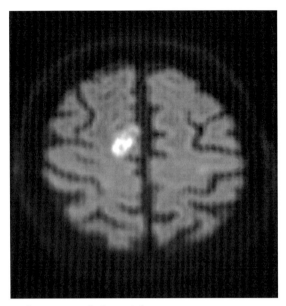

Fig. 8.7 Right anterior cerebral artery infarct.

Superior quadrantanopia is more common than inferior, because the inferior striate cortex is more susceptible to ischaemia due to poor collateral circulation. Neuropsychological manifestations are common. When the dominant hemisphere is damaged they may include: (i) transcortical sensory aphasia or anomic aphasia; (ii) alexia with or without agraphia—the lesion producing alexia without agraphia combines damage to the left calcarine cortex and to splenium of the corpus callosum or to the outflow of the callosum originating from the right visual cortex; (iii) visual or colour agnosia—infarcts causing persistent associative visual agnosia are usually large and involve the parahippocampal and fusiform gyrus. On the non-dominant side visual neglect, prosopagnosia (often transient) and topographical amnesia can be found. Both sides are associated with visual perseverations, visual illusions, hallucinations, and agitation. Declarative memory defects, concerning verbal (left side), visual (right side) material, or both are usually present. Such infarcts usually involve the hippocampus. Bilateral occipito-temporal infarcts can cause cortical blindness without or with anosognosia (Anton syndrome), associative or apperceptive visual agnosia, and severe memory defect (22, 21). Anton's syndrome with amnesia for recent events and disorientation, due to the Papez circuit involvement, is known as Dide–Botcazo syndrome (23).

PCA infarcts are due to cardioembolism in one-third of cases. Significant vertebrobasilar atheroma with occlusion or artery-to-artery embolism accounts for another one-quarter. Local PCA stenosis or occlusions are much less frequent. Infarcts associated with migraine account for a few cases.

Anterior cerebral artery infarcts

Strokes in the anterior cerebral artery (ACA) territory are uncommon (<2% in stroke registries). Left-sided infarcts cause mutism, transcortical motor aphasia, hemiparesis, and occasionally left-arm apraxia and other callosal disconnection syndromes. Right-sided infarcts cause acute confusional state, hemiparesis, and motor neglect (24) (Figure 8.7). Hemiparesis predominates in the lower limb when the precentral gyrus is involved. If the infarction extends more posteriorly sensory loss in the leg can be found. Occasionally

the paresis is proportional and indistinguishable from a MCA pattern. Proportional hemiparesis occurs when there is occlusion of the recurrent artery of Heubner that supplies the internal capsule. Abulia can be present with unilateral or bilateral infarcts that involve the cingulum and the supplementary motor area. Abulia is more prevalent in patients with bilateral lesions followed by those with left lesions (25).

Bilateral infarcts may produce akinetic mutism (26), gait apraxia (27), paraparesis, and sphincter dysfunction. Basal ganglia symptoms, including parkinsonian gait, tremor, and facial dystonia, can be observed in bilateral ACA infarcts (28).

Grasp reflex, utilization behaviour (29), and executive deficits may be present.

Combined hemispherical infarcts

Combined unilateral ACA-MCA infarcts can result from embolic occlusion of the distal ICA (carotid T). Combined MCA-PCA infarcts may be due to simultaneous embolism to the two territories, to a fetal (internal carotid) origin of the PCA or to compression of the PCA by a herniating hemisphere at the edge of the tentorial foramen.

Certain clinical syndromes are suggestive of simultaneous double ipsilateral infarction secondary to ICA occlusion: ipsilateral ocular ischaemia (retinal or anterior) plus contralateral hemispheric infarct (optocerebral syndrome); hemiplegia–hemianopia syndrome, and conduction aphasia with hemiparesis, due to combined anterior or deep MCA plus posterior MCA; mixed transcortical aphasia (isolation of the speech areas) results from the combination of anterior and posterior borderzone infarcts. Acute global aphasia without hemiparesis results from embolism to the anterior and posterior speech areas (30).

Multiple, bilateral infarcts suggest cardiembolism (31).

Combined infarcts as well as massive MCA infarcts are often complicated within 24–96 hours after onset by massive oedema with mass effect. In young and middle-aged patients this may cause clinical deterioration and death, due to brainstem compression (malignant MCA infarct). The NIHSS score typically exceeds 16–20 in dominant hemisphere MCA malignant infarcts and is more than 15–18 in non-dominant hemisphere infarcts.

Predictors of fatal brain oedema include greater than 50% MCA hypodensity, involvement of additional vascular territories (ACA, PCA, anterior choroidal artery), hypertension, heart failure, and increased white blood cell count (32). These patients are candidates for decompressive hemicraniectomy.

Brainstem infarcts

Mesencephalic infarcts

The mesencephalon has four arterial territories: anteromedial or paramedian (paramedian branches of the basilar artery) (Figure 8.8), anterolateral (branches from the P2 segment of the PCA), lateral (branches from P2 segment of PCA and from posterior choroidal arteries), and dorsal or posterior (branches from P1 segment of PCA and superior cerebellar artery). Patients with mesencephalic infarcts can be classified in four groups: (i) those with isolated mesencephalic infarcts, and those whose mesencephalic infarct is accompanied by (ii) proximal infarcts involving the medulla and the posterior-inferior cerebellar artery (PICA) territory (33), by (iii) 'middle' infarcts including the pons and the anterior inferior cerebellar artery (AICA), and by (iv) distal lesions comprising the thalamus and the PCA territory (34). 'Middle' infarcts are the most common.

Most of the pure midbrain infarctions involve the anteromedial and anterolateral midbrain territories. Patients with isolated anteromedial mesencephalic infarcts mainly present with ocular disturbances (third nerve palsy or internuclear ophthalmoplegia) followed by ataxia. Cheiro-oral sensory changes have also been described (35). Lesions usually involve the third nerve fascicles or nucleus (upper midbrain), the medial longitudinal fasciculus (lower midbrain), the red nucleus, and the median part of the cerebral peduncle. A unilateral third nerve nuclear lesion causes bilateral ptosis and superior rectus weakness, divergent strabismus and mydriasis. Fascicular lesions cause unilateral changes with divergent strabismus, unilateral ptosis and mydriasis. Claude's syndrome (ipsilesional third nerve palsy and contralateral ataxia) and Benedikt syndrome (third nerve plus contralateral involuntary movements) are very rare.

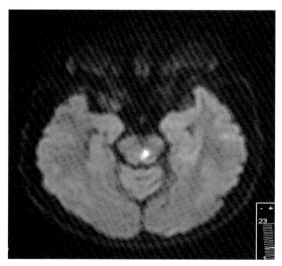

Fig. 8.8 Left paramedian tegmentum midbrain infarct.

Patients with anterolateral midbrain lesions present with ataxic hemiparesis or hypaesthesic ataxic hemiparesis due to involvement of both corticospinal tract and corticopontocerebellar fibres. Patients with lesions in both anteromedial and anterolateral areas show oculomotor disturbances and hemiparesis.

Lateral midbrain lesions cause sensory symptoms due to involvement of laterally located lemniscal sensory fibres.

'Distal' mesencephalic infarcts are associated with consciousness disturbances, gait ataxia, oculomotor disturbances, and visual field defects. 'Middle' strokes have consciousness disturbances, dysarthria, horizontal oculomotor disorders, and paresis, while 'proximal' infarcts produce acute unsteadiness, vertigo, dysphagia, dysphonia, limb ataxia, and paresis. Bilateral ataxia caused by a single lesion could be a localizing sign in patients with pure lower midbrain infarction (36) due to the involvement of crossing efferent dentatorubral fibres at the lower midbrain level.

Patients with mesencephalic infarcts can present with involuntary repetitive stereotyped movements that may be confused with seizures (37). Large artery disease, producing artery-to-artery embolism, and *in situ* thrombosis are the most common mesencephalic infarct mechanisms. Cardioembolism and small-vessel disease account for a quarter of the cases each.

Pontine infarcts

Pontine infarcts (38) have five main clinical patterns: anteromedial, anterolateral, tegmental, unilateral multiple, and bilateral. The anteromedial and anterolateral territories are supplied by the basilar artery, while the lateral territory also receives blood from the superior and anterior inferior cerebellar arteries. The posterior territory is supplied by the superior cerebellar artery.

Pontine infarcts account for 25% of lacunar strokes. The primary morphologies are wedge-shaped tegmental, basal, and tegmentobasal infarcts, caused by paramedian or circumferential basilar branch atheromatous occlusion and smaller, circumscribed lacunar infarcts attributed to lipohyalinosis. Roughly 60% of infarcts are paramedian (Figure 8.9). Pure hemiparesis is the most common presentation, followed by sensorimotor stroke and ataxic hemiparesis. Paramedian pontine infarct can present with crescendo transient ischaemic attacks similar to a capsular warning syndrome (39)

Anterolateral pontine syndromes present with motorsensory deficits associated with tegmental signs in more than half of the patients. Tegmental pontine syndromes (mild motor deficits and sensory deficits together with eye movement and vestibular symptoms and signs) are less common. Unilateral multiple pontine infarcts are always associated with severe sensory-motor deficits and tegmental signs. Bilateral infarcts cause an ominous clinical pattern of transient loss of consciousness, tetraparesis, pseudobulbar palsy, and in some cases locked-in syndrome.

Small lesion in the mediolateral tegmental pons can cause Gasperini syndrome. Main neurological signs are sixth and seventh nerve palsy of the affected side (40). The responsible artery is mainly the long circumferential branch of the anterior inferior cerebellar artery.

Palatal myoclonus and isolated hemifacial spasms can be the only manifestation of a small pontine stroke.

Medullary infarcts

Medullary infarcts can be medial, lateral, or combined. The medial territory is supplied by penetrating vessels from the anterior spinal artery and the distal vertebral artery. The lateral territory main

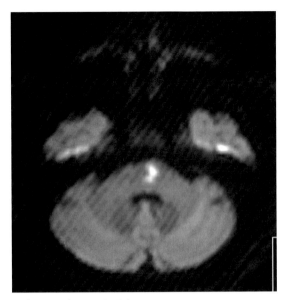

Fig. 8.9 Left paramedian pontine infarct.

arterial supply comes from penetrating arteries from the distal vertebral artery and the posterior inferior cerebellar artery. The small posterior territory is supplied by the posterior spinal artery and the posterior inferior cerebellar artery. The ratio of lateral medullary infarct and medial medullary infarct is approximately 3:1 to 4:1 (41).

Medial medullary infarcts have four major clinical patterns: (i) Dejerine's syndrome (contralateral hemiparesis and pain and thermal sensory loss plus ipsilateral lingual palsy; (ii) sensorimotor stroke without lingual palsy; (iii) hemiparesis, often combined with nystagmus; and (iv) bilateral infarcts.

Lateral infarcts produce a more or less complete Wallenberg's syndrome classically described as: ipsilateral paralysis of the ninth and tenth nerves, loss of pain and temperature sense on the face, ataxia and vestibular signs (nystagmus, ipsilesional lateropulsion) and Horner syndrome, and contralateral dissociated hemianaesthesia. This classical ipsilateral trigeminal-contralateral body pattern was only observed in a quarter of patients in a prospective study (42). Other reported sensory symptoms presentations include: bilateral trigeminal patterns in patients with large, ventrally extending lesions at the middle rostral medulla; isolated contralateral trigeminal patterns in lesions sparing the most posterolateral area of the medulla; isolated body or limb involvement in small lesions (42); isolated dermatomal sensory deficit (43). Trigeminal sensation was found to be inhomogeneously involved among the three divisions and more often of an onion-skin pattern than a divisional pattern (42). Central and peripheral (less commonly) facial palsy can occur in patients with lateral medullary infarcts (44). Nausea and vomiting, hiccups and headache are frequent. Diplopia and oscillopsia are common.

Medial medullary infarcts are often accompanied by a cerebellar infarct. The most common mechanisms are vertebral artery thrombosis or dissection and embolism.

The characteristic symptom in patients with vertebral dissections is pain, most often in the posterior part of the neck or occiput. Combined, or hemimedullary infarcts, cause Babinski–Nageotte syndrome (all the components of the Wallenberg syndrome plus ipsilateral tongue palsy and contralateral hemiplegia). They are usually secondary to occlusion of the vertebral artery.

One first negative MRI DWI on the day of stroke onset may need to be repeated in patients suspected to have medullary infarction based on neurological signs and symptoms. The infarct may only be evident in a latter MRI (45).

Stroke patterns in basilar artery occlusion

Up to 75% of patients with basilar artery occlusion (BAO) have a poor functional outcome despite the use of recanalization therapies (46). Basilar artery thrombosis may present as a locked-in syndrome, as a midbrain syndrome, a top of the basilar syndrome or as partial syndromes. BAO can occur suddenly, without warning signs. More often its onset is subacute, with heralding TIAs or a progressive course with additive neurological deficits. The final neurological picture is reached within 6 hours in about one-third of the patients, in 6–24 hours in another third, and up to 72 hours in the remaining patients. The most common initial symptoms are motor weakness, dysarthria, vertigo, nausea/vomiting, and headache. The most common initial signs, which can be bilateral, are motor deficits, facial palsies, eye movement abnormalities, pupillary abnormalities, lower cranial nerve deficits, somnolence and sometimes, stupor and bilateral extensor plantar responses (47). The outcome is invariably poor in patients with disorders of consciousness or a combination of dysarthria, pupillary disorders, and involvement of the lower cranial nerves, while if these factors are absent only 11% have a poor outcome (48). The typical syndrome of basilar artery embolism (49) is an acute loss of consciousness followed by multiple brainstem symptoms and infarcts at several levels (thalamus—PCA, midbrain, pons). Usually clinical symptoms improve quickly and even completely.

Cerebellar infarcts

Cerebellar infarcts can be territorial (superior cerebellar artery, anterior inferior cerebellar artery, posterior inferior cerebellar artery, and combined), borderzone, or lacunar. They are often combined with brainstem infarcts and with superficial PCA or thalamic infarcts. The most common isolated cerebellar infarcts are located in the superior cerebellar artery and posterior inferior cerebellar artery territories (50–52).

Superior cerebellar artery

The superior cerebellar artery (SCA) territory has two divisions: lateral and medial. Full SCA infarcts are usually accompanied by PCA or brainstem infarcts. They can be oedematous and have a malignant course. Partial infarcts are often pure cerebellar infarcts and have a benign course. Embolism is the predominant stroke mechanism in SCA territory infarction. Their clinical presentation ranges from severe patterns such as coma with quadriplegia and oculomotor disturbances, due to simultaneous brainstem infarct, or top of the basilar syndrome, with concomitant involvement of the mesencephalon and PCA territories, to more limited and benign presentations. The classical Mills–Guillain syndrome (ipsilateral cerebellar ataxia, Horner syndrome, contralateral pain, temperature sensory loss, and fourth nerve palsy) is rare and due to concomitant involvement of the pontine territory of the SCA. Tremor and other involuntary movements can be present, due to ischaemia of the superior cerebellar peduncle. Other patients have only a cerebellovestibular syndrome. Dysarthria is almost always present. Lateral SCA infarcts are the most common form of pure SCA infarcts and involve the anterior rostral cerebellum. They cause ipsilateral limb ataxia and lateropulsion and dysarthria.

Medial SCA infarcts are less well described and cause ataxia and dysarthria. They can present as an isolated body lateropulsion (53).

Patients with a SCA infarct are reported to have a lower incidence of vertigo and headache than patients with other cerebellar infarction.

Anterior inferior cerebellar artery

AICA infarcts are rarer than other cerebellar territorial infarcts. Symptoms of AICA territory infarct result from damage to the inferolateral pons, the middle cerebellar peduncle, and the flocculus. Frequently, AICA infarcts occur with other territories or are multiple. They almost always have a concomitant pontine infarct and their main cause is thrombosis superimposed on atheromatous stenosis in the distal vertebral artery or proximal basilar artery. Their clinical presentation has four major patterns: (i) coma with tetraplegia, due to pontine infarct; (ii) the classic AICA syndrome is the most frequent presenting pattern, featuring ipsilateral involvement of the fifth, seventh, and eighth cranial nerves with hearing loss, vertigo, vomiting, tinnitus, facial palsy and facial sensory loss, Horner syndrome, appendicular ataxia, contralateral temperature, and pain sensory loss; (iii) pure vestibular syndrome, with isolated vertigo; and (iv) isolated cerebellar signs.

Posterior inferior cerebellar artery

This is the common type of cerebellar stroke (Figure 8.10). If the medulla is involved, a more or less complete dorsal lateral medullary syndrome (Wallenberg syndrome) results: ipsilesional vestibular (vertigo, vomiting, nystagmus, lateropulsion), fifth, ninth, tenth cranial nerve palsies, Horner syndrome, and appendicular ataxia with contralesional loss of pain and temperature sensation. Hiccups are frequent and prolonged. If the medulla is spared, patients present with headache, vertigo, nystagmus, ipsilateral axial lateropulsion, gait, and appendicular ataxia.

Infarcts involving the nodulus can cause isolated acute vertigo, mimicking a vestibular disease. Infarcts restricted to the cerebellum are generally small and have a benign course. They can involve the

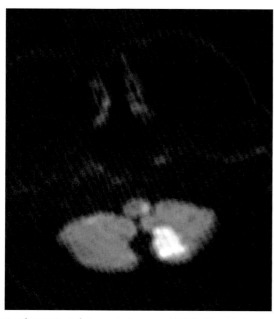

Fig. 8.10 Left posterior inferior cerebellar artery (PICA) infarct. Notice the laterobulbar extension.

medial and less often the lateral PICA subterritories. PICA infarcts combined with AICA or SCA can assume a pseudotumoural form or present as coma with tetraplegia. Medial PICA infarcts can produce: isolate vertigo; vertigo, axial lateropulsion, and dysmetria; Wallenberg syndrome, if the medulla is also involved. Lateral PICA infarcts are very rare and present with vertigo and ipsilateral dysmetria. PICA lesions but not SCA lesions can result in cognitive and affective deficits pointing to a role of posterior cerebellar regions in cognitive and affective processing (54).

Pseudotumoural cerebellar infarcts

Large cerebellar infarcts (more than one-third of the cerebellar hemisphere) can produce mass effect and lead to clinical deterioration and death. Such patients usually have combined territorial cerebellar infarcts, a full territorial PICA or SCA infarct, or infarcts confined to the medial vermian branches of the PICA or SCA. The most frequent mechanisms of infarction are large vessel occlusion, due to large artery disease or cardioembolism. These patients progress from a cerebellar syndrome to brainstem signs development and consciousness fluctuation. If untreated, coma will ensue. These infarcts with mass effect cause increased intracranial hypertension in the posterior fossa, brainstem compression, obstructive hydrocephalus, and herniation. Clinical deterioration may start hours or days after stroke onset.

Clinical stroke subtyping classification

Using clinical neurological findings the Oxfordshire Community Stroke Project (OCSP) classification divides strokes into four subgroups, locating them either to the territory of the anterior (total anterior circulation infarct, TACI; partial anterior circulation infarct, PACI; lacunar anterior circulation infarct, LACI) or posterior circulation (posterior circulation infarct, POCI) (55). The correspondence between this clinical classification and the imaging findings is not perfect, positive predictive value ranging from 71–83 (56). Nevertheless the OCSP is clinically useful. It is easy to communicate and predicts aetiology, case fatality, functional recovery, risk of stroke recurrence, complications, and average cost of hospitalization (57). TACIs have the highest mortality while LACIs have the lowest. The risk of recurrence is higher for PACI and POCI.

Other classifications such as the TOAST criteria, redefined to SSS-TOAST and the ASCO classification are mainly directed to stroke mechanism and aetiology and essentially rely on data conveyed by ancillary diagnostic tests. They have in account a smaller number of clinical data, that mainly refer to the distinction between cardioembolic and lacunar infarcts (58, 59).

Cardioembolic infarcts

Decreased consciousness at onset, sudden onset to maximal defect with rapid regression of symptoms, aphasia, neglect, and visual field defects are more common in cardioembolic than other types of stroke. Headache, seizure at onset, or onset during activity are not specific for cardioembolic stroke (60, 61). Stroke syndromes such as isolated Wernicke's aphasia, global aphasia without hemiparesis, Wallenberg syndrome, and top of the basilar syndrome are suggestive of cardioembolism.

Simultaneous or sequential strokes in different arterial territories, multilevel posterior circulation infarcts, simultaneous infarcts in the three subterritories of the MCA, and haemorrhagic transformation of an ischaemic infarct also point to a cardiac origin for the stroke (62, 63).

Lacunar syndromes

There are five main classical lacunar syndromes: pure motor, pure sensory, motorsensory, ataxic hemiparesis, and clumsy hand dysarthria. Pure motorsensory is considered the most specific lacunar syndrome (64). Although lacunar syndromes are considered suggestive of small deep infarctions (<1.5 cm) resulting from obstruction of a perforating artery, lacunar syndromes not due to lacunar infarcts can be found (65). A prospective study with MRI that evaluated the accuracy of the OCSP classification, reported a positive predictive value of 39% for the lacunar syndrome infarct (LACI) (66). In patients presenting a lacunar syndrome clinically it is important to exclude concomitant minute cortical infarcts by MRI DWI. The presence of such cortical infarcts point to embolism as the cause of stroke, while its absence indicates that small-vessel perforator occlusion was the likely mechanism of stroke (67).

References

1. Oppenheim CR, Stanescu D, Dormont S, Crozier S, Marro B, Samson Y, et al. False-negative diffusion-weighted MR findings in acute ischemic stroke. *AJNR Am J Neuroradiol.* 2000;21:1434–1440.
2. Van Overbeek EC, Knottnerus IL, van Oostenbrugge RJ. Disappearing hyperdense middle cerebral artery sign is associated with striatocapsular infarcts on follow-up CT in ischemic stroke patients treated with intravenous thrombolysis. *Cerebrovasc Dis.* 2010;30:285–289.
3. Bogousslavsky J, Caplan LR. *Stroke Syndromes* (2nd edn). Cambridge: Cambridge University Press; 2001.
4. Gorelick PB (ed). *Atlas of Cerebrovascular Disease. Philadelphia, PA: Churchill Livingstone; 1996.*
5. Heinsius T, Bogousslavsky J, van Melle G. Large infarcts in the middle cerebral artery territory. Etiology and outcome patterns. *Neurology.* 1998;50:341–350.
6. Huffman J, Stern TA. Acute psychiatric manifestations of stroke: a clinical case conference. *Psychosomatics.* 2003;44:65–75.
7. Ois A, Cuadrado-Godia E, Solano A, Perich-Alsina X, Roquer J. Acute ischemic stroke in anterior choroidal artery territory. *J Neurol Sci.* 2009;281:80–84.
8. Palomeras E, Fossas P, Cano AT, Sanz P, Floriach M. Anterior choroidal artery infarction: a clinical, etiologic and prognostic study. *Acta Neurol Scand.* 2008;118:42–47.
9. Han SW, Sohn YH, Lee PH, Suh BC, Choi IS. Pure homonymous hemianopia due to anterior choroidal artery territory infarction. *Eur Neurol.* 2000;43:35–38.
10. Leys D, Mounier-Vehier F, Lavenu I, Rondepierre P, Pruvo JP. Anteriorchoroidal artery territory infarcts. Study of presumed mechanisms. *Stroke.* 1994;25:837–842.
11. Bogousslavsky J, Regli F, Uske A. Thalamic infarcts: clinical syndromes, etiology and prognosis. *Neurology.* 1988;38:837–848.
12. Schmahmann JD. Vascular syndromes of the thalamus. *Stroke.* 2003;34:2264–2278.
13. Studer A, Georgiadis D, Baumgartner RW. Ischemic infarct involving all arterial territories of the thalamus. *Acta Neurol Scand.* 2003;107:423–425.
14. Melo TP, Bogousslavsky J, Moulin T, Nader J, Regli F. Thalamic ataxia. *J Neurol.* 1992;239:331–337.
15. Melo TP, Bogousslvasky J. Hemiataxia-hypesthesia: a thalamic stroke syndrome. *J Neurol Neurosurg Psych.* 1992;55:581–584.
16. Bogousslavsky J, Caplan LR. Vertebrobasilar occlusive disease: review of selected aspects. 3 thalamic infarcts. *Cerebrovasc Dis.* 19933:193–205.
17. Kumral E, Evyapan D, Balkir K, Kutluhan S. Bilateral thalamic infarction. Clinical, etiological and MRI correlates. *Acta Neurol Scand.* 2001;103:35–42.
18. Saeki N, Shimazaki K, Yamaura A. Isolated infarction in the territory of lateral posterior choroidal arteries. *J Neurol Neurosurg Psychiatry.* 1999;67:413–415.
19. Cals N, Devuyst G, Afsar N, Karapanayiotides T, Bogousslavsky J. Pure superficial posterior cerebral artery territory infarction in The Lausanne Stroke Registry. *J Neurol.* 2002;249:855–861.
20. Georgiadis AL, Yamamoto Y, Kwan ED, Pessin MS, Caplan LR. Anatomy of sensory findings in patients with posterior cerebral artery territory infarction. *Arch Neurol.* 1999;56:835–838.
21. Montavont A, Nighoghossian N, Hermier M, Derex L, Berthezène Y, Philippeau E, et al. Hemiplegia in posterior cerebral artery occlusion: acute MRI assessment. *Cerebrovasc Dis.* 2003;16(4) :452–453.
22. Brandt T, Steinke W, Thie A, Pessin MS, Caplan LR. Posterior cerebral artery territory infarcts: clinical features, infarct topography, causes and outcome. Multicenter results and a review of the literature. *Cerebrovasc Dis.* 2000;10:170–182.
23. Cappellari M, Tomelleri G, Di Matteo A, Carletti M, Magalini A, Bovi P, et al. Dide-Botcazo syndrome due to bilateral occlusion of posterior cerebral artery. *Neurol Sci.* 2010;31:99–101.
24. Kumral E, Bayulkem G, Evyapan D, Yunten N. Spectrum of anterior cerebral artery territory infarction: clinical and MRI findings. *Eur J Neurol.* 2002;9 :615–624.
25. Kang SY, Kim JS. Anterior cerebral artery infarction: stroke mechanism and clinical-imaging study in 100 patients. *Neurology.* 2008;70:2386–2393.
26. Wolff V, Saint Maurice JP, Ducros A, Guichard JP, Woimant F. Akinetic mutism and anterior bicerebral infarction due to abnormal distribution of the anterior cerebral artery. *Rev Neurol.* 2002;158:377–380.
27. Della Sala S, Francescani A, Spinnler H. Gait apraxia after bilateral supplementary motor area lesion. *J Neurol Neurosurg Psychiatry.* 2002;72:77–85.
28. Kobayashi S, Maki T, Kunimoto M. Clinical symptoms of bilateral anterior cerebral artery territory infarction. *J Clin Neurosci.* 2011;18:218–22.
29. Boccardi E, Della Sala S, Motto C, Spinnler H. Utilisation behaviour consequent to bilateral SMA softening. *Cortex.* 2002;38:289–308.
30. Kumral E. Multiple, multilevel and bihemispheric infarcts. In Bogousslavsky J, Caplan L (eds) *Stroke Syndromes* (pp. 499–511). Cambridge: Cambridge University Press; 2001.
31. Timsit SG, Sacco RL, Mohr JP, Foulkes MA, Tatemichi TK, Wolf PA, et al. Early clinical differentiation of cerebral infarction from severe atherosclerotic stenosis and cardioembolism. *Stroke.* 1992;23:486–491.
32. Kasner SE, Demchuk AM, Berrouschot J, Schmutzhard E, Harms L, Verro P, et al. Predictors of fatal brain edema in massive hemispheric ischemic stroke. *Stroke.* 2001;32:2117–2123.
33. Kumral E, Afsar N, Kirbas D, Balkir K, Ozdemirkiran T. Spectrum of medial medullary infarction: clinical and magnetic resonance imaging findings. *J Neurol.* 2002;249:85–93.
34. Martin PJ, Chang HM, Wityk R, Caplan LR. Midbrain infarction: associations and aetiologies in the New England Medical Center Posterior Circulation Registry. *J Neurol Neurosurg Psychiatry.* 1998;64:392–395.
35. Kim JS, Kim J. Pure midbrain infarction: clinical, radiologic, and pathophysiologic findings. *Neurology.* 2005;64:1227–1232.
36. Zhu Y, Liu HN, Zhang CD. Wernekinck commissure syndrome is a pure midbrain infarction. *J Clin Neurosci.* 2010;17:1091–1092.
37. Saposnik G, Caplan LR. Convulsive-like movements in brainstem stroke. *Arch Neurol.* 2001;58:654–657.
38. Kumral E, Bayulkem G, Evyapan D. Clinical spectrum of pontine infarction clinical-MRI correlations. *J Neurol.* 2002;249:1659–1670.
39. Muengtaweepongsa S, Singh NN, Cruz-Flores S. Pontine warning syndrome: case series and review of literature. *J Stroke Cerebrovasc Dis.* 2010;19:353–356.
40. Hayashi-Hayata M, Nakayasu H, Doi M, Fukada Y, Murakami T, Nakashima K. Gasperini syndrome, a report of two cases. *Intern Med.* 200;46:129–133.
41. Kameda W, Kawanami T, Kurita K, Daimon M, Kayama T, Hosoya T, et al. Lateral and medial medullary infarction: a comparative analysis of 214 patients. *Stroke.* 2004;35:694–699.

42. Kim JS, Lee JH, Lee MC. Patterns of sensory dysfunction in lateral medullary infarction. Clinical-MRI correlation. *Neurology*. 1997;49: 1557–1563.

43. Song IU, Kim JS, Lee DG, An JY, Ryu SY, Lee SB, *et al*. Pure sensory deficit at the t4 sensory level as an isolated manifestation of lateral medullary infarction. *J Clin Neurol*. 2007;3:112–115.

44. Park JH, Yoo HU, Shin HW. Peripheral type facial palsy in a patient with dorsolateral medullary infarction with infranuclear involvement of the caudal pons. *J Stroke Cerebrovasc Dis*. 2008;17:263–265.

45. Fukuoka T, Takeda H, Dembo T, Nagoya H, Kato Y, Deguchi I, *et al*. Clinical review of 37 patients with medullary infarction. *J Stroke Cerebrovasc Dis*. 2011; 21(7):594–599.

46. Schonewille WJ, Wijman CA, Michel P, Rueckert CM, Weimar C, Mattle HP, *et al*. Treatment and outcomes of acute basilar artery occlusion in the Basilar Artery International Cooperation Study (BASICS): a prospective registry study. *Lancet Neurol*. 2009;8:724–730.

47. von Campe G, Regli F, Bogousslavsky J. Heralding manifestations of basilar artery occlusion with lethal or severe stroke. *J Neurol Neurosurg Psychiatry*. 2003;74:1621–1626.

48. Devuyst G, Bogousslavsky J, Meuli R, Moncayo J, de Freitas G, van Melle G. Stroke or transient ischemic attacks with basilar artery stenosis or occlusion: clinical patterns and outcome. *Arch Neurol*. 2002 ;59 :567–573.

49. Schwarz S, Egelhof T, Schwab S, Hacke W. Basilar artery embolism. Clinical syndrome and neuroradiologic patterns in patients without permanent occlusion of the basilar artery. *Neurology*. 1997;49: 1346–1352.

50. Kumral E, Kisabay A, Atac C. Lesion patterns and etiology of ischemia in superior cerebellar artery territory infarcts. *Cerebrovasc Dis*. 2005;19:283–290.

51. Kumral E, Kisabay A, Ataç C. Lesion patterns and etiology of ischemia in the anterior inferior cerebellar artery territory involvement: a clinical—diffusion weighted—MRI study. *Eur J Neurol*. 2006;13(4):395–401.

52. Amarenco P, Lévy C, Cohen A, Touboul PJ, Roullet E, Bousser MG. Causes and mechanisms of territorial and nonterritorial cerebellar infarcts in 115 consecutive cases. *Stroke*. 1994;25:105–112.

53. Lee H. Isolated body lateropulsion caused by a lesion of the rostral vermis. *J Neurol Sci*. 2006;249:172–174.

54. Exner C, Weniger G, Irle E. Cerebellar lesions in the PICA but not SCA territory impair cognition. *Neurology*. 2004;63(11):2132–2135.

55. Bamford J, Sandercock P, Dennis M, Burn J, Warlow C. Classification and natural history of clinically identifiable subtypes of cerebral infarction. *Lancet*. 1991;337:1521–1526.

56. Mead GE, Lewis SC, Wardlaw JM, Dennis MS, Warlow CP. How well does Oxforshire Community Stroke Project classification predict the site and size of the infarct on brain imaging? *J Neurol Neurosurg Psychiatry*. 2000;68:558–562.

57. Pinto AN, Melo TP, Lourenço ME, Leandro MJ, Brázio A, Carvalho L, *et al*. Can a clinical classification of stroke predict complications and treatments during hospitalization? *Cerebrovasc Dis*. 1998;8:204–209.

58. Ay H, Furie KL, Singhal A, Smith WS, Sorensen AG, Koroshetz WJ. An evidence-based causative classification system for acute ischemic stroke. *Ann Neurol*. 2005;58(5):688–697.

59. Amarenco P, Bogousslavsky J, Caplan LR, Donnan GA, Hennerici MG. New approach t stroke subtyping: the A-S-C-O (phenotypic) classification of stroke. *Cerebrovasc Dis*. 2009;27:502–508.

60. Arboix A, Oliveres M, Massons J, Pujades R, Garcia-Eroles L. Early differentiation of cardioembolic from atherothrombotic cerebral infarction: a multivariate analysis. *Eur J Neurol*. 1999;6:677–683.

61. Kittner SJ, Sharkness CM, Sloan MA, Price TR, Dambrosia JM, Tuhrim S, *et al*. Infarcts with a cardiac source of embolism in the NINDS Stroke Data Bank: neurologic examination. *Neurology*. 1992;42:299–302.

62. Ramirez-Lassepas M, Cipolle RJ, Bjork RJ, Bjork RJ, Kowitz J, Snyder BD. Can embolic stroke be diagnosed on the basis of neurologic clinical criteria? *Arch Neurol*. 1987;44(1):87–89.

63. Ferro JM. Brain embolism—Answers to practical questions. *J Neurol*. 2003;250:139–147.

64. Arboix A, Massons J, García-Eroles L, Targa C, Comes E, Parra O. Clinical predictors of lacunar syndrome not due to lacunar infarction. *BMC Neurol*. 2010 May 18;10:31.

65. Ferro JM. Cardioembolic stroke: an update. *Lancet Neurol*. 2003;2:177–188.

66. Asdaghi N, Jeerakathil T, Hameed B, Saini M, McCombe JA, Shuaib A, *et al*. Oxfordshire Community Stroke Project classification poorly differentiates small cortical and subcortical infarcts. *Stroke*. 2011;42:2143–2148.

67. De Reuck J, De Groote L, VanMaele G. The classic lacunar syndromes: clinical and neuroimaging correlates. *Eur J Neurol*. 2008;15(7):681–614.

CHAPTER 9

Diagnosing transient ischaemic attack and stroke

Bruce Campbell and Stephen Davis

Transient ischaemic attack and ischaemic stroke

Recent changes to the diagnostic approach to ischaemic stroke and transient ischaemic attack (TIA) have removed the previous arbitrary distinction of stroke and TIA based on symptom duration of more or less than 24 hours. TIA is now defined as 'a transient episode of neurological dysfunction caused by focal brain, spinal cord, or retinal ischaemia, without acute infarction' (1). The identification of infarction requires brain imaging. However, accurate diagnosis depends heavily on the type of brain imaging being used as there is a major difference in sensitivity between non-contrast computed tomography (CT) and diffusion magnetic resonance imaging (MRI) (2). Nonetheless, it emphasizes the central role of imaging in the diagnosis of ischaemic syndromes.

Non-contrast CT

The introduction of non-contrast CT in the 1970s revolutionized stroke care. For the first time, the distinction between haemorrhage and infarction could be accurately made during life. Progressive technological improvements have allowed delineation of more subtle pathology than was possible with early scanners.

Early ischaemic changes

The attenuation difference between normal grey and white matter can now be visualized. Loss of this grey-white differentiation is evidence of irreversible injury (although inter-rater agreement and sensitivity in the first few hours after stroke are imperfect) (Figure 9.1A). More established infarction is hypodense due to increased water content (Figure 9.1B). Another early sign reported in ischaemic stroke is focal swelling. In contrast to loss of grey–white differentiation, focal swelling probably represents increased blood volume within ischaemic penumbra and appears to be salvageable with reperfusion (3).

Hyperdense arteries

Another early finding that can confirm the diagnosis of stroke, even if loss of grey–white differentiation has not yet occurred, is a hyperdense artery sign representing acute thrombus (Figure 9.1C, D). This has been described in the middle cerebral artery (MCA) both proximally and in the Sylvian fissure (MCA 'dot' sign), the basilar artery, the carotid artery, and the posterior cerebral arteries (4–8). Sensitivity for hyperdense arteries can be improved by reformatting the standard thick CT slices to 0.75–1.5 mm thin slices that reduce the effect of partial voluming of artery with cerebrospinal fluid (CSF) (9). This can be achieved without any extra radiation and can be a very useful indicator of arterial occlusion when intravenous contrast is contraindicated. With the exception of those patients with generalized arterial calcification, the hyperdense artery signs are strongly associated with focal arterial occlusion and generally worse outcome (depending on the success of reperfusion therapies) (10).

Diagnosing mimics

Apart from these relatively subtle signs that indicate early ischaemia, the main use of non-contrast CT has been to exclude differential diagnoses. Intracerebral haemorrhage (ICH) is hyperdense and generally obvious. Subdural haemorrhage, when acute, is hyperdense and usually obvious. However, subacute subdural blood can appear isodense to brain and evade detection by the unwary eye. Subarachnoid haemorrhage is usually obvious on CT although sensitivity does decline over time. Earlier studies quoted sensitivity of 93–95% within 24 hours dropping to 85% at 3 days and 50% at 1 week (11–13). However, a more recent large series found 100% sensitivity within 3 days of onset with modern CT scanners (14).

Focal 'convexal' subarachnoid haemorrhage is an increasingly recognized phenomenon and enters the differential diagnosis of TIA (Figure 9.2). In the elderly this generally reflects amyloid angiopathy. MRI T2*-weighted sequences, especially susceptibility-weighted imaging (SWI), often demonstrate multiple cortical cerebral microbleeds. The usual clinical presentation in these patients is transient migratory sensory phenomena in the absence of headache. This is in contrast to younger patients when convexal subarachnoid is often accompanied by thunderclap headache and warrants detailed investigation for vascular malformation, cortical vein thrombosis, or reversible cerebral vasoconstriction syndrome (15). Many tumours are hypodense although highly cellular neoplasms (e.g. lymphoma) can be hyperdense, albeit not to the degree of a haematoma. In most cases the clinical features and temporal course are sufficient to distinguish infarction from tumour.

Temporal evolution of ischaemia

Other changes can occur over time in ischaemic stroke that can sometimes confuse interpretation of non-contrast CT. Haemorrhagic transformation is part of the natural evolution of stroke. Minor haemorrhagic infarction is of no clinical consequence and very common in infarcts followed carefully over

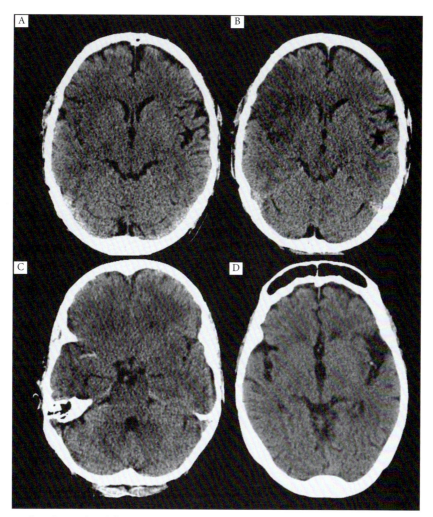

Fig. 9.1 (A) Early ischaemic change—loss of grey-white differentiation in the insular ribbon/frontal operculum. (B) Established infarction 24 hours later. (C) Hyperdense M1 segment of middle cerebral artery. (D) Hyperdense M2 segment of middle cerebral artery (Sylvian 'dot' sign).

time (16). More significant parenchymal haematoma with mass effect is more common after reperfusion, especially after thrombolysis, and can occasionally make the differentiation between haemorrhagic transformation of infarction and primary ICH difficult. MRI may be helpful in these cases. As the blood–brain barrier loses integrity in the days following stroke, contrast enhancement is observed. Occasionally, surrounding vasogenic oedema and contrast enhancement in a subacute infarct can mimic tumour, in which case MRI may indicate the true diagnosis (Figure 9.3).

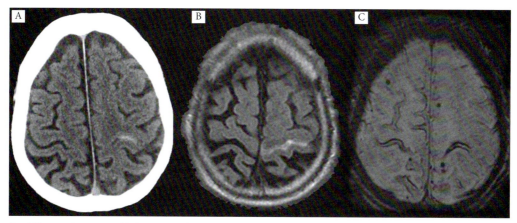

Fig. 9.2 Focal subarachnoid haemorrhage in an elderly patient with transient right arm sensory disturbance. (A) Non-contrast CT demonstrating hyperdensity in the central sulcus. (B) Fluid-attenuated inversion recovery (FLAIR) MRI. (C) Susceptibility-weighted imaging (SWI) demonstrating more widespread siderosis and cortical microbleeds consistent with amyloid angiopathy.

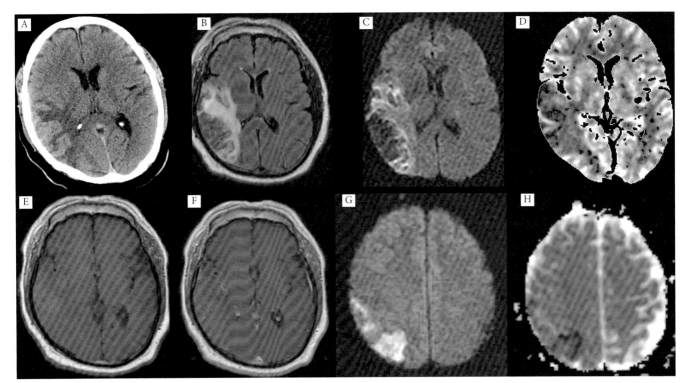

Fig. 9.3   Subacute infarct mimicking tumour. (A) Non-contrast CT. (B) Fluid attenuated inversion recovery (FLAIR) MRI. (C) Diffusion MRI. (D) Reduced cerebral blood volume in the lesion would be unusual in high-grade tumour. (E) T1. (F) T1 post-gadolinium demonstrating contrast enhancement. (G) True restricted diffusion in a higher slice confirmed by (H) reduced apparent diffusion coefficient (ADC).

'Fogging' is a phenomenon of reduced infarct conspicuity that can occur around 2–3 weeks post infarction (17). Fortunately this is not a common time for patients to present for the first time and, with modern scanners, the appearance is unlikely to be entirely normal. Finally, it is important to remember that infarcts atrophy (liquefactive necrosis) over time. After the initial oedema resolves, atrophy takes place over several weeks and is relatively stable beyond 1 month (18). This is particularly relevant to the interpretation of research where late infarct volume is measured to assess infarct growth or tissue salvage compared to baseline imaging. Delayed final infarct assessments will underestimate the volume of infarcted tissue. Volume loss is, however, also useful in distinguishing late infarction from tumours which exhibit positive mass effect.

Diffusion MRI

Diffusion MRI is an echoplanar technique that measures the natural random Brownian motion of water molecules. Cell structure can restrict this motion—often in certain directions more than others ('anisotropy')—which can be detected by measuring diffusion in several different vectors. The average diffusivity is reduced in acute ischaemic stroke, thought to be due to the extracellular to intracellular shift of water that occurs in cytotoxic oedema (19). Diffusion imaging is currently the most sensitive modality for ischaemic injury and becomes abnormal within minutes of vessel occlusion (20). Diffusion restriction is, however, not unique to ischaemia and can occur, often with a more patchy appearance, in demyelination and tumours (usually high grade). Mature cerebral abscesses exhibit

marked central diffusion restriction in the necrotic core. The directionality of diffusion anisotropy is harnessed in the technique of diffusion tensor imaging to perform white matter fibre-tracking.

Diffusion images are acquired as a B-zero (T2-weighted) image followed by application of a strong magnetic field gradient (e.g. B1000) that probes the degree of water diffusion in several directions (at least three orthogonal planes). The acquisition is rapid, generally taking 1–2 minutes, and is therefore relatively robust, even in unco-operative stroke patients. The 'diffusion-weighted image (DWI)' presented clinically is the averaged B1000 directional images. The apparent diffusion coefficient (ADC) is calculated using the B-zero and B1000 images and provides a quantitative measurement of water diffusion with low values (hypointense regions) representing ischaemic tissue. Whenever a lesion appears bright on DWI it is important to check whether the ADC is reduced in the corresponding region (Figure 9.3G, H). DWI is a T2-weighted sequence and lesions bright on T2 can 'shine through' and appear bright on DWI. They will, however, have increased ADC. This rule becomes difficult in very small lesions where the reduced visual conspicuity on ADC can prevent assessment. It is important to note that ADC increases with time after stroke onset due to increasing vasogenic oedema. This normalization of the ADC typically occurs around 3–5 days after ischaemic stroke. DWI remains bright due to the combination of true restriction and T2 signal for a variable time that relates to infarct size, ranging from days in small lesions to several weeks in large lesions (21). This can be very useful clinically to determine whether symptoms are due to acute ischaemia or exacerbation of chronic lesions.

Do diffusion lesions reverse?

Significant controversy has surrounded the potential reversibility of diffusion lesions. Although suggested as a marker of irreversible injury, several animal and human studies have reported normalization of diffusion abnormalities (22). Some of these studies have been flawed by lack of correction for the natural atrophy of infarcts over time. Others have been confounded by temporary 'reversal' that occurs in the hours following reperfusion but returns on later follow-up. This phenomenon may reflect initial restoration of energy status after reperfusion followed by secondary injury. In rats, brief periods of ischaemia of approximately 10 minutes lead to DWI lesions that undergo complete radiological reversal (23). However, histological neuronal loss is detectable even with these brief insults and human studies using highly sensitive techniques such as magnetization transfer imaging demonstrate abnormalities that extend well beyond the extent of infarction visible using conventional fluid attenuated inversion recovery (FLAIR) imaging (24). The clinical implications of milder tissue damage remain unclear. However, for clinical purposes, brain regions that have exhibited diffusion restriction very rarely return to normal (25, 26).

As the definitive histological changes of infarction take time and are not present early after stroke when imaging is usually performed to estimate the region of irreversible injury, the term 'ischaemic core' has been recommended for imaging-based estimates of ischaemic brain tissue that is irreversibly injured and will proceed to infarction even in the presence of immediate reperfusion (27). DWI is the favoured method for assessing ischaemic core.

FLAIR/T2-weighted MRI

The principle of T2-weighted MRI is that water molecules aligned in the MRI magnetic field are excited by a radiofrequency pulse. The rate of 'relaxation' back to their original position is altered by local tissue properties and provides imaging contrast. Tissues with increased water content, which conveniently includes most cerebral pathologies (e.g. stroke, tumour, demyelination, abscess), appear hyperintense on T2-weighted imaging. CSF also appears bright and, to improve delineation from pathology, an inversion pulse can be used to attenuate signal from pure water (FLAIR). Due to technical factors such as CSF motion, FLAIR is less successful in the posterior fossa. Importantly, CSF that contains blood (subarachnoid haemorrhage) or other cellular material (neutrophils in meningitis or tumour cells in leptomeningeal carcinomatosis) does not suppress with the inversion pulse and is therefore clearly visible. FLAIR is also hyperintense in slow-flowing vessels—a phenomenon described in leptomeningeal collateral vessels in ischaemic stroke (Figure 9.4).

FLAIR imaging has been proposed as a 'tissue clock'—a means of judging stroke onset time when this cannot be ascertained on history. Most infarcts develop FLAIR hyperintensity over the first few hours after stroke. Beyond 4.5 hours, most patients have visible FLAIR hyperintensity. The lack of FLAIR hyperintensity would therefore usually imply onset within 3 hours (28). However, this has limited sensitivity—in this study 58% of infarcts within 3 hours of onset had established FLAIR hyperintensity.

Perfusion imaging

Perfusion imaging can be performed with CT or MRI and tracks an intravenous contrast bolus as it circulates through the brain (see Video 9.1 online). Ischaemic stroke results from vessel occlusion and this leads to a varying degree of collateral flow through the

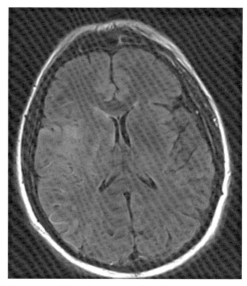

Fig. 9.4 Fluid-attenuated inversion recovery (FLAIR) imaging—CSF signal is nulled by the inversion pulse. This patient has early hyperintensity due to right middle cerebral artery infarction with hyperintense leptomeningeal vessels indicating slow collateral flow.

endogenous bypass mechanisms of the circle of Willis and leptomeningeal vessels. Collateral blood flow is delayed, dispersed, and reduced compared to the normal contralateral structures. Each image voxel in perfusion imaging has its own concentration-time curve and this can be mathematically manipulated to produce more easily interpretable maps of perfusion parameters (Figure 9.5). Time to peak (TTP) is simply the time taken for contrast to reach its peak concentration in any particular image voxel. As the absolute TTP depends on extracerebral factors such as cardiac output and injection timing, it is more meaningful to normalize TTP to the unaffected hemisphere. TTP is increased in regions of collateral flow. It is also mildly increased (usually by 1–2 seconds compared to contralateral) in severe arterial stenosis. The geographic pattern of TTP prolongation is a good indicator of the site of vessel occlusion and can direct closer scrutiny of distal branches on CT/MR angiography images. Cerebral blood volume (CBV) is the area under the concentration-time curve for each voxel. Normal CBV differs in grey matter (~4%) versus white matter (~2%) and is reduced in irreversibly damaged brain. This has been proposed to reflect collapse of ischaemic capillaries that have lost autoregulatory capacity. The evidence for this is, however, scant and it may simply reflect the marked reduction in contrast access to these severely hypoperfused regions.

Deconvolution is a complex mathematical procedure that attempts to model the concentration-time curve that would occur after an instantaneous bolus of contrast (29). In reality, the bolus is generally dispersed over 5–10 seconds but by using an 'arterial input function' (AIF) this 'tissue residue function' can be estimated. In stroke, the contralateral middle cerebral artery is usually chosen as the AIF. This, however, bears little resemblance to the true contrast bolus feeding the stroke-affected territory via collaterals. This is controversial, but the main benefit of deconvolution could therefore be argued to be normalization to the contralateral hemisphere to remove effects of extracerebral factors. There are also several variants of deconvolution

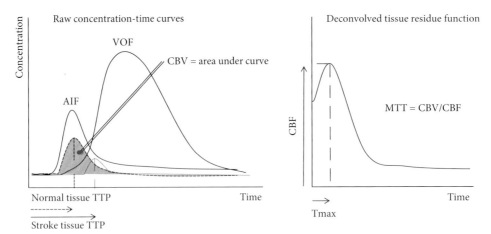

Fig. 9.5 Concentration time curve and the tissue residue function after deconvolution with an arterial input function (AIF) indicating derivation of common perfusion parameters. Time to Peak (TTP) and Tmax represent the delay to peak concentration in the raw and deconvolved curves respectively and are increased in hypoperfused regions. Cerebral blood volume (CBV) is calculated as the area under the curve. Cerebral blood flow (CBF) is proportional to the peak height of the tissue residue function. Mean transit time (MTT) is calculated as CBV/CBF. The venous outflow function (VOF) can be used to scale CT perfusion to provide quantitative CBF values.

which provide slightly different results. Parameters derived from deconvolution include Tmax (time to peak of the deconvolved tissue residue function), MTT (mean transit time), and cerebral blood flow (CBF). Much like TTP, Tmax is increased in regions of collateral flow.

Perfusion thresholds

In the DEFUSE and EPITHET studies of MR-based selection for stroke thrombolysis, Tmax was the preferred perfusion parameter (30, 31). Data from these studies and positron emission tomography (PET) research have indicated that a relatively stringent threshold (>5–6 seconds delay) is necessary to separate 'benign oligaemia' (tissue that will not infarct, even without reperfusion) from true ischaemic penumbra that will progress to infarction if timely reperfusion does not occur (32, 33). CBF is the most validated perfusion parameter in animal models of ischaemic thresholds and PET studies. As with CBV, normal CBF levels are significantly higher in grey matter compared with white matter. In CT perfusion, when ischaemic core assessment is dependent on perfusion parameters, CBF has recently been demonstrated to be the best correlate of the MRI diffusion lesion (34–36). This does, however, require careful thresholding as the visual extent of reduced CBF spreads well beyond ischaemic core into penumbra. Although less accurate in automated analyses, reduced CBV therefore provides a reasonable visual approximation of ischaemic core but is critically dependent on acquiring images for the entire transit of the contrast bolus. If this is truncated in patients with delayed perfusion, the CBV will be underestimated and the ischaemic core overestimated. MTT (CBV/CBF) is theoretically the best indicator of tissue perfusion quality and is prolonged in ischaemia. However, it is also the most prone to noise, which degrades image quality and often complicates interpretation.

Applications

TIA

For patients with suspected TIA, non-contrast CT is generally performed but has a very low diagnostic yield. However, occasional tumours and focal sub-arachnoid or other haemorrhage justify the continued use of this simple and available modality. CT angiography (CTA) has been demonstrated as a useful risk-stratification tool for recurrent events. In the absence of persistent arterial occlusion, the risk of recurrent or progressive stroke symptoms is very low (negative predictive value 96%) whereas patients with persistent arterial occlusion have a very high risk of recurrent or progressive symptoms (37). In brief neurological events, a DWI MRI has excellent prognostic value in predicting risk of recurrent ischaemia. Approximately 44% of events formerly regarded as 'TIA' have small infarcts on DWI (38). These patients are at much higher risk of recurrent stroke than those without DWI lesions and DWI is now recommended in some guidelines for all suspected TIA. To reduce access difficulties, some centres perform 'DWI-only' MR protocols for TIA (scan time <2 minutes). The presence of a DWI lesion (technically stroke under the current definition) increases the odds of recurrent stroke by a factor of 2.6 and, combined with persistent vessel occlusion, the risk is increased 8.9 times (39). Adding DWI to the commonly used ABCD² score has been proposed to improve risk stratification accuracy. Additionally, the pattern of DWI lesion may indicate the likely source of embolism. The involvement of multiple vascular territories implicates cardioembolism. When non-localizing symptoms such as dysarthria occur in the presence of significant carotid stenosis, DWI abnormalities can help indicate whether the stenosis is likely to have been symptomatic.

Ischaemic stroke

Diagnosing stroke and excluding mimics

In suspected ischaemic stroke, determining the optimal imaging protocol depends on the local access to and experience with CT versus MRI, patient factors such as renal function and implanted devices (e.g. pacemaker), the time window, the treatment options available (i.e. IV tissue plasminogen activator (tPA) and/or intra-arterial therapy), and the clinician's diagnostic confidence. Non-contrast CT remains the fastest and simplest tool for thrombolysis decisions within 4.5 hours of stroke onset. If a decision to give tPA can be made after non-contrast CT, the drug should be administered without further delay. Although early ischaemic signs and hyperdense arteries sometimes allow a positive diagnosis of stroke, inter-rater agreement is often modest. Additional imaging with CT perfusion, CTA, or MRI has the potential to make a positive diagnosis of ischaemic stroke and reveal the individual's stroke pathophysiology. This allows us to discard some traditional contraindications to tPA (e.g. seizure at onset) which were originally amongst trial exclusion criteria to reduce the risk of including stroke mimics. If the imaging demonstrates vessel occlusion and/or a perfusion lesion, the diagnosis is stroke and can be treated as such. Advanced imaging can also improve diagnostic confidence in patients where migraine or intercurrent sepsis or metabolic disturbance is a possibility (40).

Risk-stratifying 'mild' stroke

Patients with 'mild' or rapidly improving stroke are a difficult population as around 30% of patients deemed 'too good to treat' end up disabled and rapid improvement can often precede rapid deterioration (41, 42). Advanced imaging can assist in prognostication in these patients as the presence of persistent hypoperfusion or vessel occlusion indicates the potential for later deterioration whereas deterioration is very unlikely in the absence of persistent hypoperfusion. A low threshold for thrombolysis should be employed in patients with persistent hypoperfusion and mild deficits to reduce the risk of later deterioration.

Imaging selection for thrombolysis

The use of advanced imaging to select patients that should or should not receive reperfusion therapy both within and outside the 4.5-hour onset-treatment time window is an area of active investigation. Definitive results from randomized trials are currently pending. However, several themes have emerged. The volume of ischaemic core is a critical predictor of favourable clinical response to reperfusion and also of haemorrhagic transformation risk (43–45). In clinical practice, ischaemic core can be assessed using diffusion MRI or by thresholded relative CBF or reduced CBV on CT perfusion. The sensitivity of non-contrast CT is insufficient for these purposes in the early hours after stroke when reperfusion therapy decisions need to be made. One selection model is a mismatch between arterial occlusion and ischaemic core volume. CTA and MRA enable detection of vessel occlusion in the main arterial branches but lose sensitivity beyond the M2 branches of the middle cerebral arteries. The more distal occlusions that are generally not detected with non-invasive angiography tend to be the most responsive to intravenous tPA and so the vessel-core mismatch concept is not necessarily appropriate in these patients. Perfusion imaging is much more sensitive in distal vessel occlusions and can more precisely measure the volume of dead and at risk brain tissue. MR perfusion-diffusion mismatch or CT perfusion mismatch is therefore a more generalizable concept (Figure 9.6). Recent research has confirmed that diffusion lesions rarely reverse, that CT-CBF can give similar information to diffusion MR regarding ischaemic core, and that thresholding Tmax longer than 5–6 seconds best identifies potentially salvageable tissue. These refined mismatch paradigms are being incorporated into automated processing software and trialled as selection methods beyond 4.5 hours. The presence of mismatch generally indicates good collateral flow, which can also be assessed to some degree using CTA. Good collaterals buy time for reperfusion therapies and are consistently associated with improved clinical outcomes.

Risk of haemorrhagic transformation

Balanced against the potential benefit of reperfusion indicated by the volume of salvageable brain tissue is the risk of haemorrhagic transformation. Symptomatic haemorrhage generally only occurs if reperfusion is successful. Fortunately it is relatively rare (~2% after IV tPA using current definitions) but has a high mortality. In addition to ischaemic core volume, the risk of haemorrhage can be predicted by the severity of perfusion abnormality as measured by very low CBV or severely prolonged Tmax (46, 47). Although the presence of large core or severe perfusion abnormality may not dissuade us from using thrombolysis within 4.5 hours, more complete knowledge of the risk:benefit equation may be useful in more marginal cases, in the extended time window, and for counselling relatives about likely outcomes.

Considering intra-arterial rescue

If intra-arterial therapy is an option, it is worthwhile using CTA to establish the presence of a major vessel occlusion and assess the vascular access to the site of occlusion (e.g. tortuosity and upstream stenoses) before summoning the resources of the neuro-interventional team. Given the time usually required to arrange intra-arterial therapy, it is probably also worthwhile establishing the presence of reasonable collateral flow or 'mismatch'. Data suggest these patients have the greatest potential benefit from relatively delayed reperfusion.

Investigating the cause

Arterial imaging

Carotid duplex Doppler ultrasound

Carotid duplex Doppler ultrasound provides structural and blood flow information about the cervical carotid arteries and limited information about the direction of flow in the vertebral arteries. Two-dimensional (2D) images of the artery lumen and wall provide some data on the degree of stenosis and plaque characteristics. However, these measurements can be confounded by shadowing from calcific plaque and need to be interpreted in conjunction with Doppler measurements of blood flow velocity. Doppler ultrasound uses the principle of Doppler shift where echoes from fast-moving blood are shifted in frequency proportional to blood-flow velocity which is increased in the presence of haemodynamically significant stenosis. Velocity can then be converted to an estimated degree of stenosis. Another indicator of haemodynamically significant stenosis is 'spectral broadening' (Figure 9.7).

Transcranial Doppler ultrasound

Traditionally, transcranial ultrasound has utilized Doppler only, although duplex machines capable of transcranial insonation and 2D imaging are now available. The temporal bone window allows insonation of the distal internal carotid artery, proximal middle carotid artery, and anterior carotid artery in approximately 80% of stroke patients. Other windows through the foramen magnum and orbit may allow insonation of the basilar artery and ophthalmic artery respectively. As with extracranial Doppler ultrasound, the key parameter is flow velocity with stenosis initially leading to increased velocity until a point of critical stenosis where flow decreases to the point that velocity paradoxically decreases. Microembolic signals are identifiable and may indicate an increased risk of subsequent stroke, including in asymptomatic carotid stenosis (48). Intravenous injection of agitated saline ('bubble contrast')

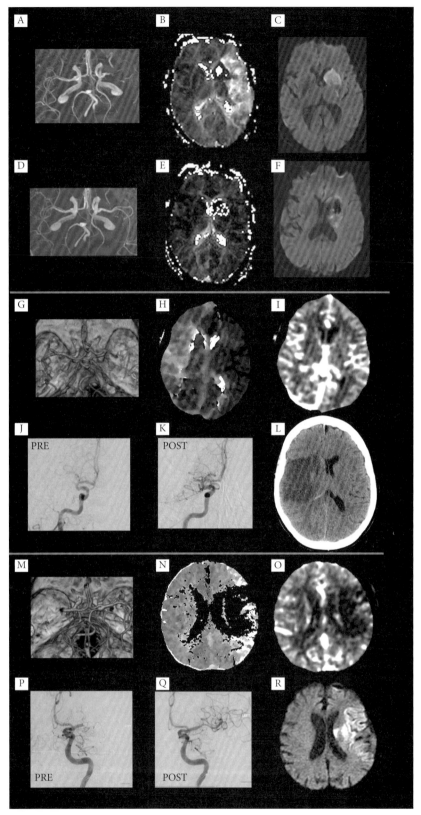

Fig. 9.6 Advanced imaging in ischaemic stroke. Top Panel: patient with left MCA occlusion on MRA (A), baseline large TTP perfusion lesion (B), and small diffusion lesion (C), i.e. 'mismatch'. Recanalization (D) and reperfusion (E) after tPA was associated with minimal infarct growth and clinically asymptomatic minor haemorrhagic transformation (F). Middle Panel: patient with right MCA occlusion on CTA (G), large CT perfusion 'mismatch' between TTP perfusion delay (H), and reduced CBV (I). Intra-arterial clot retrieval failed to recanalize (J–K) and major infarct growth was evident on follow-up CT (L). Lower Panel: patient with left MCA occlusion on CTA (M). CT perfusion showed matched TTP (N) and CBV (O). Despite rapid intra-arterial recanalization 2 hours after stroke onset (P–Q), a large infarct on follow-up DWI (R) corresponded to baseline reduced CBV representing ischaemic core.

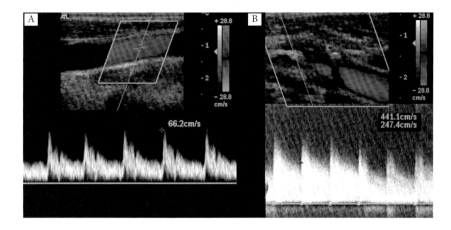

Fig. 9.7 Carotid Doppler ultrasound imaging. (A) Normal (internal carotid artery velocity 66 cm/sec). (B) High-grade stenosis—increased velocity and spectral broadening.

can be used to identify right-to-left shunts and graded using the Spencer system (49).

CTA

CTA is generally performed with a spiral acquisition after a bolus of IV iodinated contrast. The acquisition is timed to coincide with the early arterial phase. CTA provides excellent luminal delineation in 3D and can be acquired from aortic arch to vertex. The degree of stenosis can be directly measured in 3D. Many cases of arterial dissection are identifiable using CTA. Delineation of the petrous and cavernous carotid can be challenging due to surrounding bone, although subtraction technologies have the potential to improve diagnostic accuracy in these regions. There is a moderate radiation dose and the requirement for contrast can be problematic in renal and thyroid disease.

MRA

Several MR techniques can be employed to produce an angiogram. Phase-contrast angiography was the original method and provides information on flow-direction without contrast but at relatively low resolution. Time-of-flight (TOF) MRA is commonly used and visualizes the T1 signal from fast-flowing water molecules in blood without the need for contrast. TOF sequences can achieve quite high resolution but tend to overestimate the degree of stenosis due to signal drop-out in low-flow conditions. This problem can be circumvented by using dynamic contrast-enhanced MRA provided there is no contraindication to gadolinium contrast.

Digital subtraction angiography

Digital subtraction angiography (DSA) of the cerebral vessels is a minimally invasive procedure usually performed via femoral artery puncture. The risk of periprocedural stroke is less than 1%. Despite advances in non-invasive CTA and MRA, DSA remains the gold standard in luminal imaging of the extra- and intracranial vasculature. The main advantages are the high resolution and dynamic nature of the acquisition compared with traditionally static CTA and MRA. Dynamic acquisition reveals details of collateral circulation that are not clearly evident in static CTA and often invisible with TOF MRA. Another unique element of DSA is the ability to selectively catheterize an artery (e.g. internal carotid) to precisely characterize the location of occlusion which is often more distal than appreciated using static CTA due to stagnant flow in blind-ending vessels. However, newer CT scanners with large detector widths allowing dynamic CTA and contrast-enhanced MRA are rapidly approaching the quality of DSA. Even standard

CTA and MRA are perfectly adequate for demonstrating the presence of arterial occlusion in the major vessels without the small (<1%) but real risk of stroke associated with DSA. The role of DSA in stroke has therefore largely retreated to intra-arterial procedures and rare cases of suspected dissection or other vascular abnormality where the diagnosis remains unclear after non-invasive imaging.

Venous imaging

CTV

Analogous to the hyperdense artery sign in ischaemic stroke, venous sinus thrombus may also appear hyperdense on the non-contrast CT brain (Figure 9.8A) but this has limited sensitivity. The technique of CT venography (CTV) is identical to CTA except that timing of acquisition is delayed, typically 30–40 seconds after contrast bolus delivery. The so-called 'empty delta' sign indicates a filling defect due to thrombus in the sagittal sinus (Figure 9.8B). The sensitivity of CTV is relatively high in the major sinuses and comparable to MR venography (MRV) (50).

MRV

MRV can be performed using phase-contrast, TOF, or contrast-enhanced techniques (see 'MRA' section). In addition, confirmation of thrombus can be made using T2* (low signal), T1 (high signal), and T2 (loss of flow void) imaging (Figure 9.8C–F).

Cardiac imaging

Transthoracic and transoesophageal echocardiography

Although cardiac CT and MR are developing rapidly, echocardiography remains the chief cardiac investigation for stroke patients. Echocardiography can be performed via transthoracic (TTE) or transoesophageal (TOE) windows. TTE is non-invasive and more readily available. It provides information on left ventricular function, segmental wall motion abnormalities and gross valvular function. It is the optimal modality for imaging the anterior wall of the left ventricle and can often detect mural thrombus. Intravenous agitated saline 'bubble contrast' can be used to detect intracardiac shunts. Image quality is reduced in obese patients. TOE has advantages in detection of aortic arch atheroma, subtle valvular pathologies and is more sensitive for intracardiac shunts.

Applications

Large artery disease

The most common sources of thromboembolism in ischaemic stroke in Western populations are the extracranial carotid arteries

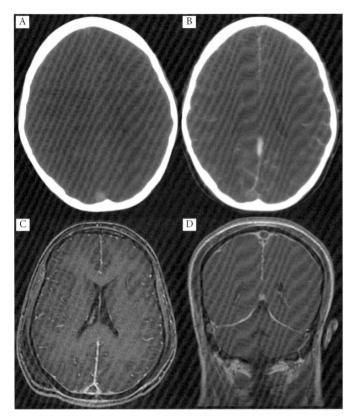

Fig. 9.8 Venous sinus thrombosis. (A) Non-contrast CT brain—hyperdense thrombus in sagittal sinus. (B) 'Empty delta' sign (absence of contrast in sinus) on CT venogram. (C, D) Contrast-enhanced T1 MRI—filling defect in sagittal sinus.

and the heart. Extracranial atherosclerosis is most common at the internal carotid bulb, immediately after the bifurcation of the common carotid. Intracranial atherosclerosis is more common in Asian populations. These factors determine the most appropriate modality for arterial imaging in a given patient population. Carotid Doppler ultrasound by an experienced operator provides reliable information about carotid bifurcation stenosis amenable to endarterectomy. It provides very limited information about more distal and intracranial stenoses or about the posterior circulation. However, as these are often not amenable to intervention, the non-invasive, radiation-free ease of carotid Doppler ultrasound makes it a popular modality. Transcranial Doppler ultrasound can often provide information about the intracranial vessels provided the skull is sufficiently thin to allow insonation (~80% of stroke patients). The technique has the advantage of being free from ionizing radiation. However, it is limited to proximal branches of the circle of Willis, usually provides only velocity data without anatomical information and is relatively operator dependent. CTA provides detailed anatomical information, not just about the carotid bifurcation, but about the entire arterial tree from aortic arch atheroma through the carotid and vertebral arteries into the intracranial vessels. It often provides sufficient anatomical detail to confirm the presence of dissection. Disadvantages of CTA include the requirement for iodinated contrast, which can create difficulties in patients with renal impairment and thyroid disease, and a moderate radiation dose. Time of flight MRA is free of contrast and radiation but tends to overestimate the degree of arterial stenosis. Contrast-enhanced MRA circumvents the overestimation of stenosis but is contraindicated in patients with poor renal function. MRI has the additional advantage of T1 fat-saturated imaging to confirm the presence of intramural methaemoglobin in cases of arterial dissection. Note that methaemoglobin takes 2–3 days to become detectable in the artery wall.

Venous sinus thrombosis

When imaging of the venous system is indicated, CTV and MRV are both reasonably sensitive for cerebral venous sinus thrombosis. CT is often more easily accessible but MR is radiation-free and has the advantage of multiple confirmatory sequences including T1 (intrinsic high signal in thrombus), T2 (loss of normal flow voids), T2* (low signal in thrombus), TOF MRV (loss of flow signal), and contrast-enhanced T1 ('empty delta' filling defect). MRI is also more sensitive to subtle parenchymal changes using diffusion and FLAIR sequences.

Cardioembolism

Cardiac imaging is most useful in the detection of segmental hypokinesis and potential mural thrombus. Other culprit valvular lesions, vegetations, and atrial myxoma are rare. It could be argued that most older patients with traditional cardiovascular risk factors and a normal electrocardiogram have such a low diagnostic yield that routine TTE is not warranted. The main advantages of TOE over TTE are in detection of intracardiac shunts, subtle valvular pathology and aortic arch atheroma. Given the current uncertainty surrounding the significance of patent foramen ovale (PFO) and the optimal management of aortic atheroma, TOE should probably be reserved for young patients (e.g. <60 years), with no other identified cause for stroke (e.g. dissection). Transcranial Doppler with bubble contrast is another option for detecting right–left cardiac (or pulmonary) shunts with similar sensitivity to echocardiography although the management implications if a shunt is discovered are often unclear.

Intracerebral haemorrhage

Diagnosis and establishing aetiology

Non-contrast CT brain

Acute haemorrhage is hyperdense on non-contrast CT brain. The location of the haematoma can often indicate the likely aetiology. In a hypertensive patient, a deep haematoma in the basal ganglia or external capsule is most likely due to chronic hypertension (Figure 9.9A). Superficial cortical 'lobar' haematomas in elderly patients are most likely due to amyloid angiopathy (Figure 9.9B). Any haematoma in the region of the Sylvian fissure or anterior, inferior frontal lobe should prompt consideration of a ruptured aneurysm or vascular malformation. The volume of the haematoma is directly related to prognosis and can be estimated using the 'ABC/2' formula. This is calculated as the axial dimensions A and B on the CT slice where the haematoma is largest, multiplied by the vertical diameter (slice thickness × number of involved slices), divided by 2 to approximate an ellipsoid (51). Haematoma volume greater than 60 mL generally indicates poor prognosis. A heterogeneous appearance to the haematoma may indicate greater likelihood of haematoma growth (52).

CT angiography

CTA can provide high-resolution imaging of the intracranial vasculature to assess for arteriovenous malformations (AVMs) and

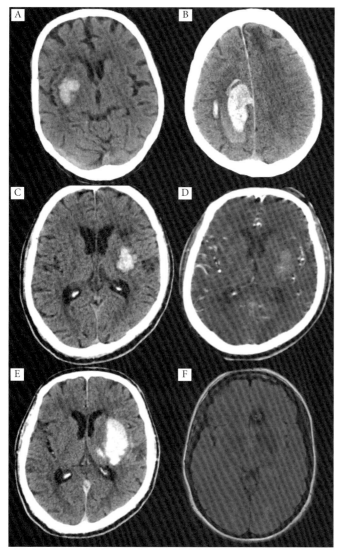

Fig. 9.9 Intracerebral haemorrhage. (A) Hypertensive basal ganglia ICH. (B) Amyloid lobar haemorrhage. (C–E) CT Angiogram 'spot sign'—active contrast extravasation acutely (D) predicts haematoma growth between baseline (C) and repeat CT 6 hours later (E). (F) Cavernous haemangioma—'popcorn' heterogeneous appearance with hypointense haemosiderin ring on T2 FLAIR.

aneurysms. It has limited sensitivity for dural arteriovenous fistulae, small peripheral AVM and mycotic aneurysms. Another potential use of CTA in ICH is the identification of ongoing active bleeding indicated by contrast extravasation within the haematoma. This so-called 'spot sign' (Figure 9.9C–E) has relatively high specificity for haematoma growth—a poor prognostic factor and potential treatment target for experimental haemostatic therapies (53).

MRI

The primary sequences used to identify haemorrhage using MRI are T2*-weighted gradient echo (GRE) and susceptibility-weighted imaging (SWI). These sequences capitalise on the susceptibility artefact induced by iron (in haemoglobin) which creates a bloom of hypointense signal drop-out in the haematoma. Calcium has a similar susceptibility effect and, when the cause is not clear on clinical grounds, CT may distinguish the cause of T2* abnormalities.

Susceptibility-weighted imaging

MRI routinely generates two sets of data called 'phase' and 'magnitude'. In general, only the magnitude image is presented clinically. However, appropriately filtered phase data carries information about local tissue susceptibility changes (e.g. due to blood products). SWI essentially multiplies the filtered phase data with the magnitude image to enhance the susceptibility effect and is significantly more sensitive than GRE (54). This is particularly evident in the number of microbleeds detected. Haemorrhage can have a varied appearance on DWI but is usually hypointense.

Temporal evolution of haematoma

Haemoglobin breakdown products are also visible on T1 and T2 images but change according to haematoma age. In the first few hours, the haematoma is predominantly oxyhaemoglobin which appears iso/hypointense on T1 and hyperintense on T2. Deoxyhaemoglobin is initially formed at the haematoma rim and is hypointense on T1 and T2. Subsequent formation of intracellular methaemoglobin, beginning in the haematoma rim and becoming most prominent after the first 1–2 days, is hyperintense on T1 and hypointense on T2. After about 7 days the methaemoglobin has become extracellular (T2 hyperintense and still T1 hyperintense). Later on, liquefaction of the haematoma creates central T1 hypointensity and T2 hyperintensity with a T2 hypointense rim due to the generation of ferritin and haemosiderin (55).

Identifying underlying lesions

Other MRI sequences can assist in identifying aetiology and underlying lesions. FLAIR sequences are sensitive to even small amounts of subarachnoid blood which presents as sulcal hyperintensity. Contrast-enhanced T1 can reveal underlying neoplasms and MRA underlying vascular malformations. Cavernous haemangiomas tend to have a typical heterogeneous 'popcorn' appearance on T2 with a circumferential hypointense haemosiderin ring (Figure 9.9F).

Applications

Although non-contrast CT is sufficient to identify haemorrhage, almost all patients warrant further imaging to refine the aetiology. As a minimum, CTA can exclude major vascular malformations and contributes diagnostic information in up to 15% of patients (56). However, caution should be exercised in peripheral bleeds where small AVMs and AVFs may evade detection by CTA and DSA should be considered. MRI in the acute phase may provide insights. However, in general, a follow-up scan after 6–8 weeks is necessary to thoroughly exclude underlying neoplasms once oedema has subsided. The pattern of microbleeds on GRE or SWI may indicate aetiology with a deep, basal ganglia predominance common in hypertensive disease and a cortical pattern common in amyloid angiopathy (Figure 9.2C).

Conclusion

In the majority of centres, non-contrast CT brain remains the primary investigation for patients with acute stroke syndromes. This is appropriate in many scenarios given its simplicity, speed, and accessibility. However, for suspected TIA, diffusion MRI can demonstrate small lesions in a significant proportion of cases. Such patients are now classified as minor stroke, and the presence of a diffusion lesion indicates a high risk of stroke recurrence. The key to mitigating this risk lies in the dual strategy of rapid institution of medical therapy and investigation (largely with imaging) of the aetiology. Carotid Doppler or CTA are the most commonly employed modalities with local experience and access generally determining the best option. Echocardiography is appropriate in selected patients. However, the clinical relevance of many cardiac abnormalities such as PFO and aortic arch atheroma remains uncertain.

In acute ischaemic stroke, non-contrast CT is often sufficient to allow thrombolysis decision-making and is usually the best modality to minimize delay to treatment. More sophisticated interpretation of subtle ischaemic signs and hyperdense arteries can derive extra diagnostic information. However, modern multimodal imaging further increases our capacity to make a positive diagnosis of ischaemic stroke. This has the ability to remove some traditional barriers to thrombolytic treatment—especially concern regarding stroke mimics and so-called 'mild' or fluctuating stroke. The pathophysiological insights also raise the possibility of pushing beyond rigid time-based patient selection towards a tissue-based assessment of the likely risk:benefit balance of reperfusion therapies.

At present, MRI remains better validated and more accurate in the identification of salvageable versus irreversibly damaged brain. However, multimodal CT can provide similar information and is currently much more readily available in most centres around the world.

In ICH, therapeutic options remain limited. Nonetheless, imaging indicates the likely aetiology and guides prognosis. Non-contrast CT plus CTA is a pragmatic strategy and identifies the majority of treatable vascular abnormalities. MRI, especially after resolution of the initial reactive changes, is strongly recommended to exclude more subtle underlying lesions. Our understanding of the significance of microbleeds remains nascent but they may aid differentiation of hypertensive and amyloid aetiologies.

Imaging is an essential complement to eliciting the clinical features of stroke and reveals otherwise unappreciated pathophysiological heterogeneity. Although the techniques and availability of different imaging modalities will continue to evolve in the years to come, the principles of imaging to identify aetiology and select optimal treatment will persist.

References

1. Easton JD, Saver JL, Albers GW, Alberts MJ, Chaturvedi S, Feldmann E, et al. Definition and evaluation of transient ischemic attack: a scientific statement for healthcare professionals from the American Heart Association/American Stroke Association Stroke Council; Council on Cardiovascular Surgery and Anesthesia; Council on Cardiovascular Radiology and Intervention; Council on Cardiovascular Nursing; and the Interdisciplinary Council on Peripheral Vascular Disease. The American Academy of Neurology affirms the value of this statement as an educational tool for neurologists. Stroke. 2009 Jun;40(6):2276–2293.

2. Schellinger PD, Bryan RN, Caplan LR, Detre JA, Edelman RR, Jaigobin C, et al. Evidence-based guideline: The role of diffusion and perfusion MRI for the diagnosis of acute ischemic stroke: report of the Therapeutics and Technology Assessment Subcommittee of the American Academy of Neurology. Neurology. 2010 Jul 13;75(2):177–185.

3. Parsons MW, Pepper EM, Bateman GA, Wang Y, Levi CR. Identification of the penumbra and infarct core on hyperacute noncontrast and perfusion CT. Neurology. 2007 Mar 6;68(10):730–736.

4. Tomsick TA, Brott TG, Chambers AA, Fox AJ, Gaskill MF, Lukin RR, et al. Hyperdense middle cerebral artery sign on CT: efficacy in detecting middle cerebral artery thrombosis. AJNR Am J Neuroradiol. 1990 May;11(3):473–477.

5. Barber PA, Demchuk AM, Hudon ME, Pexman JH, Hill MD, Buchan AM. Hyperdense sylvian fissure MCA "dot" sign: A CT marker of acute ischemia. Stroke. 2001 Jan;32(1):84–88.

6. Pressman BD, Tourje EJ, Thompson JR. An early CT sign of ischemic infarction: increased density in a cerebral artery. AJR Am J Roentgenol. 1987 Sep;149(3):583–586.

7. Bettle N, Lyden PD. Thrombosis of the posterior cerebral artery (PCA) visualized on computed tomography: the dense PCA sign. Arch Neurol. 2004 Dec;61(12):1960–1961.

8. Ehsan T, Hayat G, Malkoff MD, Selhorst JB, Martin D, Manepalli A. Hyperdense basilar artery. An early computed tomography sign of thrombosis. J Neuroimaging. 1994 Oct;4(4):200–205.

9. Riedel CH, Zimmermann P, Jensen-Kondering U, Stingele R, Deuschl G, Jansen O. The importance of size: successful recanalization by intravenous thrombolysis in acute anterior stroke depends on thrombus length. Stroke. 2009 Jun;42(6):1775–1777.

10. Tomsick T, Brott T, Barsan W, Broderick J, Haley EC, Spilker J, et al. Prognostic value of the hyperdense middle cerebral artery sign and stroke scale score before ultraearly thrombolytic therapy. AJNR Am J Neuroradiol. 1996 Jan;17(1):79–85.

11. van der Wee N, Rinkel GJ, Hasan D, van Gijn J. Detection of subarachnoid haemorrhage on early CT: is lumbar puncture still needed after a negative scan? J Neurol Neurosurg Psychiatry. 1995 Mar;58(3):357–359.

12. van Gijn J, Kerr RS, Rinkel GJ. Subarachnoid haemorrhage. Lancet. 2007 Jan 27;369(9558):306–318.

13. van Gijn J, van Dongen KJ. The time course of aneurysmal haemorrhage on computed tomograms. Neuroradiology. 1982;23(3):153–156.

14. Cortnum S, Sorensen P, Jorgensen J. Determining the sensitivity of computed tomography scanning in early detection of subarachnoid hemorrhage. Neurosurgery. 2010 May;66(5):900–902; discussion 3.

15. Kumar S, Goddeau RP, Jr, Selim MH, Thomas A, Schlaug G, Alhazzani A, et al. Atraumatic convexal subarachnoid hemorrhage: clinical presentation, imaging patterns, and etiologies. Neurology. 2010 Mar 16;74(11): 893–899.

16. Thanvi BR, Treadwell S, Robinson T. Haemorrhagic transformation in acute ischaemic stroke following thrombolysis therapy: classification, pathogenesis and risk factors. Postgrad Med J. 2008 Jul;84(993):361–367.

17. Becker H, Desch H, Hacker H, Pencz A. CT fogging effect with ischemic cerebral infarcts. Neuroradiology. 1979 Oct 31;18(4):185–192.

18. Gaudinski MR, Henning EC, Miracle A, Luby M, Warach S, Latour LL. Establishing final infarct volume: stroke lesion evolution past 30 days is insignificant. Stroke. 2008 Oct;39(10):2765–2768.

19. Moseley ME, Cohen Y, Mintorovitch J, Chileuitt L, Shimizu H, Kucharczyk J, et al. Early detection of regional cerebral ischemia in cats: comparison of diffusion- and T2-weighted MRI and spectroscopy. Magn Reson Med. 1990 May;14(2):330–346.

20. Hjort N, Christensen S, Solling C, Ashkanian M, Wu O, Rohl L, et al. Ischemic injury detected by diffusion imaging 11 minutes after stroke. Ann Neurol. 2005 Sep;58(3):462–465.

21. Schaefer PW, Grant PE, Gonzalez RG. Diffusion-weighted MR imaging of the brain. Radiology. 2000 Nov;217(2):331–345.

22. Kidwell CS, Saver JL, Starkman S, Duckwiler G, Jahan R, Vespa P, et al. Late secondary ischemic injury in patients receiving intraarterial thrombolysis. Ann Neurol. 2002 Dec;52(6):698–703.

23. Li F, Liu KF, Silva MD, Omae T, Sotak CH, Fenstermacher JD, et al. Transient and permanent resolution of ischemic lesions on diffusion-weighted imaging after brief periods of focal ischemia in rats: correlation with histopathology. Stroke. 2000 Apr;31(4):946–954.

24. Tourdias T, Dousset V, Sibon I, Pele E, Menegon P, Asselineau J, et al. Magnetization transfer imaging shows tissue abnormalities in the reversible penumbra. Stroke. 2007 Dec;38(12):3165–3171.

25. Campbell BCV, Purushotham A, Christensen S, Desmond P, Nagakane Y, Parsons MW, et al. The infarct core is well represented by the acute diffusion lesion: sustained reversal is infrequent. J Cereb Blood Flow Metab. 2012 Jan;32(1):50–56.

26. Chemmanam T, Campbell BCV, Christensen S, Nagakane Y, Desmond PM, Bladin CF, et al. Ischemic diffusion lesion reversal is uncommon and rarely alters perfusion-diffusion mismatch. Neurology. 2010 Sep 21;75(12):1040–1047.

27. Wintermark M, Albers GW, Broderick JP, Demchuk AM, Fiebach JB, Fiehler J, et al. Acute Stroke Imaging Research Roadmap II. Stroke. 2013 Sep;44(9):2628–2639.

28. Thomalla G, Rossbach P, Rosenkranz M, Siemonsen S, Krutzelmann A, Fiehler J, et al. Negative fluid-attenuated inversion recovery imaging identifies acute ischemic stroke at 3 hours or less. Ann Neurol. 2009 Jun;65(6):724–732.

29. Ostergaard L, Sorensen AG, Kwong KK, Weisskoff RM, Gyldensted C, Rosen BR. High resolution measurement of cerebral blood flow using intravascular tracer bolus passages. Part II: Experimental comparison and preliminary results. Magn Reson Med. 1996 Nov;36(5):726–736.

30. Albers GW, Thijs VN, Wechsler L, Kemp S, Schlaug G, Skalabrin E, et al. Magnetic resonance imaging profiles predict clinical response to early reperfusion: the diffusion and perfusion imaging evaluation for understanding stroke evolution (DEFUSE) study. Ann Neurol. 2006 Nov;60(5):508–517.

31. Davis SM, Donnan GA, Parsons MW, Levi C, Butcher KS, Peeters A, et al. Effects of alteplase beyond 3 h after stroke in the Echoplanar Imaging Thrombolytic Evaluation Trial (EPITHET): a placebo-controlled randomised trial. Lancet Neurol. 2008 Apr;7(4):299–309.

32. Olivot JM, Mlynash M, Thijs VN, Kemp S, Lansberg MG, Wechsler L, et al. Optimal Tmax threshold for predicting penumbral tissue in acute stroke. Stroke. 2009 Feb;40(2):469–475.

33. Zaro-Weber O, Moeller-Hartmann W, Heiss WD, Sobesky J. Maps of time to maximum and time to peak for mismatch definition in clinical stroke studies validated with positron emission tomography. Stroke. 2010 Dec;41(12):2817–2821.

34. Bivard A, McElduff P, Spratt N, Levi C, Parsons M. Defining the extent of irreversible brain ischemia using perfusion computed tomography. Cerebrovasc Dis. 2011;31(3):238–245.

35. Campbell BCV, Christensen S, Levi CR, Desmond PM, Donnan GA, Davis SM, et al. Cerebral blood flow is the optimal CT perfusion parameter for assessing infarct core. Stroke. 2011 Dec;42(12):3435–3440.

36. Kamalian S, Maas MB, Goldmacher GV, Payabvash S, Akbar A, Schaefer PW, et al. CT cerebral blood flow maps optimally correlate with admission diffusion-weighted imaging in acute stroke but thresholds vary by postprocessing platform. Stroke. 2011 May 5;42(7):1923–1928.

37. Coutts SB, Modi J, Patel SK, Demchuk AM, Goyal M, Hill MD. CT/CT angiography and MRI findings predict recurrent stroke after transient ischemic attack and minor stroke: results of the prospective CATCH study. Stroke. 2012;43(4):1013–1017.

38. Ovbiagele B, Kidwell CS, Saver JL. Epidemiological impact in the United States of a tissue-based definition of transient ischemic attack. Stroke. 2003 Apr;34(4):919–924.

39. Coutts SB, Simon JE, Eliasziw M, Sohn CH, Hill MD, Barber PA, et al. Triaging transient ischemic attack and minor stroke patients using acute magnetic resonance imaging. Ann Neurol. 2005 Jun;57(6):848–854.

40. Campbell BCV, Weir L, Desmond PM, Tu HTH, Hand PJ, Yan B, et al. CT perfusion improves diagnostic accuracy and confidence in acute ischemic stroke. J Neurol Neurosurg Psychiatry. 2013;84:613–618.

41. Barber PA, Zhang J, Demchuk AM, Hill MD, Buchan AM. Why are stroke patients excluded from TPA therapy? An analysis of patient eligibility. Neurology. 2001 Apr 24;56(8):1015–1020.

42. Smith EE, Abdullah AR, Petkovska I, Rosenthal E, Koroshetz WJ, Schwamm LH. Poor outcomes in patients who do not receive intravenous tissue plasminogen activator because of mild or improving ischemic stroke. Stroke. 2005 Nov;36(11):2497–2499.

43. Singer OC, Humpich MC, Fiehler J, Albers GW, Lansberg MG, Kastrup A, et al. Risk for symptomatic intracerebral hemorrhage after thrombolysis assessed by diffusion-weighted magnetic resonance imaging. Ann Neurol. 2008 Jan;63(1):52–60.

44. Yoo AJ, Verduzco LA, Schaefer PW, Hirsch JA, Rabinov JD, Gonzalez RG. MRI-based selection for intra-arterial stroke therapy: value of pretreatment diffusion-weighted imaging lesion volume in selecting patients with acute stroke who will benefit from early recanalization. Stroke. 2009 Jun;40(6):2046–2054.

45. Parsons MW, Christensen S, McElduff P, Levi CR, Butcher KS, De Silva DA, et al. Pretreatment diffusion- and perfusion-MR lesion volumes have a crucial influence on clinical response to stroke thrombolysis. J Cereb Blood Flow Metab. 2010 Jun;30(6):1214–1225.

46. Campbell BCV, Christensen S, Butcher KS, Gordon I, Parsons MW, Desmond PM, et al. Regional very low cerebral blood volume predicts hemorrhagic transformation better than diffusion-weighted imaging volume and thresholded apparent diffusion coefficient in acute ischemic stroke. Stroke. 2010 Jan;41(1):82–88.

47. Kim JH, Bang OY, Liebeskind DS, Ovbiagele B, Kim GM, Chung CS, et al. Impact of baseline tissue status (diffusion-weighted imaging lesion) versus perfusion status (severity of hypoperfusion) on hemorrhagic transformation. Stroke. 2010 Mar;41(3):e135–e142.

48. Markus HS, King A, Shipley M, Topakian R, Cullinane M, Reihill S, et al. Asymptomatic embolisation for prediction of stroke in the Asymptomatic Carotid Emboli Study (ACES): a prospective observational study. Lancet Neurol. 2010 Jul;9(7):663–671.

49. Spencer MP, Moehring MA, Jesurum J, Gray WA, Olsen JV, Reisman M. Power m-mode transcranial Doppler for diagnosis of patent foramen ovale and assessing transcatheter closure. J Neuroimaging. 2004 Oct;14(4):342–349.

50. Khandelwal N, Agarwal A, Kochhar R, Bapuraj JR, Singh P, Prabhakar S, et al. Comparison of CT venography with MR venography in cerebral sinovenous thrombosis. AJR Am J Roentgenol. 2006 Dec;187(6):1637–1643.

51. Kothari RU, Brott T, Broderick JP, Barsan WG, Sauerbeck LR, Zuccarello M, et al. The ABCs of measuring intracerebral hemorrhage volumes. Stroke. 1996 Aug;27(8):1304–1305.

52. Barras CD, Tress BM, Christensen S, MacGregor L, Collins M, Desmond PM, et al. Density and shape as CT predictors of intracerebral hemorrhage growth. Stroke. 2009 Apr;40(4):1325–1331.

53. Davis SM, Broderick J, Hennerici M, Brun NC, Diringer MN, Mayer SA, et al. Hematoma growth is a determinant of mortality and poor outcome after intracerebral hemorrhage. Neurology. 2006 Apr 25;66(8):1175–1181.

54. Haacke EM, Mittal S, Wu Z, Neelavalli J, Cheng YC. Susceptibility-weighted imaging: technical aspects and clinical applications, part 1. AJNR Am J Neuroradiol. 2009 Jan;30(1):19–30.

55. Bradley WG, Jr MR appearance of hemorrhage in the brain. Radiology. 1993 Oct;189(1):15–26.

56. Delgado Almandoz JE, Schaefer PW, Forero NP, Falla JR, Gonzalez RG, Romero JM. Diagnostic accuracy and yield of multidetector CT angiography in the evaluation of spontaneous intraparenchymal cerebral hemorrhage. AJNR Am J Neuroradiol. 2009 Jun;30(6):1213–1221.

CHAPTER 10

Management of stroke: general principles

Mehmet Akif Topcuoğlu and Hakan Ay

The goals of supportive care in stroke

The new age in acute stroke management calls for an immediate, dynamic, and individualized approach to patient management. Most therapeutic interventions for stroke are effective only if the patient can be treated within a few hours of the onset of stroke. (Figure 10.1) (1, 2). Given the narrow therapeutic window, timely evaluation and management is critical. The overall goal of acute stroke management is to increase survival and reduce the burden of stroke for better quality of life. Critical to achieving this goal is to provide an organized structure that links the community and the hospital's acute stroke team, a multidisciplinary approach by dedicated physicians, and a comprehensive stroke unit where timely evaluation and treatment of stroke can be achieved. Stroke management is a multidimensional concept including acute care, secondary prevention, rehabilitation, occupational therapy, and psychosocial support. This chapter introduces the general principles of acute stroke management, with particular emphasis on the specific goals of minimizing brain injury, preventing early stroke recurrence, and treating neurological and systemic complications.

Minimizing the extent of brain injury

Modern stroke management focuses on salvaging marginally perfused, electrically silent, morphologically intact, and potentially viable brain tissue from the processes that lead to tissue infarction. Any insult that reduces cerebral blood flow (CBF) below the ischaemic threshold can cause irreversible neural injury if sustained. The fate of marginally perfused tissue is determined by several factors, including the degree of ischaemia, the duration of insult, and the baseline susceptibility of brain tissue to ischaemia (Figure 10.2) (3, 4). Depending on the delicate balance between two fundamental aspects of stroke pathophysiology, that is, 'supply' (tissue perfusion) and 'demand' (cellular metabolism), the tissue may progress to necrosis or gain complete functional recovery. The primary goal of acute stroke intervention is to increase 'supply' while maintaining or decreasing 'demand'. Specific treatments that focus on the 'supply' portion of the chain such as intravenous, intra-arterial, and mechanical recanalization therapies are discussed in Chapter 11 of this book. This chapter will focus on general strategies that favourably affect the supply/demand balance. These strategies include optimal regulation of blood pressure, blood fluidity, oxygen and glucose supply, body temperature, and seizures.

Although time is critically important in the treatment of ischaemic stroke, up to 50% of patients exhibit a penumbra, as defined by diffusion-weighted/perfusion-weighted imaging mismatch detectable up to 12 hours after stroke onset (5). The existence of persistent, potentially salvageable tissue underscores the notion that optimal stroke management should carefully consider the broad variation between individual patients (6–8). This, necessitates a thorough evaluation that includes not only clinical assessment but also multimodal imaging of the brain and its vessels.

Prevention of early stroke recurrence

The risk of recurrent stroke during the first 90 days following an ischaemic stroke hovers around 5–10% (9). Approximately one out of every two recurrent strokes during 90-days occurs within the first 7 days of the index stroke (9). Early recurrent stroke is associated with longer hospitalization as well as increased neurological disability and death (10, 11). Effective prevention requires accurate identification of patients at high risk. The most important predictor of early recurrence is the underlying stroke aetiology (9, 12–14). Risk of early recurrent stroke is higher after strokes secondary to 'large artery atherosclerosis' or 'other uncommon causes' such as arterial dissection or vasculitis than in 'cardio-aortic embolism', 'cryptogenic stroke', or 'small artery occlusion'. Table 10.1 lists some known predictors of early stroke recurrence (9, 15–17). It is important to note that there is a clear distinction between 'aetiology' and 'risk factor' in regard to early stroke recurrence. Conventional stroke risk factors such as hypertension, diabetes mellitus, hypercholesterolemia, and smoking, which confer risk over the long term, do not appear to pose significant risk for recurrent stroke in the short term (9).

Diagnostic evaluation to identify the underlying aetiology of stroke should be performed in all stroke patients, and should include blood tests, brain imaging, intracranial and extracranial vascular imaging, and cardiac evaluation. Further investigations may be necessary depending on the level of suspect from a particular cause; for instance, assessment of the deep venous system should be performed for suspected paradoxical embolism. Prompt aetiological investigation requires admission to specialized stroke centres that have the infrastructure to institute timely and targeted preventive treatment.

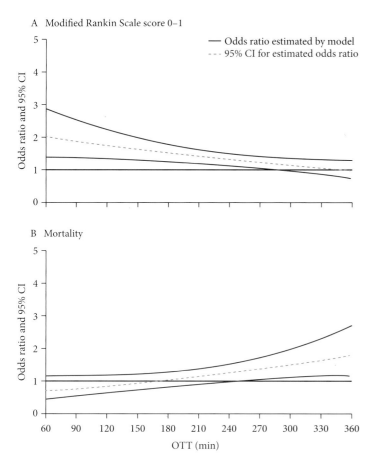

A   Modified Rankin Scale score 0–1

Odds ratio estimated by model
95% CI for estimated odds ratio

B   Mortality

OTT (min)

Fig. 10.1 Relationship between stroke onset to start of intravenous thrombolytic treatment (OTT) and treatment effect after adjustment for potential confounders. The benefit from intravenous thrombolytic treatment decreases as OTT increases; the number needed to treat for excellent outcome (modified Rankin Scale score 0 or 1) is 5 when treatment is applied within 0–90 min, 9 within 91–180 min, and 15 within 181–270 min. (Reprinted from The Lancet, 15;375(9727), Lees KR, Bluhmki E, von Kummer R, Brott TG, Toni D, Grotta JC, et al., Time to treatment with intravenous alteplase and outcome in stroke: an updated pooled analysis of ECASS, ATLANTIS, NINDS, and EPITHET trials. 1695–1703. Copyright (2010), with permission from Elsevier.).

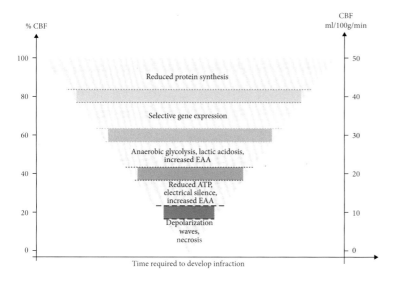

Fig. 10.2 A simplified illustration showing that the fate of the penumbra is dependent upon degree of ischaemia (vertical axis), duration of ischaemia (horizontal axis), and tissue susceptibility to ischaemia. Clinical symptoms occur almost immediately when tissue perfusion drops below the threshold for electrical silence as represented by the short dashed line. In some patients, the degree of ischaemia which is sufficient to cause electrical silence may not be sufficient to cause infarction unless sustained for a prolonged period of time. In others, the ischaemia can be so profound that brain injury occurs within a few minutes (long dashed line). EAA: excitatory amino acids, ATP: adenosine triphosphate, CBF: cerebral blood flow.

Prevention and treatment of acute neurological and systemic complications

Medical and neurological complications that arise during the acute phase of stroke are common, occurring in 40–95% of patients (Table 10.2) (18–20). Approximately 50% of stroke-related deaths during the acute period can be attributed to medical complications (20). Moreover, stroke complications can delay rehabilitation, prolong hospital stays, increase costs, and ultimately result in poorer functional outcome. Effective monitoring and early recognition of complications are vital to successful treatment. Neurological complications including cerebral oedema, brain herniation, haemorrhagic transformation, seizures, and hydrocephalus can arise as direct local effects of brain lesions. Medical complications, on the other hand, result from the remote effects of stroke on somatic and visceral functions. Presumed mechanisms of medical complications are several and include post-stroke disabilities (e.g. weakness, imbalance, dysphagia, etc.) and immobilization, impaired autonomic balance on visceral organ systems, stroke-induced changes

Table 10.1 Risk factors for complications after acute stroke

	Complication		
	Growth	**Early recurrent stroke**	**Medical complications**
Predictors of complications in ischaemic stroke	Early neurological deterioration Fluctuating non-lacunar symptoms Angiographic evidence of proximal arterial occlusion Imaging evidence of mismatch	Recent prior stroke or transient ischaemic attack Aetiological stroke subtypes of large artery atherosclerosis and other uncommon causes Multiple acute infarcts Multiple acute infarcts in both right and left anterior circulations or in both anterior and posterior circulations Multiple infarcts of different ages (combination of hyperacute, acute, or subacute infarcts) Cortical infarct location	Post-stroke disabilities (immobilization, severe weakness, dysphagia, imbalance, etc.) Infarct location (brainstem, insula, bilateral hemispheric, etc.) Infarct size (large territorial versus small) Signs and symptoms consistent with sympathoadrenal or autonomic nervous system dysfunction (sympathetic storm, fever, vomiting, tachycardia, etc.) Interventions and medications
Predictors of complications in haemorrhagic stroke	Contrast extravasation into the haematoma (spot sign) Size and number of spot signs Large haematoma volume at presentation Early presentation (within 3 hours of onset) Heterogeneity of haematoma density on admission computed tomography Prior use of warfarin or high admission international normalized ratio Prior use of antiplatelet agents Admission hyperglycaemia Uncontrolled hypertension	Lobar ICH Amyloid angiopathy related ICH Bleeding diathesis	Post-stroke disabilities (immobilization, severe weakness, dysphagia, imbalance, etc.) Intraventricular extension of haemorrhage Hydrocephalus Haematoma size (>30 mL) Haematoma location (anterior versus posterior fossa) Signs and symptoms consistent with sympathoadrenal or autonomic nervous system dysfunction (sympathetic storm, fever, vomiting, tachycardia, etc.) Interventions and medications

in immune system, activation of acute stress markers and increased concentration of circulating endothelial and homeostatic markers, acute stress response via activation of the hypothalamo–hypophyseal axis, as well as complications related to medications and

Table 10.2 Neurological and medical complications of acute stroke

Neurological complications	Medical complications
Brain oedema causing midline shift	Gastrointestinal bleeding
Brain herniation	Stress ulcers
Symptomatic haemorrhagic transformation	Cardiac arrest/life-threatening cardiac arrhythmia
Seizures	Congestive heart failure
Hydrocephalus	Takotsubo cardiomyopathy
Pneumonia	Acute coronary syndrome
Urinary tract infection	Acute pulmonary oedema
Sepsis	Dysphagia
Cellulitis	Electrolyte imbalance
Falls	Hyperglycaemia
Decubitus ulcers/pressure sores	Hypoxia/hypercapnia
Incontinence	Dehydration
Symptomatic deep venous thrombosis	Depression
Pulmonary embolism	Dementia

interventions. The following section of this chapter ('Principles of general supportive care in stroke') provides detailed discussion of the possible complications of stroke, with particular emphasis on pathophysiology, diagnosis, and treatment.

Principles of general supportive care in stroke

The primary goal of supportive acute stroke care is to maintain physiological parameters in the normal range (Tables 10.3 and 10.4). Most approaches to optimize vital physiological functions such as blood pressure, heart rate, oxygen saturation, blood glucose, and temperature have not been adequately assessed in randomized controlled trials. Therefore, the supportive measures discussed in this chapter are based largely on expert opinion and case studies.

Maintenance of tissue oxygenation

The brain is an extremely energy-dependent organ; although it accounts for approximately 2% of the total body weight, the brain consumes 20% of the oxygen in the circulation. In the absence of oxygen, neuronal death occurs in 1–3 minutes (21). Maintaining adequate oxygen supply (i.e. oxygen saturation >92%) and carbon dioxide removal is essential during the acute period to halt the progression of brain injury (22). Initial management should focus on clearing and securing the airway. Intubation and ventilatory support can be considered in patients at risk of airway compromise due to reduced consciousness. Supplemental oxygen through a nasal cannula, at 1–3 L/min, should be considered if pulse oximetry or

Table 10.3 Management of acute stroke: general issues

	Recommended actions	Actions to avoid
Airway	Secure airway Oropharyngeal suctioning and semi-upright position in patients at risk of aspiration Elective intubation in patients with Glasgow Coma Scale score <9 and signs of increased intracranial pressure	Prophylactic use of broad-spectrum antibiotic therapy in patients at risk of aspiration
Oxygenation	The goal is to maintain oxygen saturation ≥ 92% 100% oxygen through a nasal cannula at a rate of 1–3 L/min if oxygen saturation <92% Identify and treat the cause of hypoxia	Routine supplemental oxygen in patients with normal oxygen saturation Frequent blood draws and haemodilution in patients with low admission haemoglobin (<10–12 g/dL) Hyperbaric oxygen unless suspected air embolism
Breathing	Maintain PaO_2 >80 mmHg, $PaCO_2$ <45 mmHg Monitor breathing patterns particularly during sleep Ventilatory support in patients with respiratory distress or inability to protect airway due to impaired consciousness or oropharyngeal weakness	The use of medications that can cause respiratory depression in patients at risk of compromised airway due to impaired consciousness, oropharyngeal weakness, and increased intracranial pressure
Circulation	Maintain systolic blood pressure (BP) >140 mmHg and central venous pressure >5 mmHg in patients with ischaemic stroke or raised ICP 0.9% NaCl infusion at 1–3 mL/kg/h or vasopressor agents when systolic BP <140 mmHg or central venous pressure <5 mmHg	Hypotension in patients at risk of infarct growth or in those with raised ICP Indiscriminate use of vasopressor agents in ischaemic stroke to induce hypertension
Sedation/analgesia	Sedation and analgesia in patients who are agitated or delirious, connected to mechanical ventilator, or have excessive anxiety	Use of sedatives in patients in whom neurological findings need to be closely monitored
Head position	Keep head elevated at 30° in straight position (not turned to sides) in order to maximize venous outflow and minimize the risk of aspiration Keep head at neutral position (0°) in unstable infarcts (for instance, infarcts with large regions of marginally perfused tissue or infarcts that occur as a result of severe arterial stenoses) where a slight change in perfusion pressure may result in progression of ischaemic injury	Restricting devices around the neck that compromise venous outflow
Body temperature	Keep core body temperature <37°C Treat the source of fever Acetaminophen 650 mg every 4 hours if core body temperature >37°C (provides ~0.25°C drop within 4 hours) Combine acetaminophen with surface cooling if rapid and pronounced effect is desired	Routine induction of hypothermia in focal ischaemia

blood gas measures indicate hypoxia. In the absence of hypoxia, however, there is currently no convincing evidence to support the routine use of supplemental oxygen therapy (23, 24).

Hypoxia is more likely to develop in patients with large stroke, advanced age, dysphagia, and pre-existing cardiac and pulmonary disease. There are several central (neurogenic) and peripheral (non-neurogenic) causes of hypoxia in stroke. Neurogenic causes include alveolar hypoventilation due to extensive brainstem or hemispheric stroke, central obstructive sleep apnoea, central periodic breathing during sleep, and paralysis of the respiratory muscles. Peripheral causes of hypoxia include airway obstruction, aspiration pneumonia, congestive heart failure, pulmonary thromboembolism, severe anaemia, and worsening of pre-existing obstructive or restrictive lung disease (18, 23).

One important cause of hypoxia is reduced oxygen carrying capacity of the blood. Haemoglobin carries 98% of the total blood oxygen. Although tissue hypoxia generally does not develop until haemoglobin concentration falls <60 g/L, the haemoglobin threshold may be higher in cerebral ischaemia. Mathematical models

suggest that lower haemoglobin may adversely affect the energy balance within the ischaemic tissue by demonstrating an abrupt decline in tissue oxygen metabolism at haemoglobin <100 g/L (25). According to observational cohort studies, haemoglobin levels as high as 120 g/L in men, and 130 g/L in women are associated with poor functional outcome (26, 27). The risk of poor clinical outcome increases at both ends of haemoglobin scale indicating a U-shaped relationship between admission haemoglobin levels and outcome in stroke patients (26) (Figure 10.3). The clinical implication of these findings is that care should be taken to avoid further reduction of haemoglobin levels by frequent blood draws and haemodilution in patients with borderline haemoglobin levels. The safety and efficacy of corrective treatments for low haemoglobin, i.e. blood transfusion or erythropoietin therapy, have not been tested in clinical trials.

Sleep-disordered breathing (SDB), including obstructive sleep apnoea, central sleep apnoea syndrome, and Cheyne–Stokes breathing, is common after stroke, occurring in approximately 40–70% of patients (28). Patients with SDB more frequently have congestive heart failure, advanced age, and obesity (29). Significant decrease in

Table 10.4 Management of acute stroke: specific issues

	Recommended actions	Actions to avoid
Viscosity	Haemodilution in conditions in which high viscosity compromises perfusion to the ischaemic brain tissue	Haemodilution at the setting of low haematocrit (<30%), which can lead to rapid decline in oxygen delivery
Nutrition/ hydration	Screening for swallowing Behavioural intervention and diet modification in mild dysphagia Enteral feeding in severe dysphagia. Parenteral feeding if enteral feeding cannot be started within 72 hours Adequate hydration to maintain central venous pressure >5 mmHg and serum osmolality between 285–295 mOsm	Gastric distention and gastro-oesophageal reflux due to delayed gastric emptying Dehydration, which can cause reduced cerebral perfusion and increased risk of venous thromboembolism
Urinary control	External urinary catheter placement in patients who are unable to communicate or who have limited mobility Short-term indwelling urinary catheter placement when there is acute urinary retention or need for accurate monitoring of urinary output Prompted voiding, biofeedback-assisted pelvic training, and behavioural therapy in patients with incontinence	Routine use of indwelling urinary catheter placement in patients with stroke
Glycaemic control	Minimize the use of glucose containing solutions in normoglycaemic/hyperglycaemic patients during the first 24 hours Treat hypoglycaemia as an emergency in acute ischaemic stroke (30 mL IV bolus of 50% dextrose). Check blood glucose levels every 15 min Treat hyperglycaemia >180 mg/dL or >10 mmol/L with insulin infusion in non-lacunar strokes as well as before the start of thrombolytic therapy	Overcorrection of hypoglycaemia Overcorrection of hyperglycaemia with insulin treatment
Cardiac control	Cardiac assessment (ECG, cardiac enzymes, or echocardiography) to identify cardiac abnormalities that require urgent treatment, to diagnose neurocardiac abnormalities, and to rule out concurrent acute coronary syndrome Echocardiography to diagnose stunned neurogenic myocardium in patients who have ECG changes not conforming to a known coronary territory, mild troponin elevation, or signs and symptoms consistent with acute congestive heart failure Positive inotropic agents or intra-aortic balloon pump implantation in patients with severely reduced cardiac output	Medications that prolong QT interval in patients with prolonged QTc on ECG
Seizures	EEG monitoring in patients who have reduced level of consciousness or clinical deficit that is out of proportion with the extent of brain injury Anticonvulsant therapy in patients with recurrent clinical or electrographic seizures	Prophylactic administration of anticonvulsants

oxygen saturation (<90%) can develop during the apnoeic periods, negatively impacting tissue outcome. In one study, the number and duration of hypoxic episodes correlated with increased mortality at 1 year, and with functional disability measured by the Barthel index at discharge and at 1 year (30). Initial treatment should be directed at conditions that exacerbate SDB such as congestive heart failure, and use of sedative and certain hypnotic medications (e.g. opioids, benzodiazepines, barbiturates). Depending on the type of SDB, treatment with continuous positive airway pressure or non-invasive mechanical ventilation can be considered during the acute phase (31). Cheyne–Stokes breathing, characterized by a crescendo–decrescendo pattern of tidal volume with variable length episodes of apnoea, occurs in 5–10% of patients with stroke (28). Supplemental nasal oxygen therapy (1–2 L/hour) can effectively reduce the number of cycles in patients who experience Cheyne–Stokes respiration (32).

The most frequent pulmonary complication of stroke is pneumonia. It is associated with an approximately threefold increase in mortality (33, 34). Patients with decreased level of consciousness, signs of large or bilateral supratentorial infarcts, or brainstem infarcts appear to be at particularly high risk for developing aspiration pneumonia (33). Factors such as loss of clearing mechanisms and cough reflex, impaired glottic closure, intubation, recumbent position, tube feeding, dysphagia, and vomiting predispose patients to overt or micro aspiration of microorganisms from the oropharyngeal and nasopharyngeal cavities. In addition, stroke-induced immunosuppression increases the likelihood of developing aspiration pneumonia (35). Aspiration of acidic gastric contents produces chemical pneumonitis, which in turn results in accelerated microbial colonization (36). Proper respiratory therapy including postural changes (e.g. mobilization and keeping the patient in a semi-upright position), oropharyngeal care and dental hygiene, sterile nasotracheal suctioning, and aggressive chest physiotherapy are effective in reducing the risk of aspiration (37). Prophylactic broad-spectrum antibiotic treatment is not recommended for prevention of pneumonia because of its unproven efficacy, increased risk of antibiotic resistance, and pseudomembranous enterocolitis (37).

% all cause death

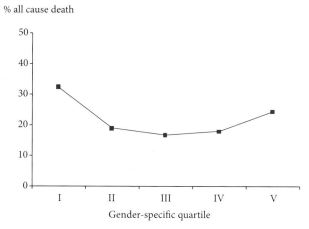

Fig. 10.3 The relationship between plasma haemoglobin levels and mortality in patients with ischaemic stroke. The figure shows outcome at 1 year according to quintiles of admission haemoglobin values. Note that there is a U-shaped relationship between haemoglobin levels and mortality where the risk of mortality increases at both ends of haemoglobin scale. (Reproduced from Tanne D, Molshatzki N, Merzeliak O, Tsabari R, Toashi M, Schwammenthal Y. Anemia status, haemoglobin concentration and outcome after acute stroke: a cohort study. *BMC Neurol.* 2010;10:22.© 2010 Tanne et al.; licensee BioMed Central Ltd.)

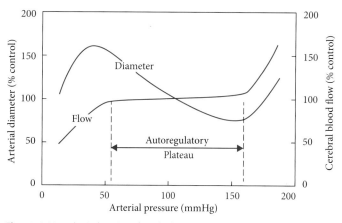

Fig. 10.4 Hypothetical tracing of cerebral arterial diameter and cerebral blood flow versus arterial pressure. Cerebral resistance arteries dilate during decreases and constrict during increases in mean arterial pressure and thus maintain relatively constant levels of cerebral blood flow over a fairly broad range of cerebral arterial pressures. (Reproduced with permission from Chillon JM, Baumbach GL. Autoregulation of cerebral blood flow. In: Welch KMA, Caplan LR, Reis DJ, et al., eds. Primer on Cerebrovascular Diseases. San Diego. CA. Academic Press, 1997, page 52. Copyright Elsevier (1997).)

Published data do not support hyperbaric oxygen therapy for routine treatment of stroke as it is not associated with improved outcome and may perhaps be harmful (38). A pilot study has suggested that high-flow oxygen therapy (normobaric hyperoxia) may be associated with transient improvement in clinical deficit and magnetic resonance imaging (MRI) abnormalities in patients with diffusion–perfusion mismatch (39). At present, there is no conclusive data on the routine use of high-flow oxygen therapy in stroke patients with normal saturation (22, 40).

Blood pressure management

Elevated blood pressure is common after ischaemic stroke. According to data from approximately 40,000 patients in the International Stroke Trial and the Chinese Acute Stroke Trial, one out of every four patients presents with systolic blood pressure greater than 180 mmHg (41, 42). Approximately 20% of stroke patients who present with high blood pressure do not have prior history of hypertension (43). Abrupt elevation in blood pressure after ischaemic stroke is often a transient phenomenon, associated with spontaneous reduction by an average of 20/10 mmHg during the following hours or days (44, 45). Increased sympathoadrenal tone has been suggested to play a role in the pathophysiology of blood pressure elevation following stroke; however, the exact mechanism is not known.

The most distinctive feature of the cerebral circulation is its capacity to maintain constant CBF in response to variations in perfusion pressure (mean arterial pressure–intracranial pressure (ICP)). In normotensive individuals, cerebral arteries and arterioles dilate as perfusion pressure decreases to 50–60 mmHg to maintain steady CBF (Figure 10.4). Further reduction in perfusion pressure below 50–60 mmHg leads to decreased CBF (46). Conversely, as perfusion pressure increases, small pial arteries and arterioles progressively constrict to keep CBF constant, until around 180 mmHg, at which point further increases in perfusion pressure cause proportional increases in CBF (46). Autoregulation protects the brain

from the threat of ischaemic injury at low perfusion pressures as well as from hyperperfusion, vasogenic oedema formation, and haemorrhage at high perfusion pressures. In cerebral ischaemia, the brain loses its capacity to maintain CBF within the autoregulatory plateau. Arteries and arterioles within the ischaemic territory are dilated to near or total capacity, with no or limited potential for further vasodilation, and as a result, CBF in the region of ischaemia becomes fully dependent upon perfusion pressure (47). Lowering high blood pressure during the acute phase of stroke may therefore be dangerous. At greatest risk for blood pressure lowering are patients with critical stenosis or occlusion in proximal arteries resulting in significant post-stenotic hypoperfusion, vasospasm, posture- or pressure-sensitive fluctuating neurological symptoms, and infarcts associated with large regions of marginally perfused tissue.

Although high blood pressure is expected to protect the brain regions with marginal tissue perfusion from progressing to infarction, it can also cause harm by increasing the risk of brain oedema, haemorrhagic transformation, early recurrent stroke, hypertensive encephalopathy, acute coronary syndrome, and worsening of heart failure. Data from recent large trials demonstrate that high blood pressure at the time of admission to the hospital is associated with poor clinical outcomes. An analysis of the International Stroke Trial shows a U-shaped relationship between systolic blood pressure assessed within 48 hours and stroke outcome (41). Systolic blood pressure higher than 140 mmHg is independently associated with increased risk of death, early (<2 week) recurrent ischaemic stroke, and combined dependency or death whereas low blood pressure is associated with increased risk of cardiovascular mortality. A subsequent pooled analysis of 32 studies confirms these findings, showing that high systolic and diastolic blood pressure during the acute phase of stroke is associated with death, combined death or disability, or combined early deterioration and death (48). Three randomized, controlled trials tested the effect of blood pressure lowering on clinical outcome during the acute phase of stroke. We briefly summarize the trials here.

The Controlling Hypertension and Hypotension Immediately Post-Stroke (CHHIPS) trial examined 179 patients with systolic blood pressure higher than 160 mmHg within 36 hours of symptom onset, randomizing them into labetalol, lisinopril, or placebo groups (49). Antihypertensive treatment resulted in an average reduction in systolic blood pressure of 10 mmHg over a 24-hour period. Ninety-day mortality was two times higher in the placebo arm, and patients in the active treatment arm showed no evidence of early neurological deterioration at 72 hours.

The Continue or Stop Post-Stroke Antihypertensives Collaborative Study (COSSACS) examined 763 patients who had taken an antihypertensive medication before their stroke; these patients were randomized into either 'continue' or 'stop' arms within 48 hours of stroke (50). In the continue group, the mean systolic and diastolic blood pressures were 13 mmHg and 8 mmHg lower than those measured in the stop group at 2 weeks. There was no difference in death or dependency between the groups at 2 weeks, but the trial was underpowered for its primary efficacy end-point.

The Scandinavian Candesartan Acute Stroke Trial (SCAST) studied 2029 patients with systolic blood pressure greater than 140 mmHg within 30 hours of symptom onset, randomly assigning them to candesartan treatment and placebo groups. At 7 days, the mean reduction in systolic and diastolic blood pressures in response to treatment was 5/2 mmHg (51). Although analysis of functional outcome at 6 months suggested marginal benefit in the placebo group, the composite endpoint of vascular death, myocardial infarction, and stroke was not different between the groups.

As evident by the results of these trials together, treatment of high blood pressure in the setting of acute ischaemic stroke remains controversial for several reasons. First, all of these trials of blood pressure lowering in acute stroke included patients with both haemorrhagic and ischaemic stroke. This raises concern that the benefit of treatment in the haemorrhagic stroke population may mask a potential harm in the ischaemic group. Second, no randomized study to date has tested the acute blood pressure reduction hypothesis a priori in patients susceptible to worsening with antihypertensive treatment. Such patients include those with fluctuating symptoms, haemodynamic stroke, or large marginally perfusing ischaemic tissue. Finally, the effect of blood pressure lowering in subsets of patients whose strokes developed as a different aetiological mechanisms (e.g. lacunar versus non-lacunar, low flow versus embolic stroke, etc.) is not known, further adding to the controversy in blood pressure lowering in acute ischaemic stroke.

Consensus guidelines recommend not to treat blood pressure in the setting of acute stroke unless systolic blood pressure is higher than 220 mmHg or diastolic blood pressure is higher than 120 mmHg; The goal of treatment is to lower blood pressure at a rate of no more than 15% during the first 24 hours of stroke onset (22, 40) (Table 10.5). To be eligible for thrombolytic therapy, patients must have systolic blood pressure of 185 mmHg or lower, and diastolic blood pressure of 110 mmHg or lower (22, 40). Blood pressure lowering during the acute phase of ischaemic stroke may also be considered in circumstances where high blood pressure poses danger to vital organs as may occur in severe cardiac insufficiency, acute renal failure, aortic dissection, or hypertensive encephalopathy. However, caution must be exercised in lowering blood pressure in patients with chronic hypertension. In these patients, the lower and upper limits of the autoregulation curve are shifted to higher levels, which render them susceptible to clinical deterioration even with subtle decrease in blood pressure.

Most protocols for managing increased blood pressure in patients with acute ischaemic stroke are empiric. General measures focus on comforting the patient, correcting hypoxia, treating pain, and emptying the bladder. Pharmacotherapy of high blood pressure in acute stroke is a complex task. The target blood pressure goal should be achieved under close monitoring for neurological deterioration. The ideal pharmacologic agent for acute stroke should be easily titratable and rapidly reversible; it should have a rapid onset of action, low risk of overshoot hypotension, predictable dose response curve, and no deleterious effect on intracranial pressure. Table 10.6 summarizes the safety, dose, and pharmacokinetic profiles of medications commonly used for treatment of high blood pressure in acute stroke.

Maintenance of optimal body temperature

Hyperthermia (>37.5°C) is not desirable in acute stroke because it increases cerebral metabolism, depletes energy reserves, and accelerates neuronal death. In a pooled analysis of 39 studies including

Table 10.5 Management of high blood pressure after acute stroke

Recommended actions	Actions to avoid
Reduce BP at a rate of no more than 15% during the first 24 hours in ischaemic stroke if systolic BP >220 mmHg or diastolic BP >120 mmHg or when high BP poses danger to vital organ functions	Administration of medications to lower BP in infarcts associated with critical stenosis/occlusion of proximal arteries, vasospasm, posture or pressure sensitive fluctuating neurological symptoms, and large regions of marginally perfused tissue unless high BP exposes thread to vital organ functions
Consider reducing BP >15% in patients who harbour large infarcts with high risk of symptomatic haemorrhagic conversion, whose brain imaging shows no or negligible amount of marginally perfused tissue, and who have stable neurological deficit with no haemodynamic lesion on vascular imaging	Pharmacotherapy to lower BP in patients who have mild hypertension (<220/120 mmHg) during the first 24 hours of stroke onset (as spontaneous decline in BP is common)
Lower systolic BP >150 mmHg to below 140 mmHg in patients with ICH	Lowering BP in increased ICP without monitoring ICP
Maintain cerebral perfusion pressure >60 mmHg in increased ICP	
Lower systolic BP ≤185 mmHg and diastolic BP ≤110 mmHg before thrombolytic therapy is started	
Maintain BP below 180/105 mmHg during the first 24 hours after thrombolytic therapy	

Table 10.6 Pharmacological agents for management of high blood pressure in patients with acute stroke

Agent	Onset of action	Elimination half life	Mechanism of action	Dose	Pros	Cons
Metoprolol	1–20 min	3–7 h	Selective beta-1 blocker	5 mg IV bolus over 5 min. Repeat to a total dose of 15 mg	–	Reduced cardiac output Overshoot hypotension
Esmolol	1–5 min	2–9 min	Selective beta-1 blocker	500 mcg/kg IV bolus over 1 minute followed by infusion at a rate of 50 mcg/kg/min	Rapid onset of action Easily titratable Rapidly reversible	Reduced cardiac output Bronchospasm
Labetalol	2–5 min	6–8 h	Selective alpha-1 + non-selective beta- (1+2) blocker	20 mg IV bolus over 2 min followed by 20–80 mg every 10 minutes to a total dose of 300 mg	Rapid onset of action Easily titratable No effect on ICP	Reduced cardiac output Orthostatic hypotension
Nicardipine	1–15 min	45 min—14 h	Dihydropyridine calcium channel blocker	5 mg IV infusion over 1 hour. Dose can be increased by 1.5 mg every 15 min to a maximum dose of 15–30 mg/h	Rapid onset of action Easily titratable Increased cardiac output Coronary and cerebral vasodilation No effect on ICP	Overshoot hypotension
Clevidipine	1–2 min	15 min	Dihydropyridine calcium channel blocker	1–2 mg IV infusion over 1 hour. Dose can be increased, to a maximum dose of 32 mg/h	Rapid onset of action Easily titratable Rapidly reversible Predictable dose response curve Increased cardiac output	Hyperlipidaemia and acute pancreatitis due to high volume infusion of lipid emulsion
Nitroglycerine	2–5 min	1–4 min	Nitric oxide donor, mixed arterial and venous dilator	5 mcg/min IV infusion. Dose can be increased by 5–20 mcg/min every 3–5 min to 200 mcg/min	Rapid onset of action Easily titratable Rapidly reversible Coronary vasodilation	Increased ICP Steal syndrome Reduced cardiac output Tolerance to antihypertensive effect
Sodium nitroprusside	<1 min	2–3 min	Nitric oxide donor, mixed arterial and venous dilator	0.3–0.5 mcg/kg/min IV infusion. Dose can be increased by 0.5 mcg/kg/min to 10 mcg/kg	Rapid onset of action Easily titratable Rapidly reversible	Increased ICP Steal syndrome Tolerance to antihypertensive effect
Enalaprilat	15 min–4 h	11 h	ACE inhibitor	1.25 mg IV bolus over 2–5 min	–	Overshoot hypotension Avoid in acute MI and renal failure
Fenoldopam	5–15 min	5 min	Dopamine D1 receptor agonist	0.1–0.3 mcg/kg/min IV infusion. Dose can be increased by 0.05–0.1 mcg/kg/min every 15 min to a maximum of 1.6 mcg/kg/min	Rapid onset of action Easily titratable Renal vasodilation	Steal syndrome Overshoot hypotension Unknown effect on ICP
Hydralazine	10–20 min	1 h	Direct arterial dilator	10–20 mg IV bolus every 4 to 6 hours to a maximum dose of 40 mg	–	Difficult to titrate Overshoot hypotension Unpredictable dose response curve Reflex sympathetic activation Avoid in aortic dissection Increased ICP

over 14,000 patients, hyperthermia was a consistent predictor of poor clinical outcome across all outcome metrics (52). Each 1°C elevation in body temperature within 6 hours of symptom onset increases the relative risk of death or disability by 2.2 (95% confidence interval (CI) 1.4–3.5) (53). Hyperthermia is also an independent predictor of infarct size and stroke severity in patients with ischaemic stroke (53).

Hypothermia, on the other hand, is neuroprotective after brain injury. For each 1°C decrease in temperature, the cerebral metabolic rate decreases by 6–7% (54, 55). Reducing body temperature from 37°C to 27°C reduces cerebral metabolic rate of oxygen consumption by 64% (56). Although mild hypothermia (~33°C) in patients with cardiac arrest (global ischaemia) is associated with improved neurological outcome (57), the effect of hypothermia in focal ischaemia is controversial. A systematic review of available data does not suggest a clinical benefit from physical cooling (58). Therapeutic hypothermia is associated with serious side effects such as infection, bleeding diathesis, hypotension, and cardiac arrhythmias, which may offset a potential benefit on clinical outcome. Furthermore, the optimal target body temperature, speed of temperature reduction, and method of cooling in focal cerebral ischaemia are not known.

Both animal studies of hypothermia-induced neuroprotection and clinical observations of hypothermia in patients with global cerebral ischaemia suggest that maintenance of normothermia (<37°C core body temperature) is a reasonable goal in acute stroke. In patients with mild hyperthermia, this could be achieved by administering antipyretic agents or applying surface cooling devices (40). Diagnosis and treatment of the source of fever is key to successful fever management. Acute hyperthermia after stroke may be central in origin, or more frequently, may result from a concurrent infection. Central fever often occurs in association with brainstem lesions, large cerebellar lesions that compress the brainstem, large hemispheric infarcts, intracerebral haemorrhage with intraventricular extension, and vasospasm due to subarachnoid haemorrhage (59). Central fever due to brainstem compression is characterized by rapid onset, significant fluctuation, absence of associated tachycardia, and extreme temperature. Elevated body temperature in the setting of acute stroke should be considered central in origin only after careful exclusion of infection or other possible causes.

Maintenance of glycaemia control

Glucose is the main substrate for energy production in the brain. Although the brain consumes approximately 25% of total body glucose, glycogen stores within the brain are very limited (barely sufficient to maintain neural function for 1–3 minutes in an event of ischaemia (21)), and hence, the brain is dependent upon continuous delivery of glucose through the bloodstream. In the brain, glucose is metabolized by glycolysis and oxidative phosphorylation. Glycolysis, a chain of reactions that occur primarily in astrocytes, results in the production of two molecules of adenosine triphosphate (ATP) and lactate. Lactate is then released into the extracellular space to be used by neurons for oxidative phosphorylation, which generates a total of 36 molecules of ATP. When oxygen supply is insufficient, the neuronal oxidative phosphorylation pathway is inhibited, causing lactate to accumulate; the resulting intracellular acidosis reduces tissue pH to approximately 6.5. Tissue acidosis in the presence of ischaemia accelerates cell death by activating a number of detrimental processes including free radical formation and excessive glutamate release (21). Experimental studies of focal and global ischaemia consistently show that elevated blood glucose in the setting of cerebral ischaemia increases lactic acid concentrations, leading to profound tissue acidosis (60, 61). Hyperglycaemia-related toxicity appears to be particularly important in experimental models in which residual circulation around the ischaemic core generates a penumbra. In models involving the complete obliteration of all the vessels supplying the ischaemic zone, hyperglycaemia appears to be non-toxic (62, 63). Hyperglycaemia accelerates the conversion of ischaemic tissue into infarction, resulting in rapid formation of larger infarcts than those seen in normoglycaemia (64). In patients who present with diffusion-perfusion MRI mismatch, blood glucose elevation from 5 to 10 mmol/L has been reported to be associated with a 56 cm^3 increase in final infarct size (65). Elevated blood glucose is also associated with increased 30-day mortality and poor functional outcome after ischaemic stroke (66), poor functional outcome after subarachnoid haemorrhage (67), poor functional outcome and symptomatic intracranial haemorrhage after thrombolysis, and reduced response to thrombolytics (68).

Admission hyperglycaemia is common after stroke, and occurs in up to approximately 60% of patients (66). In acute disorders such as stroke, hyperglycaemia may be a manifestation of underlying diabetes mellitus. According to a hospital-based study, 60% of acutely ill patients admitted to the hospital with hyperglycaemia are diagnosed with diabetes mellitus within 1 year. The distinction between diabetic and non-diabetic hyperglycaemia is important because the detrimental effect of hyperglycaemia on mortality and functional outcome after stroke is much higher in patients with non-diabetic hyperglycaemia. In a pooled analysis of 26 stroke studies, hyperglycaemia was a risk factor for mortality and poor functional outcome only in non-diabetic patients (66). The relationship between diabetes status and the effect of hyperglycaemia on outcome has also been reported after acute myocardial infarction and surgery (66, 69). It has been suggested that chronic hyperglycaemia in diabetes induces cellular conditioning that increases resistance to hyperglycaemia that may develop in response to acute illness (69). Mechanisms of hyperglycaemia other than diabetes include acute stress response via activation of neurohumoral mechanisms, acute illness-induced insulin resistance, high concentration glucose administration, and increased hepatic glucose production (69). Acute hyperglycaemia response in the absence of diabetes occurs in 10–15% of patients with stroke, depending on the glycosylated haemoglobin (HbA1c) cut-off used to exclude chronic hyperglycaemia (66); HbA1c less than 6.4% generally indicates the absence of an underlying diabetic process. The glucose level used to define hyperglycaemia in the literature ranges from 6.0–11.0 mmol/L, and admission blood glucose levels as low as 6.0 mmol/L have been linked to poor outcomes in patients with stroke (66). The cut-off values are generally lower for poor functional outcome (6.7 mmol/L) than for symptomatic intracranial haemorrhage following thrombolysis (10 mmol/L) (68). The cut-off for lacunar strokes and other end-artery strokes with little to no penumbra may be different. One study reports that hyperglycaemia up to 12 mmol/L is beneficial in lacunar strokes (70).

A reasonable approach for avoiding post-stroke hyperglycaemia is to minimize the use of glucose-containing solutions and medications, such as steroids, that can trigger hyperglycaemia within the first 24 hours after stroke. Although hyperglycaemia is associated with unfavourable clinical and tissue outcome, there is a lack of evidence to support the notion that correction of hyperglycaemia with intensive insulin therapy positively affects the clinical outcome. The largest randomized trial to date in patients with stroke was stopped early because of low enrolment, as only approximately 40% of the target sample size was reached (71). Despite the lack of evidence from randomized clinical trials, most consensus statements and guidelines recommend treatment of severe hyperglycaemia (>10–11 mmol/L) with insulin infusion (22, 72). The desired blood glucose level with treatment is in the range of 5–6.7 mmol/L. The benefit of insulin treatment can be expected to be greater in patients with large penumbra, in patients with non-lacunar strokes, and when treatment is instituted early. Frequent monitoring of blood glucose levels and proper titration of insulin dose are critical to minimizing the risk of overshoot hypoglycaemia. However, tight control of glycaemia to attain normal levels is often difficult and labour intensive (23). Intensive insulin treatment should be administered with caution in settings where resources are limited, given that hypoglycaemic episodes during intensive insulin treatment are a strong predictor of mortality in critically ill patients (73). Overcorrection of hyperglycaemia may also accelerate infarct growth in stroke patients with persistent arterial occlusion (74). The risk of hypoglycaemia with intensive insulin regimens would be expected to be higher in patients with moderate hyperglycaemia (6.7–10 mmol/L) (22). In such patients, continuous blood glucose monitoring should be considered.

Dysphagia evaluation and nutrition

Dysphagia, or impaired swallowing, is common after stroke, occurring in up to two-thirds of patients in the acute phase of stroke (75). Dysphagia is a major risk factor for developing aspiration pneumonia. Up to 20% of patients with dysphagia die from aspiration pneumonia during the first year after stroke (76). Moreover, dysphagia-related restriction of oral intake may result in undernutrition, dehydration, and metabolic abnormalities. Early management of dysphagia improves outcome and diminishes the length of hospital stay (77).

Brainstem lesions affecting the lower cranial nerve nuclei involved in swallowing are the primary cause of significant dysphagia. Unilateral supranuclear infarcts can also cause dysphagia in individuals with asymmetric supranuclear innervation of the lower cranial nerve nuclei. Most patients with supranuclear swallowing dysfunction spontaneously improve within weeks after stroke. In contrast, dysphagia caused by lesions on the brainstem often persists and causes long-lasting disability. Bilateral opercular infarcts can also cause long-lasting dysphagia with low likelihood of spontaneous recovery.

A preserved gag reflex may not be a good indicator of preserved swallowing ability. In all stroke patients, oral intake should be restricted until appropriate swallowing screening is completed. According to one estimate, institution of a formal dysphagia screening protocol early after stroke could save as many as 8300 lives, and prevent 40,000 cases of pneumonia each year in the US (78). A simple and useful bedside screening method is the water swallow test (75). The patient is given 90 mL (3 oz) water while seated in an upright position. Delayed swallowing, drooling, coughing during or right after swallowing, or dysphonia suggest

dysphagia. Patients who fail the bedside screening test should undergo more comprehensive dysphagia assessment, such as videofluoroscopic examination (76, 79), before being given food or drink. Behavioural interventions and diet modification measures can be considered to ensure safe swallowing; for instance, reducing the consistency of diet, preventing distractions during eating, eating only in the seated position, ensuring a slow feeding rate with small amounts of food per bite, breath-holding while swallowing, coughing after each swallow to clear the residual food from the hypopharynx, and airway protection strategies such as a chin tuck or head rotation along with swallowing. However, it is important to realize that although these strategies provide some protection against aspiration (80), they do not facilitate recovery of swallowing function. Early reports with transcutaneous electric stimulation of the muscles involved in swallowing suggest that such techniques may help patients regain swallowing ability after stroke (81).

In patients with severely compromised swallowing, enteral feeding via a nasogastric, nasoduodenal, or nasojejunal tube can be considered to ensure adequate intake of food, water, and medications. Early initiation of tube feeding (within the first week of stroke) appears to provide marginal reduction in the risk of death at 6 months, compared to no tube feeding (82). Compared to nasal feeding tubes, which are less comfortable and prone to dislodgement, percutaneous endoscopic gastrostomy (PEG) may be a reasonable option for prolonged enteral feeding. Still, neither feeding tubes nor PEG fully eliminate the risk of aspiration pneumonia. Delayed gastric emptying and impaired lower oesophageal sphincter function after stroke lead to gastric distension and gastro-oesophageal reflux. The risk of aspiration also increases with increased secretions due to tube irritation in nasally inserted tubes as well as with malposition or distal tip migration of the tube into the oesophagus. Head-of-bed elevation during feeding, frequent monitoring of tube location, avoidance of medications such as antacids and gastric proton pump inhibitors that can delay gastric emptying, and prevention of constipation and large bolus of food injections minimize reflux and subsequent aspiration. The use of transpyloric or small intestinal tubes does not significantly reduce reflux as compared to PEG (83, 84).

Prevention and treatment of deep venous thrombosis and pulmonary embolism

Deep vein thrombosis (DVT) in lower extremities is common after stroke, occurring in approximately 15% of patients within a month of stroke (85). According to Virchow's postulate, thrombus formation in the venous system is associated with a combination of abnormalities in the vessel wall (endothelial injury), blood flow (stasis), and blood constituents (acquired or inherited thrombophilias). Unlike arterial thrombosis, which is usually associated with endothelial injury and exposition of the subendothelial matrix to the circulating platelets, the endothelium is often intact in venous thrombosis that develops after stroke. The primary cause of venous thrombosis after stroke is stagnant venous blood flow resulting from immobilization and loss of muscle power in the lower extremities. DVT is detected contralateral to the paralytic leg in approximately 25% of stroke patients, highlighting the impact of immobilization and inherited or acquired thrombophilias in the formation of post-stroke DVT (85). Factor V Leiden mutation, prothrombin gene mutation, and hyper-homocysteinaemia are the most frequent inherited thrombophilias in patients with stroke. Common acquired causes of thrombophilia include malignancy, surgery, infection, trauma, oral contraceptive use, hormone replacement therapy, and antiphospholipid antibodies (86, 87). Other important risk factors for DVT in patients with stroke include older age, dehydration, obesity, and congestive heart failure.

In an observational study of more than 5500 immobile stroke patients, asymptomatic DVT was detected in 10% of patients, whereas symptomatic DVT was diagnosed in 5% (85). Diagnosis of symptomatic DVT can be challenging in patients with stroke due to coexisting peripheral vascular disease and impaired perception of pain in the limbs. Physical examination may reveal a palpable thrombosed vein, increased leg circumference due to ipsilateral limb oedema, superficial venous dilation, redness, warmth, pain, tenderness, and fever. DVT should be suspected in all immobilized stroke patients with unexplained fever. The differential diagnosis includes lymphangitis, lymph obstruction, cellulitis, peripheral vascular disease, and venous insufficiency (88). Measurement of D-dimer levels—almost always increased (>500 mg/dL) in patients with DVT—may be useful in suspected cases. Nonetheless, the D-dimer test has low specificity, such that although a negative test can be useful for ruling out DVT, a positive test does not provide a clear indication that DVT is present (89). In patients with high probability of DVT, compression ultrasonography can be used to substantiate the diagnosis. Ultrasonography may not detect an isolated thrombus in the external iliac vein or in the proximal portion of the common femoral vein. In such cases, pelvic magnetic resonance venography may help confirm the diagnosis of DVT (90).

The most feared complication of DVT is pulmonary embolism (PE), which occurs in 5–30% of untreated patients with proximal DVT during the first month following stroke (85). PE is the most common cause of death after stroke during the 2- to 4-week subacute period post-stroke. Given that untreated PE is associated with a mortality rate of approximately 30% (91), effective prevention and treatment of DVT is essential. Acute onset tachypnoea, tachycardia, and pleuritic pain raise concern for PE regardless of whether DVT is documented. Hypoxemia unresponsive to 100% oxygen as a result of intrapulmonary shunting supports the diagnosis. In approximately 20% of the patients ECG monitoring may reveal a classic triad of changes characterized by a large S wave in lead I, large Q wave in lead III, and inverted T wave in lead III (S1Q3T3

sign). Diagnosis of PE in the setting of stroke can be challenging, as the signs and symptoms of PE may be masked by comorbidities and systemic complications as well as by neurological deficit. Definite diagnosis can be made by direct visualization of pulmonary artery occlusion using multidetector pulmonary CT angiogram.

DVT prophylaxis should be considered for all immobile patients as well as for patients with lower extremity weakness and hereditary or acquired risk factors for DVT (Table 10.7). Early mobilization, active physical therapy, and prevention of dehydration are effective means of prophylaxis. Other measures include intermittent pneumatic compression, rotating beds, electrical stimulation, and treatment with anticoagulant agents and aspirin. One randomized trial that compared the use of thigh-length graduated compression stockings with routine care (not including medical prophylaxis) showed that graded compression stockings were not effective in reducing the risk of DVT, PE, and PE-related mortality (92). In contrast, the use of compression stockings was associated with negative effects including increased risk of skin ulcers and necrosis. Intermittent pneumatic compression, on the other hand, appears to be a modestly effective means of prophylaxis. In one study of patients with intracerebral haemorrhage, intermittent pneumatic compression reduced the risk of asymptomatic DVT to 5% compared to 16% with compression stockings (93). The major side effect of intermittent pneumatic compression is leg ischaemia, especially in patients with advanced peripheral arterial disease. It also has a potential to facilitate dislodgement of emboli from freshly formed thrombus, particularly in immobile patients with no effective means of prophylaxis. Therefore, it is important to start intermittent pneumatic compression early after acute stroke.

The mainstay of DVT prophylaxis is anticoagulant therapy. Both unfractionated heparin and low-molecular-weight heparin (LMWH) are effective in preventing DVT in patients with stroke (94). According to an open label randomized trial, low-dose LMWH (enoxaparin 40 mg/day) is more effective than subcutaneous unfractionated heparin (5000U twice daily) (95). Combination of intermittent pneumatic compression and anticoagulation treatment provides more protection than could be achieved by anticoagulation alone (96). Aspirin also provides a modest reduction in the risk of DVT, and can be considered when anticoagulation is contraindicated. Inferior vena cava filters may also be an option for patients with contraindications to anticoagulation. Limited efficacy

Table 10.7 Management of deep venous thrombosis and pulmonary embolism after acute stroke

Recommended actions	Actions to avoid
Intermittent pneumatic compression for prevention of DVT in immobilized patients with or without lower extremity weakness	Delayed application of intermittent pneumatic compression without ruling out fresh thrombus in the venous system by ultrasonography in patients with no effective means of prophylaxis
Early institution of anticoagulant therapy for prevention of DVT in immobilized patients with ischaemic stroke	
Short-term anticoagulant therapy for prevention of DVT in immobilized patients with deep ICH provided bleeding has completely ceased	Long-term anticoagulant therapy for prevention of DVT in patients with deep ICH
Full-dose anticoagulant therapy for at least 3 months for treatment of DVT or non-fatal PE after ischaemic stroke	Long-term anticoagulation for treatment of DVT or non-fatal PE in patients with lobar ICH unless absolutely necessary
Full-dose anticoagulant therapy for at least 3 months for treatment of DVT or non-fatal PE after deep ICH	
Long-term intermittent pneumatic compression, elastic stockings, adequate hydration, inferior vena cava filter with or without aspirin therapy for prevention of DVT as well as treatment of DVT or non-fatal PE in lobar ICH	

and high rate of complications such as occlusion, intraperitoneal erosion, and distal migration in patients with diminished abdominal muscle tone preclude routine use of inferior vena cava filters for the purpose of DVT prophylaxis.

Once DVT is diagnosed, full dose heparin or LMWH followed by warfarin for at least 3 months with a target international normalized ratio of 1.5–2.5, is recommended (97). The duration of treatment may be longer depending on the underlying thrombophilia and the residual thrombus on follow-up ultrasonography. Anticoagulant use requires careful assessment of risk and benefit at the individual patient level. It is critical to weigh the expected benefit from treatment against the risk of symptomatic haemorrhagic conversion or intracranial haemorrhage (ICH). Anticoagulants should be avoided during the first 24 hours after thrombolytic therapy due to elevated risk of symptomatic haemorrhagic conversion. The risk of symptomatic haemorrhagic transformation may also outweigh the benefit of anticoagulation in patients with large territorial infarcts showing signs of mass effect and oedema during the acute period.

Patients with ICH are at low but continuing risk of haematoma growth after stroke (98); therefore, it is important to confirm the cessation of bleeding, by imaging, before initiating preventive anticoagulation. Anticoagulation can be started as early as 1 day after ICH, provided bleeding has completely ceased. The major concern with anticoagulation after the acute period of ICH is recurrent ICH. ICH in deep location (hypertensive haemorrhage) recurs at a rate of about 2% per year (99). In contrast, lobar haemorrhage due to amyloid angiopathy is associated with a much higher rate of recurrence (4–6% per year). Long-term use of oral anticoagulants increases the risk of recurrent ICH approximately threefold, from approximately 2% to approximately 6% in deep ICH and approximately 5% to approximately 15% in lobar haemorrhage, while reducing the risk of DVT or PE by approximately 80% (94, 100). These estimates suggest that the risk of recurrent bleeding with long-term preventive anticoagulation outweighs the risk of symptomatic DVT or non-fatal PE regardless of the type of haemorrhage (deep versus lobar). Long-term anticoagulant therapy should therefore be avoided for DVT prophylaxis in patients with ICH. The risk of fatal PE after untreated DVT or non-fatal PE can be as high as 30%. Thus, in patients who have hypertensive ICH and established diagnosis of DVT or non-fatal PE, the benefit of full-dose anticoagulation may theoretically outweigh the risk of recurrent bleeding. In contrast, given the extremely high risk of recurrent bleeding, anticoagulation should be administered with caution, after careful assessment of individual risk, and alternative means such as inferior vena cava filters, low-intensity anticoagulation, intermittent pneumatic compression, adequate hydration, or antiplatelet therapy should be considered for non-fatal PE or proximal DVT in patients with lobar haemorrhages.

Monitoring of intracranial pressure and management of brain oedema

Brain oedema is the major cause of stroke-related mortality during the acute stroke phase. Within minutes of cerebral ischaemia, cytotoxic oedema develops due to the mobilization of water molecules from the interstitial space to the intracellular space. Cell swelling as a result of cytotoxic oedema does not cause a mass effect. As ischaemia persists, the blood–brain barrier breaks down and plasma proteins start to leak into the brain parenchyma causing vasogenic

oedema. This leads to significant expansion of the intracranial volume and traction or compression of the intracranial structures. Vasogenic oedema starts within hours of ischaemia and generally reaches a maximum volume at around 4 days. Occasionally, brain swelling peaks within 24 hours after stroke onset. The extent and rate of swelling depends on initial infarct size, time of evaluation, and reperfusion status. Large infarcts that occur secondary to persistent occlusion of the internal carotid artery or the proximal segment of the middle cerebral artery are at greater risk of developing severe oedema than are smaller infarcts (19). Lack of reperfusion and limited collateral supply to the ischaemic area further increase the risk of developing severe early swelling. In MCA infarcts, infarct volume on diffusion-weighted imaging appears to have a predictive value for development of malignant oedema. Large infarcts, i.e. greater than 82 cc (101) (approximately one-third of the MCA territory) at about 2½ hours or 145 cc (102) at around 6 h (±3.5 hours) of symptom onset predict malignant oedema formation with high (~90%) specificity, positive predictive value, and negative predictive value but with variable sensitivity changing from 50% to 100% depending on the time of assessment. Infarcts due to proximal occlusions in the presence of insufficient collateral blood flow tend to grow rapidly. Hence, the predictive accuracy of infarct volume cut-offs for malignant oedema increases as a function of time since the onset of stroke. Other imaging predictors of malignant oedema include hypodensity in greater than two-thirds of the MCA territory on the second-day brain CT and large territorial hypoperfusion on CT- or MR-perfusion images acquired within 6 hours of symptom onset (103). In settings where imaging is not available the National Institutes of Health Stroke Scale (NIHSS) score (>18 versus ≤18) can be used to predict the risk of malignant MCA infarction. However, the specificity of the NIHSS score (63%) is much lower than that is achieved by imaging (101).

Cerebral oedema is thought to be responsible for clinical deterioration in 10–20% of patients (103), and causes death in approximately 5% of patients with ischaemic stroke (104). Massive oedema in posterior circulation strokes can cause fatal transtentorial herniation and brainstem compression. The risk of herniation is higher in younger individuals, as normal aging-related cerebral atrophy can better accommodate the space-occupying cerebral swelling in older adults.

Posterior inferior cerebellar artery and sometimes superior cerebellar artery infarcts can cause space-occupying cerebellar oedema leading to brainstem compression, descending (transforaminal, tonsillar) or ascending (upward transtentorial) herniation, and obstructive hydrocephalus. Displacement of the fourth ventricle, obstructive hydrocephalus, and obliteration of the basal cisterns are the radiological signs of impending herniation in posterior circulation strokes. Compensation of the mass effect is limited in the posterior fossa due to its small volume. As a result, life-threatening brainstem compression develops rapidly. Suboccipital decompressive craniectomy or controlled external ventricular drainage may be considered before the full clinical picture develops in posterior circulation strokes (103).

Treatment options for raised intracranial pressure include supportive measures, osmotherapy, hyperventilation, ventricular drainage, and decompressive surgery (Table 10.8). The head should be kept in a neutral position to ensure proper venous drainage. Factors that provoke ICP such as hypoxia, hypercapnia, hyperthermia, hyperglycaemia, hypertension, seizures, pain, medications

Table 10.8 Management of raised intracranial pressure after acute stroke

Recommended Actions	Actions to Avoid
The goal is to keep ICP <20 mmHg and cerebral perfusion pressure >60 mmHg	Head elevation in patients with signs of downward herniation
Head elevation to 30° to increase venous outflow, intubation, sedation, hyperventilation to maintain $PaCO_2$ 25–30 mmHg, and control of hyperthermia, hyperglycaemia, and seizures	Compression of jugular veins by kinking of the neck or by external constraints
Consult with neurosurgery to assess for hemicraniectomy, decompression, external ventricular drain placement, or haematoma evacuation	Hyperventilation in patients with large regions of marginally perfused brain tissue
ICP monitoring for patients with Glasgow Coma Scale score <9, intraventricular haemorrhage and hydrocephalus, and signs of herniation	
20% mannitol 0.25–1 g/kg IV bolus, every 4–6 hours as needed to maintain blood osmolality 300–320 mOsm/L and osmolar gap <10	
23.4% NaCl 0.5–1 mL/kg IV bolus, every 4–6 hours as needed when there is high osmolar gap, renal insufficiency, high ICP despite mannitol therapy, diabetes, and hypotension or haemodynamic failure	
Metabolic suppression therapy with barbiturates or hypothermia to reduce ICP refractory to osmotherapy	
Suboccipital decompressive craniectomy or cerebellar resection in space occupying cerebellar oedema	

that cause intracranial vasodilation, and manoeuvres associated with increased intrathoracic pressure such as coughing, vomiting, shivering, and straining for bowel movements should be avoided (105). In patients with a Glasgow Coma Scale score less than 9, ICP monitoring and external ventricular drain placement can be considered (106). Elective intubation and mechanical ventilation, analgesia, sedation and paralysis may be required in cases with progressive worsening (107).

Osmotherapy with mannitol or hyperosmolar saline solutions effectively reduces ICP. Mannitol (20%) is administered at 0.25–1.0 g/kg IV over 20 minutes, and the dose can be repeated every 4–6 hours. However, the osmotic effect of mannitol diminishes with repeated doses over time because of the rebound phenomenon. In response to mannitol, cerebral blood volume and ICP initially decrease rapidly due to reflex vasoconstriction caused by mannitol-induced reduction in blood viscosity (108, 109). This effect is followed by a longer-lasting reduction in ICP, owing to its osmotic properties and inhibited CSF production. Blood and urine osmolality and osmolar gap (measured osmolality – calculated osmolarity) should be monitored during mannitol administration. Osmolality can be calculated using the following formula:

$$\text{Osmolarity} = 2 \times Na\ (mEq/L) + glucose\ (mg/dL)\ /18 + BUN\ (mg/dL)/2.8$$

The desired serum osmolality for mannitol treatment is in the range of 300–320 mOsm/L. Serum osmolality, Na, K, glucose, BUN (blood urea nitrogen), and creatinine levels should be checked 1 hour prior to each mannitol dose. Serum osmolality should be maintained <320 mOsm/L and osmolar gap <10 to avoid kidney injury (110). Possible complications of mannitol therapy include metabolic acidosis, hyponatraemia, hyperkalaemia, acute kidney injury, hypotension, and decreased cerebral perfusion pressure. Hypertonic saline, an alternative to mannitol (111), favourably affects cerebral haemodynamics, increasing cerebral perfusion pressure by augmenting cardiac output and intravascular volume while reducing ICP. It can be administered as a continuous infusion (3% NaCl, 1 mL/kg/h) or bolus (0.5–1 mL/kg 23.4% NaCl). During hypertonic saline administration, serum sodium concentration should be closely monitored to avoid excessive (>155–160 mEq/L) and rapid (12 mEq/L/day) elevation in sodium concentration.

Hyperventilation lowers ICP by reducing cerebral blood volume through hypocapneic vasoconstriction. A 10 mmHg change in $PaCO_2$ is associated with a 30% change in cerebral blood volume (112). The effect of hyperventilation on ICP is modest because cerebral blood volume accounts for only 10% of the intracranial volume. Reduction in cerebral blood flow with hyperventilation may be a concern in patients with persistent marginally perfusing brain tissue. Another concern with hyperventilation is that its effect on ICP typically fades within 6 hours due to adaptation of vasomotor reactivity to respiratory alkalosis (113). Hyperventilation should be considered as an acute treatment option to provide a temporary relief after careful assessment to identify potentially viable brain tissue in the ischaemic territory.

Although the relatively conservative measures just outlined appear to effectively reduce ICP, their effect on clinical outcome is rather dubious, particularly in patients who develop malignant infarcts, which, with conservative treatment, are associated with mortality rates as high as 80% (114, 115). For such patients, removal of the cranium, with or without resection of the underlying dead brain tissue, to accommodate the expanding (swelling) brain appears to be a viable treatment option. A pooled analyses of randomized controlled trials demonstrates that early hemicraniectomy (within 48 hours of stroke onset) results in reduced death and severe disability (modified Rankin Scale (mRS) score >4) in patients younger than 60 years (114, 115). The effectiveness of hemicraniectomy for reducing poor outcome (mRS score >3) is less certain. Survival following hemicraniectomy often comes at the expense of severe neurological disability, with the vast majority of patients who survive the procedure remaining bedridden and incontinent, and requiring constant nursing care.

Decompressive surgery may also benefit patients with large cerebellar infarcts presenting with signs and symptoms of brainstem compression, acute hydrocephalus, or imaging evidence of downward or upward herniation. Despite conservative treatment such patients often become rapidly comatose and die of cardiopulmonary arrest from medullary compression. Suboccipital decompressive craniectomy and cerebellar resection appear to benefit patients with life-threatening cerebellar oedema. Observational cohort studies have shown that suboccipital craniectomy has a marked survival advantage compared to natural history, and therefore, should be considered as a treatment option for patients with large cerebellar infarcts with early signs of acute hydrocephalus or brainstem compression (117, 118).

Monitoring of cardiac functions

Cardiac embolism is the most common cause of ischaemic stroke. There are more than 30 different cardiac conditions known to serve as an embolic source (12, 13). A thorough cardiovascular examination (including physical examination, 12-lead ECG, cardiac enzyme tests, and echocardiography) is essential for timely identification of cardiac abnormalities, some of which may require urgent treatment. Examples of such abnormalities include ruptured papillary muscles, free-floating thrombus in the left atrium, mobile intracardiac thrombus, acute myocardial infarction, and acute severe congestive heart failure. While cardiac pathologies lead to stroke, stroke can also independently lead to injury to the heart—often with serious outcomes ranging from myocardial damage to sudden death (119–121). The concept of neurogenic myocardial injury relies on three lines of evidence: ECG, cardiac enzyme, and pathological changes that occur in the absence of a clinically evident acute coronary syndrome.

ECG changes, characterized by repolarization abnormalities including cerebral T waves, transient prolongation of QT interval, inverted T waves, prominent U waves, elevated ST segments, and appearance of Q waves occur in 15–40% of patients with stroke and can sometimes fully mimic an anterolateral subendocardial ischaemia (122–123). Cardiac arrhythmias after stroke may cause recurrent stroke as well as haemodynamic perturbations that increase the risk of stroke progression. Prolongation of the QT interval and reduced heart rate variability are indicators of increased arrhythmia risk and mortality after stroke (121).

Cardiac enzyme changes are characterized by elevations in the creatine-kinase myocardial band or cardiac troponins (119, 124). The prevalence of troponin elevation is approximately 10% after ischaemic stroke (119, 125). Cardiac troponin elevation after stroke may have a prognostic value, as it is associated with greater probability of poor outcome and mortality (125, 126). Similar to ECG, cardiac biomarkers lack specificity in terms of a neurogenic mechanism. In contrast to acute coronary syndromes, in which cardiac troponin levels often exceed 1.0 mcg/L, troponin levels after stroke are often only mildly elevated, rarely exceeding 1.0 mcg/L (119). Nevertheless, even with mild troponin elevations, acute coronary syndrome can occur. Further cardiac investigations to rule out myocardial ischaemia should be considered in patients suspected of having concurrent territorial electrocardiogram (ECG) changes, relevant clinical history, or signs and symptoms of acute coronary syndrome.

Pathological changes include continuing low-grade myocardial necrosis, distinguished by foci of swollen myocytes, interstitial haemorrhage, and mononuclear infiltration in the vicinity of cardiac nerve endings (127). This characteristic tissue signature is called 'myocytolysis', 'myofibrillary degeneration', or 'contraction band necrosis' (128). Although highly specific, myocytolysis is a postmortem finding that is not available at the time of clinical evaluation. It has been suggested that the acute left ventricular dysfunction or stunning observed after subarachnoid haemorrhage is a clinical phenotype associated with myocytolysis. This syndrome is characterized by reversible, abnormal, and often non-territorial abnormalities of the left ventricular wall motion, associated with subtle elevation in cardiac troponins, non-specific ECG changes, and severely reduced ejection fraction (129). Transient cardiac ballooning syndrome, or Takotsubo cardiomyopathy syndrome (TCS), is another clinical phenotype that is associated with pathological evidence of myocytolysis (130, 131). This syndrome, which occurs mainly in postmenopausal women following emotional or physical stress, is characterized by reversible myocardial dysfunction wherein the apex, disproportionately more involved than the base of the heart, balloons during the systole. Left ventricular ejection fraction drops to as low as 10% during the acute period (132). Similar to left ventricular stunning syndrome after subarachnoid haemorrhage, ECG often shows non-specific changes, and troponin elevation is usually subtle.

TCS with typical apical ballooning has also been reported in patients with ischaemic stroke. A Japanese observational study identified seven patients with apical ballooning from among 569 consecutive patients (1.2%) with ischaemic stroke (133). The direction of association between TCS and stroke is not fully known. While stroke can cause TCS via neurocardiogenic mechanisms, TCS can also lead to stroke. Severe left ventricular dysfunction and apical akinesis in TCS provides an appropriate milieu for left ventricular thrombus formation. A systematic review reported that left ventricular thrombus can be identified in 2.5% of patients, and systemic thromboembolic complications occur in 0.8% (134). Stroke-induced left ventricular dysfunction or TCS should be considered in differential diagnosis in all stroke patients who suddenly develop haemodynamic and pulmonary symptoms consistent with acute congestive heart failure. Although the syndrome is often self-limiting and reversible within days to weeks, patients with haemodynamic instability may require supportive treatment with positive inotropic agents or implantation of an intra-aortic balloon pump. The role of central sympathetic overactivity in stroke pathophysiology suggests that empiric use of beta-adrenergic blockers may provide cardioprotection in patients with stroke-related left ventricular dysfunction. Prophylactic anticoagulant treatment may also be appropriate in some patients, until impaired left ventricular function returns to normal.

Multidisciplinary integrated stroke management

The organized structure of a primary stroke centre includes expert teams of physicians including the acute stroke team, neurosurgical team, neuroradiology team, and rehabilitation services as well as the resources and capabilities to perform timely brain imaging and cardiac and vascular evaluations on around the clock. Stroke centres that provide intensive care to severely ill stroke patients and can perform neurointerventional procedures are referred to comprehensive stroke centres (135, 136). Focused care in dedicated acute stroke units led by a multidisciplinary team of physicians is associated with improved overall outcome for patients with ischaemic stroke. According to a meta-analysis of 6936 patient data from 31 studies, management of acute stroke patients in dedicated units leads to reductions in the odds of death at 1 year (odds ratio (OR) 0.86; 95% confidence interval (CI) 0.76–0.98), the odds of death or institutionalized care (OR 0.82; 95% CI 0.73–0.92), and death or dependency (OR 0.82; 95% CI 0.73–0.92) (137). According to another study, organized multidisciplinary stroke approach increases the number of patients who can be treated by intravenous tissue plasminogen activator by approximately sevenfold within the prerequisite of 3 hours (138). The effectiveness of stroke units in improving stroke outcome is robust. There are several factors that can explain the success of stroke units. Stroke centres are staffed by physicians, nurses, and ancillary personnel experienced in stroke management who are able to provide specialized care for acute stroke patients (136). In addition, such units allow continuous monitoring of vital signs (blood pressure, pulse, respiration, and oxygenation) (22, 139), regular assessment of the neurological status, better communication between health care professionals, early detection and treatment of medical complications, timely diagnosis of the underlying aetiology, and acute rehabilitation (22, 139). Organized stroke centre approach requires strict adherence to standardized stroke management protocols as well as incorporation of registry systems that allow recording of adherence metrics to standard protocols. One can thus measure the degree of compliance with standard protocols and identify the sources of protocol deviations. This information, in turn, could be used to further improve the system. Published guidelines strongly encourage medical centres to implement primary or comprehensive stroke centres. The guidelines also advocate certification of all stroke centres by external and independent.

References

1. Lees KR, Bluhmki E, von Kummer R, Brott TG, Toni D, Grotta JC, et al. Time to treatment with intravenous alteplase and outcome in stroke: an updated pooled analysis of ECASS, ATLANTIS, NINDS, and EPITHET trials. Lancet. 2010 May 15;375(9727):1695–1703.
2. Saver JL. Time is brain—quantified. Stroke. 2006 Jan;37(1):263–266.
3. Astrup J, Siesjo BK, Symon L. Thresholds in cerebral ischemia—the ischemic penumbra. Stroke. 1981 Nov-Dec;12(6):723–725.
4. Hossmann KA. Viability thresholds and the penumbra of focal ischemia. Ann Neurol. 1994 Oct;36(4):557–565.
5. Darby DG, Barber PA, Gerraty RP, Desmond PM, Yang Q, Parsons M, et al. Pathophysiological topography of acute ischemia by combined diffusion-weighted and perfusion MRI. Stroke. 1999 Oct;30(10):2043–2052.
6. Lees KR, Hankey GJ, Hacke W. Design of future acute-stroke treatment trials. Lancet Neurol. 2003 Jan;2(1):54–61.
7. Copen WA, Rezai Gharai L, Barak ER, Schwamm LH, Wu O, Kamalian S, et al. Existence of the diffusion-perfusion mismatch within 24 hours after onset of acute stroke: dependence on proximal arterial occlusion. Radiology. 2009 Mar;250(3):878–886.
8. Schellinger PD, Fiebach JB, Hacke W. Imaging-based decision making in thrombolytic therapy for ischemic stroke: present status. Stroke. 2003 Feb;34(2):575–583.
9. Ay H, Gungor L, Arsava EM, Rosand J, Vangel M, Benner T, et al. A score to predict early risk of recurrence after ischemic stroke. Neurology. 2010 Jan 12;74(2):128–135.
10. Sacco RL, Foulkes MA, Mohr JP, Wolf PA, Hier DB, Price TR. Determinants of early recurrence of cerebral infarction. The Stroke Data Bank. Stroke. 1989 Aug;20(8):983–989.
11. Moroney JT, Bagiella E, Paik MC, Sacco RL, Desmond DW. Risk factors for early recurrence after ischemic stroke: the role of stroke syndrome and subtype. Stroke. 1998 Oct;29(10):2118–2124.
12. Ay H, Furie KL, Singhal A, Smith WS, Sorensen AG, Koroshetz WJ. An evidence-based causative classification system for acute ischemic stroke. Ann Neurol. 2005 Nov;58(5):688–697.
13. Ay H, Benner T, Arsava EM, Furie KL, Singhal AB, Jensen MB, et al. A computerized algorithm for etiologic classification of ischemic stroke: the Causative Classification of Stroke System. Stroke. 2007 Nov;38(11):2979–2984.
14. Arsava EM, Ballabio E, Benner T, Cole JW, Delgado-Martinez MP, Dichgans M, et al. The Causative Classification of Stroke system: an international reliability and optimization study. Neurology. 2010 Oct 5;75(14):1277–1284.
15. Sylaja PN, Coutts SB, Subramaniam S, Hill MD, Eliasziw M, Demchuk AM. Acute ischemic lesions of varying ages predict risk of ischemic events in stroke/TIA patients. Neurology. 2007 Feb 6;68(6):415–419.
16. Wen HM, Lam WW, Rainer T, Fan YH, Leung TW, Chan YL, et al. Multiple acute cerebral infarcts on diffusion-weighted imaging and risk of recurrent stroke. Neurology. 2004 Oct 12;63(7):1317–1319.
17. Bang OY, Lee PH, Heo KG, Joo US, Yoon SR, Kim SY. Specific DWI lesion patterns predict prognosis after acute ischaemic stroke within the MCA territory. J Neurol Neurosurg Psychiatry. 2005 Sep;76(9):1222–1228.
18. Kumar S, Selim MH, Caplan LR. Medical complications after stroke. Lancet Neurol. 2010 Jan;9(1):105–118.
19. Langhorne P, Stott DJ, Robertson L, MacDonald J, Jones L, McAlpine C, et al. Medical complications after stroke: a multicenter study. Stroke. 2000 Jun;31(6):1223–1229.
20. Johnston KC, Li JY, Lyden PD, Hanson SK, Feasby TE, Adams RJ, et al. Medical and neurological complications of ischemic stroke: experience from the RANTTAS trial. RANTTAS Investigators. Stroke. 1998 Feb;29(2):447–453.
21. Siesjo BK. Pathophysiology and treatment of focal cerebral ischemia. Part I: Pathophysiology. J Neurosurg. 1992 Aug;77(2):169–184.
22. Adams HP, Jr, del Zoppo G, Alberts MJ, Bhatt DL, Brass L, Furlan A, et al. Guidelines for the early management of adults with ischemic stroke: a guideline from the American Heart Association/American Stroke Association Stroke Council, Clinical Cardiology Council, Cardiovascular Radiology and Intervention Council, and the Atherosclerotic Peripheral Vascular Disease and Quality of Care Outcomes in Research Interdisciplinary Working Groups: the American Academy of Neurology affirms the value of this guideline as an educational tool for neurologists. Stroke. 2007 May;38(5):1655–1711.
23. Lukovits TG, Goddeau RP, Jr Critical care of patients with acute ischemic and hemorrhagic stroke: update on recent evidence and international guidelines. Chest. 2011 Mar;139(3):694–700.
24. Ronning OM, Guldvog B. Should stroke victims routinely receive supplemental oxygen? A quasi-randomized controlled trial. Stroke. 1999 Oct;30(10):2033–2037.
25. Dexter F, Hindman BJ. Effect of haemoglobin concentration on brain oxygenation in focal stroke: a mathematical modelling study. Br J Anaesth. 1997 Sep;79(3):346–351.
26. Tanne D, Molshatzki N, Merzeliak O, Tsabari R, Toashi M, Schwammenthal Y. Anemia status, hemoglobin concentration and outcome after acute stroke: a cohort study. BMC Neurol. 2010;10:22.
27. Kellert L, Martin E, Sykora M, Bauer H, Gussmann P, Diedler J, et al. Cerebral oxygen transport failure?: decreasing hemoglobin and hematocrit levels after ischemic stroke predict poor outcome and mortality: STroke: RelevAnt Impact of hemoGlobin, Hematocrit and Transfusion (STRAIGHT)—an observational study. Stroke. 2011 Oct;42(10):2832–2837.
28. Johnson KG, Johnson DC. Frequency of sleep apnea in stroke and TIA patients: a meta-analysis. J Clin Sleep Med. 2010 Apr 15;6(2):131–137.
29. Budhiraja R, Budhiraja P, Quan SF. Sleep-disordered breathing and cardiovascular disorders. Respir Care. 2010 Oct;55(10):1322–1332; discussion 30-2.
30. Good DC, Henkle JQ, Gelber D, Welsh J, Verhulst S. Sleep-disordered breathing and poor functional outcome after stroke. Stroke. 1996 Feb;27(2):252–259.
31. Tsivgoulis G, Zhang Y, Alexandrov AW, Harrigan MR, Sisson A, Zhao L, et al. Safety and tolerability of early noninvasive ventilatory correction using bilevel positive airway pressure in acute ischemic stroke. Stroke. 2011 Apr;42(4):1030–1034.
32. Hanly PJ, Millar TW, Steljes DG, Baert R, Frais MA, Kryger MH. The effect of oxygen on respiration and sleep in patients with congestive heart failure. Ann Intern Med. 1989 Nov 15;111(10):777–782.

33. Finlayson O, Kapral M, Hall R, Asllani E, Selchen D, Saposnik G. Risk factors, inpatient care, and outcomes of pneumonia after ischemic stroke. *Neurology*. 2011 Oct 4;77(14):1338–1345.

34. Ingeman A, Andersen G, Hundborg HH, Svendsen ML, Johnsen SP. In-hospital medical complications, length of stay, and mortality among stroke unit patients. *Stroke*. 2011 Nov;42(11):3214–3218.

35. Klehmet J, Harms H, Richter M, Prass K, Volk HD, Dirnagl U, et al. Stroke-induced immunodepression and post-stroke infections: lessons from the preventive antibacterial therapy in stroke trial. *Neuroscience*. 2009 Feb 6;158(3):1184–1193.

36. Varkey AB, Naderi S, Stearns DA, Swaminathan A, Varkey B. *Aspiration Pneumonia*. 2011. <http://emedicine.medscape.com/article/296198-overview> (accessed 11 April 2012).

37. Rello J, Lode H, Cornaglia G, Masterton R. A European care bundle for prevention of ventilator-associated pneumonia. *Intensive Care Med*. 2010 May;36(5):773–780.

38. Rusyniak DE, Kirk MA, May JD, Kao LW, Brizendine EJ, Welch JL, et al. Hyperbaric oxygen therapy in acute ischemic stroke: results of the Hyperbaric Oxygen in Acute Ischemic Stroke Trial Pilot Study. *Stroke*. 2003 Feb;34(2):571–574.

39. Singhal AB, Benner T, Roccatagliata L, Koroshetz WJ, Schaefer PW, Lo EH, et al. A pilot study of normobaric oxygen therapy in acute ischemic stroke. *Stroke*. 2005 Apr;36(4):797–802.

40. Guidelines for management of ischaemic stroke and transient ischaemic attack 2008. *Cerebrovasc Dis*. 2008;25(5):457–507.

41. Leonardi-Bee J, Bath PM, Phillips SJ, Sandercock PA. Blood pressure and clinical outcomes in the International Stroke Trial. *Stroke*. 2002 May;33(5):1315–1320.

42. CAST: randomised placebo-controlled trial of early aspirin use in 20,000 patients with acute ischaemic stroke. CAST (Chinese Acute Stroke Trial) Collaborative Group. *Lancet*. 1997 Jun 7;349(9066):1641–1649.

43. Rodriguez-Yanez M, Castellanos M, Blanco M, Garcia MM, Nombela F, Serena J, et al. New-onset hypertension and inflammatory response/poor outcome in acute ischemic stroke. *Neurology*. 2006 Dec 12;67(11):1973–1978.

44. Wallace JD, Levy LL. Blood pressure after stroke. *JAMA*. 1981 Nov 13;246(19):2177–2180.

45. Aslanyan S, Fazekas F, Weir CJ, Horner S, Lees KR. Effect of blood pressure during the acute period of ischemic stroke on stroke outcome: a tertiary analysis of the GAIN International Trial. *Stroke*. 2003 Oct;34(10):2420–2425.

46. Kontos HA, Wei EP, Navari RM, Levasseur JE, Rosenblum WI, Patterson JL, Jr Responses of cerebral arteries and arterioles to acute hypotension and hypertension. *Am J Physiol*. 1978 Apr;234(4):H371–H383.

47. Agnoli A, Fieschi C, Bozzao L, Battistini N, Prencipe M. Autoregulation of cerebral blood flow. Studies during drug-induced hypertension in normal subjects and in patients with cerebral vascular diseases. *Circulation*. 1968 Oct;38(4):800–812.

48. Willmot M, Leonardi-Bee J, Bath PM. High blood pressure in acute stroke and subsequent outcome: a systematic review. *Hypertension*. 2004 Jan;43(1):18–24.

49. Potter JF, Robinson TG, Ford GA, Mistri A, James M, Chernova J, et al. Controlling hypertension and hypotension immediately post-stroke (CHHIPS): a randomised, placebo-controlled, double-blind pilot trial. *Lancet Neurol*. 2009 Jan;8(1):48–56.

50. Robinson TG, Potter JF, Ford GA, Bulpitt CJ, Chernova J, Jagger C, et al. Effects of antihypertensive treatment after acute stroke in the Continue or Stop Post-Stroke Antihypertensives Collaborative Study (COSSACS): a prospective, randomised, open, blinded-endpoint trial. *Lancet Neurol*. 2010 Aug;9(8):767–775.

51. Sandset EC, Bath PM, Boysen G, Jatuzis D, Korv J, Luders S, et al. The angiotensin-receptor blocker candesartan for treatment of acute stroke (SCAST): a randomised, placebo-controlled, double-blind trial. *Lancet*. 2011 Feb 26;377(9767):741–750.

52. Greer DM, Funk SE, Reaven NL, Ouzounelli M, Uman GC. Impact of fever on outcome in patients with stroke and neurologic injury: a comprehensive meta-analysis. *Stroke*. 2008 Nov;39(11):3029–3035.

53. Reith J, Jorgensen HS, Pedersen PM, Nakayama H, Raaschou HO, Jeppesen LL, et al. Body temperature in acute stroke: relation to stroke severity, infarct size, mortality, and outcome. *Lancet*. 1996 Feb 17;347(8999):422–425.

54. Rosomoff HL. Hypothermia and cerebral vascular lesions. I. Experimental interruption of the middle cerebral artery during hypothermia. *J Neurosurg*. 1956 Jul;13(4):244–255.

55. Rosomoff HL. Interruption of the middle cerebral artery during hypothermia. *Trans Am Neurol Assoc*. 1956(81st Meeting):64–65.

56. Rosomoff HL. Some effects of hypothermia on the normal and abnormal physiology of the nervous system. *Proc R Soc Med*. 1956 Jun;49(6):358–364.

57. Bernard SA, Gray TW, Buist MD, Jones BM, Silvester W, Gutteridge G, et al. Treatment of comatose survivors of out-of-hospital cardiac arrest with induced hypothermia. *N Engl J Med*. 2002 Feb 21;346(8):557–563.

58. Den Hertog HM, van der Worp HB, Tseng MC, Dippel DW. Cooling therapy for acute stroke. *Cochrane Database Syst Rev*. 2009(1):CD001247.

59. Saper CB, Breder CD. The neurologic basis of fever. *N Engl J Med*. 1994 Jun 30;330(26):1880–1886.

60. Gisselsson L, Smith ML, Siesjo BK. Hyperglycemia and focal brain ischemia. *J Cereb Blood Flow Metab*. 1999 Mar;19(3):288–297.

61. de Courten-Myers G, Myers RE, Schoolfield L. Hyperglycemia enlarges infarct size in cerebrovascular occlusion in cats. *Stroke*. 1988 May;19(5):623–630.

62. Ginsberg MD, Prado R, Dietrich WD, Busto R, Watson BD. Hyperglycemia reduces the extent of cerebral infarction in rats. *Stroke*. 1987 May–Jun;18(3):570–574.

63. Kraft SA, Larson CP, Jr, Shuer LM, Steinberg GK, Benson GV, Pearl RG. Effect of hyperglycemia on neuronal changes in a rabbit model of focal cerebral ischemia. *Stroke*. 1990 Mar;21(3):447–450.

64. Piironen K, Putaala J, Rosso C, Samson Y. Glucose and acute stroke: evidence for an interlude. *Stroke*. 2012 Mar;43(3):898–902.

65. Parsons MW, Barber PA, Desmond PM, Baird TA, Darby DG, Byrnes G, et al. Acute hyperglycemia adversely affects stroke outcome: a magnetic resonance imaging and spectroscopy study. *Ann Neurol*. 2002 Jul;52(1):20–28.

66. Capes SE, Hunt D, Malmberg K, Pathak P, Gerstein HC. Stress hyperglycemia and prognosis of stroke in nondiabetic and diabetic patients: a systematic overview. *Stroke*. 2001 Oct;32(10):2426–2432.

67. Kruyt ND, Biessels GJ, de Haan RJ, Vermeulen M, Rinkel GJ, Coert B, et al. Hyperglycemia and clinical outcome in aneurysmal subarachnoid hemorrhage: a meta-analysis. *Stroke*. 2009 Jun;40(6):e424–e430.

68. Ahmed N, Davalos A, Eriksson N, Ford GA, Glahn J, Hennerici M, et al. Association of admission blood glucose and outcome in patients treated with intravenous thrombolysis: results from the Safe Implementation of Treatments in Stroke International Stroke Thrombolysis Register (SITS-ISTR). *Arch Neurol*. 2010 Sep;67(9):1123–1130.

69. Dungan KM, Braithwaite SS, Preiser JC. Stress hyperglycaemia. *Lancet*. 2009 May 23;373(9677):1798–1807.

70. Uyttenboogaart M, Koch MW, Stewart RE, Vroomen PC, Luijckx GJ, De Keyser J. Moderate hyperglycaemia is associated with favourable outcome in acute lacunar stroke. *Brain*. 2007 Jun;130(Pt 6):1626–1630.

71. Gray CS, Hildreth AJ, Sandercock PA, O'Connell JE, Johnston DE, Cartlidge NE, et al. Glucose-potassium-insulin infusions in the management of post-stroke hyperglycaemia: the UK Glucose Insulin in Stroke Trial (GIST-UK). *Lancet Neurol*. 2007 May;6(5):397–406.

72. Clement S, Braithwaite SS, Magee MF, Ahmann A, Smith EP, Schafer RG, et al. Management of diabetes and hyperglycemia in hospitals. *Diabetes Care*. 2004 Feb;27(2):553–591.

73. Finfer S, Chittock DR, Su SY, Blair D, Foster D, Dhingra V, et al. Intensive versus conventional glucose control in critically ill patients. *N Engl J Med*. 2009 Mar 26;360(13):1283–1297.

74. McCormick M, Hadley D, McLean JR, Macfarlane JA, Condon B, Muir KW. Randomized, controlled trial of insulin for acute poststroke hyperglycemia. *Ann Neurol*. 2010 May;67(5):570–578.

75. Miller EL, Murray L, Richards L, Zorowitz RD, Bakas T, Clark P, et al. Comprehensive overview of nursing and interdisciplinary rehabilitation

care of the stroke patient: a scientific statement from the American Heart Association. *Stroke*. 2010 Oct;41(10):2402–2448.

76. Teasell R, Murie-Fernandez M, McClure M, Foley N. *Medical Complications*. 2011. <http://www.ebrsr.com/~ebrsr/uploads/E_Medical_Complications_(Questions_and_Answers).pdf> (accessed 16 October 2011).

77. Smithard DG, O'Neill PA, Parks C, Morris J. Complications and outcome after acute stroke. *Does dysphagia matter? Stroke*. 1996 Jul;27(7):1200–1204.

78. Hinchey JA, Shephard T, Furie K, Smith D, Wang D, Tonn S. Formal dysphagia screening protocols prevent pneumonia. *Stroke*. 2005 Sep;36(9):1972–1976.

79. Summers D, Leonard A, Wentworth D, Saver JL, Simpson J, Spilker JA, et al. Comprehensive overview of nursing and interdisciplinary care of the acute ischemic stroke patient: a scientific statement from the American Heart Association. *Stroke*. 2009 Aug;40(8):2911–2944.

80. Carnaby G, Hankey GJ, Pizzi J. Behavioural intervention for dysphagia in acute stroke: a randomised controlled trial. *Lancet Neurol*. 2006 Jan;5(1):31–37.

81. Shaw GY, Sechtem PR, Searl J, Keller K, Rawi TA, Dowdy E. Transcutaneous neuromuscular electrical stimulation (VitalStim) curative therapy for severe dysphagia: myth or reality? *Ann Otol Rhinol Laryngol*. 2007 Jan;116(1):36–44.

82. Dennis MS, Lewis SC, Warlow C. Effect of timing and method of enteral tube feeding for dysphagic stroke patients (FOOD): a multicentre randomised controlled trial. *Lancet*. 2005 Feb 26-Mar 4;365(9461):764–772.

83. Neumann DA, DeLegge MH. Gastric versus small-bowel tube feeding in the intensive care unit: a prospective comparison of efficacy. *Crit Care Med*. 2002 Jul;30(7):1436–1438.

84. Anderson CS, Huang Y, Arima H, Heeley E, Skulina C, Parsons MW, et al. Effects of early intensive blood pressure-lowering treatment on the growth of hematoma and perihematomal edema in acute intracerebral hemorrhage: the Intensive Blood Pressure Reduction in Acute Cerebral Haemorrhage Trial (INTERACT). *Stroke*. 2010 Feb;41(2):307–312.

85. Dennis M, Mordi N, Graham C, Sandercock P. The timing, extent, progression and regression of deep vein thrombosis in immobile stroke patients: observational data from the CLOTS multicenter randomized trials. *J Thromb Haemost*. 2011 Nov;9(11):2193–2200.

86. Goldhaber SZ, Tapson VF. A prospective registry of 5,451 patients with ultrasound-confirmed deep vein thrombosis. *Am J Cardiol*. 2004 Jan 15;93(2):259–262.

87. Goldhaber SZ. Risk factors for venous thromboembolism. *J Am Coll Cardiol*. 2010 Jun 29;56(1):1–7.

88. Hull R, Hirsh J, Sackett DL, Taylor DW, Carter C, Turpie AG, et al. Clinical validity of a negative venogram in patients with clinically suspected venous thrombosis. *Circulation*. 1981 Sep;64(3):622–625.

89. Stein PD, Hull RD, Patel KC, Olson RE, Ghali WA, Brant R, et al. D-dimer for the exclusion of acute venous thrombosis and pulmonary embolism: a systematic review. *Ann Intern Med*. 2004 Apr 20;140(8):589–602.

90. Spritzer CE, Arata MA, Freed KS. Isolated pelvic deep venous thrombosis: relative frequency as detected with MR imaging. *Radiology*. 2001 May;219(2):521–525.

91. Horlander KT, Mannino DM, Leeper KV. Pulmonary embolism mortality in the United States, 1979-1998: an analysis using multiple-cause mortality data. *Arch Intern Med*. 2003 Jul 28;163(14):1711–1717.

92. Dennis M, Sandercock PA, Reid J, Graham C, Murray G, Venables G, et al. Effectiveness of thigh-length graduated compression stockings to reduce the risk of deep vein thrombosis after stroke (CLOTS trial 1): a multicentre, randomised controlled trial. *Lancet*. 2009 Jun 6;373(9679):1958–1965.

93. Lacut K, Bressollette L, Le Gal G, Etienne E, De Tinteniac A, Renault A, et al. Prevention of venous thrombosis in patients with acute intracerebral hemorrhage. *Neurology*. 2005 Sep 27;65(6):865–869.

94. Kamphuisen PW, Agnelli G. What is the optimal pharmacological prophylaxis for the prevention of deep-vein thrombosis and pulmonary embolism in patients with acute ischaemic stroke? *Thromb Res*. 2007;119(3):265–274.

95. Sherman DG, Albers GW, Bladin C, Fieschi C, Gabbai AA, Kase CS, et al. The efficacy and safety of enoxaparin versus unfractionated heparin for the prevention of venous thromboembolism after acute ischaemic stroke (PREVAIL Study): an open-label randomised comparison. *Lancet*. 2007 Apr 21;369(9570):1347–1355.

96. Kamran SI, Downey D, Ruff RL. Pneumatic sequential compression reduces the risk of deep vein thrombosis in stroke patients. *Neurology*. 1998 Jun;50(6):1683–1688.

97. Agnelli G, Becattini C. Acute pulmonary embolism. *N Engl J Med*. 2010 Jul 15;363(3):266–274.

98. Fujii Y, Tanaka R, Takeuchi S, Koike T, Minakawa T, Sasaki O. Hematoma enlargement in spontaneous intracerebral hemorrhage. *J Neurosurg*. 1994 Jan;80(1):51–57.

99. Bailey RD, Hart RG, Benavente O, Pearce LA. Recurrent brain hemorrhage is more frequent than ischemic stroke after intracranial hemorrhage. *Neurology*. 2001 Mar 27;56(6):773–777.

100. Eckman MH, Rosand J, Knudsen KA, Singer DE, Greenberg SM. Can patients be anticoagulated after intracerebral hemorrhage? A decision analysis. *Stroke*. 2003 Jul;34(7):1710–1716.

101. Thomalla G, Hartmann F, Juettler E, Singer OC, Lehnhardt FG, Kohrmann M, et al. Prediction of malignant middle cerebral artery infarction by magnetic resonance imaging within 6 hours of symptom onset: A prospective multicenter observational study. *Ann Neurol*. 2010 Oct;68(4):435–445.

102. Oppenheim C, Samson Y, Manai R, Lalam T, Vandamme X, Crozier S, et al. Prediction of malignant middle cerebral artery infarction by diffusion-weighted imaging. *Stroke*. 2000 Sep;31(9):2175–2181.

103. Balami JS, Chen RL, Grunwald IQ, Buchan AM. Neurological complications of acute ischaemic stroke. *Lancet Neurol*. 2011 Apr;10(4):357–371.

104. Hacke W, Kaste M, Fieschi C, von Kummer R, Davalos A, Meier D, et al. Randomised double-blind placebo-controlled trial of thrombolytic therapy with intravenous alteplase in acute ischaemic stroke (ECASS II). Second European-Australasian Acute Stroke Study Investigators. *Lancet*. 1998 Oct 17;352(9136):1245–1251.

105. Dunn LT. Raised intracranial pressure. *J Neurol Neurosurg Psychiatry*. 2002 Sep;73 Suppl 1:i23–i27.

106. Balami JS, Buchan AM. Complications of intracerebral haemorrhage. *Lancet Neurol*. 2012 Jan;11(1):101–118.

107. Mednick AS, Mayer SA. Critical care management of neurologic catastrophes. *Adv Neurol*. 2002;90:87–101.

108. Diringer MN, Scalfani MT, Zazulia AR, Videen TO, Dhar R, Powers WJ. Effect of mannitol on cerebral blood volume in patients with head injury. *Neurosurgery*. 2012;70:1215–1218.

109. Muizelaar JP, Wei EP, Kontos HA, Becker DP. Mannitol causes compensatory cerebral vasoconstriction and vasodilation in response to blood viscosity changes. *J Neurosurg*. 1983 Nov;59(5):822–828.

110. Mayer SA, Chong JY. Critical care management of increased intracranial pressure. *Journal of Intensive Care Medicine*. 2002;17(2):55–67.

111. Mortazavi MM, Romeo AK, Deep A, Griessenauer CJ, Shoja MM, Tubbs RS, et al. Hypertonic saline for treating raised intracranial pressure: literature review with meta-analysis. *J Neurosurg*. 2011 Sep 23.

112. McLone D. *Pediatric Neurosurgery: Surgery of the Developing Nervous System*. Philadelphia: W.B. Saunders; 2001.

113. Newell DW, Weber JP, Watson R, Aaslid R, Winn HR. Effect of transient moderate hyperventilation on dynamic cerebral autoregulation after severe head injury. *Neurosurgery*. 1996 Jul;39(1):35–43; discussion -4.

114. Vahedi K, Hofmeijer J, Juettler E, Vicaut E, George B, Algra A, et al. Early decompressive surgery in malignant infarction of the middle cerebral artery: a pooled analysis of three randomised controlled trials. *Lancet Neurol*. 2007 Mar;6(3):215–222.

115. Berrouschot J, Sterker M, Bettin S, Koster J, Schneider D. Mortality of space-occupying ('malignant') middle cerebral artery infarction under conservative intensive care. *Intensive Care Med*. 1998 Jun;24(6):620–623.

116. Cruz-Flores S, Berge E, Whittle IR. Surgical decompression for cerebral oedema in acute ischaemic stroke. *Cochrane Database Syst Rev*. 2012;1:CD003435.

117. Pfefferkorn T, Eppinger U, Linn J, Birnbaum T, Herzog J, Straube A, et al. Long-term outcome after suboccipital decompressive craniectomy for malignant cerebellar infarction. *Stroke.* 2009 Sep;40(9):3045–3050.

118. Chen HJ, Lee TC, Wei CP. Treatment of cerebellar infarction by decompressive suboccipital craniectomy. *Stroke.* 1992 Jul;23(7):957–961.

119. Ay H, Koroshetz WJ, Benner T, Vangel MG, Melinosky C, Arsava EM, et al. Neuroanatomic correlates of stroke-related myocardial injury. *Neurology.* 2006 May 9;66(9):1325–1329.

120. Oppenheimer SM, Wilson JX, Guiraudon C, Cechetto DF. Insular cortex stimulation produces lethal cardiac arrhythmias: a mechanism of sudden death? *Brain Res.* 1991 May 31;550(1):115–121.

121. Tokgozoglu SL, Batur MK, Top uoglu MA, Saribas O, Kes S, Oto A. Effects of stroke localization on cardiac autonomic balance and sudden death. *Stroke.* 1999 Jul;30(7):1307–1311.

122. Burch GE, Meyers R, Abildskov JA. A new electrocardiographic pattern observed in cerebrovascular accidents. *Circulation.* 1954 May;9(5):719–723.

123. Cheung RT, Hachinski V. The insula and cerebrogenic sudden death. *Arch Neurol.* 2000 Dec;57(12):1685–1688.

124. Norris JW, Hachinski VC, Myers MG, Callow J, Wong T, Moore RW. Serum cardiac enzymes in stroke. *Stroke.* 1979 Sep–Oct;10(5):548–553.

125. Jensen JK, Kristensen SR, Bak S, Atar D, Hoilund-Carlsen PF, Mickley H. Frequency and significance of troponin T elevation in acute ischemic stroke. *Am J Cardiol.* 2007 Jan 1;99(1):108–112.

126. James P, Ellis CJ, Whitlock RM, McNeil AR, Henley J, Anderson NE. Relation between troponin T concentration and mortality in patients presenting with an acute stroke: observational study. *BMJ.* 2000 Jun 3;320(7248):1502–1504.

127. Connor RC. Heart damage associated with intracranial lesions. *Br Med J.* 1968 Jul 6;3(5609):29–31.

128. Virmani R, Farb A, Burke A. Contraction-band necrosis: new use for an old friend. *Lancet.* 1996 Jun 22;347(9017):1710–1711.

129. Mayer SA, Lin J, Homma S, Solomon RA, Lennihan L, Sherman D, et al. Myocardial injury and left ventricular performance after subarachnoid hemorrhage. *Stroke.* 1999 Apr;30(4):780–786.

130. Dote K, Sato H, Tateishi H, Uchida T, Ishihara M. Myocardial stunning due to simultaneous multivessel coronary spasms: a review of 5 cases (Japanese). *J Cardiol.* 1991;21(2):203–214.

131. Wittstein IS, Thiemann DR, Lima JA, Baughman KL, Schulman SP, Gerstenblith G, et al. Neurohumoral features of myocardial stunning due to sudden emotional stress. *N Engl J Med.* 2005 Feb 10;352(6):539–548.

132. Gupta R, Sech C, Lazzara R. Transient cardiac ballooning—the syndrome. *Clin Cardiol.* 2009 Nov;32(11):614–620.

133. Yoshimura S, Toyoda K, Ohara T, Nagasawa H, Ohtani N, Kuwashiro T, et al. Takotsubo cardiomyopathy in acute ischemic stroke. *Ann Neurol.* 2008 Nov;64(5):547–554.

134. de Gregorio C, Grimaldi P, Lentini C. Left ventricular thrombus formation and cardioembolic complications in patients with Takotsubo-like syndrome: a systematic review. *Int J Cardiol.* 2008 Dec 17;131(1):18–24.

135. Alberts MJ, Latchaw RE, Selman WR, Shephard T, Hadley MN, Brass LM, et al. Recommendations for comprehensive stroke centers: a consensus statement from the Brain Attack Coalition. *Stroke.* 2005 Jul;36(7):1597–1616.

136. Alberts MJ, Latchaw RE, Jagoda A, Wechsler LR, Crocco T, George MG, et al. Revised and updated recommendations for the establishment of primary stroke centers: a summary statement from the brain attack coalition. *Stroke.* 2011 Sep;42(9):2651–2665.

137. Stroke Unit Trialists' Collaboration. Organised inpatient (stroke unit) care for stroke. *Cochrane Database Syst Rev.* 2007(4):CD000197.

138. Lattimore SU, Chalela J, Davis L, DeGraba T, Ezzeddine M, Haymore J, et al. Impact of establishing a primary stroke center at a community hospital on the use of thrombolytic therapy: the NINDS Suburban Hospital Stroke Center experience. *Stroke.* 2003 Jun;34(6):e55–e57.

139. Leifer D, Bravata DM, Connors JJ, 3rd, Hinchey JA, Jauch EC, Johnston SC, et al. Metrics for measuring quality of care in comprehensive stroke centers: detailed follow-up to Brain Attack Coalition comprehensive stroke center recommendations: a statement for healthcare professionals from the American Heart Association/American Stroke Association. *Stroke.* 2011 Mar;42(3):849–877.

CHAPTER 11

Acute phase therapy in ischaemic stroke

Krassen Nedeltchev and Heinrich P. Mattle

Introduction

Ischaemic stroke is associated with significant morbidity and mortality, ranking as the most important cause of long-term disability in adults, second most common cause of dementia, and third most common cause of death in industrialized countries. In addition, stroke is a frequent cause of depression and the most common cause of epilepsy in the elderly. Despite better control of preventable risk factors, the global burden of stroke is expected to rise in the future due to the ageing of the world's population. Reducing morbidity and mortality by evidence-based acute therapies is essential to avoid the increase in the health, economic, and social burdens of stroke.

The main goal of the acute phase therapies is to improve the clinical outcome. The effect of most therapies, and particularly of thrombolysis, is strongly time-dependent: the sooner the treatment is administered, the greater the impact on the clinical outcome.

This chapter summarizes thrombolytic and other revascularization techniques, neuroprotection, and other acute stroke therapies. Treatment recommendations adhere to current international standards and particularly to the European Stroke Organisation (ESO) *Guidelines for Management of Ischemic Stroke* (1). General stroke treatment is extensively covered in Chapter 10.

Thrombolytic treatment

Intravenous thrombolysis

The goal of the thrombolytic treatment is to remove the occlusion and to restore blood flow to the hypoperfused brain tissue. Typically, the hypoperfused area consists of irreversibly damaged brain tissue (infarct core) that is surrounded by viable and potentially salvageable brain parenchyma (ischaemic penumbra). The ischaemic penumbra can be salvaged by a timely vessel recanalization.

The publication of the results of the landmark National Institute of Neurological Disorders and Stroke (NINDS) Recombinant Tissue Plasminogen Activator (rtPA) Study in December 1995 put an end to the 'pre-thrombolytic era' in the management of acute stroke (2). In 1996, based on the strength of the NINDS report, the US Food and Drug Administration (FDA) approved rtPA for use in early acute ischaemic stroke. For the first time in history, stroke was recognized and treated as a time-critical emergency.

Alteplase (rtPA) is an enzyme that converts plasminogen to plasmin. It binds to fibrin within the thrombus, forming an active thrombolytic complex. The recommended alteplase dose for patients with acute ischaemic stroke is 0.9 mg/kg (maximum 90 mg), with a bolus of 10% of the dose administered over 1 minute, and the remainder infused over 60 minutes.

Table 11.1 summarizes the indications and contraindications for intravenous rtPA in acute ischaemic stroke (2, 3).

Efficacy

The NINDS rtPA study established the efficacy of alteplase administered within 3 hours of stroke onset. It was conducted in two parts. The primary endpoint of part 1 included a comparison of the proportion of patients with neurologic improvement as defined by an increase of 4 or more points on the NIHSS score or resolution of neurological deficit at 24 hours after stroke onset based on time to treat (0–90 min, 90–180 min). There was no statistically significant difference between groups in the primary end point (47% in the treatment group vs 39% in the placebo group, p <0.21). Part 2

Table 11.1 Indications and contraindications for IV rtPA in acute ischaemic stroke

Indications
Age >18 years
Time window <4.5 hours
National Institutes of Health Stroke Study (NIHSS) score: 4–25 points
Symptoms persisting for ≥30 minutes without significant improvement

Contraindications
Evidence of intracranial haemorrhage on pretreatment CT or MRI
Recent (within 3 months) intracranial or intraspinal surgery, serious head trauma, or previous stroke
History of intracranial haemorrhage
Uncontrolled hypertension at time of treatment (>185 mmHg systolic or >110 mmHg diastolic blood pressure)
Seizure at the onset of stroke
Active internal bleeding
Intracranial neoplasm, arteriovenous malformation, or aneurysm
Known bleeding diathesis including but not limited to the following:
• Current use of oral anticoagulants (e.g. warfarin) or an international normalized ratio >1.7 or a prothrombin time >15 seconds
• Administration of heparin within 48 hours before the onset of stroke and an elevated activated partial thromboplastin time at presentation
• Platelet count <100 × 10^3/mm^3

of the trial evaluated the odds for favourable functional outcome at 3 months. The combination of the Barthel Index (BI), modified Rankin Scale (mRS), Glasgow Outcome Scale (GOS), and NIHSS was used to assess the functional outcome (4). All four scales indicated statistically significant improvements in 3-month outcomes in the alteplase group compared with the placebo group. Patients receiving rtPA were at least 30% more likely than those in the placebo group to have minimal or no disability at 3 months.

Despite this clear proof of efficacy, intravenous thrombolysis (IVT) remained underutilized, with less than 3% of all acute stroke patients receiving adequate treatment. Major obstacles for the implementation of IVT were the narrow therapeutic time window and the fear of intracranial haemorrhage (i.e. its safety).

Initial attempts to widen the 3-hour time window failed. The rtPA (Alteplase) 0- to 6-Hour Acute Stroke Trial, Part A (A0276g) was designed to assess the efficacy and safety of IVT in patients with acute ischaemic stroke who were treated within 6 hours of symptom onset (5). This phase II trial was stopped prematurely due to an increased frequency of adverse events in the 5–6-hour group. In the successor phase III study, the Alteplase Thrombolysis for Acute Noninterventional Therapy in Ischemic Stroke (ATLANTIS), IV rtPA or placebo was administered within 3–5 hours of symptom onset (6). The primary efficacy endpoint was the proportion of patients with excellent functional outcome (NIHSS 0 or 1) at 3 months; it was missed in both the intention-to-treat (ITT) and the per-protocol analyses. The ECASS (7) and the ECASS II (8) enrolled patients within 6 hours of stroke onset; both trials failed to demonstrate the efficacy of IV rtPA within the extended time window.

The first randomized controlled trial (RCT) that demonstrated the efficacy of IVT beyond 3 hours of symptom onset was the ECASS III trial (4). The study employed both ITT and per-protocol analyses and followed strict inclusion and exclusion criteria. The primary efficacy endpoint was favourable functional outcome (mRS score 0 or 1) at 3 months. The median time from symptom onset to IV rtPA was 3 hours 59 minutes. In the ITT analysis, 52.4% patients in the alteplase and 45.2% in the placebo group reached the primary efficacy endpoint (odds ratio (OR) 1.34, 95% confidence interval (CI) 1.02–1.76, p=0.04). The per-protocol analysis indicated that 54.9% in the treatment group versus 45.4% in the placebo group reached a mRS score of 0 or 1 with a reported OR of 1.47 (95% CI 1.10–1.97, p <0.01).

Based on the results of ECASS III, the American Heart Association/American Stroke Association (AHA/ASA), and the European Stroke Organisation (ESO) recommended to expand the window of treatment from 3 to 4.5 hours (1, 9).

A recent pooled analysis of the ECASS, ATLANTIS, NINDS, and EPITHET trials examined the effect of time to treatment with IVT on the clinical outcome at 3 months (10). Treatment was started within 360 min of stroke onset in 3670 patients randomly allocated to alteplase (n=1850) or to placebo (n=1820). Odds of a favourable 3-month outcome increased as OTT decreased (p=0.0269) and no benefit of alteplase treatment was seen after around 270 min. Adjusted odds of a favourable 3-month outcome were 2.55 (95% CI 1.44–4.52) for 0–90 min, 1.64 (1.12–2.40) for 91–180 min, 1.34 (1.06–1.68) for 181–270 min, and 1.22 (0.92–1.61) for 271–360 min in favour of the alteplase group.

In the largest thrombolysis trial to date, the third International Stroke Trial (IST-3), treatment within 6 hours of symptom onset improved the functional outcome (11). The study enrolled 3035

patients, of whom 1617 (53%) were older than 80 years of age. At 6 months, 554 (37%) patients in the rtPA group versus 534 (35%) in the control group were alive and independent (Oxford Handicap Score, OHS 0–2; adjusted OR 1.13, 95% CI 0.95—1.35, p=0.181). An ordinal analysis showed a significant shift in OHS scores; common OR 1.27 (95% CI 1.10–1.47, p=0.001). More deaths occurred within 7 days in the rtPA group than in the control group, but between 7 days and 6 months there were fewer deaths in the rtPA group than in the control group, so that by 6 months, similar numbers, in total, had died (408 (27%) in the rtPA group versus 407 (27%) in the control group). Overall benefit did not appear to be diminished among elderly patients over 80, and benefit was greatest amongst those randomized within 3 hours.

The most recent meta-analysis included 7012 patients from 12 trials and showed that for every 1000 patients allocated to rtPA up to 6 hours after a stroke, 42 additional patients are alive and independent, and 55 were alive with a favourable outcome at the end of follow-up.

To summarize, patients with ischaemic stroke benefit from IV rtPA when treated within 4.5 hours. To increase the benefit to a maximum, efforts should be made to shorten delay in initiation of treatment. Beyond 4.5 hours, the risks might outweigh the benefit.

Safety

The most feared complication of thrombolysis is *intracranial haemorrhage* (ICH). With IVT, about 5% of patients experience ICH associated with early worsening (i.e. symptomatic ICH) (11), and half of them have their functional outcome altered as a result. ICH is considered symptomatic if it is not seen on pre-treatment imaging and if it results in any decline in neurological status.

In NINDS rtPA study, symptomatic ICH occurred in 6.4% of patients receiving alteplase versus 0.6% of patients in the placebo group (P <0.001) (3). Part A of the A0276g was prematurely terminated due to an increased rate of symptomatic ICH in the 5–6 hours stratum in patients treated with alteplase (6). Reanalysis of the baseline data showed a higher prevalence of moderate to severe strokes (NIHSS > 20) in the alteplase (23%) compared with the placebo group (8%, P < 0.05). Overall, patients with NIHSS higher than 20 were more likely to experience a symptomatic ICH and to have an unfavourable outcome at 3 months. Similar findings were demonstrated in the ATLANTIS, ECASS, and ECASS II studies: the prevalence of symptomatic (fatal and non-fatal) ICH was significantly increased in the alteplase group (7–9).

In 2007, the Safe Implementation of Thrombolysis in Stroke–MOnitoring STudy (SITS-MOST) reported safety results in 6483 patients receiving alteplase within 0–3 hours of symptom onset in the clinical practice (i.e. outside of RCT) (12). The frequency of symptomatic ICH at 7 days after treatment was 7.3% in SITS-MOST, compared with 8.6% in the pooled randomized trials. It was concluded that IVT is safe and effective, when used within 3 hours of stroke onset. The same group of investigators compared the safety of IV rtPA in 664 patients treated 3–4.5 hours after symptom onset with that in 11,865 patients who received treatment within 3 hours of symptom onset (13). The rate of symptomatic ICH was 8% in the extended window group versus 7.3% in the 0–3 hours group (adjusted OR 1.13, 95% CI 0.097–1.32, p=0.11).

Another crucial safety endpoint in the described studies was *mortality*. There was no significant difference in the mortality rates between treatment and placebo in the NINDS, in the per-protocol population of ECASS, and in the ECASS II and II trials (3, 4, 8, 9). Increased mortality following IVT was observed in A0276g, ATLANTIS, and in the ITT population of ECASS, mostly in patients with symptomatic ICH and in those with major protocol violations (6–8).

Intra-arterial thrombolysis and mechanical thrombectomy

The intra-arterial application of fibrinolytic agents was initially motivated by considerations for improving the risk:benefit ratio and extending the time window. Compared with intravenous therapy, intra-arterial thrombolysis (IAT) offers several advantages, including a higher concentration of fibrinolytic agent delivered to the clot, a lower systemic exposure to drug, and higher recanalization rates. Disadvantages include additional time required to initiate therapy and availability only at highly specialized centres.

The Prolyse in Acute Cerebral Thromboembolism II (PROACT II) study randomized 180 patients with occlusion of the main stem of the middle cerebral artery within 6 hours of stroke onset to receive either 9 mg of intra-arterial pro-urokinase (pro-UK) and heparin or intravenous heparin alone (14). The recanalization rate was significantly greater in the pro-UK group than in the control group. More importantly, more subjects treated with pro-UK had a favourable functional outcome at 3 months after stroke. Although this phase III trial demonstrated a 15% absolute risk reduction of dependency and mortality, the evidence was not considered sufficient by the FDA to gain approval. In the early 2000s, large case series reported favourable outcomes with IA fibrinolytic agents (e.g. rtPA, urokinase, reteplase) and corroborated the findings of the PROACT II trial (15).

The Middle Cerebral Artery Embolism Local Fibrinolytic Intervention Trial (MELT) aimed at reproducing the findings of the PROACT II study and gaining FDA approval for IAT (16). The study widely implemented the PROACT II design and randomized patients with acute (0–6 hours) M1 and M2 occlusions to either IA urokinase or placebo. The primary endpoint did not reach statistical significance. Nevertheless, the secondary analyses suggested that IAT has the potential to increase the likelihood of favourable functional outcome. As a result, IAT is commonly administered as an off-label therapy for stroke at tertiary centres within 6 hours of onset in the anterior circulation and up to 12–24 hours after onset in the posterior circulation.

Because recanalization of large vessel occlusions is less likely with pharmacological (both intravenous and intra-arterial) means only, thrombectomy offers an alternative method to restore blood flow in this population. In 2007, the Merci Retriever (Concentric Medical, Mountain View, CA) was recognized by the AHA/ASA guidelines for management of acute ischaemic stroke as a mechanical thrombectomy device with benefits in carefully selected patients (17). The Multi Mechanical Embolus Removal in Cerebral Ischemia (Multi MERCI) trial was an international, multicenter, prospective, single-arm trial of thrombectomy within 8 hours of symptom onset in patients with large-vessel occlusion (18). Patients with persistent large vessel occlusion after IV alteplase treatment were included. Treatment with the newer generation retriever (L5 Retriever) resulted in successful recanalization in 57.3% treatable vessels and in 69.5% after adjunctive therapy (intra-arterial tissue plasminogen activator, mechanical). Overall, favourable clinical outcomes (mRS score 0 to 2) occurred in 36% and mortality was

34%; both outcomes were significantly related to vascular recanalization. Symptomatic intracerebral haemorrhage occurred in 9.8%. Clinically significant procedural complications occurred in 5.5% of patients. Patients in this trial had severe baseline neurological deficits (NIHSS score 19), which is an independent risk factor for mortality. This trial established the importance of recanalization in decreasing mortality rates in patients with large-vessel disease.

A recently approved device called the Penumbra System (Penumbra, Inc., Alameda, CA) is designed to remove the clot by placement of a clot disrupter centrally into the clot (19). The Penumbra System also uses vacuum to remove the fragmented thrombus. Most recently, retrievable stents (e.g. Enterprise, Codman Neurovascular, Raynham, MA; Solitaire FR, ev3, Inc., Irvine, CA) have been shown to significantly reduce time to recanalization and further increase the recanalization rates (20).

Next-generation mechanical clot retrievers—the Solitaire flow restoration device and the Trevo retriever—outperformed the Merci Retriever in two recent randomized comparison trials (21, 22). Both devices were significantly better in restoring the blood flow in the occluded arteries and had similar or even better safety profiles. Trials comparing the next-generation clot retrievers with medical therapy are still lacking.

Combination of IVT and IAT (bridging therapy)

Efforts to combine the advantages of IVT (wide availability, fast administration) and IAT (higher recanalization rates, extended time window) resulted in the so-called 'bridging therapy' that was first tested in the Interventional Management of Stroke Part 1 (IMS 1) (23). The study administered IA alteplase on top of low-dose IV alteplase and achieved better efficacy and similar rates of ICH compared with the results of the NINDS rtPA study. The second part of the same study (IMS 2) used the same setting, and, in addition, allowed the utilization of the EKOS micro-infusion system (EKOS Corp., Bothell, WA). EKOS is a low-energy ultrasound device that may reversibly alter the structure of the thrombus and accelerate thrombolysis. Again, efficacy and safety were comparable with those of the NINDS rtPA study. The Interventional Management of Stroke Part 3 (IMS III) was a phase 3, randomized, open-label international trial comparing a combined IV and IA stroke treatment with standard IV rtPA alone within 3 hours of stroke onset (24). Endovascular therapy included a choice of catheters and devices or IA rtPA based on the lesion characteristics, the experience and training of the investigator. However, at the outset, only one device was available, the Concentric Merci retriever. There was no difference in safety between the combination therapy and the standard IV rtPA: the mortality at 90 days ranked 19.1% and 21.6%, respectively (P=0.52), and the proportion of patients with symptomatic intracerebral haemorrhage within 30 hours after initiation of rtPA was 6.2% and 5.9%, respectively (P=0.83). However, there was no signal of additional efficacy either: the proportion of participants with a mRS score of 2 or less at 90 days did not differ significantly according to treatment (40.8% with endovascular therapy and 38.7% with IV rtPA). Subgroup analyses showed non-significant trends that patients treated early and patients with very severe strokes might derive a benefit. The main shortcomings of IMS III are twofold: firstly, only four patients were treated with stent retrievers, and secondly, endovascular therapy was achieved on average only after 6 hours after stroke onset, at a time point when the average stroke patient does not benefit any longer from treatment. New studies will have to treat patients in a time window when there is still a realistic chance of a benefit.

Neuroprotective therapy

Neuroprotective therapies are used to prevent irreversible injury in potentially viable neurons within the ischaemic area. Neuroprotection comprises both pharmacological (drugs) and non-pharmacological (i.e. physical, e.g. hypothermia) interventions.

One action of neuroprotective agents aims at prevention of early ischaemic injury. Many of these agents modulate neuronal receptors to reduce release of excitatory neurotransmitters, which contribute to deleterious effects of ischaemia on cells. The most commonly studied drugs block the N-methyl-D-aspartate (NMDA) receptor (e.g. dextrorphan, selfotel, GV150526). Magnesium is another agent with actions on the NMDA receptor that may reduce ischaemic injury by increasing regional blood flow and antagonizing voltage-sensitive calcium channels. The ongoing Field Administration of Stroke Therapy—Magnesium Phase III (FAST-MAG) trial is studying the effectiveness and safety of field-initiated magnesium sulphate in improving the long-term functional outcome of patients with acute stroke (25).

Calcium channel blockers (e.g. nimodipine), gamma-aminobutyric acid (GABA) agonists (clomethiazole), nitric oxide antagonists (lubelozole), free radical scavenger (tirilazad), or trapping agents (NXY-059) produced promising results in animal studies but failed in phase III studies.

Another group of neuroprotective agents attempts to prevent reperfusion injury. Agents that prevent white blood cells from adhering to vessel walls, limit formation of free radicals, or promote neuronal repair may protect the brain from additional injury during reperfusion. Citicolin, an exogenous form of cytidine-5'-diphosphocholine (CDP-choline) used in membrane biosynthesis, may reduce ischaemic injury by stabilizing membranes and decreasing free radical formation. A large international trial, the International Citicoline Trial on acUte Stroke (ICTUS), was stopped for futility after enrolling 2078 patients (26).

Hypothermia is being evaluated for its neuroprotective capabilities. Extracorporeal physical, pharmacological, and endovascular methods are employed to maintain controlled normo- and hypothermia in the acute phase after ischaemic stroke (27). Ice packs, water- or air-circulating blankets and mattresses, and water circulating gel-coated ice pads are commercially available for temperature management. The efficacy of the extracorporeal physical methods is limited by the relatively slow cooling rates, especially in obese patients. Complications like skin erosions or even necroses as well as vasoconstriction in patients taking vasoactive drugs represent further disadvantages of the extracorporeal cooling.

During the last decade, endovascular cooling devices have gained importance for induction of mild hypothermia. A central venous catheter is inserted into the inferior vena cava via a femoral vein. Normal saline is pumped through balloons mounted on the catheter and returned to a central system in a closed loop. The saline flow within the balloons is in close contact with the patient's blood flow and serves as heat exchange system. An automatic temperature control device adjusts the temperature of the circulating saline based on the patient's rectal temperature. Using the endovascular

approach, the body temperature can be reduced to 33°C within less than 3 hours. To prevent shivering, patients are given warm blankets, meperidine, or buspirone.

The invasive character of endovascular cooling raises concerns over the possibility of infection through the catheter. Complications may occur during the insertion of the catheter and include arterial or venous embolism, puncture site haematoma, balloon rupture, or infection.

Induced hypothermia to protect the brain in patients with stroke was studied in a recent RCT (ICTuS-L) (28). The study demonstrated the feasibility and the safety of combining endovascular hypothermia after stroke with IVT, but the efficacy needs to be confirmed in a larger trial. Pneumonia was more frequent after hypothermia. At 3 months, 18% of patients treated with hypothermia had a favourable outcome (mRS score 0 or 1) versus 24% in the normothermia group (non-significant).

Devices have added to the non-pharmacological means of neuroprotection. The NEST 2 and 3 trials are based on delivering laser energy to the mitochondrial cytochrome c oxidase-photoreceptors within 24 hours of stroke onset. SENTIS evaluated balloon occlusion of the aorta above and below the renal arteries to increase cerebral blood flow in patients treated up to 14 hours from symptom onset. IMPACT 24 applied stimulation of the sphenopalatinum (pterygopalatine) ganglion to increase brain perfusion.

Ongoing studies will determine whether these drugs and interventions are indeed effective in preventing early ischaemic or delayed reperfusion neuronal injury.

Antiplatelet therapy

The results of two randomized, non-blinded, intervention studies demonstrated a modest but statistically significant benefit of aspirin when initiated within 48 hours (29, 30). For every 1000 patients treated, 13 more were independent and alive at the end of follow-up. Aspirin therapy was associated with a small excess of two symptomatic ICH for every 1000 patients treated, but this was more than offset by a reduction of seven recurrent ischaemic strokes and about one pulmonary embolism for every 1000 patients treated.

Other antiplatelets such as clopidogrel, dipyridamole, or combinations thereof have not been evaluated in the acute phase of ischaemic stroke.

Early anticoagulation

Anticoagulation has failed to demonstrate a net benefit in improving the functional outcome, when started within 24–48 hours of stroke onset. Improvements in outcome or reductions in stroke recurrence rates were mostly counterbalanced by an increased number of haemorrhagic complications. The anticoagulants tested were standard unfractionated heparin, low-molecular-weight heparins, heparinoids, oral anticoagulants, and thrombin inhibitors (31). In one study, patients with non-lacunar stroke anticoagulated within 3 hours had more self-independence (38.9% vs 28.6%; P=0.025), fewer deaths (16.8% vs 21.9%; P=0.189), and more symptomatic brain haemorrhages (6.2% vs 1.4%; P=0.008) (32).

Despite the lack of conclusive evidence, some centres administer full-dose heparin in patients with cardiac sources of embolism with high risk of re-embolism, arterial dissection or high-grade arterial stenosis prior to surgery. Contraindications for heparin treatment include large infarcts (e.g. >50% of MCA territory), uncontrollable arterial hypertension, and advanced microvascular changes in the brain.

Management of brain oedema and elevated intracranial pressure

Medical therapy

Intravenous glycerol (4 × 250 mL of 10% glycerol over 30–60 minutes) or mannitol (25–50 g every 3–6 hours) is first-line medical treatment if clinical or radiological signs of space-occupying oedema occur (33, 34). However, glycerol and mannitol have only a short-term effect. Dexamethasone and corticosteroids are not useful (35).

Decompressive surgery

Malignant middle cerebral infarction

A pooled analysis of the DECIMAL (decompressive craniectomy in malignant middle cerebral artery infarcts), DESTINY (decompressive surgery for the treatment of malignant infarction of the middle cerebral artery), and HAMLET (hemicraniectomy after middle cerebral artery infarction with life-threatening oedema trial) trials demonstrated the benefit of decompressive surgery in both reducing the mortality and improving the functional outcome at 1 year after stroke (36). The analysis included 93 patients aged 18–60 years, with NIHSS score greater than 15, infarct signs on CT of 50% or more of the MCA territory or greater than 145 cm^3 on DWI, and inclusion less than 45 hours after onset (surgery <48 hours).

Cerebellar infarction

Ventriculostomy and decompressive surgery are considered treatments of choice for space-occupying cerebellar infarctions, although RCTs are lacking. The prognosis among survivors can be very good, even in patients who are comatose before surgery.

References

1. European Stroke Organisation. *Guidelines for Management of Ischemic Stroke*. 2008, updated 2009. <http://www.eso-stroke.org/recommendations.php?cid=9&sid=1> (accessed 16 October 2011).
2. The National Institute of Neurological Disorders and Stroke rt-PA Stroke Study Group. Tissue plasminogen activator for acute ischemic stroke. *N Engl J Med*. 1995;333:1581–1587.
3. Hacke W, Kaste M, Bluhmki E, Brozman M, Dávalos A, Guidetti D, *et al.*; ECASS Investigators. Thrombolysis with alteplase 3 to 4.5 hours after acute ischemic stroke. *N Engl J Med*. 2008;359:1317–1329.
4. The Internet Stroke Centre. *Stroke Assessment Scales*. <http://www.strokecenter.org/professionals/stroke-diagnosis/stroke-assessment-scales/> (accessed November 2011).
5. Clark WM, Albers GW, Madden KP, Hamilton S, for the Thromblytic Therapy in Acute Ischemic Stroke Study Investigators. The rtPA (alteplase) 0- to 6-hour acute stroke trial, part A (A0276g): results of a double-blind, placebo-controlled, multicenter study. *Stroke* 2000;31:811–816.
6. Clark WM, Wissman S, Albers GW, Jhamandas JH, Madden KP, Hamilton S. Recombinant tissue-type plasminogen activator (alteplase) for ischemic stroke 3 to 5 hours after symptom onset: the ATLANTIS study—a randomized controlled trial (alteplase thrombolysis for acute noninterventional therapy in ischemic stroke). *JAMA* 1999;282:2019–2026.
7. Hacke W, Kaste M, Fieschi C, Toni D, Lesaffre E, von Kummer R, *et al.* Intravenous thrombolysis with recombinant tissue plasminogen activator for acute hemispheric stroke. The European Cooperative Acute Stroke Study (ECASS). *JAMA*. 1995;274:1017–1025.
8. Hacke W, Kaste M, Fieschi C, von Kummer R, Davalos A, Meier D, *et al.* Randomised double-blind placebo-controlled trial of thrombolytic therapy with intravenous alteplase in acute ischaemic stroke (ECASS II). Second European-Australasian Acute Stroke Study Investigators. *Lancet*. 1998;352:1245–1251.
9. Del Zoppo GJ, Saver JL, Jauch EC, Adams HP Jr. American Heart Association Stroke Council. Expansion of the time window for treatment of acute ischemic stroke with intravenous tissue plasminogen activator: a science advisory from the American Heart Association/American Stroke Association. *Stroke*. 2009; 40:2945–2948.
10. Lees KR, Bluhmki E, von Kummer R, Brott TG, Toni D, Grotta JC, *et al.* Time to treatment with intravenous alteplase and outcome in stroke: an updated pooled analysis of ECASS, ATLANTIS, NINDS, and EPITHET trials. *Lancet*. 2010;375:1695–1703.
11. IST-3 collaborative group, Sandercock P, Wardlaw JM, Lindley RI, Dennis M, Cohen G, *et al.* The benefits and harms of intravenous thrombolysis with recombinant tissue plasminogen activator within 6 h of acute ischaemic stroke (the third international stroke trial [IST-3]): a randomised controlled trial. *Lancet*. 2012;379: 2352–2363.
12. Wahlgren N, Ahmed N, Dávalos A, Ford GA, Grond M, Hacke W, *et al.*; SITS-MOST investigators. Thrombolysis with alteplase for acute ischaemic stroke in the Safe Implementation of Thrombolysis in Stroke-Monitoring Study (SITS-MOST): an observational study. *Lancet*. 2007;369:275–282.
13. Wahlgren N, Ahmed N, Dávalos A, Hacke W, Millán M, Muir K, *et al.*; SITS investigators. Thrombolysis with alteplase 3-4.5 h after acute ischaemic stroke (SITS-ISTR): an observational study. *Lancet*. 2008;372:1303–1309.
14. Furlan A, Higashida R, Wechsler L, Gent M, Rowley H, Kase C, *et al.* Intra-arterial prourokinase for acute ischemic stroke. The PROACT II study: a randomized controlled trial. Prolyse in Acute Cerebral Thromboembolism. *JAMA*. 1999;282:2003–2011.
15. Arnold M, Schroth G, Nedeltchev K, Loher T, Remonda L, Stepper F, *et al.* Intra-arterial thrombolysis in 100 patients with acute stroke due to middle cerebral artery occlusion. *Stroke*. 2002;33:1828–1833.
16. Randomized trial of intraarterial infusion of urokinase within 6 hours of middle cerebral artery stroke: the middle cerebral artery embolism local fibrinolytic intervention trial (MELT) Japan. *Stroke*. 2007;38:2633–2639.
17. Adams HP Jr, del Zoppo G, Alberts MJ, Bhatt DL, Brass L, Furlan A, *et al.*; Guidelines for the early management of adults with ischemic stroke: a guideline from the American Heart Association/American Stroke Association Stroke Council, Clinical Cardiology Council, Cardiovascular Radiology and Intervention Council, and the Atherosclerotic Peripheral Vascular Disease and Quality of Care Outcomes in Research Interdisciplinary Working Groups: the American Academy of Neurology affirms the value of this guideline as an educational tool for neurologists. *Stroke*. 2007;38:1655–1711.
18. Smith WS, Sung G, Saver J, Budzik R, Duckwiler G, Liebeskind DS, *et al.* Mechanical thrombectomy for acute ischemic stroke: final results of the Multi MERCI trial. *Stroke*. 2008;39:1205–1212.
19. Bose A, Henkes H, Alfke K, Reith W, Mayer TE, Berlis A, *et al.*; Penumbra Phase 1 Stroke Trial Investigators. The Penumbra System: a mechanical device for the treatment of acute stroke due to thromboembolism. *AJNR Am J Neuroradiol*. 2008; 29:1409–1413.
20. Brekenfeld C, Schroth G, Mordasini P, Fischer U, Mono ML, Weck A, *et al.* Impact of retrievable stents on acute ischemic stroke treatment. *AJNR Am J Neuroradiol*. 2011;32:1269–1273.
21. Saver JL, Jahan R, Levy EI, Jovin TG, Baxter B, Nogueira RG, *et al.*; SWIFT Trialists. Solitaire flow restoration device versus the Merci Retriever in patients with acute ischaemic stroke (SWIFT): a randomised, parallel-group, non-inferiority trial. *Lancet*. 2012;380:1241–1249.
22. Nogueira RG, Lutsep HL, Gupta R, Jovin TG, Albers GW, Walker GA, *et al*; TREVO 2 Trialists. Trevo versus Merci retrievers for thrombectomy

revascularisation of large vessel occlusions in acute ischaemic stroke (TREVO 2): a randomised trial. *Lancet*. 2012;380:1231–1240.

23. The IMS Study Investigators. Combined intravenous and intraarterial recanalization for acute ischemic stroke: the interventional management of stroke study. *Stroke*. 2004;35:904–911.

24. Broderick JP, Palesch YY, Demchuk AM, Yeatts SD, Khatri P, Hill MD, *et al*. Interventional Management of Stroke (IMS) III Investigators. Endovascular therapy after intravenous t-PA versus t-PA alone for stroke. *N Engl J Med*. 2013;368:893–903.

25. The Internet Stroke Center. *Field Administration of Stroke Therapy – Magnesium (FAST-MAG) Trial*. <http://www.strokecenter.org/trials/clinicalstudies/449> (accessed 19 May 2013).

26. Dávalos A, Alvarez-Sabín J, Castillo J, Díez-Tejedor E, Ferro J, Martínez-Vila E, *et al*. International Citicoline Trial on acUte Stroke (ICTUS) trial investigators. Citicoline in the treatment of acute ischaemic stroke: an international, randomised, multicentre, placebo-controlled study (ICTUS trial). *Lancet*. 2012 Jul 28;380(9839): 349–357.

27. Schwab S, Schellinger PD, Werner C, Unterberger A, Hacke W. *Neurointensiv*. Heidelberg: Springer Medizin Verlag; 2008.

28. Hemmen TM, Raman R, Guluma KZ, Meyer BC, Gomes JA, Cruz-Flores S, *et al*. ICTuS-L Investigators. Intravenous thrombolysis plus hypothermia for acute treatment of ischemic stroke (ICTuS-L): final results. *Stroke*. 2010;41:2265–2270.

29. International-Stroke-Trial-Collaborative-Group. The International Stroke Trial (IST): a randomised trial if aspirin, subcutaneous heparin, both, or neither among 19435 patients with acute ischaemic stroke. *Lancet*. 1997;349:1569–1581.

30. CAST-Collaborative-Group. CAST: randomised placebo-controlled trial of early aspirin use in 20000 patients with acute ischaemic stroke. *Lancet*. 1997;349:1641–1649.

31. Gubitz G, Sandercock P, Counsell C. Anticoagulants for acute ischaemic stroke. *Cochrane Database Syst Rev*. 2004;3:CD000024.

32. Camerlingo M, Salvi P, Belloni G, Gamba T, Cesana BM, Mamoli A. Intravenous heparin started within the first 3 hours after onset of symptoms as a treatment for acute nonlacunar hemispheric cerebral infarctions. *Stroke*. 2005;36:2415–2420.

33. Righetti E, Celani MG, Cantisani TA, Sterzi R, Boysen G, Ricci S. Glycerol for acute stroke: a Cochrane systematic review. *J Neurol*. 2002;249:445–451.

34. Bereczki D, Liu M, do Prado GF, Fekete I. Mannitol for acute stroke. *Cochrane Database Syst Rev*. 2001;1:CD001153.

35. Qizilbash N, Lewington SL, Lopez-Arrieta JM. Corticosteroids for acute ischaemic stroke. *Cochrane Database Syst Rev*. 2002;2:CD000064.

36. Vahedi K, Hofmeijer J, Jüttler E, Vicaut E, George B, Algra A, *et al*. Early decompressive surgery in malignant infarction of the middle cerebral artery: a pooled analysis of three randomised controlled trials. *Lancet Neurol*. 2007;6:215–222.

CHAPTER 12

Acute management and treatment of intracerebral haemorrhage

Marek Sykora, Jennifer Diedler, and Thorsten Steiner

Introduction

Spontaneous intracerebral haemorrhage (ICH) is a devastating condition accounting for approximately 10–15% of all strokes. Despite recent advances in understanding of its pathophysiology and novel therapeutic approaches, ICH still remains the least treatable type of stroke with overall mortality ranging from 35–50%. Around one-half of the ICH patients die within the first 24 hours after symptom onset. The functional outcome of the survivors remains poor, with less than 20% being independent at 6 months (1). However, at least a part of the high mortality is attributable to the traditional therapeutic nihilism, early do not resuscitate orders, and self-fulfilling prophecies (2).

General management

Medical therapies for ICH are based mainly on expert opinions. Evidence from randomized controlled trials for almost all aspects of ICH management is missing or inconclusive. Nevertheless, outcomes after ICH seem to be better when patients are treated in specialized stroke units or intensive care units (ICUs). Studies by Diringer et al. and Mirski et al. demonstrated that admission to the neurological ICU (NICU) is associated with decreased mortality as compared to the general ICU (3, 4). Observation and treatment in a stroke unit or an NICU is therefore strongly recommended for at least the first 24–48 hours as the risk for further neurological deterioration and complications requiring critical care measures is highest in this period.

Intubation and mechanical ventilation

Initial management includes urgent stabilization of cardiac and respiratory functions. Approximately one-third of ICH patients require mechanical ventilation. The indications for intubations and mechanical ventilation include impaired consciousness (Glasgow Coma Scale (GCS) score ≤8), decreased or missing protective airway reflexes, aspiration, impaired central respiratory drive, respiratory failure, or planned neurosurgical intervention as placement of ventricle drainage or haematoma evacuation. Maintenance of adequate oxygenation is essential in patients with acute stroke. Avoidance of hypercapnia is of importance, as it promotes cerebral vasodilation and thus increases intracranial pressure (ICP). Mechanical ventilation should be initiated at PaO_2 lower than 60–70 mmHg and/or $PaCO_2$ higher than 50–60 mmHg. Pressure- or volume-controlled ventilation modes might be both used. Positive end-expiratory pressure (PEEP) levels may increase intrathoracic pressure and reduce venous return and thereby theoretically promote an increase in ICP. Stepwise elevation of PEEP to 15 mmHg resulted in an increase in central venous pressure and a significant decrease of mean arterial pressure (MAP) and regional cerebral blood flow (CBF) (5). However, reduction of CBF depended on MAP changes as a result of disturbed cerebrovascular autoregulation and normalization of MAP restored regional CBF to baseline values. Likewise, PEEP levels up to 12 mmHg did not increase ICP in patients with acute stroke (6). Equally, it was shown that alterations of the inspiratory:expiratory ratio from 1:2 to 1:1 do not influence ICP or CPP, and could therefore be readily applied in patients with acute stroke (7). In summary, PEEP application seems to be safe, provided that MAP is maintained. Monitoring of MAP, ICP, and CPP is desirable.

Blood pressure management

The riddle of optimal blood pressure (BP) management in acute ICH remains still unsolved. Two main pathophysiological concepts have to be considered. The rationale for lowering BP is to avoid haemorrhagic expansion associated with high BP. On the other hand, aggressive lowering of BP bears the theoretical risk of inducing ischaemia in the oedematous region adjacent to the haemorrhage (8). Studies underlining and mitigating the importance of both principles have been published so far. However, recent studies have challenged the concept of major ischaemia in the perihaematomal oedema (9). A recent randomized pilot trial (INTERACT) investigated intensive BP reduction in acute ICH (10). Patients with spontaneous ICH were included within 6 hours of onset and randomly assigned to early intensive lowering of BP with target systolic BP of 140 mmHg (n=203) or standard-based management (n=201) with target systolic BP of 180 mmHg. Mean BP in the first hour was 153 mmHg in the intensive group versus 167 mmHg in the guideline group. Within the first 24 hours, BP was 146 mmHg versus 157 mmHg. At 24 hours, mean proportional haematoma growth was 36.3% in the guideline group versus 13.7% in the intensive group. The mean absolute difference in haematoma volume between both groups was 1.7 mL at 24 hours. This pilot study established the safety of decreasing BP acutely after ICH by absence of significant adverse events or increased mortality and showed a trend toward reduced haematoma growth. The ongoing follow-up study INTERACT-2 has been designed to prove outcome effects of BP lowering in 2800 patients. Another randomized, controlled trial (ATACH) confirmed the feasibility and safety of BP lowering in ICH using intravenous nicardipine. Systolic BP reduction to 110–140 mmHg in the first 24 hours was well tolerated and associated with a trend to reduced haematoma expansion and neurological deterioration (11). Ongoing ATACH-2 aims to test outcome effects of BP lowering to systolic BP 140 mmHg or lower in 1280 patients.

Current guidelines recommend maintaining systolic BP at less than 180 mmHg and diastolic BP below 105 mmHg. MAP should not exceed 120–130 mmHg (12, 13). Acute lowering of the systolic BP to 140 mmHg is probably safe. However, the importance is outlined to select a target BP on the basis of individual patient factors, such as baseline BP, history of hypertension, presumed cause of haemorrhage, age, elevated ICP, and state of autoregulation.

Haemostatic therapy

Recombinant activated factor VII (rFVIIa) acts locally at the site of tissue injury and vascular wall disruption. At higher doses, rFVIIa directly activates factor X on the surface of activated platelets, leading to a thrombin burst and acceleration of coagulation. In a phase II trial including 399 patients with spontaneous ICH, patients were randomized to treatment with 40, 80, or 160 mcg/kg rFVIIa within 4 hours of ictus (14). Compared to placebo, treatment with rFVIIa limited haematoma expansion, decreased mortality and improved 3 month clinical outcome; a 5% increase in arterial thromboembolic events was found within the group receiving the highest dose. These results lead to initiation of a larger phase III trial including 841 patients; patients with a GCS score less than 5 were excluded (FAST-trial) (15). Two hundred and sixty-eight patients were randomized to placebo, 276 patients had 20 mcg/kg rFVIIa, and 297 patients had 80 mcg/kg rFVIIa within 4 hours of stroke. At 24 hours, treatment with 80 mcg/kg significantly reduced haemorrhage growth as compared with placebo (26% versus 11%), corresponding to a moderate but statistically significant reduction of 3.8 mL in the growth in volume as compared to placebo. Total final lesion volumes at 72 hours were similar in the three groups. There was no significant difference regarding survival or functional outcome between the three groups. The overall frequency of thromboembolic serious adverse events was similar in the three groups; however, arterial events were significantly more frequent in the 80 mcg/kg group compared to the placebo group. The investigators point out imbalances between groups with a higher rate of intraventricular extension in the treatment group; moreover, they attribute the disappointing results to the fact that the placebo group had a more favourable outcome compared to the placebo group of the previous phase-II trial (mortality 19% vs 29%, modified Rankin Scale (mRS) score 5 and 6 24% vs 45%). Post hoc analysis of the FAST trial suggests specific subgroups that may benefit from rFVIIa treatment. Patient under 70 years of age, with ICH volumes less than 60 mL and IVH less than 5 mL treated within 2.5 hours may have improved outcome when treated with rFVIIa (odds ratio for poor outcome 0.28; 95% confidence interval 0.08–1.06) (16). Another promising approach to select patients for rFVIIa treatment may be identification of patients at high risk for haematoma growth by

using the spot-sign. Spot-sign, contrast extravasation into the haematoma, has been repeatedly shown to be a very strong predictor of haematoma growth. The ongoing STOP-IT trial is investigating this issue. This randomized, prospective, controlled study includes ICH patients within 6 hours of onset and compares rFVIIa versus placebo for patients with ICH and positive spot-sign on computed tomography (CT) angiography.

Reversal of anticoagulation

Early assessment and correction of the coagulation status of a patient with ICH are particularly important, because it may affect both the progression of cerebral bleeding and the incidence of early rebleeding. A therapeutic dilemma arises in patients with anticoagulant-associated ICH and an underlying condition associated with a high risk of recurrent embolism. Between 0.3% to 0.6% of patients on warfarin anticoagulation suffer from ICH, risk factors including age, intensity of anticoagulation, and leucoaraiosis. However, the annual risk of 5–10% of a thromboembolic complication without anticoagulation in patients with prosthetic valves can be translated as a 2-week risk of 0.2–0.4% that should be weighed against a rather high risk of early rebleeding (13, 17).

Patients with a prolonged activated partial thromboplastin time because of heparin therapy should be treated with protamine sulphate, adjusted to the time since last heparin use (30–60 minutes 0.5–0.75 mg/IU; 60–120 minutes 0.375–0.5 mg/IU; >120 minutes 0.25–0.375 mg/IU, according to (12)). The total dose should not exceed 50 mg and infusion rate should be below 5mg/min; eventually prothrombin complex concentrate (PCC) or fresh frozen plasma (FFP) may be added. Low-molecular-weight heparins (LMWHs) are increasingly employed for anticoagulation in clinical practice. However, there is no uniformly effective or specific antidote to reverse bleeding complications. Protamine sulphate only partially antagonizes the anticoagulant effects of LMWHs. PCC have been proven more efficient (18).

A prolonged prothrombin time due to phenprocoumon or warfarin therapy should be reversed with intravenous PCC, FFP, or both. Dosages and composition of factors of PCC largely vary between products and details should be obtained from the manufacturer. For FFP, the following approximation can be applied: 10 mL/kg will reduce an international normalized ratio (INR) of 4.2 to 2.4, an INR of 3.0 to 2.1, or an INR of 2.4 to 1.8; reducing an INR of 4.2 to 1.4 would therefore require 40 mL/kg (13). Treatment must be combined with vitamin K_1 (1–2 × 5–10 mg IV), since half-lives of phenprocoumon (7 days) and warfarin (24 hours) exceed that of vitamin K-dependent factors. Currently, there are no randomized clinical trials comparing PCC versus FFP. However, PCC seems to reverse anticoagulation faster than FFP. In one retrospective study with 55 patients the use of PCC as compared to FFP showed faster effect and reduced haematoma growth (19). The use of FFP may require infusion of relatively large volumes of plasma. The necessary time for infusion may give place to haematoma enlargement and can lead to volume overload, at worst provoking heart failure. Moreover, concentration of factors varies between different batches, making the degree of effectiveness somewhat unpredictable (12). PCC concentrates can correct coagulopathy faster with smaller volumes, at the price of a higher risk for thromboembolic complications. Repeated measurements of coagulation status are necessary; INR should be re-evaluated 15 minutes after application of PCC. The ongoing randomized comparison between PCC and

FFP in oral anticoagulant treatment (OAT)-related ICH (INCH trial) has been designed to resolve these questions (20).

The efficacy of novel direct oral anticoagulants (DOACs) dabigatran (factor II-inhibitor), apixaban, and rivaroxaban (factor Xa-inhibitors) for stroke prevention in non-valvular atrial fibrillation has been demonstrated in three non-inferiority trials against warfarin (21–23). The rate of ICH in all three studies was significantly lower as compared to warfarin (0.2–0.5% vs 0.7–0.8%). The substantial issue in DOAC-related haemorrhages is the fact that routine haemocoagulation tests (Quick, PTT) are not sufficient to detect and measure the anticoagulatory activity of these drugs and that until now no specific antidote is known. Existing tests for dabigatran—the ecarin clotting time (ECT), thrombin time (TT), and the Hemoclot-test, for rivaroxaban and apixaban—the antifactor Xa levels, are mostly not available for the clinical routine. In DOAC-related ICH, off-label PCC, factor VIIa, or FFP administration may be tried (24, 25). However, no data on reversal of DOAC in patients with ICH has been published so far.

Resumption of anticoagulation

Resumption of anticoagulation primarily concerns patients with a high risk of cardiogenic embolism associated with mechanical heart valves or atrial fibrillation. Current guidelines summarize the available data as follows: in 114 patients from three clinical series, antagonizing anticoagulation with FFP and discontinuation of warfarin for a mean of 7–10 days was associated with embolism in 5% of patients. Rebleeding upon reinstitution of anticoagulation between day 7 and 10 occurred in one patient (0.8%). Seven additional clinical series including 78 patients used PCC for reversal of anticoagulation, resulting in 5% of thromboembolic events; haematoma expansion occurred in 6% (12). These limited data suggest reversal of anticoagulation with FFP or PCC seems to be safe in patients with high risk for cardioembolic events; re-initiation of warfarin appears to be safe within the first 7–14 days.

Recent American guidelines recommend resumption of OAT in indicated cases 7–10 days after symptom onset, the European guidelines suggest waiting 10–14 days after ICH.

Blood glucose management

Post-stroke hyperglycaemia is common. Several clinical trials have found an association between post-stroke hyperglycaemia, higher mortality, and poor functional outcome (26). In a study including critically ill surgical patients, intensive insulin therapy with target blood glucose levels between 80–110 mg/dL lowered in-hospital mortality from 10.9% to 7.2% (27). However, these results could not be confirmed in a follow-up study in medical ICU patients (28). Moreover, a larger randomized trial comparing conventional and intensive glycaemic control (target 80–110 mg/dL) in general ICU patients (NICE-SUGER trial) showed increased mortality in the arm with intensive glycaemic control (29). A recent microdialysis study in patients with severe brain injury demonstrated that tight glycaemic control might be associated with increased prevalence of brain metabolic crises defined as glucose less than 0.7 mmol/L and lactate/pyruvate ratio greater than 40, which was in turn associated with increased mortality (30).

The so far largest randomized trial of blood glucose management in stroke patients (GIST-UK) found no difference in mortality or functional outcome between patients with mild-to-moderate glucose elevations (median 137 mg/dL) compared to those under intensive insulin therapy with target glucose levels between 72–126 mg/dL (31). Current guidelines therefore do not recommend the routine use of insulin infusion in ICH patients with moderate hyperglycaemia and refer to the common practice to lower blood glucose at levels higher than 180 mg/dL (32).

Body temperature management and hypothermia

Hyperthermia in acute stroke is associated with poor outcome and increased mortality. High incidences of fever were reported in a retrospective study including ICH patients, especially for patients with ventricular haemorrhage; the duration of fever was associated with poor outcome (33). Possible mechanisms by which hyperthermia affects outcome include release of neurotransmitters, oxygen radical production, blood–brain barrier breakdown, increase of ischaemic depolarizations and impaired recovery of energy metabolism, inhibition of protein kinases, and propagation of cytoskeletal proteolysis (34). A raise in body temperature should prompt a search for an infectious focus and treatment should aim to maintain body temperature below 37.5°C. A frequently used agent is paracetamol; external cooling with cooling blankets may be more effective. Some centres employ intravascular cooling catheters. However, outcome effects of temperature control are unproven. A recent small pilot study using historical controls showed that mild hypothermia is feasible in ICH and may reduce perihaematomal oedema (35).

Seizure control

Around 8% of ICH-patients develop clinical seizures within 30 days after ictus. Subclinical seizures as seen in continuous EEG monitoring may be, however, present up to 30% of patients (36). Although prophylactic antiepileptic drugs may reduce the incidence of seizures in lobar ICH (37), their routine use is not recommended. If seizures occur, they should be treated aggressively. Non-convulsive seizures might be associated with progressive midline shift and poor outcome (38). Continuous EEG should be considered in ICH patients with otherwise unexplained impairment of consciousness.

Prevention of pulmonary embolism and deep vein thrombosis

Incidences of pulmonary embolism and deep vein thrombosis after acute stroke vary largely between studies (39, 40). One study reports sudden death as the first symptom of pulmonary embolism in 50% of the cases; in the remaining cases, clinical diagnosis was based on the occurrence of sudden dyspnoea, pleuritic pain, or tachycardia (41). The risk of deep vein thrombosis and pulmonary embolism can be reduced by hydration and early mobilization, if possible. Compression stockings have been found effective in surgical patients, however, their efficacy after stroke remains unproven (42, 43). Intermittent pneumatic compression combined with elastic stockings has been shown to be more effective than stockings alone in patients with ICH (44). Studies in ischaemic stroke patients have shown that administration of LMWH reduced the incidence of deep venous thrombosis and pulmonary embolism without increasing the risk of intracerebral haemorrhage (45, 46). Current guidelines recommend the use of low-dose subcutaneous heparin or LMWHs for patients with stroke at high risk for deep vein thrombosis or pulmonary embolism (32, 47). Because of the fear to trigger re-bleeding, thromboembolism prophylaxis is frequently withheld from haemorrhagic stroke patients during the first days after ICH, or administered at half of the normal dose in patients at high risk for deep venous thrombosis. A small randomized trial compared early versus late application of low-dose subcutaneous heparin in patients with haemorrhagic stroke. The authors found a significant reduction of pulmonary embolism when prophylaxis was started on the second day after ictus, compared to patients where treatment was initiated on day 4–10 (48). No overall increase of rebleeding was observed in any of the groups. It has been recommended that in neurologically stable patients low-dose heparin can be started on the second day after onset of ICH (13). Other guidelines recommend starting after day 3 and 4 (12).

Neuromonitoring, cerebral perfusion pressure, and intracranial pressure management

In sedated patients, the clinical monitoring of the neurostatus in order to detect secondary deterioration due to brain oedema or secondary ischaemia is of limited value. The main goals of neuromonitoring are therefore to detect deterioration before irreversible secondary brain injury develops, to monitor the effect of therapeutic measures, and to predict outcome. The benefit of extensive brain monitoring in terms of clinical outcome has yet to be determined. Basic monitoring in sedated and ventilated stroke patients at risk for secondary brain injury comprises placement of an ICP probe. It is recommended that ICH patients with GCS score less than 8, with clinical and/or radiological evidence of raised ICP, or those with intraventricular extension and hydrocephalus should be considered for ICP monitoring and treatment (49). There is only limited evidence on monitoring and treatment of increased ICP in ICH. In one study of surgically treated ICH patients, ICP and cerebral perfusion pressure (CPP) levels were significantly associated with outcome at discharge, but not at 6 months (50). Likewise, there is no evidence to guide CPP after ICH. The data on CPP management are mostly extrapolated from patients with traumatic brain injury (TBI) and applied to ICH patients which might not necessarily be accurate. In ICH patients it is recommended to target CPP levels of 50–70 mmHg (49). However, a recent study showed that CPP levels above 60 mmHg or even above 70 mmHg may still be associated with hypoxia and metabolic crisis the perihaemorrhagic zone as measured by PtO_2 and microdialysis (51). Moreover, it seems that an individually tailored CPP management based on the actual state of cerebral autoregulation might be useful (optimal CPP concept) (52, 53). Case series exist describing the use of brain tissue oxygen monitoring and microdialysis in patients with ICH, however, the small numbers preclude any recommendation on these technologies at this time (51, 54, 55).

Treatment of elevated intracranial pressure

Basic conservative measures to combat raised ICP are elevated head position to 30 degrees and adequate analgesia and sedation. Further options to lower ICP include osmotherapy, tromethamine, barbiturates, hyperventilation, and cerebrospinal fluid (CSF) drainage and decompressive hemicranietomy. However, it has to be noted, that for all ICP treatments in ICH, the evidence for improved outcome is until now scarce and inconclusive.

Osmotherapy

Osmotherapeutic agents are hypertonic solutions of low molecular weight that increase serum osmolarity, thus creating an osmotic gradient between blood and brain tissue. An intact blood–brain barrier is essential for this osmotic gradient. Theoretically, migration of osmotic substances through the damaged blood–brain barrier in ICH can reverse the osmotic gradient and aggravate brain oedema (rebound effect) (56).

Mannitol is the most commonly used osmotherapeutic agent. However, there is only limited data on clinical usefulness of Mannitol. In a meta-analysis based on three trials, the effectiveness of mannitol in patients with acute ischaemic and haemorrhagic stroke was evaluated and neither beneficial nor harmful effects could be proven (57). In another study including ICH patients, mannitol was not found to improve outcome (58). The data suggest that mannitol can be efficiently employed to manage an acute ICP crisis and to bridge the time until further interventions such surgery or placement of external ventricular drainage (EVD) can be initiated.

The effectiveness of hypertonic saline solutions in the treatment of intracranial hypertension after head trauma has been documented in several studies. In contrast, Qureshi and co-workers reported ICP reduction after infusion of 3% saline/acetate in patients with head trauma or postoperative oedema, but not in patients with non-traumatic intracranial haemorrhage or ischaemic stroke (59). However, hypertonic saline was shown to decrease ICP in eight mixed stroke patients in whom mannitol had been without effect. Maximal ICP decrease was observed 20 minutes after the end of the infusion (60). More recently, in a small study with historical control group, continuous hypertonic saline has been shown to reduce perihaematomal oedema in ICH (61). The optimum concentration of hypertonic saline remains controversial; multiple concentrations ranging from 3–23.4% have been tested with different application schedules in patients with TBI (62). Side effects include severe hypernatremia, congestive heart failure and pulmonary oedema.

Regardless of the therapeutic regimen, it is vital to monitor serum electrolyte levels and osmolarity closely while osmotic agents are used. We initially use mannitol (100 mL of a 20% mannitol solution over 15 minutes) to control ICP, preferably through a central line. Because the half-life of mannitol is short (approximately 1 hour), up to four or six administrations per day are necessary. In predisposed patients, a cumulative dose of 300 g may already be nephrotoxic and induce tubular necrosis. Therefore, mannitol accumulation in the serum has to be monitored by simultaneous calculation and measurement of serum osmolality (63). Usually, both values should be identical. If mannitol accumulates, an osmolar gap will occur with serum osmolality exceeding the calculated osmolality. We target a serum osmolarity of 320 mOsm/L. If mannitol therapy is not sufficient for ICP control, we use 10% hypertonic saline or a combination of hypertonic saline hydroxyethyl starch (HS-HES) and hypertonic saline.

Tromethamine

THAM (tris-hydroxy-methyl-aminomethan) leads to a reduction of ICP via vasoconstriction. A prospective randomized clinical trial in 149 patients with TBI receiving either THAM or placebo demonstrated that the use of THAM was associated with a significantly lower incidence of ICP values exceeding 20 mmHg during the first

2 treatment days and a significantly lower number of patients with barbiturate coma requiring treatment (64). Nevertheless, evidence for ICH patients is missing. THAM should always be infused via a central line, because extravasation leads to severe tissue necrosis. Initially, the effectiveness of THAM should be assessed by infusing 1 mmol/kg over 45 minutes. Continuous THAM infusion should be initiated only if the first application leads to significant ICP reduction. The dose is adapted so as to achieve and then maintain blood pH between 7.5 and 7.55.

Barbiturates

The main effect of barbiturates is a decrease in cerebral metabolism and CBF. Schwartz and colleagues found no differences in efficacy between barbiturate coma and mannitol in 95 patients with head injury (65). In contrast, in another study only five of 60 patients treated with barbiturates survived and sustained ICP control was only achieved in the five survivors (66). It must be noted, however, that barbiturates were mostly used as the last line of treatment, after failure of other treatment options; thus, outcome in some patients treated with barbiturates may already have been predetermined by the extent of brain lesions. In another series comprising 21 patients with elevated ICP after large middle cerebral artery infarction, ICP was temporarily decreased in every case by barbiturate treatment, but this effect was associated with a reduction in cerebral oxygen pressure and CPP (67). Because of several potentially severe side effects including marked arterial hypotension, myocardial damage, electrolyte disturbances, impairment of liver function, and predisposition to infection, this treatment should only be used as a therapy of last choice. Application of barbiturates should be accompanied by invasive monitoring of MAP and frequent evaluations of serum electrolyte and liver enzyme levels. Thiopental is the barbiturate used most in neurocritical care unit. It is advisable to cautiously apply a bolus injection of 100 mg and to only proceed with further applications if a marked ICP reduction is observed. Barbiturate effects can be monitored via electroencephalogram on the basis of the appearance of a burst-suppression pattern. Serum drug levels are not reliable.

Hyperventilation

Hyperventilation leads to reduction of $PaCO_2$ which causes vasoconstriction, thus reducing CBF, cerebral blood volume, and, subsequently, ICP. This effect usually occurs within minutes of initiation of hyperventilation. It must be noted that metabolic autoregulation is not intact in perihaemorrhagic brain regions, where brain arterioles are maximally dilated. Vasoconstriction is therefore limited to vessels supplying unaffected brain tissue, a feature that could theoretically lead to redistribution of CBF (reverse steal phenomenon). The applicability of hyperventilation is limited by the following major factors: (i) cerebral vasoconstriction can result in cerebral ischaemia and (ii) the induced elevation of CSF pH is compensated by the choroid plexus within hours, in contrast to the much slower compensation of blood pH, which can require several days. This latter finding implies that the effect of hyperventilation lasts for only a few hours, after which cerebral vessels regain their normal diameter. Termination of hyperventilation at this stage results in an increase of $PaCO_2$ in both blood and CSF, which in turn causes cerebral vasodilation, potentially leading to a rebound effect on ICP. Several clinical studies reported deleterious effects of hyperventilation on cerebral oxygenation and metabolism and outcome (68). While long-term hyperventilation cannot be recommended for stroke patients (69), it may be an option for short interventions to counteract sudden ICP elevations. Under these conditions, the risk of rebound is minimal. Hyperventilation is easily induced through an approximate 10% increase in tidal volume, target levels are 30–35 mmHg arterial $PaCO_2$.

Surgical management

The underlying origin, the location of haemorrhage as well as the neurological status on presentation have to be carefully considered in the decision for or against surgical treatment. With respect to surgery, one classically separates between supra- and infratentorial ICH.

Haematoma evacuation in supratentorial intracranial haemorrhage

The rationale for haematoma evacuation is to reduce the pressure and metabolic effects of the haematoma on the surrounding tissue. Large haematomas result in elevated intracranial pressure, followed by midline shift, brainstem compression and herniation; smaller haematomas may compromise perfusion and/or metabolism in the surrounding tissue and thereby promote secondary brain injury. Experimental studies have shown that removal of the mass lesion improved perfusion in the surrounding brain tissue (70, 71). More recently, a concept of metabolic, rather the ischaemic penumbra has been proposed in secondary injury of adjacent perihaematomal brain tissue (72, 73). Despite completion of a large, multicentre randomized trial, the indication for surgery in supratentorial ICH itself, the optimal technique and best timing are still unknown. The largest trial so far has been the International Surgical Trial in Intracerebral Hemorrhage (STICH) which has been published in 2005 (74). Patients were eligible for inclusion if they had spontaneous, supratentorial ICH with onset of symptoms within 72 hours and the responsible neurosurgeon was uncertain about the benefit of either medical or surgical treatment (the 'uncertainty-principle'). This trial included 1033 patients from 83 centres, 503 were randomized to early surgery and 530 to initial best conservative treatment. Upon inclusion, haematoma evacuation by the method of choice of the responsible neurosurgeon had to be undertaken within 24 hours. Primary outcome measures were mortality and disability at 6 months as measured by the extended Glasgow Outcome Scale (GOS), using a parallel-group trial design dividing patients into good and poor prognosis groups with differing definitions of favourable outcome. In the intention-to-treat analysis, no significant difference regarding favourable outcome between the surgical (26% favourable outcome) and conservative (24% favourable outcome) group was found. Surgery within 96 hours was associated with a statistically insignificant absolute benefit of 2.3% in 6-month outcome. The same statistically insignificant trend in favour for surgery was found for the other outcome parameters mortality, mRS score and Barthel Index. Thus, patients had no benefit from early surgery when compared with initial conservative treatment. However, a subgroup analysis identified patients with superficial, lobar haematomas (≤1 cm from cortical surface) and those with GCS score of 9–12 that were more likely to benefit from surgery; however, this did not reach statistical significance. In contrast, patients presenting in coma with initial GCS score of 8 or lower, nearly all had unfavourable outcomes; early surgery even raised the relative risk of poor outcome by 8%, suggesting that surgery is probably harmful in this subgroup of patients. A recent meta-analysis pooling the data from eight randomized controlled trials since 1985 suggest that there may be improved outcome with surgery if performed within 8 hours of ictus, in haematomas between 20 to 50 mL, in GCS between 9 and 12 and in patients between 50 and 69 years. In addition, there was some evidence that more superficial haematomas with no intraventricular haemorrhage might also benefit (75). Unfortunately, proper evidence from randomized, controlled trials is still missing. Prospective randomized controlled STICH II trial is currently ongoing. This study, based on the results from STICH, focuses on early surgery of lobar superficial (within 1 cm of the cortical surface) haematomas without intraventricular haemorrhage.

Taking the available evidence into account, current treatment strategies largely depend on (i) haemorrhage size and location and (ii) clinical impairment and course of neurological symptoms. Table 12.1 summarizes our current procedure regarding surgical or nonsurgical treatment in special subgroups of patients.

Other approaches apart from standard craniotomy—chosen by the majority of surgeons in the STICH trial—comprise stereotactic or endoscopic aspiration of haematomas. Two studies in non-comatose patients showed impact on levels of consciousness and outcome parameters when compared to craniotomy (76, 77). Combinations of stereotactic haematoma removal with thrombolytic therapy of intracerebral blood clots offer promise (78, 79) and is currently under prospective investigation (MISTIE trial). Summarized, for patients with supratentorial ICH, the decision whether to operate or not remains controversial and is made usually upon consensus. The results of STICH II and MISTIE should clarify more this important issue (80).

As for indication and surgical technique, the question about the ideal timing of intervention remains unresolved. Despite promising results of an early report (81) on clot extraction of putaminal haemorrhages within 7 hours of ictus, a subsequent single-centre randomized trail provided evidence for an increased risk of rebleeding

in four of 11 patients who underwent ultra-early surgery less than 4 hours after ictus. Results in the same study were better for patients operated in the 12-hour time-frame (82). Mortality rate in these patients was 18% compared to 29% in the conservative arm. However, this did not translate into improved functional outcome. In another small study, patients randomized to surgery had clot evacuation during the first 9 hours after symptom onset. No difference regarding outcome and mortality was found compared to medically treated patients (83). In the STICH trial, the average time from the onset of symptoms to surgery was 30 hours and only 16% of patients were treated within 12 hours. Interestingly, recombinant factor VII given pre- or perioperatively may decrease the rebleeding rate associated with ultra-early surgery and may represent an attractive adjunct option (84).

In summary, no clear evidence indicates that ultra-early surgery improves functional outcome. In contrast, delayed evacuation by craniotomy seems to offer little benefit, even more so in comatose patients with deep seated haemorrhage.

Hemicraniectomy for supratentorial intracranial haemorrhage

Only little evidence has been published about decompressive surgery following ICH. Murphy et al. report 12 patients with supratentorial hypertensive ICH who underwent haematoma evacuation and decompressive hemicraniectomy (85). Of 11 surviving patients, six had a good functional outcome (mRS score ≤3) at a mean follow-up time of 17 months. In another small study on clot evacuation in patients with primary supratentorial haemorrhage, in 15 patients in whom progression of brain swelling was anticipated, decompressive craniectomy was performed after clot removal. The combination of decompressive craniectomy and haematoma evacuation showed promising results in a subgroup of severely compromised patients (86).

An uncontrolled retrospective series of 23 patients who underwent hemicraniectomy without haematoma removal in putaminal haemorrhages was published in 2009. At 3 months, 13 patients had good outcome and ten had poor outcome including three deaths. However, included patients had also small haemorrhages and 16 patients had admission GCS score above 9 indicating relatively good admission status. Moreover, the indication for hemicraniectomy was not defined clearly.

Hemicraniectomy for cerebral sinus thrombosis

In patients with large haemorrhagic venous infarcts, midline shift and impending transtentorial herniation may mean decompressive hemicraniectomy has beneficial effect. Until now, only case reports and small series indicate the advantage of this procedure. However, recent series including a literature review states that among all published cases taken together, 11 patients of 13 patients had an excellent outcome (mRS score ≤3) (88). Thus, this promising approach is being prospectively analysed as a part of the ongoing ISCVT-2 trial.

Surgery for cerebellar ICH

Unlike with supratentorial haematomas, the indication for surgery in cerebellar haematomas is undisputed, despite the complete lack of prospective trials. A class I recommendation of the current AHA-guidelines states that patients with cerebellar haemorrhage larger than 3 cm and neurological deterioration or brainstem

Table 12.1 Recommendations for surgical or conservative treatment of ICH

ICH localization	Clinical or CT features	Treatment
BG/thalamus	GCS score >12, ICH volume <30 mL	Conservative
	GCS score <9, ICH volume >60 mL	Conservative
	GCS score 9–12, ICH volume 30–60 mL, and/or deteriorating	Consider evacuation
BG/thalamus + IVH 3rd, 4th ventricle		Additionally EVD
Lobar	GCS score 9–12, ICH volume 20–60 mL, and/or deteriorating	Consider evacuation
Cerebellum	ICH >3 cm and/or expansive behaviour or hydrocephalus	Evacuation and/or EVD
Pons, midbrain, medulla	–	Conservative

BG: basal ganglia, EVD: external ventricular drainage; ICH: intracerebral haemorrhage, IVH: intraventricular haemorrhage.

compression and/or hydrocephalus from ventricular obstruction should have surgical removal of the haemorrhage as soon as possible (12). This recommendation is based on non-randomized series of patients reporting good outcomes for surgically treated patients with cerebellar haemorrhages larger than 3 cm, hydrocephalus, or brainstem compression. Conservative management of patients with smaller haemorrhages without signs of brainstem compression as decrease in vigilance seems to be justified (89, 90).

No recommendation can be made for surgical evacuation of brainstem haematomas, because the tissue destruction caused by the initial bleeding precludes any benefit.

Intraventricular haemorrhage and hydrocephalus

IVH occurs in up to 40% of all patients with ICH. Amount of intraventricular blood, time to clearance of the ventricles, and development of hydrocephalus were identified as independent predictors of poor outcome or death (91, 92). EVD is the treatment of choice. Intraventricular thrombolysis was proposed as an effective measure to hasten the resolution of the intraventricular blood clot, reduce the duration of EVD, decrease the severity and incidence of communicating hydrocephalus, and reduce IVH-associated mortality. At the moment, a prospective phase III study on intraventricular thrombolysis with rtPA is ongoing (CLEARIII).

Conclusion

Medical treatments of ICH target mainly BP optimization and haematoma growth. Surgical treatment may represent an attractive and conclusive option to remove clotted blood, derive CSF, or combat intracranial pressure. Outcome effects of both medical and surgical approaches rely substantially on the follow-up neurocritical care. Despite great efforts in the last 10 years, effective evidence-based treatment for ICH remains still undefined. However, even with a scarcity of evidence, our understanding of ICH including definition of novel clinical targets is progressing rapidly.

References

1. Bamford J, Sandercock P, Dennis M, Burn J, Warlow C. A prospective study of acute cerebrovascular disease in the community: The Oxfordshire community stroke project—1981–86. 2. Incidence, case fatality rates and overall outcome at one year of cerebral infarction, primary intracerebral and subarachnoid haemorrhage. *J Neurol Neurosurg Psychiatry*. 1990;53:16–22.

2. Hemphill JC, 3rd, Newman J, Zhao S, Johnston SC. Hospital usage of early do-not-resuscitate orders and outcome after intracerebral hemorrhage. *Stroke*. 2004;35:1130–1134.

3. Diringer MN, Edwards DF. Admission to a neurologic/neurosurgical intensive care unit is associated with reduced mortality rate after intracerebral hemorrhage. *Crit Care Med*. 2001;29:635–640.

4. Mirski MA, Chang CW, Cowan R. Impact of a neuroscience intensive care unit on neurosurgical patient outcomes and cost of care: evidence-based support for an intensivist-directed specialty ICU model of care. *J Neurosurg Anesthesiol*. 2001;13:83–92.

5. Muench E, Bauhuf C, Roth H, Horn P, Phillips M, Marquetant N, *et al.* Effects of positive end-expiratory pressure on regional cerebral blood flow, intracranial pressure, and brain tissue oxygenation. *Crit Care Med*. 2005;33:2367–2372.

6. Georgiadis D, Schwarz S, Baumgartner RW, Veltkamp R, Schwab S. Influence of positive end-expiratory pressure on intracranial pressure and cerebral perfusion pressure in patients with acute stroke. *Stroke*. 2001;32:2088–2092.

7. Georgiadis D, Schwarz S, Kollmar R, Baumgartner RW, Schwab S. Influence of inspiration:expiration ratio on intracranial and cerebral perfusion pressure in acute stroke patients. *Intensive Care Med*. 2002;28:1089–1093.

8. Kidwell CS, Saver JL, Mattiello J, Warach S, Liebeskind DS, Starkman S, *et al.* Diffusion-perfusion mr evaluation of perihematomal injury in hyperacute intracerebral hemorrhage. *Neurology*. 2001;57:1611–1617.

9. Herweh C, Juttler E, Schellinger PD, Klotz E, Jenetzky E, Orakcioglu B, *et al.* Evidence against a perihemorrhagic penumbra provided by perfusion computed tomography. *Stroke*. 2007;38:2941–2947.

10. Anderson CS, Huang Y, Wang JG, Arima H, Neal B, Peng B, *et al.* Intensive blood pressure reduction in acute cerebral haemorrhage trial (interact): A randomised pilot trial. *Lancet Neurol*. 2008;7:391–399.

11. Robinson TG, Dawson SL, Eames PJ, Panerai RB, Potter JF. Cardiac baroreceptor sensitivity predicts long-term outcome after acute ischemic stroke. *Stroke*. 2003;34:705–712.

12. Broderick J, Connolly S, Feldmann E, Hanley D, Kase C, Krieger D, *et al.* Guidelines for the management of spontaneous intracerebral hemorrhage in adults: 2007 update: a guideline from the American Heart Association/American Stroke Association Stroke Council, High Blood Pressure Research Council, and the Quality of Care and Outcomes in Research Interdisciplinary Working Group. *Circulation*. 2007;116:e391–413.

13. Steiner T, Kaste M, Forsting M, Mendelow D, Kwiecinski H, Szikora I, *et al.* Recommendations for the management of intracranial haemorrhage—part I: spontaneous intracerebral haemorrhage. The European Stroke Initiative Writing Committee and the Writing Committee for the EUSI Executive Committee. *Cerebrovasc Dis*. 2006;22:294–316.

14. Mayer SA, Brun NC, Begtrup K, Broderick J, Davis S, Diringer MN, *et al.* Recombinant activated factor VII for acute intracerebral hemorrhage. *N Engl J Med*. 2005;352:777–785.

15. Mayer SA, Brun NC, Begtrup K, Broderick J, Davis S, Diringer MN, *et al.* Efficacy and safety of recombinant activated factor VII for acute intracerebral hemorrhage. *N Engl J Med*. 2008;358:2127–2137.

16. Mayer SA, Davis SM, Skolnick BE, Brun NC, Begtrup K, Broderick JP, *et al.* Can a subset of intracerebral hemorrhage patients benefit from hemostatic therapy with recombinant activated factor VII? *Stroke*. 2009;40:833–840.

17. Flibotte JJ, Hagan N, O'Donnell J, Greenberg SM, Rosand J. Warfarin, hematoma expansion, and outcome of intracerebral hemorrhage. *Neurology*. 2004;63:1059–1064.

18. Firozvi K, Deveras RA, Kessler CM. Reversal of low-molecular-weight heparin-induced bleeding in patients with pre-existing hypercoagulable states with human recombinant activated factor VII concentrate. *Am J Hematol*. 2006;81:582–589.

19. Huttner HB, Schellinger PD, Hartmann M, Kohrmann M, Juettler E, Wikner J, *et al.* Hematoma growth and outcome in treated neurocritical care patients with intracerebral hemorrhage related to oral anticoagulant therapy: Comparison of acute treatment strategies using vitamin K, fresh frozen plasma, and prothrombin complex concentrates. *Stroke*. 2006;37:1465–1470.

20. Steiner T, Freiberger A, Griebe M, Husing J, Ivandic B, Kollmar R, *et al.* International normalised ratio normalisation in patients with coumarin-related intracranial haemorrhages—the INCH trial: a randomised controlled multicentre trial to compare safety and preliminary efficacy of fresh frozen plasma and prothrombin complex—study design and protocol. *Int J Stroke*. 2011;6:271–277.

21. Connolly SJ, Ezekowitz MD, Yusuf S, Eikelboom J, Oldgren J, Parekh A, *et al.* Dabigatran versus warfarin in patients with atrial fibrillation. *N Engl J Med*. 2009;361:1139–1151.

22. Patel MR, Mahaffey KW, Garg J, Pan G, Singer DE, Hacke W, *et al.* Rivaroxaban versus warfarin in nonvalvular atrial fibrillation. *N Engl J Med*.365:883–891.

23. Granger CB, Alexander JH, McMurray JJ, Lopes RD, Hylek EM, Hanna M, *et al.* Apixaban versus warfarin in patients with atrial fibrillation. *N Engl J Med*.365:981–992.

24. Zhou W, Zorn M, Nawroth P, Butehorn U, Perzborn E, Heitmeier S, Veltkamp R. Hemostatic therapy in experimental intracerebral hemorrhage associated with rivaroxaban. *Stroke*. 2013 Mar;44(3):771–778.

25. Zhou W, Schwarting S, Illanes S, Liesz A, Middelhoff M, Zorn M, *et al*. Hemostatic therapy in experimental intracerebral hemorrhage associated with the direct thrombin inhibitor dabigatran. *Stroke*.42:3594–3599.

26. Capes SE, Hunt D, Malmberg K, Pathak P, Gerstein HC. Stress hyperglycemia and prognosis of stroke in nondiabetic and diabetic patients: a systematic overview. *Stroke*. 2001;32:2426–2432.

27. van den Berghe G, Wouters P, Weekers F, Verwaest C, Bruyninckx F, Schetz M, *et al*. Intensive insulin therapy in the critically ill patients. *N Engl J Med*. 2001;345:1359–1367.

28. Van den Berghe G, Wilmer A, Hermans G, Meersseman W, Wouters PJ, Milants I, *et al*. Intensive insulin therapy in the medical ICU. *N Engl J Med*. 2006;354:449–461.

29. Finfer S, Chittock DR, Su SY, Blair D, Foster D, Dhingra V, *et al*. Intensive versus conventional glucose control in critically ill patients. *N Engl J Med*. 2009;360:1283–1297.

30. Oddo M, Schmidt JM, Carrera E, Badjatia N, Connolly ES, Presciutti M, *et al*. Impact of tight glycemic control on cerebral glucose metabolism after severe brain injury: a microdialysis study. *Crit Care Med*. 2008;36:3233–3238.

31. Gray CS, Hildreth AJ, Sandercock PA, O'Connell JE, Johnston DE, Cartlidge NE, *et al*. Glucose-potassium-insulin infusions in the management of post-stroke hyperglycaemia: the UK glucose insulin in stroke trial (GIST-UK). *Lancet Neurol*. 2007;6:397–406.

32. Guidelines for management of ischaemic stroke and transient ischaemic attack 2008. *Cerebrovasc Dis*. 2008;25:457–507.

33. Schwarz S, Hafner K, Aschoff A, Schwab S. Incidence and prognostic significance of fever following intracerebral hemorrhage. *Neurology*. 2000;54:354–361.

34. Ginsberg MD, Busto R. Combating hyperthermia in acute stroke: a significant clinical concern. *Stroke*. 1998;29:529–534.

35. Kollmar R, Staykov D, Dorfler A, Schellinger PD, Schwab S, Bardutzky J. Hypothermia reduces perihemorrhagic edema after intracerebral hemorrhage. *Stroke*. 2010;41:1684–1689.

36. Claassen J, Jette N, Chum F, Green R, Schmidt M, Choi H, *et al*. Electrographic seizures and periodic discharges after intracerebral hemorrhage. *Neurology*. 2007;69:1356–1365.

37. Passero S, Rocchi R, Rossi S, Ulivelli M, Vatti G. Seizures after spontaneous supratentorial intracerebral hemorrhage. *Epilepsia*. 2002;43:1175–1180.

38. Vespa PM, O'Phelan K, Shah M, Mirabelli J, Starkman S, Kidwell C, *et al*. Acute seizures after intracerebral hemorrhage: a factor in progressive midline shift and outcome. *Neurology*. 2003;60:1441–1446.

39. Kamphuisen PW, Agnelli G, Sebastianelli M. Prevention of venous thromboembolism after acute ischemic stroke. *J Thromb Haemost*. 2005;3:1187–1194.

40. Kelly J, Rudd A, Lewis RR, Coshall C, Moody A, Hunt BJ. Venous thromboembolism after acute ischemic stroke: a prospective study using magnetic resonance direct thrombus imaging. *Stroke*. 2004;35:2320–2325.

41. Wijdicks EF, Scott JP. Pulmonary embolism associated with acute stroke. *Mayo Clin Proc*. 1997;72:297–300.

42. Mazzone C, Chiodo GF, Sandercock P, Miccio M, Salvi R. Physical methods for preventing deep vein thrombosis in stroke. *Cochrane Database Syst Rev*. 2004;4:CD001922.

43. Dennis M, Sandercock PA, Reid J, Graham C, Murray G, Venables G, *et al*. Effectiveness of thigh-length graduated compression stockings to reduce the risk of deep vein thrombosis after stroke (CLOTS trial 1): a multicentre, randomised controlled trial. *Lancet*. 2009;373:1958–1965.

44. Lacut K, Bressollette L, Le Gal G, Etienne E, De Tinteniac A, Renault A, *et al*. Prevention of venous thrombosis in patients with acute intracerebral hemorrhage. *Neurology*. 2005;65:865–869.

45. Diener HC, Ringelstein EB, von Kummer R, Landgraf H, Koppenhagen K, Harenberg J, *et al*. Prophylaxis of thrombotic and embolic events

46. in acute ischemic stroke with the low-molecular-weight heparin certoparin: results of the protect trial. *Stroke*. 2006;37:139–144.

46. Sherman DG, Albers GW, Bladin C, Fieschi C, Gabbai AA, Kase CS, *et al*. The efficacy and safety of enoxaparin versus unfractionated heparin for the prevention of venous thromboembolism after acute ischaemic stroke (PREVAIL study): an open-label randomised comparison. *Lancet*. 2007;369:1347–1355.

47. Adams HP, Jr, del Zoppo G, Alberts MJ, Bhatt DL, Brass L, Furlan A, *et al*. Guidelines for the early management of adults with ischemic stroke. *Circulation*. 2007;115:e478–534.

48. Boeer A, Voth E, Henze T, Prange HW. Early heparin therapy in patients with spontaneous intracerebral haemorrhage. *J Neurol Neurosurg Psychiatry*. 1991;54:466–467.

49. Morgenstern LB, Hemphill JC, 3rd, Anderson C, Becker K, Broderick JP, Connolly ES, Jr, *et al*. Guidelines for the management of spontaneous intracerebral hemorrhage: a guideline for healthcare professionals from the American Heart Association/American Stroke Association. *Stroke*. 2010;41: 2108–2129.

50. Fernandes HM, Siddique S, Banister K, Chambers I, Wooldridge T, Gregson B, *et al*. Continuous monitoring of ICP and CPP following ICH and its relationship to clinical, radiological and surgical parameters. *Acta Neurochir Suppl*. 2000;76:463–466.

51. Ko SB, Choi HA, Parikh G, Helbok R, Schmidt JM, Lee K, *et al*. Multimodality monitoring for cerebral perfusion pressure optimization in comatose patients with intracerebral hemorrhage. *Stroke*. 2011;42:3087–3092.

52. Steiner LA, Czosnyka M, Piechnik SK, Smielewski P, Chatfield D, Menon DK, *et al*. Continuous monitoring of cerebrovascular pressure reactivity allows determination of optimal cerebral perfusion pressure in patients with traumatic brain injury. *Crit Care Med*. 2002;30:733–738.

53. Diedler J, Sykora M, Rupp A, Poli S, Karpel-Massler G, Sakowitz O, Steiner T. Impaired cerebral vasomotor activity in spontaneous intracerebral hemorrhage. *Stroke*. 2009;40:815–819.

54. Hemphill JC, 3rd, Morabito D, Farrant M, Manley GT. Brain tissue oxygen monitoring in intracerebral hemorrhage. *Neurocrit Care*. 2005;3: 260–270.

55. Diedler J, Karpel-Massler G, Sykora M, Poli S, Sakowitz OW, Veltkamp R, *et al*. Autoregulation and brain metabolism in the perihematomal region of spontaneous intracerebral hemorrhage: an observational pilot study. *J Neurol Sci*. 2010;295:16–22.

56. Kaufmann AM, Cardoso ER. Aggravation of vasogenic cerebral edema by multiple-dose mannitol. *J Neurosurg*. 1992;77:584–589

57. Bereczki D, Liu M, do Prado GF, Fekete I. Mannitol for acute stroke. *Stroke*. 2008;39:512–513.

58. Misra UK, Kalita J, Ranjan P, Mandal SK. Mannitol in intracerebral hemorrhage: a randomized controlled study. *J Neurol Sci*. 2005;234:41–45.

59. Qureshi AI, Suarez JI. Use of hypertonic saline solutions in treatment of cerebral edema and intracranial hypertension. *Crit Care Med*. 2000;28: 3301–3313.

60. Schwarz S, Georgiadis D, Aschoff A, Schwab S. Effects of hypertonic (10%) saline in patients with raised intracranial pressure after stroke. *Stroke*. 2002;33:136–140.

61. Wagner I, Hauer EM, Staykov D, Volbers B, Dorfler A, Schwab S, Bardutzky J. Effects of continuous hypertonic saline infusion on perihemorrhagic edema evolution. *Stroke*. 2011;42:1540–1545.

62. Ogden AT, Mayer SA, Connolly ES, Jr Hyperosmolar agents in neurosurgical practice: the evolving role of hypertonic saline. *Neurosurgery*. 2005;57:207–215.

63. Dorman HR, Sondheimer JH, Cadnapaphornchai P. Mannitol-induced acute renal failure. *Medicine (Baltimore)*. 1990;69:153–159.

64. Wolf AL, Levi L, Marmarou A, Ward JD, Muizelaar PJ, Choi S, *et al*. Effect of THAM upon outcome in severe head injury: a randomized prospective clinical trial. *J Neurosurg*. 1993;78:54–59.

65. Schwartz ML, Tator CH, Rowed DW, Reid SR, Meguro K, Andrews DF. The University of Toronto head injury treatment study: a prospective,

randomized comparison of pentobarbital and mannitol. *Can J Neurol Sci.* 1984;11:434–440.

66. Schwab S, Spranger M, Schwarz S, Hacke W. Barbiturate coma in severe hemispheric stroke: Useful or obsolete? *Neurology.* 1997;48: 1608–1613.

67. Steiner T, Pilz J, Schellinger P, Wirtz R, Friederichs V, Aschoff A, *et al.* Multimodal online monitoring in middle cerebral artery territory stroke. *Stroke.* 2001;32:2500–2506.

68. Muizelaar JP, Marmarou A, Ward JD, Kontos HA, Choi SC, Becker DP, *et al.* Adverse effects of prolonged hyperventilation in patients with severe head injury: a randomized clinical trial. *J Neurosurg.* 1991;75: 731–739.

69. Bardutzky J, Schwab S. Antiedema therapy in ischemic stroke. *Stroke.* 2007;38:3084–3094.

70. Nehls DG, Mendelow DA, Graham DI, Teasdale GM. Experimental intracerebral hemorrhage: early removal of a spontaneous mass lesion improves late outcome. *Neurosurgery.* 1990;27:674–682.

71. Kingman TA, Mendelow AD, Graham DI, Teasdale GM. Experimental intracerebral mass: time-related effects on local cerebral blood flow. *J Neurosurg.* 1987;67:732–738.

72. Zazulia AR, Videen TO, Powers WJ. Transient focal increase in perihematomal glucose metabolism after acute human intracerebral hemorrhage. *Stroke.* 2009;40:1638–1643.

73. Vespa PM. Metabolic penumbra in intracerebral hemorrhage. *Stroke.* 2009;40:1547–1548.

74. Mendelow AD, Gregson BA, Fernandes HM, Murray GD, Teasdale GM, Hope DT, *et al.* Early surgery versus initial conservative treatment in patients with spontaneous supratentorial intracerebral haematomas in the international Surgical Trial in Intracerebral Haemorrhage (STICH): a randomised trial. *Lancet.* 2005;365:387–397.

75. Gregson BA, Broderick JP, Auer LM, Batjer H, Chen XC, Juvela S, *et al.* Individual patient data subgroup meta-analysis of surgery for spontaneous supratentorial intracerebral hemorrhage. *Stroke.*43:1496–1504.

76. Marquardt G, Wolff R, Sager A, Janzen RW, Seifert V. Subacute stereotactic aspiration of haematomas within the basal ganglia reduces occurrence of complications in the course of haemorrhagic stroke in non-comatose patients. *Cerebrovasc Dis.* 2003;15:252–257.

77. Cho DY, Chen CC, Chang CS, Lee WY, Tso M. Endoscopic surgery for spontaneous basal ganglia hemorrhage: comparing endoscopic surgery, stereotactic aspiration, and craniotomy in noncomatose patients. *Surg Neurol.* 2006;65:547–555.

78. Teernstra OP, Evers SM, Lodder J, Leffers P, Franke CL, Blaauw G. Stereotactic treatment of intracerebral hematoma by means of a plasminogen activator: a multicenter randomized controlled trial (SICHPA). *Stroke.* 2003;34:968–974.

79. Vespa P, McArthur D, Miller C, O'Phelan K, Frazee J, Kidwell C, *et al.* Frameless stereotactic aspiration and thrombolysis of deep intracerebral hemorrhage is associated with reduction of hemorrhage volume and neurological improvement. *Neurocrit Care.* 2005;2:274–281.

80. Morgan T, Zuccarello M, Narayan R, Keyl P, Lane K, Hanley D. Preliminary findings of the minimally-invasive surgery plus rtPA for intracerebral hemorrhage evacuation (MISTIE) clinical trial. *Acta Neurochir Suppl.* 2008;105:147–151.

81. Kaneko M, Tanaka K, Shimada T, Sato K, Uemura K. Long-term evaluation of ultra-early operation for hypertensive intracerebral hemorrhage in 100 cases. *J Neurosurg.* 1983;58:838–842.

82. Morgenstern LB, Demchuk AM, Kim DH, Frankowski RF, Grotta JC. Rebleeding leads to poor outcome in ultra-early craniotomy for intracerebral hemorrhage. *Neurology.* 2001;56:1294–1299.

83. Zuccarello M, Brott T, Derex L, Kothari R, Sauerbeck L, Tew J, *et al.* Early surgical treatment for supratentorial intracerebral hemorrhage: a randomized feasibility study. *Stroke.* 1999;30:1833–1839.

84. Sutherland CS, Hill MD, Kaufmann AM, Silvaggio JA, Demchuk AM, Sutherland GR. Recombinant factor VIIa plus surgery for intracerebral hemorrhage. *Can J Neurol Sci.* 2008;35:567–572.

85. Murthy JM, Chowdary GV, Murthy TV, Bhasha PS, Naryanan TJ. Decompressive craniectomy with clot evacuation in large hemispheric hypertensive intracerebral hemorrhage. *Neurocrit Care.* 2005;2:258–262.

86. Maira G, Anile C, Colosimo C, Rossi GF. Surgical treatment of primary supratentorial intracerebral hemorrhage in stuporous and comatose patients. *Neurol Res.* 2002;24:54–60.

87. Ramnarayan R, Anto D, Anilkumar TV, Nayar R. Decompressive hemicraniectomy in large putaminal hematomas: an Indian experience. *J Stroke Cerebrovasc Dis.* 2009;18:1–10.

88. Coutinho JM, Majoie CB, Coert BA, Stam J. Decompressive hemicraniectomy in cerebral sinus thrombosis: consecutive case series and review of the literature. *Stroke.* 2009;40:2233–2235.

89. van Loon J, Van Calenbergh F, Goffin J, Plets C. Controversies in the management of spontaneous cerebellar haemorrhage. A consecutive series of 49 cases and review of the literature. *Acta Neurochir (Wien).* 1993;122:187–193

90. Da Pian R, Bazzan A, Pasqualin A. Surgical versus medical treatment of spontaneous posterior fossa haematomas: a cooperative study on 205 cases. *Neurol Res.* 1984;6:145–151.

91. Diringer MN, Edwards DF, Zazulia AR. Hydrocephalus: a previously unrecognized predictor of poor outcome from supratentorial intracerebral hemorrhage. *Stroke.* 1998;29:1352–1357.

92. Tuhrim S, Horowitz DR, Sacher M, Godbold JH. Volume of ventricular blood is an important determinant of outcome in supratentorial intracerebral hemorrhage. *Crit Care Med.* 1999;27:617–621.

CHAPTER 13

Acute treatment in subarachnoid haemorrhage

Katja E. Wartenberg

Prognosis

Current developments in neurocritical care including advanced continuous monitoring techniques, a shift of focus to immediate real-time normalization of pathophysiological states, and better recognition and management of complications following subarachnoid haemorrhage (SAH) have improved the level of care for SAH patients and their clinical outcome. The mortality rate has been reduced from 50% to 25–35% (1–3). Of all SAH patients 12% die before they reach medical attention (4, 5). Of the two-thirds of patients who survive, approximately 50% are permanently disabled, mainly due to neurocognitive deficits (20%), anxiety, and depression which occur in up to 80%. Many patients do not return to work or they retire early, and their relationships are affected (6, 7). Advanced age, poor clinical status, recurrent haemorrhage, larger aneurysm size, global cerebral oedema, delayed cerebral ischaemia, and medical complications impact functional outcome after SAH. Of all these factors, the clinical condition upon arrival in the hospital appears to be the single most important risk factor for poor outcome (8–11). The poor-grade patients (Hunt–Hess or World Federation of Neurological Surgeons Scale (WFNS) grade IV and V), 18–24% of the entire SAH population, present the greatest challenge. They have worse long-term functional outcomes and higher mortality rates (11–13). However, early and aggressive treatment of patients with severe SAH resulted in unexpected improvements of long-term outcome (14–16). In a Japanese study of 283 poor-grade SAH patients, 34% achieved afavourableoutcome (good recovery, moderate disability on Glasgow Outcome Scale (GOS 4 and 5)) at discharge. Improvement in WFNS grade was associated with favourable outcome (17). In another retrospective study of 47 WFNS grade 4 and 5 SAH patients who underwent coiling of the ruptured aneurysm and aggressive neurocritical care, good outcome (GOS 4 and 5) at 6 months was achieved in 53% (3). Of 70 vigorously treated patients with Hunt and Hess grade V SAH, 35 (50%) died. Of 26 patients with neurocognitive testing at 1 year, half of the patients, mainly young and highly educated individuals, all employed in full-time jobs prior to SAH, had mild cognitive deficits and were able to live a normal life (12).

Furthermore, mortality rates are substantially higher and good long-term functional outcomes less often achieved at medical centres that treat less than 18 patients with SAH per year (18–20).

Clinical scores

The clinical condition upon admission of a patient is most commonly rated with the Glasgow Coma Scale (GCS) (21), Hunt–Hess scale (22), or the WFNS scale (23). The scales are listed in Tables 13.1–13.3. The reports about intra- and interobserver agreements are sparse and highly variable. However, obtaining a score on admission is recommended to have an estimate of long-term outcome (24).

The Fisher scale is a radiological scale based on the amount and distribution of blood on computed tomography (CT) used to predict the future occurrence of delayed cerebral ischaemia (Figure 13.1) (25). A modification of the original Fisher scale with attention to thick cisternal and ventricular blood resulted in a more accurate association with symptomatic vasospasm (Figure 13.2) (26, 27).

General emergency and critical care management

In acute SAH, the sudden rise of intracranial pressure (ICP) up to levels of the mean arterial pressure (MAP) results in an arrest of cerebral circulation which is clinically seen as loss of consciousness (28), and in development of global cerebral oedema as well as acute ischaemic injury on neuroimaging (Figure 13.3) (8, 29–31).

While diagnosing the cause of SAH and preparing for aneurysm repair initial care should focus on:

◆ Stabilization of systemic oxygenation and haemodynamics to optimize cerebral perfusion and oxygen supply

◆ Control of ICP caused by hydrocephalus and/or global cerebral oedema

◆ Blood pressure control

◆ Seizure control

◆ Antifibrinolytic agents to prevent aneurysm rebleeding.

The resuscitation goals for SAH are presented in Table 13.4. The treatment of SAH starts with management of airway, respiration, and circulation, followed by evaluation of the level of consciousness. A complete blood count (CBC), metabolic panel, coagulation studies, troponin I, creatine kinase, urine analysis, urine toxicology screen, blood for type and crossmatch, an electrocardiogram, and a chest x-ray should be obtained.

The next step is aimed at prevention of rebleeding which occurs in 9–17% of patients in the first 72 hours, 40–87% of those within the first 6 hours. Patients with high-grade SAH, loss of consciousness at index bleed, larger aneurysms, sentinel bleeds, angiography within 3–6 hours of symptom onset, delay to treatment, and incomplete

Table 13.1 Glasgow Coma Scale (21)

Eye opening response	Spontaneous eye opening with blinking at baseline	4 points
	Eye opening to verbal command, speech, or shout	3 points
	Eye opening to painful stimuli	2 points
	None	1 point
Verbal response	Oriented	5 points
	Confused conversation, but able to answer questions	4 points
	Inappropriate responses, words discernible	3 points
	Incomprehensible speech	2 points
	None	1 point
Motor response	Following commands for movement	6 points
	Purposeful movement to painful stimuli (localizing pain)	5 points
	Withdrawal from pain (non-localizing)	4 points
	Abnormal flexion response to pain, decorticate posture	3 points
	Extension response to pain, decerebrate posture	2 points
	None	1 point

From Teasdale and Jennett (21).

aneurysm repair are at higher risk for recurrent haemorrhage (15, 32–34). The available data are not sufficient for specific recommendations regarding blood pressure reduction, administration of antifibrinolytic therapy with tranexamic acid or aminocaproic acid prior to cerebral angiography or aneurysm repair. Lowering blood pressure to a systolic value of 140–160 mmHg is usually practised. A MAP of 110 mmHg can be tolerated. However, care should be taken to adjust the MAP and cerebral perfusion pressure (CPP) to maintain cerebral blood flow (CBF).

A short course of antifibrinolytic therapy may be undertaken until aneurysm repair for a maximum of 72 hours. This therapy should be discontinued 2 hours prior to endovascular aneurysm repair. Thromboembolic events present a contraindication, and the

Table 13.2 Hunt–Hess scale

		Hospital mortality (%)[a]	
Grade	Clinical findings	1968	1997
I	Asymptomatic or mild headache	11	1
II	Moderate to severe headache, or oculomotor palsy	26	5
III	Confused, drowsy, or mild focal signs	37	19
IV	Stupor (localizes to pain)	71	42
V	Coma (posturing or no motor response to pain)	100	77
Total		35	18

[a] Data from 275 patients reported by Hunt and Hess in 1968, and 214 patients reported by Oshiro et al in 1997; mortality figures do not include out-of-hospital deaths.
From Hunt and Hess (22) and Oshiro et al. (164).

Table 13.3 World Federation of Neurological Surgeons Scale

Grade	Glasgow Coma Scale score	Motor deficit
I	15	Absent
I	13–14	Absent
III	13–14	Present
IV	8–12	Absent or present
V	<8	Absent or present

From Report of World Federation of Neurological Surgeons Committee on a Universal Subarachnoid Hemorrhage Grading Scale (23).

patients should be monitored closely for deep venous thrombosis (34, 35). The use of steroids is not supported by any controlled trials.

The patients diagnosed with SAH should be treated at high-volume centres with appropriate specialty neurointensive care units, neurointensivists, vascular neurosurgeons, and interventional neuroradiologists (18–20).

Treatment of intracranial hypertension

Subarachnoid haemorrhage is associated with intracranial hypertension caused by hydrocephalus, space-occupying intracerebral haemorrhage, global and focal cerebral oedema. The development of acute hydrocephalus is primarily related to the volume of intraventricular and subarachnoid blood in the basal cisterns. Hydrocephalus occurs in 20–30% after SAH (36–38). Clinical findings of hydrocephalus are lethargy, psychomotor slowing, impaired short-term memory, limitation of upgaze, abducens palsies, and lower extremity hyperreflexia.

When hydrocephalus leads to increased ICP, the patient may be found stuporous or comatose with signs of brainstem compression. Insertion of an extraventricular drain (EVD) is life saving with a prompt clinical response such as improvement of consciousness (39), but is complicated by a high risk of infection (up to 15%). If there is no improvement in 36–48 hours and the ICP is low, a poor neurological state is likely due to primary brain injury related to the acute effects of haemorrhage. Weaning of the EVD should begin after ICP is controlled for 48 hours either by trials of intermittent clamping or raising the EVD level with ICP monitoring. Serial lumbar puncture (40) or placement of a lumbar drain (41) present alternatives to prolonged or repeated EVD placement if the basal cisterns are open. Late hydrocephalus after SAH creates a clinical syndrome indistinguishable from normal pressure hydrocephalus, and is closely correlated with a prolonged duration of EVD treatment. The symptoms encompass dementia, gait disturbance, and urinary incontinence which respond to shunting. About 18–26% of all SAH patients require a ventriculoperitoneal shunt for persistent hydrocephalus (37, 42).

Beside drainage of CSF for ICP control and monitoring, space-occupying intraparenchymal haemorrhages should be treated by craniotomy and surgical decompression. Decompressive craniectomy is indicated in patients with life-threatening cerebral oedema with and without intracerebral haemorrhage, due to infarction or rebleeding and should be performed rapidly to avoid herniation (43).

Apart from head-of-bed elevation, sedation, temperature control, administration of isotonic fluids, maintaining CPP >60 mmHg,

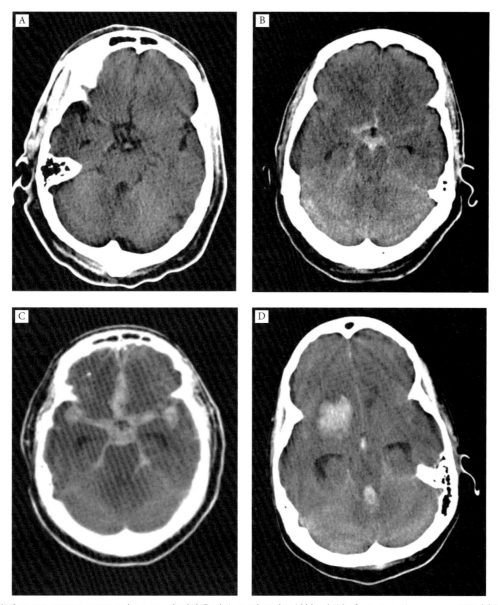

Fig. 13.1 Fisher scale (25) on non-contrast computed tomography. (A) Grade I: no subarachnoid blood, risk of symptomatic vasospasm 21%. (B) Grade II: diffuse, thin subarachnoid blood <1 mm thick, risk of symptomatic vasospasm 25%. (C) Grade III: diffuse or focal, thick subarachnoid blood >1 mm, risk of symptomatic vasospasm 37%. (D) Grade IV: no or diffuse, thin subarachnoid blood with ventricular haemorrhage, risk of symptomatic vasospasm 31%.

and an arterial partial pressure of carbon dioxide of 35 mmHg, bolus administration of hypertonic saline may be the preferred treatment for ICP crisis. Hypertonic saline (23.5%) given for ICP control resulted in an increase in CBF in ischaemic regions and in augmentation of brain tissue oxygenation as well as in a decrease in ICP (44, 45).

Multimodal monitoring including ICP, MAP, CPP, partial pressure of cerebral tissue oxygen (PbtO$_2$), cerebral lactate, pyruvate, glucose, glycerol, and glutamate by microdialysis and reactivity indices may help to determine the optimal CPP threshold. The pressure reactivity index is calculated as the correlation coefficient between ICP and MAP to reflect cerebral autoregulation states. If autoregulation is disturbed, MAP changes are directly transmitted passively through a non-reactive vasculature to ICP (see Figure 13.4). The optimal CPP was defined as the CPP at the

lowest pressure reactivity index observed within a range of CPP (50–90 mmHg usually) (46).

Management of volume status

Intravascular volume status should be monitored as reduced intravascular volume regulation resulting in hypovolaemia may increase the frequency of cerebral ischaemia and infarction (47–50). Although placement of a central venous catheter is recommended for large-volume access and monitoring, central venous pressure (CVP) is an unreliable marker of intravascular volume (51, 52). Assessment of fluid status should not be based solely on CVP. Clinical examination of the patient, records of in- and output, hourly urine output, and stroke volume variation in intubated patients may be helpful variables. Routine placement of pulmonary artery catheters is not recommended (35). In general, intravenous

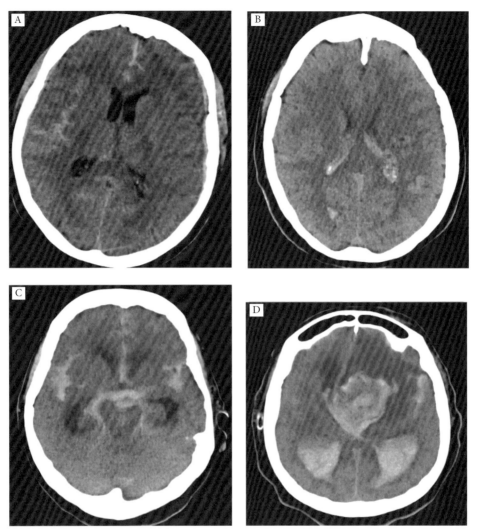

Fig. 13.2 Modified Fisher Scale (26, 27) on non-contrast computed tomography. (A) Grade I: no or minimal subarachnoid blood, no intraventricular haemorrhage risk of symptomatic vasospasm 24%. (B) Grade II: minimal subarachnoid blood with intraventricular haemorrhage, risk of symptomatic vasospasm 33%. (C) Grade III: diffuse or focal, thick subarachnoid blood, no intraventricular haemorrhage, risk of symptomatic vasospasm 33%. (D) Grade IV: diffuse or focal, thick subarachnoid blood with intraventricular haemorrhage, risk of symptomatic vasospasm 40%.

fluid management for patients with SAH should target euvolaemia (24, 35). Prophylactic hypervolaemia may be harmful (53–56). Isotonic fluids such as 0.9% saline at 1–1.5 mL/kg/hour can be used. Supplemental 250 ml boluses of crystalloid (0.9% saline) or colloid (5% albumin) solution can be given every 2 hours. However, crystalloids are preferred (35). Hypertonic saline solutions (2% or 3% sodium chloride/acetate, 1 mL/kg/hour) are an alternative to normal saline for patients suffering from refractory intracranial hypertension or symptomatic intracranial mass effect. The infusion is adjusted to maintain a sodium level of 150–155 mEq/L and serum osmolality of 310–320 mOsms/L. Hypotonic fluids should be avoided (24).

Prevention and treatment of seizures

The frequency of seizures in SAH has been reported to be 1–7% at onset, although many of these events may represent tonic posturing. Approximately 5% experience seizures during hospitalization, and 7% will develop epilepsy during the first year after discharge (57, 58). The most important trigger for seizure is focal pathology such as large subarachnoid clots, subdural haematoma, or cerebral infarction. A seizure at the onset of SAH does not predict an increased risk for epilepsy (57). Routine use of phenytoin or fosphenytoin may worsen functional and cognitive outcome after SAH (59, 60) and is no longer recommended (24, 35). If seizure prophylaxis with other antiepileptic drugs such as levetiracetam is warranted to prevent rebleeding, they should be administered for 3–7 days only (35).

Comatose patients may have non-convulsive seizures or status epilepticus (8–19%) (61–63). Therefore, continuous electroencephalographic monitoring (cEEG) is recommended in poor-grade SAH patients in stupor or coma. The effect of treatment of non-convulsive seizures in these patients is less clear (35).

Aneurysm repair

Craniotomy and aneurysm clipping with microsurgical technique and preservation of the parent artery and its branches has long been considered the gold standard of aneurysm therapy. Clipping within 48–72 hours of presentation and safer microsurgical

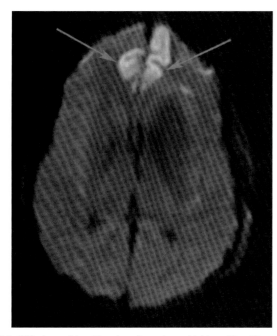

Fig. 13.3 Diffusion-weighted Imaging of a patient with Hunt–Hess IV subarachnoid haemorrhage, obtained on admission, showing acute ischaemic injury in the distribution of the bilateral anterior cerebral artery territory.

techniques result in permanent aneurysm obliteration in over 90% confirmed by intra- or postoperative angiograms as well as in low morbidity and mortality (5–15%) excluding giant aneurysms (64–67). The complication rate of clipping is highest when the aneurysm is large or located on the basilar artery (68–70). Aneurysms on the middle cerebral artery may be more amendable to surgery (71, 72).

With the introduction of Guglielmi Detachable Coils (soft thrombogenic detachable platinum coils, GDC, Target Therapeutics, Fremont, CA) for endovascular therapy of aneurysms in 1991 (73, 74), coil embolization became an important alternative to craniotomy and aneurysm clipping. Obliteration of small-necked aneurysms is achieved in 80–90% of the cases with a complication rate up to 9% including perforation and cerebral ischaemia (75). For a short-term period endovascular coiling seems to be safer than clipping as demonstrated by the International Subarachnoid Hemorrhage Aneurysm Trial (ISAT). The ISAT study enrolled 2134 good-grade patients with mostly small aneurysms smaller than 10 mm in the anterior circulation in a randomized fashion to undergo aneurysm clipping or coiling. At 1 year, death and dependency was 23.5% after coiling and 30.9% after clipping (absolute risk reduction of death and dependence at 1 year 7.4% with coiling) which may be attributed to decreased brain retraction injury or intraprocedural rebleeding with coiling compared to clipping. This finding is further substantiated by previous and follow-up studies. There is a decreased risk of epilepsy with coiling after 1 year (14% vs 24%) as well. The main concern about endovascular therapy is an increased rate of rebleeding after several years due to coil compaction and aneurysm re-growth at the residual neck (recurrent haemorrhage 7% after coiling versus 2% with clipping after 1 year) (58, 76).

The decision between surgical clipping and endovascular coiling should be made by a team of neurological, surgical, and interventional cerebrovascular experts and based on clinical and radiological characteristics such as:

- Clinical status of the patient
- Anticipated surgical difficulty based on anatomical location
- Anatomy of the access vessels (tortuosity, extent of arteriosclerotic change)
- Width of aneurysm neck in comparison to the dome and the parent artery (wide neck aneurysms are difficult to completely obliterate with coils, coils may migrate and be a source for emboli)
- Presence of an intracerebral haematoma with mass effect (24, 69).

Recent advances in technique including the balloon remodelling technique that holds the coils in the aneurysm cavity, liquid polymer coils and embolic agents, and endovascular stents through which coils can be employed into the aneurysm make treatment of broad neck aneurysm feasible. The skills of the treating interventionalist or neurosurgeon as well as the institution may have a great impact on outcome (24).

Delayed cerebral ischaemia

Delayed cerebral ischaemia (DCI) is defined as development of new focal neurological signs, deterioration in level of consciousness, lasting for more than 1 hour, or the appearance of new infarction on CT or magnetic resonance imaging (MRI) when the underlying pathophysiology is thought to be vasospasm and other causes are excluded (77, 78). This definition has been found to be more meaningful than symptomatic vasospasm (new focal deficit and/or decrease in level of consciousness due to vasospasm), especially in poor-grade patients whose neurological deterioration may happen unrecognized. Arterial narrowing can be demonstrated angiographically in 50–70% and leads to delayed ischaemia in 19–46% after SAH (angiographic vasospasm, see Figure 13.5). Development of vasospasm begins on day 3 after SAH, is maximal at 5–14 days, and resolves by day 21. Presence of thick subarachnoid blood seen on admission CT and severe intraventricular haemorrhage are strongly associated with higher risk for vasospasm (Figures 13.1 and 13.2) (25–27, 79, 80). Prevention and management of DCI are listed in Table 13.4.

Monitoring for delayed cerebral ischaemia

Observation in a neurointensive care unit with expertise (GCS exam hourly, National Institute of Health Stroke Scale (NIHSS) (81) 6-hourly), and daily transcranial Doppler ultrasonography (TCD) are simple and helpful monitoring tools (35). Decreased level of consciousness and focal signs such as aphasia or hemiparesis in a good grade SAH patient should prompt the clinician to take immediate action such as a confirmatory test (35).

TCD is a non-invasive method used to diagnose vasospasm in the larger cerebral arteries with high specificity and variable sensitivity, dependent on the operator and other systemic conditions (82, 83). A mean flow velocity (Vm) of greater than 120 cm/second in the middle cerebral artery (MCA) is concerning for vasospasm, Vm above 200 cm/second is considered to be predictive, but dynamic changes of the mean flow velocities such as a twofold increase might be more sensitive for the diagnosis of vasospasm (82, 84). The Lindegaard index (Vm of the middle cerebral artery in relation to Vm in the extracranial internal carotid artery) above 6 also indicates the presence of arterial vasospasm (84–86). A high suspicion for DCI

Table 13.4 Acute management and resuscitation goals of subarachnoid haemorrhage

Blood pressure	Invasive monitoring
	Goal: systolic <160 mmHg, diastolic <110 mmHg, mean blood pressure <110 mmHg, CPP >60 mmHg until aneurysm repair
	Drugs: IV urapidil 5–40 mg/h, IV labetalol 5-150 mg/h, IV nicardipine 5–15 mg/h, IV clevidipine 1-32 mg/h, IV esmolol 50–100 mcg/kg/min, IV metoprolol 1–5 mg/h, IV hydralazine 1.5–7.5 mg/h, IV clonidine 0.03—0.12 mg/h
Prevention of rebleeding	Aneurysm repair through coiling or clipping
	Option: epsilon aminocaproic acid 4 g IV, followed by 1 g/h for a maximum of 72 hours, up to 4 hours prior to angiogram
Fluid balance	Monitoring through internal jugular or subclavian central line (CVP), urine output, stroke volume variation, and clinically
	Isotonic fluids only: 0.9% NaCl at 1.0–1.5 mL/kg/h
Oxygenation	Goal: oxygen saturation >93%
	Intubation and mechanical ventilation if Glasgow coma scale <8
Fever control	Goal: temperature ≤37°C
	Methods: IV or PO acetaminophen or metamizol 500–1000 mg, if not successful ice packs, cold wraps, surface or endovascular temperature control systems with management of shivering
Glucose control	Goal: 4.5–7.0 mmol/L
	Methods: continuous insulin infusion
	Adjust to cerebral glucose level if microdialysis is used
Nutrition	Enteral nutrition should be started and be at goal (25-30 kcal/kg/day) within 48 hours of admission
DVT prophylaxis	Sequential compression devices
	Heparin 5000 U SC every 8 hours or enoxaparin 30–40 mg SC daily within 24 hours after aneurysm repair, withhold 24 hours before and after intracranial procedures
Aspiration prophylaxis	Head-of-bed elevation 30°C
Gastric protection	Pantoprazole 20–40 mg IV or PO daily
Laboratory	Admission: electrolytes, CBC, coagulation, D-dimer, troponin I, creatine kinase, type and crossmatch blood, urine analysis, toxicology screening
	Daily: CBC, electrolytes, creatinine, blood gas
Other tests	Electrocardiogram
	Chest radiograph
	Option: transthoracic echocardiography
Hyponatraemia	Isotonic fluids: 0.9% NaCl at 1.0–1.5 mL/kg/h
	Limit free water intake
	Options: 2–20% hypertonic saline solutions, NaCl tablets, fludrocortisone or hydrocortisone for negative fluid balance
Seizure prophylaxis	Prophylaxis for patients with initial seizure, focal intracerebral clot or focal cerebral oedema prior to aneurysm clipping with levetiracetam 500–2000 mg IV daily
	Maximum 3–7 days without evidence of seizures
	EEG monitoring of patients with Hunt and Hess grade 4 and 5
Extraventricular drainage	Emergent EVD placement for all patients with Hunt and Hess grade IV and V and patients with decreased mental status and hydrocephalus
	Raising the EVD level or clamping dependent on EVD output as soon as possible
	No antibiotic prophylaxis
	CSF for cell count and differential, glucose, lactate, protein every other day; culture if cell count increases
Neurogenic stunned myocardium with pulmonary oedema	Haemodynamic monitoring (PICCO, Flowtrac, pulmonary artery catheter)
	Goal MAP: 70–90 mmHg
	Inotropic support: milrinone 0.25–0.75 mcg/kg/min or dobutamine 3–15 mcg/kg/min
	Vasopressors: noradrenaline 0.03–0.6 mcg/kg/min (first choice), phenylephrine 2–10 mcg/kg/min, dopamine 5–30 mcg/kg/min
	Diuresis
	Increase FiO_2 and PEEP
	Transthoracic echocardiography

Table 13.4 continued

Vasospasm prophylaxis and diagnosis	Nimodipine 60 mg PO every 4 hours until SAH day 21
	Option: simvastatin 40–80 mg PO or pravastatin 40 mg PO daily until SAH day 14
	Avoid hypomagnesaemia
	Daily transcranial Doppler sonography including Lindegaard index
	CT angiography, CT perfusion, or MR perfusion imaging on SAH day 4-12 (mean 9) in high risk patients (Hunt and Hess grade 4, 5; modified Fisher grade 3, 4)
Vasospasm therapy	Trendelenburg position (head down)
	Infusion of 500–1000 mL 0.9% saline or 5% albumin over 15 min
	Start vasopressors (noradrenaline, phenylephrine, dopamine) to raise systolic blood pressure to 160–220 mmHg (20 mmHg above current) until deficits resolve
	Consider milrinone or dobutamine in patients with congestive heart failure or myocardial ischaemia
	Refractory vasospasm:
	Angiographic angioplasty and/or intra-arterial papaverine, verapamil, or nicardipine
	Haemodynamic monitoring with PICCO or Flowtrac, augmentation for goal cardiac index ≥4.0 L/min/m² end diastolic pulmonary artery pressure >14 mmHg with dobutamine or milrinone

CBC: complete blood count; CPP: cerebral perfusion pressure; CSF: cerebrospinal fluid; CT: computed tomography; CVP: central venous pressure; DVT: deep vein thrombosis; EEG: electroencephalography; EVD: extraventricular drainage; FiO_2: inspired fraction of oxygen; MAP: mean arterial pressure; MR: magnetic resonance tomography; PEEP: positive end-expiratory pressure; NaCl: sodium chloride; SAH: subarachnoid haemorrhage.
Modified after (165).

due to vasospasm should trigger an imaging study, such as CT with CT angiography (CTA) and/or CT perfusion (CTP), MRI with MR angiography (MRA), or the gold standard, a cerebral angiogram (35). CTA was found to have a high negative predictive value of 95–100%, a good correlation with cerebral angiography, and a tendency to overestimate the degree of arterial narrowing (87, 88). CTP may add information about brain tissue perfusion status with mean transit time (MTT) and CBF. Both correlate well with cerebral angiography, MTT greater than 6.4 seconds is more sensitive, and CBF more specific for vasospasm (89, 90). These imaging tests should be repeated if the clinician is uncertain about the change in clinical status being caused by DCI, if an endovascular intervention is considered, and if the risks of the planned therapy may outweigh the benefits (35).

Poor-grade patients in stupor or coma require different monitoring techniques to identify DCI. Multimodal monitoring may be helpful in these patients by providing direct and real-time information about $PbtO_2$ (by polarographic technique through Clark electrode) and metabolism (cerebral lactate, pyruvate, glucose, glycerol, and glutamate by microdialysis), cerebral perfusion (MAP – ICP=CPP, cerebral blood flow by thermal diffusion microprobe), and depression of brain activity (alpha variability or alpha/delta ratio) by cEEG or intracortical electrodes. Quantitative cEEG analysis demonstrated sensitive and specific detection of DCI by reductions in alpha variability or alpha/delta ratio (91, 92). $PbtO_2$ monitoring allows for early detection of DCI showing a decrease in cerebral oxygenation

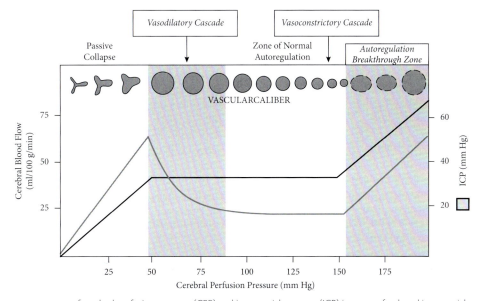

Fig. 13.4 Relationship between extremes of cerebral perfusion pressure (CPP) and intracranial pressure (ICP) in states of reduced intracranial compliance. In the vasodilatory cascade zone, CPP insufficiency and intact pressure autoregulation leads to reflex cerebral vasodilation and increased ICP: the treatment is to raise CPP. In the autoregulation breakthrough zone, pressure and volume overload which overwhelms the brain's capacity to autoregulate leads to increased cerebral blood volume and ICP: the treatment is to lower CPP. Reproduced from (151).

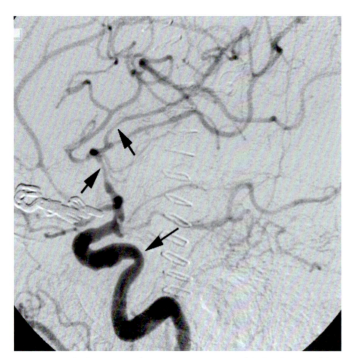

Fig. 13.5 Cerebral angiogram demonstrates vasospasm of the basilar artery (black arrow), the right vertebral artery (arrowhead), and branches of the left posterior cerebral artery (arrowhead). Reproduced from *The Stroke Book*, Cambridge University Press, first edition, 2007.

(93). Elevations of glycerol, glutamate, and lactate/pyruvate ratios as markers of ischaemia were correlated with reductions of CBF on positron emission tomography and DCI (94–96). When used, these parameters should be interpreted taking into account their limited region of capture and their location in relation to blood and other pathology. Moreover, screening for perfusion deficits and arterial narrowing with CTA and CTP may be reasonable in poor-grade patients (35).

Prevention of delayed cerebral ischaemia

Aside from high vigilance for symptoms of DCI, several pharmacological interventions have been investigated for their effect on the incidence of DCI.

Nimodipine, a calcium channel blocker was found to improve neurological outcome after SAH based on neuroprotection rather than an effect on the vasculature. Oral nimodipine (60 mg every 4 hours) should be administered from day 1 through day 21 (24, 35, 97).

Magnesium blocks voltage-gated calcium channels and reduces release of glutamate and calcium entry into cells. Its vasodilatative effect and safety in SAH was repeatedly confirmed. The IMASH trial enrolled 327 patients to be randomized to receive magnesium or placebo within 48 hours of symptom onset for 10–14 days. A difference in primary outcome, defined as favourable outcome at 6 months according to the extended GOS could not be demonstrated (98). Only one trial with 107 patients showed a reduction of DCI defined as ischaemic infarction by 29% in the magnesium group (64 mmol/day for 14 days) which did not result in better long-term outcome or reduced mortality at 6 months (99). Therefore, administration of additional magnesium is not recommended at this point. However, hypomagnesaemia should be treated (35).

Statins have been evaluated in small randomized controlled trials for safety, their neuroprotective effect, and their potential to diminish the incidence of DCI after SAH. A small effect on mortality could be shown, the remainder of the results were heterogeneous (100). A multicentre trial, STASH, is ongoing. As the use of statins is safe in SAH, patients already on statins prior to SAH should continue their medication and starting statins may be considered in patients presenting with SAH (35).

Clot removal and intrathecal administration of recombinant tissue plasminogen activator (rtPA) or urokinase during craniotomy to promote fibrinolysis as well as head shaking aimed at clot dissolution are still under investigation (101, 102). Endothelin receptor antagonists such as clazosentan did not succeed in reduction of DCI (103).

Management of delayed cerebral ischaemia

The treatment of DCI includes haemodynamic and endovascular management.

Haemodynamic augmentation encompasses aggressive volume expansion with crystalloid or colloid solutions as well as elevation of blood pressure and cardiac output in order to improve CBF through arteries in spasm and without autoregulatory capacity. This management strategy is often referred to as 'triple H therapy': hypervolaemia, hypertension, haemodilution, and is considered the standard therapy of DCI. However, only limited data is available about its effect (104–109). Most of these small studies report safety of hypervolaemia and/or administration of vasopressors such as dopamine or noradrenaline with variable effects on CBF and DCI. Phenylephrine was found to be safe to elevate the MAP by 20–35% in the setting of DCI (110). In presence of cardiac dysfunction, dobutamine or milrinone infusions are alternatives to maintain sufficient cardiac output as measured by cardiac index (109–113). However, dobutamine may lower the MAP and require an increase in vasopressor dosage (35). Haemodilution is not recommended because of a reduction of oxygen delivery to the brain (114). If DCI is suspected, saline bolus administration and a trial of stepwise induced hypertension with a vasopressor or inotropic drug should be undertaken with periodic neurological assessments of the patient to define the MAP target. If nimodipine administration leads to temporary hypotension, the dosing intervals may be changed or the drug discontinued (24, 35).

If DCI is refractory to maximized induced hypertension and hypervolaemia or limited by complications such as congestive heart failure, myocardial ischaemia, or pulmonary oedema, cerebral balloon angioplasty and/or administration of intra-arterial papaverine, nicardipine, or verapamil may lead to reversal of neurological deterioration. Intracranial pressure and arterial blood pressure should be monitored during administration of intra-arterial vasodilators. The timing of endovascular therapy should take into account the level and tolerance of haemodynamic augmentation, prior evidence of vasospasm, and the availability of endovascular procedures (24, 35, 115–117).

Electrolyte disturbances

Hyponatraemia occurs in 20–40% of SAH patients. Hypomagnesaemia (40%), hypokalaemia (25%), and hypernatremia (20%) are also common after SAH (11, 119–121). Hyponatraemia is usually the result of inappropriate secretion of antidiuretic hormone (SIADH) and free-water retention and/or excessive renal sodium excretion due to increased atrial natriuretic factor, so called 'cerebral salt wasting syndrome', or both (11, 122). Intravascular volume depletion and sodium loss may increase the risk of DCI and infarction (48, 50). In 124 WFNS grade IV and V patients, hyponatraemia (serum sodium <135 mmol/L) developed in 63%, caused by cerebral salt wasting syndrome in 55%. Late onset hyponatraemia (between SAH day 4 and 9) correlated with a higher occurrence of cerebral infarction in this patient population. Nevertheless, hyponatraemia did not have an association with poor outcome at 3 months (GOS 1–3) (123).

Fludrocortisone and hydrocortisone were studied for prevention of hyponatraemia in SAH (124–128). If started early, the corticosteroids are effective in prevention of natriuresis and hyponatraemia. However, their use was complicated by hyperglycaemia and hypokalaemia.

Administration of large volume isotonic crystalloids and restriction of free water intake should be applied to counteract potential hypovolaemia and to prevent inappropriate water retention. Hypertonic saline (3%) may be used to correct hyponatraemia (35, 129).

Conivaptan is an arginine vasopressin receptor antagonist (V_{1A}/V_2) approved for the treatment of euvolaemic and hypervolaemic hyponatraemia (130). Initial reports of its use in neurocritical care patients with hyponatraemia have yielded promising results (131). Caution should be taken to avoid hypovolaemia with the use of conivaptan (35).

Treatment of medical complications

In addition to the direct effects of the initial haemorrhage and secondary neurological complications, SAH also predisposes to medical complications that may have an impact on outcome (11) and increase the length of stay in the neurocritical care unit (NICU) and in the hospital (132).

Fever

Fever (≥38.3°C) is a frequent event in patients with SAH (41–72%) (11, 133–138) and associated with an increased risk of symptomatic vasospasm (137), an increased length of NICU and hospital stay (132), with poor outcome (modified Rankin Scale (mRS) score 4–6), dependence in activities of daily living, and cognitive impairment at 3 months (11, 137, 138). Normothermia should be the target in every SAH patient (see Table 13.4). In a case–control study of advanced fever control with surface or endovascular cooling devices for 40 SAH patients, advanced fever control resulted in a lower daily fever burden and in better outcomes at 12 months (mRS score 4–6 in 21%) compared to conventional fever management of 80 SAH patients (mRS score 4–6 in 46%, P=0.03) (133). In SAH patients, the temperature should be monitored frequently. With a new occurrence of fever, infections need to be sought for and treated. Fever control should be attempted with antipyretics as first-line therapy, followed by surface cooling or intravascular devices along with treatment for shivering (35).

Hyperglycaemia

Admission or persistent hyperglycaemia was associated with DCI as well as poor short and long-term outcome (GOS 1–3, mRS score 4–6) after SAH in several investigations (11, 95, 139–143).

Depending on the definition, hyperglycaemia can be found in 30–100% of SAH patients (11, 139, 142, 144).

A small trial of 55 patients with SAH demonstrated feasibility and safety of continuous insulin infusion for glucose values exceeding 7 mmol/L (126 mg/dL) with glucose assessments performed every 2 hours (145). The first randomized trial of intensive glucose control (target glucose 80–120 mg/dL= 4.4–6.7 mmol/L) versus standard insulin therapy (target glucose 80–220 mg/dL = 4.4–12.2 mmol/L) in 78 SAH patients showed a reduced rate of infection from 42% to 27% in the intensive group. Mortality at 6 months and the frequency of vasospasm were comparable in the two groups (146). Retrospective studies reflecting changes of clinical practice (introduction of insulin protocols) demonstrated that good glycaemic control (mean glucose burden above 7.8 mmol/L (140 mg/dL) <1.1 mmol/L (20 mg/dL)) significantly reduced the likelihood of poor outcome at 3–6 months (147) and identified hypoglycaemia (<60 mg/dL=3.3 mmol/L) as powerful independent predictor of mortality at discharge (148). Hypoglycaemia resulting from tight glucose control was linked to an increased risk of DCI and infarction (149). This may be seen as a decrease of cerebral glucose as well as an increase in lactate/pyruvate ratio and glycerol as a markers for cell stress when utilizing microdialysis (143, 150–152). Clinical signs of systemic and cerebral hypoglycaemia may not be obvious in poor-grade SAH patients. Therefore, hypoglycaemia should be avoided while applying tight glucose control. If microdialysis is used, the serum glucose level can be titrated according to the cerebral glucose measurements (35).

Anaemia

Anaemia treated with blood transfusions is linked to an increased risk of delayed infarction, mortality, and poor functional outcome at 3 months after SAH (11, 153) as well as brain tissue hypoxia ($PbtO_2$ ≤15 mmHg) and metabolic distress (lactate/pyruvate ratio ≥40) (154). In a safety study, 44 SAH patients were randomized to haemoglobin targets of 10 g/dL (6.2 mmol/L) or 11.5 g/dL (7.1 mmol/L). Achieving the higher haemoglobin target by transfusion of packed red blood cells was found to be safe and feasible (155). It remains uncertain whether anaemia after SAH reflects general illness severity, impacts outcome directly, or whether the treatment for anaemia—blood transfusions—contribute to poor outcome (153, 156, 157). To minimize the frequency of anaemia, the number of blood drawings should be reduced. Maintenance of haemoglobin levels between 8 and 10 g/dL (5.0–6.2 mmol/L) is recommended (35).

Neurogenic stunned myocardium and pulmonary oedema

Subarachnoid haemorrhage may be further complicated by cardiac dysfunction and pulmonary oedema due to a catecholamine surge, resulting in neurogenic 'stunned myocardium' or 'neurogenic stress cardiomyopathy' and neurogenic pulmonary oedema. Cardiac dysfunction is accompanied by transient electrocardiographic abnormalities, troponin leaks, reversible wall motion abnormalities on echocardiogram, hypotension, and reduction of cardiac output. Neurogenic pulmonary oedema is caused by increased permeability of the pulmonary vasculature and may occur isolated or in conjunction with neurogenic cardiac injury. Hypotension, reduced cardiac output, and impaired oxygenation may impair cerebral perfusion in the setting of increased ICP or DCI (158–160). Troponin

I elevations are found in about 35% of SAH patients (161, 162), cardiac arrhythmias in 35% (11). A recent meta-analysis showed that cardiac abnormalities on electrocardiogram, echocardiography, and troponin measurements are linked to DCI, poor outcome, and death after SAH (discharge—6-month follow-up period) (163). Thus, baseline evaluation with serial cardiac enzymes and electrocardiogram is recommended. Patients with evidence of depressed myocardial function and pulmonary oedema should receive echocardiography and monitoring of cardiac output. Standard management for heart failure is applied with meticulous attention to cerebral perfusion status. In pulmonary oedema, lung protective ventilation and euvolaemia are the targets of therapy (35).

Outlook

The majority of the recommendations for management of patients with SAH are based on consensus opinions of experts in the field (35). There are many open-ended questions such as the efficacy of antifibrinolytic therapy, the optimal blood pressure goal prior to aneurysm repair, the efficacy of intensive glucose control and its target range, the impact of maintained normothermia on outcome, the target range for haemoglobin after SAH and during DCI, and the optimal therapy regimen for neurogenic stunned myocardium. New endovascular techniques such as intra-aortic balloon pumps and counterpulsation entered the field of DCI management. Current prevention of DCI and neuroprotection trials include intracisternal application of thrombolytic therapy to decrease the clot burden, early placement of lumbar drainage, randomized, controlled outcome studies of statins, magnesium, and human albumin. The best monitoring technique and triggers for neuroimaging and intervention for DCI in poor-grade SAH patients need to be defined.

References

1. Feigin VL, Lawes CM, Bennett DA, Barker-Collo SL, Parag V. Worldwide stroke incidence and early case fatality reported in 56 population-based studies: a systematic review. *Lancet Neurol.* 2009;8:355–369.
2. Lichtman JH, Jones SB, Leifheit-Limson EC, Wang Y, Goldstein LB. 30-day mortality and readmission after hemorrhagic stroke among medicare beneficiaries in joint commission primary stroke center-certified and noncertified hospitals. *Stroke.* 2011;42(12):3387–3391.
3. Taylor CJ, Robertson F, Brealey D, O'Shea F, Stephen T, Brew S, *et al.* Outcome in poor grade subarachnoid hemorrhage patients treated with acute endovascular coiling of aneurysms and aggressive intensive care. *Neurocrit Care.* 2011;14(3):341–347.
4. Ingall T, Asplund K, Mahonen M, Bonita R. A multinational comparison of subarachnoid hemorrhage epidemiology in the WHO MONICA stroke study. *Stroke.* 2000;31:1054–1061.
5. Schievink WI. Intracranial aneurysms. *N Engl J Med.* 1997;336:28–40.
6. Mayer SA, Kreiter KT, Copeland D, Bernardini GL, Bates JE, Peery S, *et al.* Global and domain-specific cognitive impairment and outcome after subarachnoid hemorrhage. *Neurology.* 2002;59:1750–1758.
7. Springer MV, Schmidt JM, Wartenberg KE, Frontera JA, Badjatia N, Mayer SA. Predictors of global cognitive impairment 1 year after subarachnoid hemorrhage. *Neurosurgery.* 2009;65:1043–1050.
8. Claassen J, Carhuapoma JR, Kreiter KT, Du EY, Connolly ES, Mayer SA. Global cerebral edema after subarachnoid hemorrhage: frequency, predictors, and impact on outcome. *Stroke.* 2002;33:1225–1232.
9. Claassen J, Vu A, Kreiter KT, Kowalski RG, Du EY, Ostapkovich N, *et al.* Effect of acute physiologic derangements on outcome after subarachnoid hemorrhage. *Crit Care Med.* 2004;32:832–838.
10. Frontera JA, Fernandez A, Schmidt JM, Claassen J, Wartenberg KE, Badjatia N, *et al.* Impact of nosocomial infectious complications after subarachnoid hemorrhage. *Neurosurgery.* 2008;62:80–87.
11. Wartenberg KE, Schmidt JM, Claassen J, Temes RE, Frontera JA, Ostapkovich N, *et al.* Impact of medical complications on outcome after subarachnoid hemorrhage. *Crit Care Med.* 2006;34:617–623;quiz 624.
12. Haug T, Sorteberg A, Finset A, Lindegaard KF, Lundar T, Sorteberg W. Cognitive functioning and health-related quality of life 1 year after aneurysmal subarachnoid hemorrhage in preoperative comatose patients (Hunt and Hess Grade V patients). *Neurosurgery.* 2010;66:475–484.
13. Huang AP, Arora S, Wintermark M, Ko N, Tu YK, Lawton MT. Perfusion computed tomographic imaging and surgical selection with patients after poor-grade aneurysmal subarachnoid hemorrhage. *Neurosurgery.* 2010;67:964–974.
14. Bailes JE, Spetzler RF, Hadley MN, Baldwin HZ. Management morbidity and mortality of poor-grade aneurysm patients. *J Neurosurg.* 1990;72:559–566.
15. Laidlaw JD, Siu KH. Ultra-early surgery for aneurysmal subarachnoid hemorrhage: outcomes for a consecutive series of 391 patients not selected by grade or age. *J Neurosurg.* 2002;97:250–258.
16. Le Roux PD, Elliott JP, Newell DW, Grady MS, Winn HR. Predicting outcome in poor-grade patients with subarachnoid hemorrhage: a retrospective review of 159 aggressively managed cases. *J Neurosurg.* 1996;85:39–49.
17. Shirao S, Yoneda H, Kunitsugu I, Ishihara H, Koizumi H, Suehiro E, *et al.* Preoperative prediction of outcome in 283 poor-grade patients with subarachnoid hemorrhage: a project of the Chugoku-Shikoku Division of the Japan Neurosurgical Society. *Cerebrovasc Dis.* 2010;30:105–113.
18. Berman MF, Solomon RA, Mayer SA, Johnston SC, Yung PP. Impact of hospital-related factors on outcome after treatment of cerebral aneurysms. *Stroke.* 2003;34:2200–2207.
19. Cowan JA Jr, Dimick JB, Wainess RM, Upchurch GR Jr, Thompson BG. Outcomes after cerebral aneurysm clip occlusion in the United States: the need for evidence-based hospital referral. *J Neurosurg.* 2003;99:947–952.
20. Cross DT 3rd, Tirschwell DL, Clark MA, Tuden D, Derdeyn CP, Moran CJ, *et al.* Mortality rates after subarachnoid hemorrhage: variations according to hospital case volume in 18 states. *J Neurosurg.* 2003;99:810–817.
21. Teasdale G, Jennett B. Assessment of coma and impaired consciousness. A practical scale. *Lancet.* 1974;2:81–84.
22. Hunt WE, Hess RM. Surgical risk as related to time of intervention in the repair of intracranial aneurysms. *J Neurosurg.* 1968;28:14–20.
23. Report of World Federation of Neurological Surgeons Committee on a Universal Subarachnoid Hemorrhage Grading Scale. *J Neurosurg.* 1988;68:985–986.
24. Bederson JB, Connolly ES Jr, Batjer HH, Dacey RG, Dion JE, Diringer MN, *et al.* Guidelines for the management of aneurysmal subarachnoid hemorrhage: a statement for healthcare professionals from a special writing group of the Stroke Council, American Heart Association. *Stroke.* 2009;40:994–1025.
25. Fisher CM, Kistler JP, Davis JM. Relation of cerebral vasospasm to subarachnoid hemorrhage visualized by computerized tomographic scanning. *Neurosurgery.* 1980;6:1–9.
26. Claassen J, Bernardini GL, Kreiter K, Bates J, Du YE, Copeland D, *et al.* Effect of cisternal and ventricular blood on risk of delayed cerebral ischemia after subarachnoid hemorrhage: the Fisher scale revisited. *Stroke.* 2001;32:2012–2020.
27. Frontera JA, Claassen J, Schmidt JM, Wartenberg KE, Temes R, Connolly ES Jr, *et al.* Prediction of symptomatic vasospasm after subarachnoid hemorrhage: the modified fisher scale. *Neurosurgery.* 2006;59:21–27.
28. Nornes H. The role of intracranial pressure in the arrest of hemorrhage in patients with ruptured intracranial aneurysm. *J Neurosurg.* 1973;39:226–234.
29. Hadeishi H, Suzuki A, Yasui N, Hatazawa J, Shimosegawa E. Diffusion-weighted magnetic resonance imaging in patients with subarachnoid hemorrhage. *Neurosurgery.* 2002;50:741–747.
30. Sato K, Shimizu H, Fujimura M, Inoue T, Matsumoto Y, Tominaga T. Acute-stage diffusion-weighted magnetic resonance imaging for predicting outcome of poor-grade aneurysmal subarachnoid hemorrhage. *J Cereb Blood Flow Metab.* 2010;30:1110–1120.
31. Wartenberg KE, Sheth SJ, Michael Schmidt J, Frontera JA, Rincon F, Ostapkovich N, *et al.* Acute ischemic injury on diffusion-weighted

magnetic resonance imaging after poor grade subarachnoid hemorrhage. *Neurocrit Care.* 2011;14:407–415.

32. Fujii Y, Takeuchi S, Sasaki O, Minakawa T, Koike T, Tanaka R. Ultra-early rebleeding in spontaneous subarachnoid hemorrhage. *J Neurosurg.* 1996;84:35–42.

33. Hillman J, Fridriksson S, Nilsson O, Yu Z, Saveland H, Jakobsson KE. Immediate administration of tranexamic acid and reduced incidence of early rebleeding after aneurysmal subarachnoid hemorrhage: a prospective randomized study. *J Neurosurg.* 2002;97:771–778.

34. Starke RM, Connolly ES Jr. Rebleeding after aneurysmal subarachnoid hemorrhage. *Neurocrit Care.* 2011;5:241–246.

35. Diringer MN, Bleck TP, Claude Hemphill J 3rd, Menon D, Shutter L, Vespa P, et al. Critical care management of patients following aneurysmal subarachnoid hemorrhage: recommendations from the Neurocritical Care Society's Multidisciplinary Consensus Conference. *Neurocrit Care.* 2011;15:211–240.

36. Mehta V, Holness RO, Connolly K, Walling S, Hall R. Acute hydrocephalus following aneurysmal subarachnoid hemorrhage. *Can J Neurol Sci.* 1996;23:40–45.

37. Sheehan JP, Polin RS, Sheehan JM, Baskaya MK, Kassell NF. Factors associated with hydrocephalus after aneurysmal subarachnoid hemorrhage. *Neurosurgery.* 1999;45:1120–1127.

38. Suarez-Rivera O. Acute hydrocephalus after subarachnoid hemorrhage. *Surg Neurol.* 1998;49:563–565.

39. Hasan D, Vermeulen M, Wijdicks EF, Hijdra A, van Gijn J. Management problems in acute hydrocephalus after subarachnoid hemorrhage. *Stroke.* 1989;20:747–753.

40. Hasan D, Lindsay KW, Vermeulen M. Treatment of acute hydrocephalus after subarachnoid hemorrhage with serial lumbar puncture. *Stroke.* 1991;22:190–194.

41. Murad A, Ghostine S, Colohan AR. Role of controlled lumbar CSF drainage for ICP control in aneurysmal SAH. *Acta Neurochir Suppl.* 2011;110:183–187.

42. Gruber A, Reinprecht A, Bavinzski G, Czech T, Richling B. Chronic shunt-dependent hydrocephalus after early surgical and early endovascular treatment of ruptured intracranial aneurysms. *Neurosurgery.* 1999;44:503–509.

43. Guresir E, Schuss P, Vatter H, Raabe A, Seifert V, Beck J. Decompressive craniectomy in subarachnoid hemorrhage. *Neurosurg Focus.* 2009;26:E4.

44. Al-Rawi PG, Zygun D, Tseng MY, Hutchinson PJ, Matta BF, Kirkpatrick PJ. Cerebral blood flow augmentation in patients with severe subarachnoid haemorrhage. *Acta Neurochir Suppl.* 2005;95:123–127.

45. Tseng MY, Al-Rawi PG, Pickard JD, Rasulo FA, Kirkpatrick PJ. Effect of hypertonic saline on cerebral blood flow in poor-grade patients with subarachnoid hemorrhage. *Stroke.* 2003;34:1389–1396.

46. Bijlenga P, Czosnyka M, Budohoski KP, Soehle M, Pickard JD, Kirkpatrick PJ, et al. "Optimal cerebral perfusion pressure" in poor grade patients after subarachnoid hemorrhage. *Neurocrit Care.* 2010;13:17–23.

47. Hasan D, Vermeulen M, Wijdicks EF, Hijdra A, van Gijn J. Effect of fluid intake and antihypertensive treatment on cerebral ischemia after subarachnoid hemorrhage. *Stroke.* 1989;20:1511–1515.

48. Hasan D, Wijdicks EF, Vermeulen M. Hyponatremia is associated with cerebral ischemia in patients with aneurysmal subarachnoid hemorrhage. *Ann Neurol.* 1990;27:106–108.

49. Solomon RA, Post KD, McMurtry JG 3rd. Depression of circulating blood volume in patients after subarachnoid hemorrhage: implications for the management of symptomatic vasospasm. *Neurosurgery.* 1984;15:354–361.

50. Wijdicks EF, Vermeulen M, Hijdra A, van Gijn J. Hyponatremia and cerebral infarction in patients with ruptured intracranial aneurysms: is fluid restriction harmful? *Ann Neurol.* 1985;17:137–140.

51. Moretti R, Pizzi B. Inferior vena cava distensibility as a predictor of fluid responsiveness in patients with subarachnoid hemorrhage. *Neurocrit Care.* 2010;13:3–9.

52. Mutoh T, Ishikawa T, Nishino K, Yasui N. Evaluation of the FloTrac uncalibrated continuous cardiac output system for perioperative hemodynamic monitoring after subarachnoid hemorrhage. *J Neurosurg Anesthesiol.* 2009;21:218–225.

53. Egge A, Waterloo K, Sjoholm H, Solberg T, Ingebrigtsen T, Romner B. Prophylactic hyperdynamic postoperative fluid therapy after aneurysmal subarachnoid hemorrhage: a clinical, prospective, randomized, controlled study. *Neurosurgery.* 2001;49:593–605.

54. Lennihan L, Mayer SA, Fink ME, Beckford A, Paik MC, Zhang H, et al. Effect of hypervolemic therapy on cerebral blood flow after subarachnoid hemorrhage: a randomized controlled trial. *Stroke.* 2000;31:383–391.

55. Muench E, Horn P, Bauhuf C, Roth H, Philipps M, Hermann P, et al. Effects of hypervolemia and hypertension on regional cerebral blood flow, intracranial pressure, and brain tissue oxygenation after subarachnoid hemorrhage. *Crit Care Med.* 2007;35:1844–1851;quiz 1852.

56. Mutoh T, Ishikawa T, Suzuki A, Yasui N. Continuous cardiac output and near-infrared spectroscopy monitoring to assist in management of symptomatic cerebral vasospasm after subarachnoid hemorrhage. *Neurocrit Care.* 2010;13:331–338.

57. Claassen J, Peery S, Kreiter KT, Hirsch LJ, Du EY, Connolly ES, et al. Predictors and clinical impact of epilepsy after subarachnoid hemorrhage. *Neurology.* 2003;60:208–214.

58. Molyneux AJ, Kerr RS, Yu LM, Clarke M, Sneade M, Yarnold JA, et al. International subarachnoid aneurysm trial (ISAT) of neurosurgical clipping versus endovascular coiling in 2143 patients with ruptured intracranial aneurysms: a randomised comparison of effects on survival, dependency, seizures, rebleeding, subgroups, and aneurysm occlusion. *Lancet.* 2005;366:809–817.

59. Naidech AM, Kreiter KT, Janjua N, Ostapkovich N, Parra A, Commichau C, et al. Phenytoin exposure is associated with functional and cognitive disability after subarachnoid hemorrhage. *Stroke.* 2005;36:583–587.

60. Rosengart AJ, Huo JD, Tolentino J, Novakovic RL, Frank JI, Goldenberg FD, et al. Outcome in patients with subarachnoid hemorrhage treated with antiepileptic drugs. *J Neurosurg.* 2007;107:253–260.

61. Claassen J, Mayer SA, Hirsch LJ. Continuous EEG monitoring in patients with subarachnoid hemorrhage. *J Clin Neurophysiol.* 2005;22:92–98.

62. Dennis LJ, Claassen J, Hirsch LJ, Emerson RG, Connolly ES, Mayer SA. Nonconvulsive status epilepticus after subarachnoid hemorrhage. *Neurosurgery.* 2002;51:1136–1143.

63. Little AS, Kerrigan JF, McDougall CG, Zabramski JM, Albuquerque FC, Nakaji P, et al. Nonconvulsive status epilepticus in patients suffering spontaneous subarachnoid hemorrhage. *J Neurosurg.* 2007;106:805–811.

64. David CA, Vishteh AG, Spetzler RF, Lemole M, Lawton MT, Partovi S. Late angiographic follow-up review of surgically treated aneurysms. *J Neurosurg.* 1999;91:396–401.

65. Kassell NF, Torner JC. Aneurysmal rebleeding: a preliminary report from the Cooperative Aneurysm Study. *Neurosurgery.* 1983;13:479–481.

66. Kassell NF, Torner JC, Haley EC Jr, Jane JA, Adams HP, Kongable GL. The International Cooperative Study on the Timing of Aneurysm Surgery. Part 1: Overall management results. *J Neurosurg.* 1990;73:18–36.

67. Raaymakers TW, Rinkel GJ, Ramos LM. Initial and follow-up screening for aneurysms in families with familial subarachnoid hemorrhage. *Neurology.* 1998;51:1125–1130.

68. Gruber DP, Zimmerman GA, Tomsick TA, van Loveren HR, Link MJ, Tew JM Jr. A comparison between endovascular and surgical management of basilar artery apex aneurysms. *J Neurosurg.* 1999;90:868–874.

69. Johnston SC, Higashida RT, Barrow DL, Caplan LR, Dion JE, Hademenos G. Recommendations for the endovascular treatment of intracranial aneurysms: a statement for healthcare professionals from the Committee on Cerebrovascular Imaging of the American Heart Association Council on Cardiovascular Radiology. *Stroke.* 2002;33:2536–2544.

70. Johnston SC, Wilson CB, Halbach VV, Higashida RT, Dowd CF, McDermott MW, et al. Endovascular and surgical treatment of unruptured cerebral aneurysms: comparison of risks. *Ann Neurol.* 2000;48:11–19.

71. Regli L, Dehdashti AR, Uske A, de Tribolet N. Endovascular coiling compared with surgical clipping for the treatment of unruptured

middle cerebral artery aneurysms: an update. *Acta Neurochir Suppl.* 2002;82:41–46.

72. Regli L, Uske A, de Tribolet N. Endovascular coil placement compared with surgical clipping for the treatment of unruptured middle cerebral artery aneurysms: a consecutive series. *J Neurosurg.* 1999;90:1025–1030.

73. Guglielmi G, Vinuela F, Dion J, Duckwiler G. Electrothrombosis of saccular aneurysms via endovascular approach. Part 2: Preliminary clinical experience. *J Neurosurg.* 1991;75:8–14.

74. Guglielmi G, Vinuela F, Sepetka I, Macellari V. Electrothrombosis of saccular aneurysms via endovascular approach. Part 1: Electrochemical basis, technique, and experimental results. *J Neurosurg.* 1991;75:1–7.

75. Brilstra EH, Rinkel GJ. Treatment of ruptured intracranial aneurysms by embolization with controlled detachable coils. *Neurologist.* 2002;8:35–40.

76. Molyneux A, Kerr R, Stratton I, Sandercock P, Clarke M, Shrimpton J, Holman R. International Subarachnoid Aneurysm Trial (ISAT) of neurosurgical clipping versus endovascular coiling in 2143 patients with ruptured intracranial aneurysms: a randomised trial. *Lancet.* 2002;360:1267–1274.

77. Frontera JA, Fernandez A, Schmidt JM, Claassen J, Wartenberg KE, Badjatia N, *et al.* Defining vasospasm after subarachnoid hemorrhage: what is the most clinically relevant definition? *Stroke.* 2009;40:1963–1968.

78. Vergouwen MD, Vermeulen M, van Gijn J, Rinkel GJ, Wijdicks EF, Muizelaar JP, *et al.* Definition of delayed cerebral ischemia after aneurysmal subarachnoid hemorrhage as an outcome event in clinical trials and observational studies: proposal of a multidisciplinary research group. *Stroke.* 2010;41:2391–2395.

79. Fisher CM, Roberson GH, Ojemann RG. Cerebral vasospasm with ruptured saccular aneurysm—the clinical manifestations. *Neurosurgery.* 1977;1:245–248.

80. Heros RC, Zervas NT, Varsos V. Cerebral vasospasm after subarachnoid hemorrhage: an update. *Ann Neurol.* 1983;14:599–608.

81. Brott T, Adams HP Jr, Olinger CP, Marler JR, Barsan WG, Biller J, *et al.* Measurements of acute cerebral infarction: a clinical examination scale. *Stroke.* 1989;20:864–870.

82. Carrera E, Schmidt JM, Oddo M, Fernandez L, Claassen J, Seder D, *et al.* Transcranial Doppler for predicting delayed cerebral ischemia after subarachnoid hemorrhage. *Neurosurgery.* 2009;65:316–323.

83. Lysakowski C, Walder B, Costanza MC, Tramer MR. Transcranial Doppler versus angiography in patients with vasospasm due to a ruptured cerebral aneurysm: a systematic review. *Stroke.* 2001;32:2292–2298.

84. Sloan MA, Alexandrov AV, Tegeler CH, Spencer MP, Caplan LR, Feldmann E, *et al.* Assessment: transcranial Doppler ultrasonography: report of the Therapeutics and Technology Assessment Subcommittee of the American Academy of Neurology. *Neurology.* 2004;62:1468–1481.

85. Lindegaard KF, Bakke SJ, Sorteberg W, Nakstad P, Nornes H. A non-invasive Doppler ultrasound method for the evaluation of patients with subarachnoid hemorrhage. *Acta Radiol Suppl.* 1986;369:96–98.

86. Lindegaard KF, Nornes H, Bakke SJ, Sorteberg W, Nakstad P. Cerebral vasospasm after subarachnoid haemorrhage investigated by means of transcranial Doppler ultrasound. *Acta Neurochir Suppl (Wien).* 1988;42:81–84.

87. Chaudhary SR, Ko N, Dillon WP, Yu MB, Liu S, Criqui GI, *et al.* Prospective evaluation of multidetector-row CT angiography for the diagnosis of vasospasm following subarachnoid hemorrhage: a comparison with digital subtraction angiography. *Cerebrovasc Dis.* 2008;25:144–150.

88. Yoon DY, Choi CS, Kim KH, Cho BM. Multidetector-row CT angiography of cerebral vasospasm after aneurysmal subarachnoid hemorrhage: comparison of volume-rendered images and digital subtraction angiography. *AJNR Am J Neuroradiol.* 2006;27:370–377.

89. Wintermark M, Dillon WP, Smith WS, Lau BC, Chaudhary S, Liu S, *et al.* Visual grading system for vasospasm based on perfusion CT imaging: comparisons with conventional angiography and quantitative perfusion CT. *Cerebrovasc Dis.* 2008;26:163–170.

90. Wintermark M, Ko NU, Smith WS, Liu S, Higashida RT, Dillon WP. Vasospasm after subarachnoid hemorrhage: utility of perfusion CT and CT angiography on diagnosis and management. *AJNR Am J Neuroradiol.* 2006;27:26–34.

91. Claassen J, Hirsch LJ, Kreiter KT, Du EY, Connolly ES, Emerson RG, *et al.* Quantitative continuous EEG for detecting delayed cerebral ischemia in patients with poor-grade subarachnoid hemorrhage. *Clin Neurophysiol.* 2004;115:2699–2710.

92. Vespa PM, Nuwer MR, Juhasz C, Alexander M, Nenov V, Martin N, *et al.* Early detection of vasospasm after acute subarachnoid hemorrhage using continuous EEG ICU monitoring. *Electroencephalogr Clin Neurophysiol.* 1997;103:607–615.

93. Vath A, Kunze E, Roosen K, Meixensberger J. Therapeutic aspects of brain tissue pO2 monitoring after subarachnoid hemorrhage. *Acta Neurochir Suppl.* 2002;81:307–309.

94. Nilsson OG, Saveland H, Boris-Moller F, Brandt L, Wieloch T. Increased levels of glutamate in patients with subarachnoid haemorrhage as measured by intracerebral microdialysis. *Acta Neurochir Suppl.* 1996;67:45–47.

95. Sarrafzadeh A, Haux D, Kuchler I, Lanksch WR, Unterberg AW. Poor-grade aneurysmal subarachnoid hemorrhage: relationship of cerebral metabolism to outcome. *J Neurosurg.* 2004;100:400–406.

96. Saveland H, Nilsson OG, Boris-Moller F, Wieloch T, Brandt L. Intracerebral microdialysis of glutamate and aspartate in two vascular territories after aneurysmal subarachnoid hemorrhage. *Neurosurgery.* 1996;38:12–19.

97. Allen GS, Ahn HS, Preziosi TJ, Battye R, Boone SC, Chou SN, *et al.* Cerebral arterial spasm—a controlled trial of nimodipine in patients with subarachnoid hemorrhage. *N Engl J Med.* 1983;308:619–624.

98. Wong GK, Poon WS, Chan MT, Boet R, Gin T, Ng SC, *et al.* Intravenous magnesium sulphate for aneurysmal subarachnoid hemorrhage (IMASH): a randomized, double-blinded, placebo-controlled, multicenter phase III trial. *Stroke.* 2010;41:921–926.

99. Westermaier T, Stetter C, Vince GH, Pham M, Tejon JP, Eriskat J, *et al.* Prophylactic intravenous magnesium sulfate for treatment of aneurysmal subarachnoid hemorrhage: a randomized, placebo-controlled, clinical study. *Crit Care Med.* 2010;38:1284–1290.

100. Tseng MY. Summary of evidence on immediate statins therapy following aneurysmal subarachnoid hemorrhage. *Neurocrit Care.* 2011;15:298–301.

101. Kawamoto S, Tsutsumi K, Yoshikawa G, Shinozaki MH, Yako K, Nagata K, *et al.* Effectiveness of the head-shaking method combined with cisternal irrigation with urokinase in preventing cerebral vasospasm after subarachnoid hemorrhage. *J Neurosurg.* 2004;100:236–243.

102. Zabramski JM, Spetzler RF, Lee KS, Papadopoulos SM, Bovill E, Zimmerman RS, *et al.* Phase I trial of tissue plasminogen activator for the prevention of vasospasm in patients with aneurysmal subarachnoid hemorrhage. *J Neurosurg.* 1991;75:189–196.

103. Macdonald RL, Higashida RT, Keller E, Mayer SA, Molyneux A, Raabe A, *et al.* Clazosentan, an endothelin receptor antagonist, in patients with aneurysmal subarachnoid haemorrhage undergoing surgical clipping: a randomised, double-blind, placebo-controlled phase 3 trial (CONSCIOUS-2). *Lancet Neurol.* 2011;10:618–625.

104. Brown FD, Hanlon K, Mullan S. Treatment of aneurysmal hemiplegia with dopamine and mannitol. *J Neurosurg.* 1978;49:525–529.

105. Kassell NF, Peerless SJ, Durward QJ, Beck DW, Drake CG, Adams HP. Treatment of ischemic deficits from vasospasm with intravascular volume expansion and induced arterial hypertension. *Neurosurgery.* 1982;11:337–343.

106. Kosnik EJ, Hunt WE. Postoperative hypertension in the management of patients with intracranial arterial aneurysms. *J Neurosurg.* 1976;45:148–154.

107. Mori K, Arai H, Nakajima K, Tajima A, Maeda M. Hemorheological and hemodynamic analysis of hypervolemic hemodilution therapy for cerebral vasospasm after aneurysmal subarachnoid hemorrhage. *Stroke.* 1995;26:1620–1626.

108. Otsubo H, Takemae T, Inoue T, Kobayashi S, Sugita K. Normovolaemic induced hypertension therapy for cerebral vasospasm after subarachnoid haemorrhage. *Acta Neurochir (Wien)*. 1990;103:18–26.

109. Muizelaar JP, Becker DP. Induced hypertension for the treatment of cerebral ischemia after subarachnoid hemorrhage. Direct effect on cerebral blood flow. *Surg Neurol*. 1986;25:317–325.

110. Miller JA, Dacey RG, Jr, Diringer MN. Safety of hypertensive hypervolemic therapy with phenylephrine in the treatment of delayed ischemic deficits after subarachnoid hemorrhage. *Stroke*. 1995;26:2260–2266.

111. Arakawa Y, Kikuta K, Hojo M, Goto Y, Ishii A, Yamagata S. Milrinone for the treatment of cerebral vasospasm after subarachnoid hemorrhage: report of seven cases. *Neurosurgery*. 2001;48:723–728.

112. Fraticelli AT, Cholley BP, Losser MR, Saint Maurice JP, Payen D. Milrinone for the treatment of cerebral vasospasm after aneurysmal subarachnoid hemorrhage. *Stroke*. 2008;39:893–898.

113. Levy ML, Rabb CH, Zelman V, Giannotta SL. Cardiac performance enhancement from dobutamine in patients refractory to hypervolemic therapy for cerebral vasospasm. *J Neurosurg*. 1993;79:494–499.

114. Ekelund A, Reinstrup P, Ryding E, Andersson AM, Molund T, Kristiansson KA, et al. Effects of iso- and hypervolemic hemodilution on regional cerebral blood flow and oxygen delivery for patients with vasospasm after aneurysmal subarachnoid hemorrhage. *Acta Neurochir (Wien)*. 2002;144:703–712.

115. Bejjani GK, Bank WO, Olan WJ, Sekhar LN. The efficacy and safety of angioplasty for cerebral vasospasm after subarachnoid hemorrhage. *Neurosurgery*. 1998;42:979–986.

116. Feng L, Fitzsimmons BF, Young WL, Berman MF, Lin E, Aagaard BD, et al. Intraarterially administered verapamil as adjunct therapy for cerebral vasospasm: safety and 2-year experience. *AJNR Am J Neuroradiol*. 2002;23:1284–1290.

117. Hoh BL, Ogilvy CS. Endovascular treatment of cerebral vasospasm: transluminal balloon angioplasty, intra-arterial papaverine, and intra-arterial nicardipine. *Neurosurg Clin N Am*. 2005;16:501–516, vi.

118. Rosenwasser RH, Armonda RA, Thomas JE, Benitez RP, Gannon PM, Harrop J. Therapeutic modalities for the management of cerebral vasospasm: timing of endovascular options. *Neurosurgery*. 1999;44:975–979.

119. Fisher LA, Ko N, Miss J, Tung PP, Kopelnik A, Banki NM, et al. Hypernatremia predicts adverse cardiovascular and neurological outcomes after SAH. *Neurocrit Care*. 2006;5:180–185.

120. McGirt MJ, Blessing R, Nimjee SM, Friedman AH, Alexander MJ, Laskowitz DT, et al. Correlation of serum brain natriuretic peptide with hyponatremia and delayed ischemic neurological deficits after subarachnoid hemorrhage. *Neurosurgery*. 2004;54:1369–1373.

121. Qureshi AI, Suri MF, Sung GY, Straw RN, Yahia AM, Saad M, et al. Prognostic significance of hypernatremia and hyponatremia among patients with aneurysmal subarachnoid hemorrhage. *Neurosurgery*. 2002;50:749–755.

122. Audibert G, Steinmann G, de Talance N, Laurens MH, Dao P, Baumann A, et al. Endocrine response after severe subarachnoid hemorrhage related to sodium and blood volume regulation. *Anesth Analg*. 2009;108:1922–1928.

123. Zheng B, Qiu Y, Jin H, Wang L, Chen X, Shi C, Zhao S. A predictive value of hyponatremia for poor outcome and cerebral infarction in high-grade aneurysmal subarachnoid haemorrhage patients. *J Neurol Neurosurg Psychiatry*. 2011;82(2):213–217.

124. Hasan D, Lindsay KW, Wijdicks EF, Murray GD, Brouwers PJ, Bakker WH, et al. Effect of fludrocortisone acetate in patients with subarachnoid hemorrhage. *Stroke*. 1989;20:1156–1161.

125. Katayama Y, Haraoka J, Hirabayashi H, Kawamata T, Kawamoto K, Kitahara T, et al. A randomized controlled trial of hydrocortisone against hyponatremia in patients with aneurysmal subarachnoid hemorrhage. *Stroke*. 2007;38:2373–2375.

126. Mori T, Katayama Y, Kawamata T, Hirayama T. Improved efficiency of hypervolemic therapy with inhibition of natriuresis by fludrocortisone in patients with aneurysmal subarachnoid hemorrhage. *J Neurosurg*. 1999;91:947–952.

127. Moro N, Katayama Y, Kojima J, Mori T, Kawamata T. Prophylactic management of excessive natriuresis with hydrocortisone for efficient hypervolemic therapy after subarachnoid hemorrhage. *Stroke*. 2003;34:2807–2811.

128. Woo MH, Kale-Pradhan PB. Fludrocortisone in the treatment of subarachnoid hemorrhage-induced hyponatremia. *Ann Pharmacother*. 1997;31:637–639.

129. Suarez JI, Qureshi AI, Parekh PD, Razumovsky A, Tamargo RJ, Bhardwaj A, et al. Administration of hypertonic (3%) sodium chloride/acetate in hyponatremic patients with symptomatic vasospasm following subarachnoid hemorrhage. *J Neurosurg Anesthesiol*. 1999;11:178–184.

130. Zeltser D, Rosansky S, van Rensburg H, Verbalis JG, Smith N. Assessment of the efficacy and safety of intravenous conivaptan in euvolemic and hypervolemic hyponatremia. *Am J Nephrol*. 2007;27:447–457.

131. Wright WL, Asbury WH, Gilmore JL, Samuels OB. Conivaptan for hyponatremia in the neurocritical care unit. *Neurocrit Care*. 2009;11(1):6–13.

132. Naidech AM, Bendok BR, Tamul P, Bassin SL, Watts CM, Batjer HH, et al. Medical complications drive length of stay after brain hemorrhage: a cohort study. *Neurocrit Care*. 2009;10:11–19.

133. Badjatia N, Fernandez L, Schmidt JM, Lee K, Claassen J, Connolly ES, et al. Impact of induced normothermia on outcome after subarachnoid hemorrhage: a case-control study. *Neurosurgery*. 2010;66:696–700.

134. Dorhout Mees SM, Luitse MJ, van den Bergh WM, Rinkel GJ. Fever after aneurysmal subarachnoid hemorrhage: relation with extent of hydrocephalus and amount of extravasated blood. *Stroke*. 2008;39:2141–2143.

135. Fernandez A, Schmidt JM, Claassen J, Pavlicova M, Huddleston D, Kreiter KT, et al. Fever after subarachnoid hemorrhage: risk factors and impact on outcome. *Neurology*. 2007;68:1013–1019.

136. Kilpatrick MM, Lowry DW, Firlik AD, Yonas H, Marion DW. Hyperthermia in the neurosurgical intensive care unit. *Neurosurgery*. 2000;47:850–855.

137. Naidech AM, Bendok BR, Bernstein RA, Alberts MJ, Batjer HH, Watts CM, et al. Fever burden and functional recovery after subarachnoid hemorrhage. *Neurosurgery*. 2008;63:212–217.

138. Todd MM, Hindman BJ, Clarke WR, Torner JC, Weeks JB, Bayman EO et al. Perioperative fever and outcome in surgical patients with aneurysmal subarachnoid hemorrhage. *Neurosurgery*. 2009;64:897–908.

139. Alberti O, Becker R, Benes L, Wallenfang T, Bertalanffy H. Initial hyperglycemia as an indicator of severity of the ictus in poor-grade patients with spontaneous subarachnoid hemorrhage. *Clin Neurol Neurosurg*. 2000;102:78–83.

140. Frontera JA, Fernandez A, Claassen J, Schmidt M, Schumacher HC, Wartenberg et al. Hyperglycemia after SAH: predictors, associated complications, and impact on outcome. *Stroke*. 2006;37:199–203.

141. Kruyt ND, Biessels GJ, de Haan RJ, Vermeulen M, Rinkel GJ, Coert B, et al. Hyperglycemia and clinical outcome in aneurysmal subarachnoid hemorrhage. A meta-analysis. *Stroke*. 2009;40(6):e424–430.

142. Lanzino G, Kassell NF, Germanson T, Truskowski L, Alves W. Plasma glucose levels and outcome after aneurysmal subarachnoid hemorrhage. *J Neurosurg*. 1993;79:885–891.

143. Schlenk F, Vajkoczy P, Sarrafzadeh A. Inpatient hyperglycemia following aneurysmal subarachnoid hemorrhage: relation to cerebral metabolism and outcome. *Neurocrit Care*. 2009;11:56–63.

144. Lanzino G. Plasma glucose levels and outcome after aneurysmal subarachnoid hemorrhage. *J Neurosurg*. 2005;102:974–975.

145. Bell DA, Strong AJ. Glucose/insulin infusions in the treatment of subarachnoid haemorrhage: a feasibility study. *Br J Neurosurg*. 2005;19:21–24.

146. Bilotta F, Spinelli A, Giovannini F, Doronzio A, Delfini R, Rosa G. The effect of intensive insulin therapy on infection rate, vasospasm,

neurologic outcome, and mortality in neurointensive care unit after intracranial aneurysm clipping in patients with acute subarachnoid hemorrhage: a randomized prospective pilot trial. *J Neurosurg Anesthesiol.* 2007;19:156–160.

147. Latorre JG, Chou SH, Nogueira RG, Singhal AB, Carter BS, Ogilvy CS, *et al.* Effective glycemic control with aggressive hyperglycemia management is associated with improved outcome in aneurysmal subarachnoid hemorrhage. *Stroke.* 2009;40:1644–1652.

148. Thiele RH, Pouratian N, Zuo Z, Scalzo DC, Dobbs HA, Dumont AS, *et al.* Strict glucose control does not affect mortality after aneurysmal subarachnoid hemorrhage. *Anesthesiology.* 2009;110:603–610.

149. Naidech AM, Levasseur K, Liebling S, Garg RK, Shapiro M, Ault ML, *et al.* Moderate Hypoglycemia is associated with vasospasm, cerebral infarction, and 3-month disability after subarachnoid hemorrhage. *Neurocrit Care.* 2010;12:181–187.

150. Oddo M, Schmidt JM, Carrera E, Badjatia N, Connolly ES, Presciutti M, *et al.* Impact of tight glycemic control on cerebral glucose metabolism after severe brain injury: a microdialysis study. *Crit Care Med.* 2008;36:3233–3238.

151. Schlenk F, Graetz D, Nagel A, Schmidt M, Sarrafzadeh AS. Insulin-related decrease in cerebral glucose despite normoglycemia in aneurysmal subarachnoid hemorrhage. *Crit Care.* 2008;12(1):R9.

152. Schlenk F, Sarrafzadeh AS. Is continuous insulin treatment safe in aneurysmal subarachnoid hemorrhage? *Vasc Health Risk Manag.* 2008;4:885–891.

153. Kramer AH, Gurka MJ, Nathan B, Dumont AS, Kassell NF, Bleck TP. Complications associated with anemia and blood transfusion in patients with aneurysmal subarachnoid hemorrhage. *Crit Care Med.* 2008;36:2070–2075.

154. Kurtz P, Schmidt JM, Claassen J, Carrera E, Fernandez L, Helbok R, *et al.* Anemia is associated with metabolic distress and brain tissue hypoxia after subarachnoid hemorrhage. *Neurocrit Care.* 2010;13:10–16.

155. Naidech AM, Shaibani A, Garg RK, Duran IM, Liebling SM, Bassin SL, *et al.* Prospective, randomized trial of higher goal hemoglobin after subarachnoid hemorrhage. *Neurocrit Care.* 2010;13(3):313–320.

156. Broessner G, Lackner P, Hoefer C, Beer R, Helbok R, Grabmer C, *et al.* Influence of red blood cell transfusion on mortality and long-term functional outcome in 292 patients with spontaneous subarachnoid hemorrhage. *Crit Care Med.* 2009;37:1886–1892.

157. Wartenberg KE SJ, Fernandez A, Frontera JA, Claassen J, Ostapkovich ND, Palestrant D, *et al.* Impact of red blood cell transfusion on outcome after subarachnoid hemorrhage. *Crit Care Med.* 2007;34:A124.

158. Banki NM, Kopelnik A, Dae MW, Miss J, Tung P, Lawton MT, *et al.* Acute neurocardiogenic injury after subarachnoid hemorrhage. *Circulation.* 2005;112:3314–3319.

159. Lee VH, Oh JK, Mulvagh SL, Wijdicks EF. Mechanisms in neurogenic stress cardiomyopathy after aneurysmal subarachnoid hemorrhage. *Neurocrit Care.* 2006;5:243–249.

160. Mayer SA, Fink ME, Homma S, Sherman D, LiMandri G, Lennihan L, *et al.* Cardiac injury associated with neurogenic pulmonary edema following subarachnoid hemorrhage. *Neurology.* 1994;44:815–820.

161. Deibert E, Barzilai B, Braverman AC, Edwards DF, Aiyagari V, Dacey R, *et al.* Clinical significance of elevated troponin I levels in patients with nontraumatic subarachnoid hemorrhage. *J Neurosurg.* 2003;98:741–746.

162. Hravnak M, Frangiskakis JM, Crago EA, Chang Y, Tanabe M, Gorcsan J 3rd, *et al.* Elevated cardiac troponin I and relationship to persistence of electrocardiographic and echocardiographic abnormalities after aneurysmal subarachnoid hemorrhage. *Stroke.* 2009;40:3478–3484.

163. van der Bilt IA, Hasan D, Vandertop WP, Wilde AA, Algra A, Visser FC, *et al.* Impact of cardiac complications on outcome after aneurysmal subarachnoid hemorrhage: a meta-analysis. *Neurology.* 2009;72:635–642.

164. Oshiro EM, Walter KA, Piantadosi S, Witham TF, Tamargo RJ. A new subarachnoid hemorrhage grading system based on the Glasgow Coma Scale: a comparison with the Hunt and Hess and World Federation of Neurological Surgeons Scales in a clinical series. *Neurosurgery.* 1997;41:140–147.

165. Wartenberg KE. Critical care of poor-grade subarachnoid hemorrhage. *Curr Opin Crit Care.* 2011;17:85–93.

CHAPTER 14

Less common causes of stroke: diagnosis and management

Turgut Tatlisumak, Jukka Putaala, and Stephanie Debette

Introduction

The Trial of Org 10172 in Acute Stroke Treatment (TOAST) is the most commonly used aetiological classification system for ischaemic stroke (1) and denotes five subtypes (please see Chapter 4, Table 4.3). The first three aetiologies, namely large-artery atherosclerosis, cardioembolism, and small-vessel occlusion are common and considered conventional. This chapter will deal with the TOAST 4 group (ischaemic stroke of other determined aetiology), which accounts for less than 5% of unselected ischaemic stroke patients (2) whereas it amounts to one-fourth among the young (3–6) and even more in paediatric strokes (7).

Those with non-conventional causes of stroke are younger than ischaemic stroke patients in general, but gender distribution, stroke severity, mortality, and recurrence rates, as well as functional outcome, are similar to those of unselected stroke patients (2). However, their length of stay in hospitals is significantly longer, probably reflecting a more complex diagnostic workup and management (2). Thus, this group requires a wide range of diagnostic testing (Table 14.1) and demands special expertise. Occurrence rates of ischaemic stroke due to uncommon aetiology decrease or remain constant with age, but their proportion of all strokes falls because the prevalence of conventional aetiologies increase steeply with age.

Approximately 200 different conditions causing or associated with ischaemic stroke have been reported (Tables 14.2–14.8). Of note, some of these are based on individual case reports or small series of patients only, making the causal relationship uncertain. This chapter will discuss all but conventional recognized aetiological causes (TOAST categories 1–3) and aims at delivering hints useful for the aetiological diagnosis, including patient and family history as well as specific features in clinical examination. We will discuss more thoroughly the most common of these uncommon causes of ischaemic stroke and provide a brief overview of specific treatment approaches. Readers are referred to more comprehensive textbooks specifically covering the unusual aetiologies of ischaemic stroke (8).

Patient and family history

Demographic features

Ethnicity and geography have implications for stroke aetiology. African Americans and Hispanics have a higher stroke incidence, individuals of African or Asian origin more often have intracranial stenoses. Sickle cell disease and thalassemia are more common among individuals of African origin or from Mediterranean countries, whereas moyamoya and Takayasu disease are severalfold more common among Asians. Behçet disease is more frequently found in eastern Mediterranean and Japanese people, and Kawasaki disease is common in Asians. Human immunodeficiency virus (HIV) infection is a particularly important cause in endemic areas, especially in Sub-Saharan Africa. Neurocysticercosis and Chagas disease are frequent causes in endemic regions, particularly in Latin America. Cerebral autosomal recessive arteriopathy with subcortical infarcts and leucoencephalopathy (CARASIL) was described in Asian (Japanese) patients mainly. Within the same continent and country, aetiologies can differ widely according to the area and surroundings. For instance, in certain geographic regions in the urban US illicit drug use amounted to 5% of the causes of all young ischaemic stroke patients.

Medical history

Hearing loss is common in mitochondrial diseases, Cogan syndrome, Kawasaki syndrome, and retinocochleocerebral arteriolopathy (Susac syndrome). *Epistaxis* is a usual finding in hereditary haemorrhagic telangiectasia (HHT, also called Osler–Weber–Rendu disease), which paradoxically can lead to arterial thrombosis. *Painful paraesthesias* (acroparesthesia) of the extremities should remind of Fabry disease. *Spontaneous miscarriages* may indicate antiphospholipid syndrome. History of *asthma* is an essential component of Churg–Strauss syndrome.

Clues to the diagnosis of *thrombophilias* include a history of a prior thrombo-occlusive event, recurrent fetal loss, thrombocytopenia, livedo reticularis, skin necrosis during initiation of oral anticoagulant therapy with warfarin, absence of conventional risk factors, malignancy, sepsis, recurrent thrombosis despite treatment, venous thrombosis after minimal injury, and thrombosis at unusual sites.

Recent immobilization associated with conditions such as long travel, ongoing pregnancy, or recent delivery precipitates to pelvic or leg deep venous thrombosis, which in association with Valsalva immediately before stroke onset may indicate right-to-left shunt (e.g. in patent foramen ovale).

Recent trauma may underlie a dissection, cerebral venous thrombosis, *in situ* arterial thrombosis, or arteriovenous fistula. Recently

Table 14.1 Specific diagnostic tests and examples of target diagnoses

Diagnostic tests	Target diagnoses
Arterial biopsy	Temporal (giant cell) arteritis, Sneddon syndrome
Cerebromeningeal biopsy	Primary cerebral vasculitides
Muscle biopsy	Mitochondrial disease, CADASIL
Skin biopsy	Sometimes in CADASIL and CARASIL. Sneddon syndrome, pseudoxanthoma elasticum, and whenever an unexplained skin lesion is present
Fluorescein angiography	Vasculitides
GLA activity	Fabry disease
Lumbar puncture	Vasculitides, sarcoidosis, CNS infections
TPHA, VDRL, FTA	Syphilis
Serum titres	Specific infections (viral, bacterial)
ANA-, ENA-, and anti-DNA-antibodies, Complement	SLE, connective tissue diseases
ANCA, MPOAbG, Pr3AbG	Systemic vasculitides
Rheumatoid factors	Rheumatic disease
Protein electrophoresis	Paraproteinaemia
Hb electrophoresis	Sickle cell anaemia (HbS), thalassemia
Blood and urine toxicology	Illicit drug use
Ammonium	Glutaric aciduria type 1 and 2, urea cycle disorders
Lactic acidosis in blood	Branch-chained organic acidurias, glutaric acidaemia type 1 and 2, mitochondrial diseases
Acidosis in CSF	Branch-chained organic acidurias, glutaric acidaemia type 1 and 2, mitochondrial diseases
Thrombophilia	Antithrombin, protein C, and protein S levels, antiphospholipid antibodies (lupus anticoagulant, anticardiolipin antibodies, β2-glycoprotein antibodies), homocysteine, factor V Leiden mutation (FVR506Q), prothrombin gene mutation (G20210A), methylenetetrahydrofolate gene mutation (C677T), factor XII gene mutation (C46T)

Table 14.2 Monogenic disorders causing ischaemic stroke

Monogenic disorders with ischaemic stroke as the primary manifestation
Cerebral autosomal dominant arteriopathy with subcortical infarcts and leucoencephalopathy (CADASIL)—*NOTCH3* mutation, AD
Cerebral autosomal recessive arteriopathy with subcortical infarcts and leucoencephalopathy (CARASIL)—*HTRA1* mutation, AR
Hereditary endotheliopathy, retinopathy, nephropathy and strokes (HERNS)—*TREX* mutation, AD
Hereditary angiopathy, nephropathy, aneurysm, and muscle cramps (HANAC)—COL4A1, AD'
Autosomal dominant *TREX1* angiopathy[a]—TREX mutation, AD
Cerebroretinal vasculopathy (CRV)—*TREX* mutation, AD
Moyamoya—*ACTA2, MTCP1,* or *RNF213* mutation, AD or AR
Cerebral amyloid angiopathies
Monogenic disorders with ischaemic stroke as a recognized but not primary manifestation
Sickle cell disease—*HBB* mutation, recessive
Fabry disease—*GLA* mutation, X-linked recessive
Homocystinuria—*CBS* mutation (most common), AR
Familial hemiplegic migraine—*CACNA1A, ATP1A2* or *SCNA1* mutation, AD
Hereditary haemorrhagic telangiectasia or (Osler–Weber–Rendu syndrome) *ACVRL1* or *ENG* mutation (most common), AD
Vascular Ehlers–Danlos syndrome—*COL3A1* mutation, AD
Marfan syndrome—*Fibrillin 1* mutation, AD
Pseudoxanthoma elasticum—*ABCC6* mutation, AR
Loeys–Dietz syndrome—*TGFBR1* or *TGFBR2* mutation, AD
Arterial tortuosity syndrome—*SLC2A10* mutation, AR
Neurofibromatosis type 1 (von Recklinghausen disease)—*NF1* mutation, AD
Carney syndrome (Facial lentiginosis and myxoma)

[a] synonyms of autosomal dominant *TREX1* angiopathy include HERNS, CRV, RCVL, and CHARIOT.

AD, autosomal dominant; AR, autosomal recessive,

developed uni- or bilateral intracranial systolic bruit may indicate dissection or arteriovenous fistula.

Family history

Family history may disclose heritable diseases, especially with a dominant trait, which may underlie a stroke. Patients should be asked for a history of stroke, dementia, or other vascular events in the family, events occurring at a young age and in several family members being particularly suggestive of an inherited disorder. History of venous thromboembolisms in the family, particularly at younger age, may indicate hereditary thrombotic tendency.

Symptoms at admission

Headache is a common feature in stroke patients, and migraine with aura specifically is associated with an increased risk of stroke. Migraine-like headaches are particularly frequent and characteristic in antiphospholipid syndrome, Sneddon syndrome, systemic lupus erythematosus (SLE), mitochondrial encephalopathy, lactic acidosis, and stroke-like episodes (MELAS), cerebral autosomal dominant arteriopathy with subcortical infarcts and leucoencephalopathy (CADASIL), and hereditary endotheliopathy, retinopathy, nephropathy, and strokes (HERNS). Thunderclap headache is commonly associated with dissections of brain supplying arteries and reversible cerebral vasoconstriction syndrome (RCVS). Differential diagnoses include subarachnoid haemorrhage, sentinel headache (warning leak headache), and cerebral venous thrombosis (CVT). Ischaemic strokes preceded by an unusual headache, with an onset hours of days before (not necessarily

Table 14.3 Non-atherosclerotic non-inflammatory causes of ischaemic stroke

Dissections of brain-supplying arteries: extracranial (carotid, vertebral), intracranial
Fibromuscular dysplasia (FMD)
Moyamoya disease and syndrome
Cerebral amyloid angiopathies
Tumoral encasement of cervicocerebral arteries
Divry and Van Bogaert syndrome (diffuse meningocerebral angiomatosis and leucoencephalopathy)
Eosinophil-induced neurotoxicity
Endovascular lymphoma
Epidermal nevus syndrome
Dolichoectatic basilar artery, arterial kinking
Coiling and hypoplasia of cervical arteries
Radiation-induced angiopathy
Retinocochleocerebral arteriolopathy (Susac syndrome)
Sturge–Weber syndrome (encephalotrigeminal angiomatosis)
SAMHD1 gene mutation-associated cerebral vasculopathy

Table 14.4 Non-atherosclerotic inflammatory arteriopathies

Primary vasculitis
Isolated angiitis of the CNS (primary CNS vasculitis)
Secondary vasculitis in association with systemic diseases
Takayasu arteritis
Eales disease
Buerger disease (thromboangiitis obliterans)
Giant cell arteritis (temporal arteritis, Horton disease)
Kawasaki disease
Sweet syndrome (acute febrile neutrophilic dermatosis)
Kohlmeier–Degos disease (malignant atrophic papulosis)
Acute posterior multifocal placoid pigment epitheliopathy
Vogt–Koyanagi–Harada syndrome
Systemic disorders with possible cerebrovascular involvement, but cerebral vasculitis is usually not the most prominent feature: Wegener's granulomatosis, polyarteritis nodosa, Churg–Strauss syndrome, Sjögren's syndrome, Behçet's disease, systemic lupus erythematosus, sarcoidosis, ulcerative colitis, Crohn's disease, mixed connective tissue disease, rheumatoid arthritis, scleroderma, Cogan's syndrome, dermatomyositis and polymyositis, Henoch–Schönlein purpura (HSP)
Secondary vasculitis in association with infectious diseases
Virus: herpes zoster, varicella zoster, HIV, hepatitis B and C, cytomegalovirus, Coxsackie-9 virus, California encephalitis virus, mumps, paramyxovirus, Epstein–Barr virus if X-linked lymphoproliferative disease
Bacteria: bacterial meningitis, syphilis, Lyme disease, tuberculosis, mycoplasma pneumoniae, brucellosis
Parasites: leptospirosis, cysticercosis, malaria, Chagas disease
Mycotic infections
Other inflammatory arteriopathies
Neoplastic and paraneoplastic vasculitis (lymphomas, malign histiocytosis, hairy-cell leukaemia)
Radiation vasculitis
Hypersensitivity vasculitides (Henoch–Schönlein purpura, drug-induced, chemical, and essential mixed cryoglobulinaemia)

abruptly), are suggestive of dissection or vasculitis, CVT being the major differential diagnosis. *Seizure* at stroke onset is common and is frequently associated with cortical infarcts, CVT, mitochondrial disease, SLE, Divry–van Boagert syndrome, Menkes disease, Sturge–Weber syndrome, and organic acid disorders. Seizures may also indicate alcohol or drug abstinence, hypoglycaemia, or severe electrolyte imbalance.

Physical examination

General hints

Complete physical examination is a crucial step in the search for the cause of ischaemic stroke. In patients without an obvious aetiology for their stroke, particular emphasis should be put on evaluation of skin, head, neck, mucous membranes, eyes, hands, and joints. Patients should be undressed for the examination.

Tall stature may indicate Marfan syndrome, acromegaly or gigantism, homocystinuria, or Loeys–Dietz syndrome. Short stature may be found in mitochondrial diseases, progeria (premature aging and atherosclerosis), and hypothyroidism.

Fever is usually caused by infections, sometimes by inflammatory diseases, and rarely by hyperthyroidism. A large difference of systolic blood pressures between the arms or lack of pulses in the arms, or both, may indicate Takayasu disease.

Skin

Café au laut changes indicate neurofibromatosis type 1 (von Recklinghausen disease). Erythema chronicum migrans can be found in Lyme disease (borreliosis). Lymphadenopathy is a frequent sign of infection or malignancy, particularly lymphoma. Recurrent genital and oral ulcers are present in syphilis, SLE, and Behçet disease. Painful genital ulcers may point out herpes

simplex, whereas painless ulcers may refer to syphilis or Behçet disease.

Relapsing erythema on the body (frequently around buttocks) together with a febrile disease indicate Sweet syndrome. Maculopapular lesions around the umbilicus should alert for Fabry disease (angiokeratoma). Erythema nodosum is seen in connective tissue disorders, Behçet disease, SLE, sarcoidosis, tuberculosis, and post-streptococcic infections (e.g. acute rheumatic fever).

Presence of fixed deep bluish-red reticular skin lesions on the legs (livedo racemosa) is typical to Sneddon syndrome. Divry and van Bogaert syndrome is associated with livedo reticularis. Generalized purpura may indicate Henoch–Schönlein disease in children. Widespread telangiectasias are a fundamental feature of hereditary haemorrhagic telangiectasia.

Table 14.5 Vasospastic disorders

Migrainous infarction
Stroke-like migraine attacks after radiation therapy (SMART)
Paroxysmal hypertension
Reversible cerebral vasoconstriction syndromes (RCVS)
Subarachnoid haemorrhage (SAH)
Post-carotid endarterectomy syndrome
Hypercalcaemia
Hyperparathyroidism
Neck procedures
Cerebral angiography
Systemic or specific infections
Illicit drugs:
Amphetamine
Cocaine
Crack
Ergot intoxication
Sympathomimetics
Heroin
Phencyclidine (PCP, angel dust)
Anabolic steroids
Ecstasy (3,4-methylenedioxymethamphetamine)
Methylphenidate (IV use)
Pentazocine (IV use)

Table 14.6 Haematological disorders

Hyperviscosity states
Plasma abnormalities (paraproteinaemia, Waldenström's macroglobulinemia, congenital hyperfibrinogenemia)
Increased cellularity (polycythemia vera, stress polycythemia, erythrocytosis, myeloproliferative syndromes, hyperleucocytic leukaemias)
Decreased deformability (Sickle cell anaemia [drepanocytosis], spherocytosis, haemoglobinopathies)
Coagulopathies
Homocysteinuria
Sneddon syndrome
Antiphospholipid antibodies
Systemic lupus erythematosus
Nephrotic syndrome
Deficiencies of protein S, protein C, antithrombin III, plasminogen, prekallikrein, factors VIII and XII, heparin cofactor II
Platelet hyperaggregability
Fibrinolytic insufficiency
Factor V Leiden mutation
Prothrombin G20210A mutation
Vitamin K treatment
Antifibrinolytic therapy
Disseminated intravascular coagulation
Essential thrombocytosis
Paroxysmal nocturnal haemoglobinuria
Moschcowitz syndrome (thrombotic thrombocytopenic purpura)
Snakebite
Anaemias
Microcytic anaemias (iron deficiency, thalassaemias, chronic disease, sideroblastic anaemias)
Normocytic anaemias (acute haemorrhage or haemolysis, anaplastic anaemia, chronic disease, combined iron and folate deficiencies)
Macrocytic anaemias (vitamin B_{12} deficiency, folic acid deficiency, alcohol-induced, chronic disease)

Skin is extremely elastic and may be pulled up to 20 cm in pseudoxanthoma elasticum. A typical cobblestone-like skin lesion present at the neck and axillary regions becoming lax and excessive over time is pathognomonic to pseudoxanthoma elasticum.

Needle punctures may indicate illicit drug use. Skin tattoos may prompt consideration of blood-borne infections such as hepatitis or HIV, but may also be hiding injection sites for illicit drug use. The linear marks of thrombosed veins caused by intravenous drug injection in addicts are characteristic.

Head and neck

A beaked nose with stretched face skin is typical of scleroderma. Recent hair loss may be caused by SLE, temporal arteritis, hyperthyroidism, iron deficiency, CARASIL, or may be drug-induced. Butterfly erythema in the face is typical to SLE. Corneal arcus and xanthelasma indicate hyperlipidaemia. Sturge–Weber syndrome presents with large portwine stains on the face.

Mouth

High-arched palate is common in Marfan syndrome, but may also be present in homocysteinuria, Ehlers–Danlos, and pseudoxanthoma elasticum. A cleft palate is, in turn, common in Loeys–Dietz's syndrome. Frequent oral ulcers may indicate syphilis, Behçet disease, SLE, ulcerative colitis, Crohn disease, or herpes infection.

Strawberry tongue and cervical lymphadenopathy are frequently found in Kawasaki disease. Enlarged orange-coloured tonsils are typical to Tangier disease.

Eyes

Visual loss is common in mitochondrial disease, retinocochleocerebral arteriolopathy (Susac syndrome), temporal arteritis, acute posterior multifocal placoid-pigment epitheliopathy, Vogt–Koyanagi–Harada disease, Cogan syndrome, pseudoxanthoma elasticum, HERNS, and Eales disease. Horner syndrome, especially when occurring in a young or middle-aged person, and when associated with headache or neck pain, is highly suggestive of carotid dissection. Argyll Robertson pupils (pinpoint irregular pupils constricting only on convergence) are typical for neurosyphilis.

Table 14.7 Metabolic disorders

Mitochondrial disorders associated with cerebrovascular events or stroke-like episodes:
Mitochondrial encephalopathy, lactic acidosis, and stroke-like episodes (MELAS)
Myoclonic epilepsy with ragged-red fibres (MERRF)
Leigh's disease (subacute necrotizing encephalomyelopathy)
Kearns–Sayre
Mitochondrial recessive ataxia syndrome (MIRAS)
Hyperornithinaemia–hyperammonaemia–homocitrullinuria syndrome (HHH)
Menkes disease
Homocystinuria
Tangier's disease
Branched-chain organic acidurias (isovaleric-, propionic-, and methylmalonic-aciduria)
Glutaric aciduria type 1 and type 2
Urea cycle disorders (ornithine transcarbamylase deficiency, carbamoyl phosphate synthatase 1 deficiency, citrullinaemia, argininosuccinic aciduria, argininaemia)
Purine nucleoside phosphorylase deficiency

Table 14.8 Miscellaneous causes of stroke

Cerebral venous thrombosis
Pulmonary diseases:
Arteriovenous fistulas
Osler–Weber–Rendu syndrome (hereditary haemorrhagic telangiectasia)
AV-malformations
Pulmonary vein thrombosis
Pulmonary tumours
Mechanical or systemic:
Traumas
Mediastinal mass
Cervical rib or atlanto-axial subluxation
Iatrogenic (cardiac and vascular procedures)
Decompression sickness
Eagles syndrome (styloid process compressing internal carotid artery)
Transplantation
Unconventional embolic phenomena:
Fat embolism
Air embolism
Fibrocartilaginous embolism
Tumour embolism
Iatrogenic or foreign body embolism
Aneurysm-borne embolus
Rare syndromes:
Adult progeria (specifically Werner's syndrome)
von Hippel–Lindau syndrome
Malign neuroleptic syndrome

Dry eyes are common in Sjögren syndrome. A bluish colour of scleras is caused by thinning and reflects the colour of underlying venous net. Blue sclera is seen in osteogenesis imperfecta, and Ehlers–Danlos syndrome, both risking to arterial dissections. Scleritis appears red and presence of white patches refers to systemic vasculitides. Recurrent iritis may indicate Behçet disease. Hamartoma of the iris, also called Lisch spots, is specific for neurofibromatosis type 1. Dislocation and ectopia of the lens can be seen in Marfan syndrome, leading to severe myopia. Retinitis pigmentosa (pigmentary retinopathy) is found in Fabry disease and mitochondrial diseases. Retinal arteriovenous malformations are found in Wyburn–Mason's syndrome. Angioid streaks, reddish or gravy in colour, radiating from the optic disk and being wider than veins are common in pseudoxanthoma elasticum and sickle cell disease. Roth's spots refer to flame-shaped retinal haemorrhages with a cotton-wool centre resulting from septic emboli in infective endocarditis. Retinal haemorrhages are often associated with Eales syndrome, in which chronic retinal ischaemia presumably resulting from vasculitic mechanism. Moreover, retinal haemorrhages may indicate other types of vasculitides.

Hands and joints

Clubbing fingers are typical in chronic heart and lung disease. Long, thin fingers (arachnodactyly) are found in Marfan syndrome, whereas hands are large in acromegaly. In iron deficiency, the nails become brittle, flat, and eventually spoon-shaped (koilonychias). White nails (leuconychia) are signs of shortage of proteins (hypoalbuminaemia). Splinter haemorrhages under the nails may indicate infective endocarditis. Vasculitides and SLE may cause small necrotic lesions at the base of the nail and on the pulps.

Raynaud phenomenon is usually associated with connective tissue disorders, atherosclerosis, malignancy, and hyperviscosity syndromes. The joints show hypermobility in Marfan and Loeys–Dietz syndromes. Deformations in finger joints, particularly in metacarpophalangeal and proximal interphalangeal joints, suggest rheumatoid disease.

Diagnostic investigations

Imaging

Imaging is the cornerstone of stroke diagnostics. When thrombolysis or other hyperacute interventions are considered, selection and extent of imaging modality should follow institutional guidelines. Otherwise, brain imaging aims at visualizing ischaemia and characterizing lesion location, size, age, and multiplicity. Brain imaging reveals also other pathological changes, excludes causes mimicking stroke, and describes associated features such as leucoaraiosis, microbleeds, and silent brain infarcts. The most appropriate brain imaging modality for ischaemic stroke is magnetic resonance imaging (MRI) when available. In particular, patients without a conventional aetiology and young patients with a suspicion of stroke should undergo MRI.

Vascular imaging aims at detecting pathologies in the vasculature and excluding certain changes, and thus, guides in aetiological diagnosis as well as treatment choices. The most appropriate and practical vascular imaging approach is combining MRI along with magnetic resonance angiography (MRA) of cervical and intracranial vasculature including the venous phase. In cases with suspicion of dissection, T1-weighted fat suppression imaging of the neck region can be added to visualize mural haematoma.

MRA brings versatile information of the underlying stroke aetiology. For instance, intracranial artery aneurysms may be associated with fibromuscular dysplasia, polycystic renal disease, Ehlers–Danlos syndrome, pseudoxanthoma elasticum, coarctation of aorta, and probably in Marfan syndrome. Arteriovenous malformations are found in Sturge–Weber syndrome, hereditary haemorrhagic telangiectasia, and Wyburn–Mason syndrome. Beading of cerebral arteries is common in vasculitides, RCVS, subarachnoid haemorrhage, intracranial atherosclerosis, and mitochondrial-disease-associated angiopathy. However, beading of cerebral arteries is not specific to any particular aetiology. Dolichoectasia is common in Fabry disease, sickle cell disease, acquired immunodeficiency syndrome, and Ehlers–Danlos syndrome. Pseudoxanthoma elasticum patients have widespread tortuosity and ectasia of the neck vessels.

Digital subtraction angiography used to be the preferred investigation for evaluating cerebral arteries, but advances in computed tomography (CT) and MRA have enabled non-invasive evaluation of cervical and intracranial arteries with good sensitivity and specificity and have become the gold standard. Digital subtraction angiography is still useful when these techniques cannot bring a definite answer, providing superior spatial and temporal resolution. Digital subtraction angiography is useful particularly in the diagnosis of vasculitides, and some intracranial dissections, but should be used only when yielding a demonstrable benefit, given the invasiveness of the technique that exposes the patient to serious adverse events.

Ultrasound examination provides a rapid and non-invasive assessment of the carotid (duplex ultrasound) and intracerebral (transcranial Doppler) arteries. Both are excellent screening tests and useful in patient follow-up, but can suffer from operator or technology-dependent limitations. In determining rare aetiologies for ischaemic stroke, MRA and CT angiography techniques are clearly superior to ultrasound examination.

New imaging technologies are currently under development and may be helpful in some cases. Such methods include, for example, delayed post-contrast vascular imaging that can directly detect endothelial inflammation.

Characteristics of ischaemic lesions in brain imaging can give clues regarding the underlying stroke aetiology. Multiple infarcts in different arterial territories should raise the suspicion for cardiac or aortic source of embolism, vasculitis, moyamoya disease, MELAS, Kohlmeier–Degos syndrome, and CADASIL. Haemorrhagic infarcts, on the other hand, support cardiac embolism or CVT. Presence of both intracerebral haemorrhage and infarcts of different ages support endocarditis, vasculitides, moyamoya, CVT, or illicit drug use. Basal ganglia calcification on CT or MRI may suggest MELAS, but is a fairly frequent and nonspecific finding. Temporal arteritis, Behçet disease, and Fabry disease all have a predilection for vertebral artery territory infarctions. Migraneous infarcts are usually located in the occipital lobes. Involvement of

anterior temporal lobes together with widespread leucoaraiosis and multiple lacunar infarcts is rather typical to CADASIL.

Laboratory testing

Routine and advanced laboratory tests aim at detecting stroke mimics such as hypoglycaemia or hyponatraemia, simultaneous disorders complicating stroke (uraemia, liver dysfunction), well-documented stroke risk factors (diabetes, dyslipidaemia), or aetiology of stroke (antiphospholipid syndrome, single-gene disorders). All ischaemic stroke patients should undergo a routine package of testing including complete blood count, erythrocyte sedimentation rate, C-reactive protein, kidney and liver function tests, thyroid tests, myocardial enzymes (troponin T and/or creatine phosphokinase), activated partial thromboplastin time, international normalized ratio, blood electrolytes, glucose, blood lipid profile, urine analysis, 12-lead electrocardiogram, and chest x-ray. Advanced tests (Table 14.1) should be used in selected cases as they are costly, their yield may be modest, and some bring discomfort (lumbar puncture, muscle biopsy) or even risky (brain biopsy) to the patient. Cardiac testing is dealt elsewhere in this book.

Blood and urine toxicology tests are helpful in known illicit drug use, suspicion of drug abuse, or intoxication. Blood samples can also be stored for later testing. D-dimer, blood ethanol, ammonium, amylase, haemoglobin glucose, arterial blood gas analysis, blood lactate, thiamine, blood typing, homocysteine, B_{12} vitamin, folic acid, pregnancy test, and others may be useful in selected cases.

Clotting tests should be considered in young patients without an obvious aetiology and those with a personal or family history of tendency to thromboembolic disease (Table 14.1). However, as mentioned earlier, association between coagulation abnormalities and arterial stroke is not well established and routine testing on all patients with ischaemic stroke does not seem reasonable or cost-effective. Testing for vasculitis should be considered in those with features of vasculitides and in young patients without an obvious aetiology (Table 14.1).

Other specific blood tests include, for example, Venereal Disease Research Laboratory test and fluorescent treponemal antibody test for syphilis, antibody measurements for infectious agents, Sickle cell preparation and haemoglobin electrophoresis for sickle cell disease. All HIV-positive patients should be tested for syphilis and vice versa. Pregnancy test should be taken in females of child-bearing age.

Lumbar puncture brings information when inflammatory or infectious causes are considered. Vasculitides are usually associated with a non-specific mild inflammatory response in the cerebrospinal fluid. Lactate level in the cerebrospinal fluid is usually increased in mitochondrial disease, but lactate measurement should be done immediately while the sample is kept on ice to avoid artificial increase of lactate.

Genetic testing

Genetic testing is available for several conditions (Table 14.2) and should be performed in specialized centres (<http://www.orpha.net>).

Advanced testing

Any unusual skin changes detected during physical examination must be recorded and may serve as potential biopsy sites. Skin biopsies are used to be taken in CADASIL and Fabry disease in the past and are still useful whenever an unexplained skin lesion is present in an ischaemic stroke patient. Mitochondrial disease diagnostics may necessitate muscle biopsy. Ragged red fibres in muscle biopsy are seen in MELAS, myoclonic epilepsy with ragged-red fibres (MERRF), and Menkes disease.

Histopathological confirmation is the gold standard and is essential for accurate diagnosis of CNS vasculitides. Leptomeningeal specimen along with brain parenchymal biopsy from a damaged area is preferred. If no clear reachable non-eloquent brain area is found, right frontal lobe biopsy is usually suggested. Biopsy is clearly underused in vasculitis diagnostics because of the fear of serious complications and because negative biopsy results are not uncommon. Similarly, a biopsy is needed when intravascular lymphoma or other neoplastic changes in brain are suspected.

A temporal artery biopsy should be performed whenever a diagnosis of giant cell arteritis is suspected, but this should not delay the initiation of treatment; a bilateral biopsy is seldom necessary. An adequate sample length of at least 1 cm is important when a biopsy is carried out which will enable the pathologist to look at multiple sections of the artery over a wide area.

Genetic disorders

A large number of single-gene disorders have been linked to ischaemic stroke. However, ischaemic stroke is the principal manifestation in few (CADASIL, CARASIL, HERNS), a recognized feature in some (sickle cell disease, Fabry disease, MELAS, homocystinuria), and an occasional phenomenon in most (Ehlers–Danlos, Marfan, pseudoxanthoma elasticum, hereditary haemorrhagic telangiectasia) of these single-gene disorders. Only the most common genetic disorders are discussed in the text, other genetic diseases potentially causing stroke are listed in Table 14.2.

CADASIL is a rare autosomal dominant disease caused by mutations in the *NOTCH3* gene on chromosome 19.9. *NOTCH3* encodes a cell-surface receptor involved in vascular smooth muscle cell survival and vascular remodelling. The prevalence of this disorder has been estimated at about 1/24,000, which is probably an underestimation (<http://www.orpha.net>). CADASIL patients suffer from recurrent lacunar strokes. The phenotype also includes progressive cognitive impairment, psychiatric disturbances—especially mood disturbances—and migraine with aura, with an onset between the third and sixth decade. The underlying vascular lesion is a non-arteriosclerotic, amyloid-negative angiopathy involving small arteries and capillaries. MRI shows multiple infarcts and severe leucoaraiosis with a typical involvement of temporal poles. The definitive diagnostic test is the molecular genetic analysis of the *NOTCH3* gene. Skin biopsy can reveal characteristic granular osmiophilic material within the vascular basal lamina on electron microscopic examination (9).

Fabry disease is an X-linked lysosomal storage disease where deficiency of alpha-galactosidase enzyme leads to accumulation of globotriaosylceramide in several visceral tissues (10). Cardiac and renal failure, hypohydrosis, acroparaesthesia, painful polyneuropathy, corneal and lenticular opacities, and red angiokeratomas that appear in periumbilical area and extensor surfaces are common findings. The disease is less severe and diagnosis is somewhat troublesome in females. Death occurs mostly of renal or cardiac failure. Ischaemic strokes are more common in posterior circulation.

Less than 1% of all young patients with ischaemic stroke harbour Fabry disease which commonly manifests with oligosymptomatic features (5).

In *sickle cell disease*, a genetic abnormality causes alterations in the haemoglobin molecule leading to easy sickling of the erythrocytes (HbS). Factors such as fever, infection, hypoxia, dehydration, and acidosis may lead to sickling of erythrocytes resulting in haemolysis, thrombosis formation within the vasculature, and anaemia. HbS increases erythrocyte adhesion to endothelium. A slowly progressing vasculopathy resembling that in moyamoya disease can cause bilateral stenosis and gradual obstruction of middle cerebral arteries. Neurological complications are particularly common the homozygote form of sickle cell disease (HbSS). Both overt and silent brain infarcts are frequent in HbSS patients (approximately in 20%).

Homocystinuria is a genetic disease caused by homozygosity of the defective *MTHFR* gene. The disease is associated with high plasma levels of homocysteine, increased urinary homocysteine, long stature with Marfan-like features, and premature atherosclerosis.

Non-atherosclerotic non-inflammatory arteriopathies

Cervical artery dissection is the most common of unusual stroke aetiologies in Western countries, especially in young and middle-aged adults. Fibromuscular dysplasia and moyamoya are also classical rare causes of ischaemic stroke. Other, less frequent conditions in the group of non-atherosclerotic non-inflammatory arteriopathies are detailed in Table 14.3.

Cervical artery dissection (CEAD) is one of the most common causes of ischaemic stroke in young and middle aged adults occurring at a mean age of 44–46 years, and very seldom beyond the age of 65 (11). Pathologically, CEAD corresponds to a haematoma in the wall of a cervical artery (carotid or vertebral), which can lead to intra-luminal thrombus formation, causing cerebral or, seldomly, retinal ischaemia. Patients with an ischaemic stroke due to CEAD often have accompanying signs, including headache, cervical pain, Horner syndrome (ipsilateral to a carotid dissection, by compression of sympathetic fibres), and sometimes cranial nerve palsies (also ipsilateral to a carotid dissection). These 'local signs' are often present several hours or days before the ischaemic stroke. Characteristic radiological features of CEAD include an enlarged artery with a mural haematoma (which appears as a hyperintense rim on T1-weighted axial cervical MRI scans with the fat-saturation technique), long tapering stenosis, and dissecting aneurysms. Cervical trauma is an important predisposing factor for CEAD, but a causal relationship is often difficult to establish, and many cases of CEAD occur spontaneously, without any trauma. Hypertension seems to be associated with a moderately increased risk of CEAD, while hypercholesterolemia and overweight appear to be inversely associated with the disease. Other putative risk factors include recent infection, migraine, and fibromuscular dysplasia.

Fibromuscular dysplasia (FMD) affects mostly middle-aged women and is characterized by non-atherosclerotic segmental non-inflammatory arteriopathy that affects renal and cervical arteries (12). FMD leads to arterial stenosis, which typically has a string-of-beads appearance in angiography. Cerebral symptoms seem to occur in a minority of the patients, but precise estimates of the occurrence of ischaemic cerebrovascular events are lacking. Dissections and intracranial aneurysms are frequently encountered. Renal arteries should be imaged and screened for FMD in patients in whom cervical FMD is discovered during stroke workup.

Moyamoya is characterized by chronic progressive stenosis and eventually occlusion of distal intracranial internal carotid artery and proximal middle, anterior, and rarely of other cerebral arteries (13). Simultaneously, a compensatory network of thin collateral arteries develops in the basal regions of the brain visualized as a hazy puff of smoke (moyamoya in Japanese language) on angiographic imaging. If idiopathic, the finding is called moyamoya disease, whereas if there is an underlying disease such as neurofibromatosis type 1, Down syndrome, irradiation of the head, meningitis, sickle cell disease, hydrocephalus, brain tumours, the condition is called moyamoya syndrome. Conventionally the radiologic findings should be bilateral; unilateral findings sometimes progress to bilateral disease over years. Moyamoya is more frequent in Asians than in Caucasians. Moyamoya is at least twice as frequent in females. Moyamoya presents typically bimodally; in children around 5–10 years of age and in adults in their 40s. Ischaemic stroke and transient ischaemic attack are common manifestations of moyamoya. It seems that intracerebral haemorrhage is also a common manifestation in Asians, but probably not in Caucasians.

Non-atherosclerotic inflammatory arteriopathies

Vasculitides are a heterogeneous group of disorders (Table 14.4) characterized by inflammation and occasionally necrotic changes of blood vessel walls including arteries and veins of differing calibre resulting in stenotic, occlusive, or aneurysmal changes in the vessels (14). They manifest clinically with mostly ischaemic and seldom haemorrhagic events, which are often multifocal. Vasculitides can be classified in various ways, but most commonly classified as small-, medium-, and large-vessel vasculitis. Major symptoms of central nervous system vasculitides are headache, stroke, and encephalopathy. Increased erythrocyte sedimentation rate and C-reactive protein level are common findings in blood tests. Cerebrospinal fluid studies reveal mild non-specific inflammatory response. Anaemia, thrombocytosis, elevated liver enzymes, and low complement levels are also frequent. Survival from all forms of vasculitides has improved since the introduction of corticosteroids and later with the continuously widening arsenal of cytostatic agents.

Large-vessel vasculitides involving central nervous system include *Takayasu's disease* affecting the aorta and its major branches in adolescent girls and young females. The disease typically leads to lack of pulse in upper extremities and causes inflammation of temporal and ophthalmic arteries that manifest as headache, malaise, jaw claudication, hair loss, increased erythrocyte sedimentation rate and C-reactive protein, and visual impairment (that can eventually lead to blindness). A normal erythrocyte sedimentation rate and C-reactive protein value should raise suspicion of an alternate diagnosis. Pathology demonstrates vascular wall inflammation with granuloma and giant cell formation.

Medium-sized arteries are involved in *Kawasaki syndrome* in childhood and in classic *polyarteritis nodosa*. Cerebral involvement

is frequent in polyarteritis nodosa but is unusual in Kawasaki syndrome.

Small vessel vasculitides can be separated into anti-neutrophilic cytoplasmic antibody (ANCA) -positive and ANCA-negative vasculitides. A positive test for cytoplasmic ANCA (cANCA) targeted to proteinase 3 (PR3), or perinuclear ANCA (pANCA) against myeloperoxidase (MPO) has a high sensitivity and specificity for the diagnosis of ANCA-associated vasculitis. ANCA-positive vasculitides include (1) *Churg–Strauss syndrome* presenting with asthma and eosinophilia, (2) *Wegener granulomatosis* presenting with granulomas in the upper airways and renal involvement, and (3) *microscopic polyangiitis*, the microscopic variant of polyarteritis nodosa, which presents without asthma or granulomas. Churg–Strauss syndrome and microscopic angiitis are associated with pANCA/MPO. cANCA/PR3 are present in Wegener's disease. *Primary angiitis* of the central nervous system (PACNS) involves primarily small arteries, but also medium-sized arteries, arterioles, capillaries, venules, and veins. No other organ is involved. The disease is multifocal and usually has a remitting and relapsing course. Antibodies and other specific tests are normal with C-reactive protein being usually elevated.

Immune complex deposits are seen in vasculitic variants of connective tissue diseases such as SLE, rheumatoid arthritis, and Behçet disease. SLE increases stroke risk by tenfold and majority of SLE patients have at least some neurological involvement. These include strokes, seizures, chorea, dementia, psychosis, neuropathy, and myelopathy. SLE-associated stroke occurs by several mechanisms, namely by increased thrombotic tendency due to antiphospholipid antibodies or thrombogenic cytokines, accelerated atherosclerosis, heart valve disease, Libmann–Sacks endocarditis, and vasculitis. However, only a small fraction of SLE patients with central nervous system involvement have a real vasculitis.

Vasospastic syndromes

Vasospasm in cerebral arteries can be demonstrated with angiographic procedures and may be found in a number of underlying conditions (Table 14.5). Vasospasm may lead to cerebral ischaemia when it substantially interferes with blood circulation and is sufficiently long-standing. In all cases, the cause should be explored and treatment should be started quickly in order to inhibit or limit ischaemic damage.

Patients with migraine with aura have a doubled risk for ischaemic stroke whereas the association between migraine without aura (common migraine) and ischaemic stroke is less clear (15). Presence of other risk factors, such as smoking and oral contraceptive use increase the risk to approximately tenfold in women with aural migraine. Migraine was associated with a fourfold increase in the risk of white matter abnormalities; the risk correlates with burden of migraine attacks, suggesting a dose-response relationship. The mechanisms(s) of ischaemic stroke in patients with migraine, however, remain speculative as a typical migraneous infarction fulfilling the International Headache Society definition, is rare. Further mechanisms may include repeated cortical spreading depressions, the association with dissections and patent foramen ovale, use of vasoconstrictor agents in highly sensitive individuals, and an increased prevalence of vascular risk factors among patients with migraine (15). Migraine is also associated with several diseases and conditions which have a well-recognized increased frequency for ischaemic stroke (e.g. CADASIL, MELAS, antiphospholipid syndrome, SLE). Nevertheless, long-standing aura-like symptoms with a new ischaemic lesion are very suggestive of a vasospastic migraneous infarction.

New light has recently been shed on another cause of vasospasm in cerebral arteries, namely RCVS (16, 17). RCVS comprises a large group of overlapping prolonged cerebral vasospastic disorders such as Call–Fleming syndrome, pregnancy- and puerperium-related angiopathy, migraneous vasospasm, benign angiopathies, drug-induced vasospastic conditions, illicit-drug-related 'vasculitis', vasospasm attributable to neurosurgical procedures, and cerebral vasospasm following sympathomimetic use.

The general feature of RCVS is a sudden severe headache (thunderclap) and demonstration of widespread cerebral artery vasospasm with alternating areas of arterial constriction and dilatation in multiple vascular beds, so-called string and beads appearance. Neurological symptoms and signs differ or may be absent. Hypertension is a frequent feature. Most patients are young to middle-aged females. Other causes of thunderclap headache (subarachnoid haemorrhage, dissection, or CVT) must be ruled out. Beading of cerebral arteries is common and lasts several days to weeks, but disappears usually within 12 weeks. CSF examination is almost always normal or near normal and helps in distinguishing RCVS from vasculitis. The course of RCVS is usually benign, but severe neurological syndromes and even death have been reported. In addition to ischaemic changes, intracerebral haemorrhages are also frequent, particularly in patients with extreme blood pressures.

Of note, while illicit drug use is a classical cause of vasospasm in cerebral arteries, it can also cause ischaemic stroke by other mechanisms, including foreign body embolism, infective endocarditis, increased platelet aggregation, and vasculitis. Cocaine and amphetamine use are most commonly linked to both haemorrhagic and ischaemic strokes.

Haematological disorders

Abnormalities in viscosity alter cerebral blood flow. Haematocrit levels above 60% may predispose to clotting. Polycythemia increases blood viscosity, decreases cerebral blood flow, and increases thrombosis. Leukaemia with high white blood cell values increases viscosity. Thrombocytosis causes hypercoagulability after thrombocyte count exceeds one million. Low platelet counts are found in antiphospholipid syndrome, SLE, vasculitides, heparin treatment, and thrombotic thrombocytopenic purpura. Severe anaemia also predisposes to thrombosis.

Numerous haematological disorders (Table 14.6) increase the risk of ischaemic stroke via various mechanisms, most importantly by increased tendency of clotting and by hyperviscosity. Most of these factors lack, however, well-documented causality with ischaemic stroke. Nevertheless, their contribution alone may be rather modest, but becomes significant when other risk factors coexist. Conversely, sickle cell anaemia that occurs mainly in black people and among people from the Mediterranean region has been extensively studied and is frequently associated with ischaemic stroke as discussed earlier in this chapter.

Coagulation abnormalities are usually firmly linked to venous thrombosis, but only modestly to arterial thrombosis. A recent meta-analysis showed that deficiencies of antithrombin, protein C, and protein S, mutations in Factor V Leiden, Factor II prothrombin, and the methylenetetrahydrofolate gene, presence of antiphospholipid antibodies and combined thrombophilias, and finally elevated levels of lipoprotein(a) were all strongly associated with an increased risk for arterial thrombosis or CVT, or both, in neonates and children (18). However, the link appears to be less certain in adult patients.

Other causes

Metabolic diseases which might be complicated with ischaemic stroke are rare and frequency of ischaemic stroke in individuals suffering from these diseases is also low (Table 14.7). A study on young ischaemic stroke patients reported only one MELAS patient among over 1000 consecutively recruited patients (3). A number of miscellaneous disorders may be associated with ischaemic stroke (Table 14.8). However, again most of these are rare occasions and seen only rarely in clinical practice. Among these causes, relatively commonly encountered are CVT and iatrogenic ischaemic strokes, mainly appearing during or immediately after cardiac and vascular procedures. We will briefly review CVT in this chapter.

Cerebral venous thrombosis is diagnosed in approximately one person in 200,000 annually and forms less than 1% of all strokes (19). CVT is mainly seen in young individuals with a clear female predominance (~75%). Numerous causes and risk factors have been described including genetic and acquired thrombophilias and several haematological diseases (Table 14.6), local and systemic infections, cytostatic and hormonal medications, surgical procedures of the head, cancer, dehydration, pregnancy, and puerperium. Most common sites of thrombosis are the superior sagittal and transverse sinuses, but any sinus or vein may be involved. The disease may manifest either with general intracranial pressure increase syndrome due to impaired venous drainage or with focal symptoms and signs due to parenchymal injury (oedema, haemorrhage, or sometimes venous infarction usually with a haemorrhagic component). Multiple and bilateral lesions are frequent. Headache and seizures are common presentations. Papilloedema is a common finding. D-dimer levels are increased in most patients, but are not reliable enough for excluding the disease. Diagnosis is based on imaging findings. Most commonly MRI and MRA are used. Demonstration of clot material within a sinus or a cortical vein on imaging is the preferred method. Most patients make good recovery with adequate management and mortality is now lesser than 10% with most patients achieving complete recovery.

Treatment
Acute phase treatment

Evidence-based data from randomized trials are usually lacking and therapeutic decisions are based on expert opinions in most situations of ischaemic stroke of uncommon cause. Immediate evaluation, diagnosis, and supportive care are important first steps. Only limited data exist on safety and efficacy of thrombolysis or mechanical thrombectomy in patients with ischaemic stroke of unconventional aetiologies. It seems that patients with dissection are not harmed by thrombolysis (20, 21). Probably, acute recanalization approaches should be tried in most patients with unconventional aetiologies, but should be limited to those with a visible acute arterial occlusion proved on non-invasive angiographic procedures.

Young patients with space-occupying ischaemic lesions are good candidates for decompressive craniectomy independent of aetiology.

Almost all patients will benefit and probably almost none will be harmed with long-term aspirin or other antiplatelet treatments. However, the exact target population, the most appropriate antiplatelet agent, dose, or duration of treatment are yet unknown. European moyamoya patients may be treated with antiplatelet agents as bleeding is rare unlike in Asian moyamoya patients. CVT patients should be started on long-term anticoagulants, even in the presence of intracranial haemorrhage. Patients with dissections are usually treated either with full-dose anticoagulation or antiplatelet agents, each approach associated with low rates of recurrences or complications.

Treatment of the underlying cause

The underlying disease should be treated according to the best available evidence in order to restrict symptom progression and to prevent recurrent cerebrovascular events. Some examples of specific tailored treatments are discussed here.

Repeated blood transfusions with a target reduction of sickled haemoglobin to less than 30% has successfully prevented ischaemic strokes and reversed moyamoya-like changes in children with sickle cell disease. Hydroxyurea decreases painful episodes in these patients. Extracranial-intracranial bypass surgery has been widely applied to patients with moyamoya-like vascular stenosis. These procedures are reported to have low rate of serious complications, but their benefit is not clear.

L-arginine (0.5 g/kg IV for one or several days followed by oral treatment for several weeks) is an inexpensive and well-tolerated treatment in MELAS patients. Although not an evidence-based approach, several cases with dramatic improvement shortly after receiving L-arginine have been reported. Enzyme replacement is beneficial and may even reverse ceramide accumulation in Fabry disease, although it is not yet known whether enzyme replacement treatment can prevent future strokes. Calcium channel antagonists such as nimodipine can be considered in patients with a vasospastic phenomenon of cerebral arteries.

Corticosteroids are the drug of choice in vasculitides often started alone in large vessel vasculitides at a high dose and later tapered slowly to a maintenance dose. In case of progression of the disease, corticosteroids are typically combined with cytostatic agents. Low-dose aspirin is recommended in large vessel vasculitides as an adjunctive medication. Corticosteroids and cytostatics in combination are recommended in small vessel vasculitides. Patients with SLE require both corticosteroids and oral anticoagulation. Importantly, long-term corticosteroid treatment necessitates osteoporosis prevention both pharmacologically and in form of increased exercise.

References

1. Adams HP Jr, Bendixen BH, Kappelle LJ, Biller J, Love BB, Gordon DL, et al. Classification of subtype of acute ischemic stroke. Definitions for use in a multicenter clinical trial. TOAST. Trial of Org 10172 in Acute Stroke Treatment. *Stroke.* 1993;24:35–41.

2. Grau AJ, Weimar C, Buggle F, Heinrich A, Goertler M, Neumaier S, *et al.* Risk factors, outcome, and treatment in subtypes of ischemic stroke: the German Stroke Data Bank. *Stroke.* 2001;32:2559–2566.

3. Putaala J, Metso AJ, Metso TM, Konkola N, Kraemer Y, Haapaniemi E, *et al.* Analysis of 1008 consecutive patients aged 15 to 49 with first-ever ischemic stroke: the Helsinki Young Stroke Registry. *Stroke.* 2009;40:1195–1203.

4. Ferro JM, Massaro AR, Mas JL. Aetiological diagnosis of ischaemic stroke in young adults. *Lancet Neurol.* 2010;9:1085–1096.

5. Rolfs A, Fazekas F, Grittner U, Dichgans M, Martus P, Holzhausen M, *et al.*, on behalf of The Stroke in Young Fabry Patients (sifap) Investigators. Acute cerebrovascular disease in the young: The Stroke in Young Fabry Patients Study. *Stroke.* 2013;44:340–349.

6. Yesilot N, Putaala J, Waje-Andreasson U, Vassilopoulou S, Nardi K, Odier C, *et al.* Etiology of first-ever ischemic stroke in the young between geographic regions in Europe: The 15-Cities Young Stroke Study. *Eur J Neurol.* 2013;20:1431–1439.

7. Roach ES, Golomb MR, Adams R, Biller J, Daniels S, deVeber G, *et al.* Management of stroke in infants and children. A scientific statement from a special writing group of the American Heart Association Stroke Council and the Council on Cardiovascular Disease in the Young. *Stroke.* 2008;39:2644–2691.

8. Caplan LR. *Uncommon Causes of Stroke* (2nd edn). Cambridge: Cambridge University Press; 2008.

9. Chabriat H, Joutel A, Dichgans M, Tournier-Lasserve E, Bousser MG. CADASIL. *Lancet Neurol.* 2009;8:643–653.

10. Zarate YA, Hopkin RJ. Fabry's disease. *Lancet.* 2008;372:1427–1435.

11. Debette S, Leys D. Cervical-artery dissections: predisposing factors, diagnosis, and outcome. *Lancet Neurol.* 2009;8:668–678.

12. Touze E, Oppenheim C, Trystram D, Nokam G, Pasquini M, Alamowitch S, *et al.* Fibromuscular dysplasia of cervical and intracranial arteries. *Int J Stroke.* 2010;5:296–305.

13. Scott RM, Smith ER. Moyamoya disease and moyamoya syndrome. *N Engl J Med.* 2009;360:1226–1237.

14. Berlit P. Diagnosis and treatment of cerebral vasculitis. *Ther Adv Neurol Disord.* 2010;3:29–42.

15. Kurth T, Chabriat H, Bousser MG. Migraine and stroke: a complex association with clinical implications. *Lancet Neurol.* 2012;11:92–100.

16. Calabrese LH, Dodick DW, Schwedt TJ, Singhal AB. Narrative review: reversible cerebral vasoconstriction syndromes. *Ann Intern Med.* 2007;146:34–44.

17. Ducros A. Reversible cerebral vasoconstriction syndrome. *Lancet Neurol.* 2012;11:906–917.

18. Kenet G, Lutkhoff LK, Albisetti M, Bernard T, Bonduel M, Brandao L, *et al.* Impact of thrombophilia on risk of arterial ischemic stroke or cerebral sinovenous thrombosis in neonates and children. A systematic review and meta-analysis of observational studies. *Circulation.* 2010;121:1838–1847.

19. Saposnik G, Barinagarrementeria F, Brown RD, Bushnell CD, Cucchiara B, Cushman M, *et al.* Diagnosis and management of cerebral venous thrombosis. *Stroke.* 2011;42:1158–1192.

20. Zinkstok SM, Vergouwen MD, Engelter ST, Lyrer PA, Bonati LH, Arnold M, *et al.* Safety and functional outcome of thrombolysis in dissection-related ischemic stroke: A meta-analysis of individual patient data. *Stroke.* 2011;42:2515–2520.

21. Engelter ST, Dallongeville J, Kloss M, Metso TM, Leys D, Brandt T, *et al.*; Cervical Artery Dissection and Ischaemic Stroke Patients-Study Group. Thrombolysis in cervical artery dissection – data from the Cervical Artery Dissection and Ischaemic Stroke Patients (CADISP) database. *Eur J Neurol.* 2012;19:1199–1206.

CHAPTER 15

Secondary prevention of stroke

Thalia S. Field and Oscar R. Benavente

Introduction

Stroke is the second leading cause of death worldwide and the commonest cause of adult-acquired disability in most nations (1, 2). Recurrent strokes in particular account for a large proportion of morbidity and mortality, as repeat events tend to be more severe and more likely to result in disability and dementia (3).

The risk of recurrent stroke has diminished considerably in the context of medical, surgical, and administrative advances over the past three decades, and their widespread application. Namely, the introduction of antiplatelet agents, anticoagulation for atrial fibrillation (AF), blood pressure control, statin use, endarterectomy and stenting for symptomatic carotid disease, and rapid assessment after minor stroke and transient ischaemic attack (TIA), have all contributed to a reduced burden of recurrent stroke (4). In 1982, data from the population-based Framingham study found a 5-year risk of recurrent stroke of 42% in males and 24% in females; 5-year recurrence rate from the South London Stroke Register in 2003 was 16.6% (5, 6). In the Oxfordshire Community Stroke Project, the 5-year risk of recurrent stroke decreased by half between 1981–1986 (30% recurrence rate) and 2002–2010 (4, 7).

Rapid assessment of TIA and minor stroke is addressed in chapters 9 and 10; in this chapter we address major medical and surgical management for secondary prevention of ischaemic stroke and primary intracranial haemorrhage (ICH).

Antiplatelet therapy for non-cardioembolic ischaemic stroke

Antiplatelet therapy remains the mainstay of antithrombotic therapy for secondary prevention of non-cardioembolic ischaemic stroke. Currently, monotherapy with aspirin or clopidogrel or combination aspirin plus extended-release dipyridamole are all appropriate options for patients with non-cardioembolic ischaemic events. Though long-term use of combination aspirin–clopidogrel have not shown a significant benefit for secondary prevention and are associated with an excess risk of intracranial and systemic bleeding, the role of short-term combination antiplatelet therapy after minor stroke or TIA is currently under investigation. Major antiplatelet trials for secondary stroke prevention from 1995 onwards are summarized in Table 15.1.

Antiplatelets versus oral anticoagulation

Large randomized trials have not demonstrated superiority of warfarin over aspirin for secondary prevention of non-cardioembolic stroke (Table 15.2). There are no trials to date comparing the efficacy of novel oral anticoagulants to antiplatelet agents for secondary prevention of non-cardioembolic stroke.

Aspirin

Aspirin remains the most widely used antiplatelet agent for secondary prevention of ischaemic events. Aspirin was associated with a 22% reduction in stroke in a meta-analysis of secondary prevention trials, with a non-significant increase in intracranial haemorrhage with aspirin as compared to placebo (8). Aspirin has demonstrated efficacy for secondary stroke prevention for doses ranging from 30 mg to 1300 mg daily. Higher doses are associated with an increased risk of gastrointestinal bleeding and upset (9–13).

Aspirin plus dipyridamole

Combination aspirin plus dipyridamole demonstrated a small but significant benefit over aspirin monotherapy for secondary prevention in both the ESPS-2 and ESPRIT trials (12, 14). There was no excess of major bleeding in the combination antiplatelet group in either trial, though a large proportion (34%) of the combination group discontinued therapy in the ESPRIT trial, mostly due to headache.

Clopidogrel

There were no significant differences in stroke occurrence between the aspirin and clopidogrel groups in the CAPRIE trial, which randomized over 19,000 patients with a history of stroke, myocardial infarction (MI), or peripheral vascular disease to one of the two antiplatelet agents (15). There was a small but significant reduction of overall recurrent vascular events, however, in the clopidogrel group, which also had a lower rate of gastric side effects than the aspirin group.

Aspirin plus dipyridamole versus clopidogrel

Aspirin-dipyridamole and clopidogrel were compared directly in the PRoFESS trial, which was designed as a non-inferiority trial assessing the efficacy of one agent against the other for secondary stroke prevention in over 20,000 patients (16). Though there was no significant difference between groups with respect to stroke recurrence, aspirin–dipyridamole failed to meet non-inferiority due to an increased rate of major systemic haemorrhage and higher rates of discontinuation, mostly due to headache.

Aspirin plus clopidogrel

The efficacy of combination aspirin plus clopidogrel is yet to be fully clarified in clinical trials. Long-term studies of the agents in combination for secondary prevention have failed to demonstrate a significant benefit over antiplatelet monotherapy. Short-term

Table 15.1 Major randomized trials of antiplatelet therapy for long-term secondary prevention of non-cardioembolic stroke

Trial	n, patient population	Intervention (doses in mg)	Stroke mechanism	Time to enrolment after event	Follow-up	Primary endpoint	Efficacy	Major safety/ adverse event
ESPS-2 (12) 1996	**6602** with prior ischaemic stroke or TIA	Placebo; ASA 25 bid; ERDP 200 bid; ASA-ERDP 25/200 bid	–	Within 3 months	2 years	Stroke, death, and stroke or death together	ASA-ERDP vs ASA: 12.9% RRR (95% CI ±6.0%)	Rates of discontinuation due to bleeding highest in ASA (absolute rate, any bleeding 11.2%) and ASA-ERDP (1.3%) Rates of discontinuation due to headache highest in ERDP (8.0%) and ASA-ERDP (8.1%)
ESPRIT (14) 2006	**2739** with recent minor stroke or TIA	ASA 30–325 bid; ASA-ERDP 30–325/200 bid	Large vessel 30%; Small vessel 50%; Unspecified 20%	Within 6 months	Mean 3.5 years (SD 2.0)	All-cause vascular death, non-fatal stroke, non-fatal MI, major bleed	20% hazard reduction (95% CI, 2–34)	No significant difference in major bleeding, 34% in combination group discontinued treatment due to headache
CAPRIE (15) 1996	19,185 with history of stroke, MI, or PVD	ASA 325; Clopidogrel 75	History of stroke 33.5% History of MI 32.8% History of PVD 33.7%	1 week to 6 months	Mean 1.91 years	Ischaemic stroke, MI, or vascular death	All patients: 8.7% RRR (95% CI, 0.3–16.5); Stroke subgroup: 7.3% (–5.7 to 18.7)	No significant difference in major haemorrhage
PRoFESS (16) 2008	20,332	ASA-ERDP 25/200 bid; Clopidogrel 75	LA 28% CE 2% Small vessel 52% Other 2% Undetermined 16%	Within 90 days (median 15 days)	Mean 2.5 years	First recurrence of stroke	1% hazard reduction (95% CI, –8 to 11)	Major haemorrhage increased in DP group (HR, 1.15; 95% CI, 1.00–1.32), rates of discontinuation higher in DP group (6.5% absolute difference; 95% CI, 5.3–7.7), mostly due to headache
MATCH (17) 2004	**7599** with recent IS or TIA and at least one additional vascular risk factor who were already taking daily clopidogrel	Clopidogrel 75; ASA-C 81–162/75	1.8% CE 41.4% Small vessel 26.8% LA 0.9% Other 7.8% Unk	Within 3 months (median 15 days)	18 months	Composite of ischaemic stroke, MI, vascular death, or rehospitalisation for acute ischaemia	6.4% RRR (95% CI, –4.6 to 16.3); Ischaemic stroke: 7.1% (95% CI, –8.5 to 20.4)	1.3% absolute risk increase (1.3% vs 2.6%, 95% CI, 0.6–1.9) in major and life-threatening bleeding in combination group, no difference in fatal bleeding
CHARISMA (18) 2006	15,603 with clinically evident cardiovascular disease, documented cerebrovascular disease or multiple vascular risk factors	ASA 75–162; ASA-C 75/162/75	24% of participants with prior stroke	Symptomatic cerebrovascular disease criteria: stroke/TIA within 5 y	28 months	Composite of MI, stroke, or death from cardiovascular causes	Primary endpoint 6.8 % ASA-C vs 7.3 % ASA (RR, 0.93; 95% CI 0.83–1.05; P=0.22)	Non-significant increase in severe and fatal bleeding, significant increase in moderate bleeding in combination group (1.3% vs 2.1%, RR, 1.62; 95% CI, 1.27–2.08)
SPS3 (19) 2012	**3020** with MRI-proven clinically evident subcortical stroke	ASA 81; ASA-C 81/75	Small vessel disease	180 days (median 62)	Mean 3.4 y	Any recurrent stroke (ischaemic and haemorrhagic)	2.5%/yr ASA-C vs 2.7% ASA: HR 0.92% 95% CI 0.72–1.16	Mortality 77 deaths ASA vs 113 ASA-C, HR 1.52; 95% CI, 1.14 to 2.04; P=0.004. Major haemorrhage 1.1% ASA vs 2.1 % ASA-C, HR 1.97, 95% CI 1.41–2.71, p<0.001

AF: atrial fibrillation; ASA: aspirin; ASA-C: aspirin and clopidogrel; CE: cardioembolic; ICH: intracranial haemorrhage; IS: ischaemic stroke; LA: large artery; Lac: lacunar; MCA: middle cerebral artery; MI: myocardial infarction; RF: risk factor; TIA: transient ischaemic attack; Unk: unknown.

Table 15.2 Randomized trials comparing warfarin to antiplatelet therapy for secondary prevention of non-cardioembolic stroke (191)

Trial	Year	Patient population, n	Follow-up	Comparison	Primary outcome	Efficacy	Safety
SPIRIT	1997	1316 with stroke or TIA	14 months	ASA 30 mg/day Warfarin target INR 3.0–4.5	Vascular death, non-fatal stroke non-fatal MI or non-fatal major bleeding	4.1% in both groups (HR 1.03, 95% CI 0.6–0.71)	Major haemorrhage 8.1% warfarin and 1.0% ASA (HR 9.3, 95% CI 4.0–22)
WARSS	2001	2206 with ischaemic stroke	2 years	ASA 325 mg/day Warfarin target INR 1.4–2.8	Recurrent ischaemic stroke or death	17.8% warfarin, 16.0% ASA (HR 1.13, 95% CI 0.92–1.38)	No significant difference in major haemorrhage 2.22/100,000 pt-yrs warfarin, 1.49 ASA (RR 1.48, 95% CI 0.93–2.44)
WASID	2005	569 with stroke or TIA and intracranial stenosis 50–99%	1.8 years	ASA 1300 mg/day Warfarin target INR 2.0–3.0	Ischaemic and haemorrhagic stroke, vascular death	22.1% ASA, 21.8% warfarin (HR 1.04, 95% CI 0.73–1.48)	Major haemorrhage 3.2% ASA, 8.3% warfarin (HR 0.39, 95% CI 0.18–0.84), MI and sudden death 2.9% ASA, 7.3% warfarin (HR 0.40, 95% CI 0.18–0.91)
ESPRIT	2007	1068 with recent stroke or TIA	Mean 4.6 years (SD 2.2)	ASA 30–325 mg/day Warfarin target INR 2.0–3.0	Vascular death non-fatal stroke. Non-fatal MI, or major bleeding complication	18% ASA, 19% warfarin (HR 1.02, 95% CI 0.77–1.35) Post hoc ASA-EDRP vs warfarin (HR 1.31, 95% CI 0.98–1.75)	Major bleeding 8.4% warfarin, 3.4% ASA (HR 2.56, 95% CI 1.48–4.43)

ASA acetylsalicylic acid; ERDP extended-release dipyridamole; ESPRIT European/Australasian Stroke Prevention in Reversible Ischemia Trial; MI myocardial infarction; SPIRIT Stroke Prevention in Reversible Ischemia Trial; WARSS Warfarin-Aspirin Recurrent Stroke Study; WASID Warfarin-Aspirin Symptomatic Intracranial Disease study.

use (<3 months) of combination aspirin plus clopidogrel is still under investigation for secondary prevention in the acute post-stroke phase.

Both the MATCH and the CHARISMA trials failed to demonstrate superiority of combination antiplatelet therapy over clopidogrel (MATCH) or aspirin (CHARISMA) monotherapy for secondary prevention of recurrent ischaemic events (17, 18). The MATCH trial, which randomized 7599 patients with previous stroke/TIA to aspirin/clopidogrel versus clopidogrel alone, found no overall benefit for dual antiplatelet therapy for prevention of the primary endpoint, a composite of ischaemic stroke, MI, vascular death, or hospitalization for ischemia. Though there was an increased bleeding risk in the combination antiplatelet group, this did not become apparent until the third month of therapy. The CHARISMA trial compared aspirin plus clopidogrel to aspirin alone in 15,603 patients with symptomatic vascular disease or asymptomatic patients with multiple vascular risk factors. There were no differences between groups with respect to the primary event, a combination of stroke, MI, and vascular death. In contrast to MATCH, there was no difference in major intracranial or systemic haemorrhage between the monotherapy and combination antiplatelet groups.

The SPS3 trial found no benefit of combination aspirin plus clopidogrel over aspirin alone for prevention of recurrent ischaemic events in over 3000 patients with symptomatic lacunar infarcts (19). A non-significant reduction of recurrent ischaemic events was offset by a non-significant increase of intracranial haemorrhage in the dual antiplatelet group. There was an increase of all-cause mortality and increased risk of systemic haemorrhage in the dual antiplatelet group.

Based on results from the MATCH, CHARISMA, and SPS3 trials, which incorporated patients with multiple non-cardioembolic stroke types (MATCH and CHARISMA) and lacunar stroke (SPS3),

there is no indication for long-term use of combination aspirin and clopidogrel for secondary prevention of recurrent ischaemic stroke. Whether dual antiplatelet therapy may confer additional benefits for secondary prevention in the case of intracranial large vessel disease, which has the highest early recurrence rate, is uncertain.

In two small randomized trials, CLAIR and CARESS, single versus dual antiplatelet therapy were compared for reduction of microembolic signals on transcranial Doppler after recent symptomatic large artery disease. It is unclear as to whether the number, presence, or timing of detectable microemboli serve as a reliable marker for risk of recurrent ischemia (20, 21). Thus, the clinical implications of these trials are unclear.

In the SAMMPRIS trial (see 'Intracranial atherosclerotic disease' section), patients with symptomatic stenosis of at least 70% of a major intracranial artery were randomized to percutaneous stenting versus best medical therapy, consisting of 90 days of combination aspirin plus clopidogrel followed by aspirin alone, and aggressive management of blood pressure, hypercholesterolaemia, and lifestyle modification (22). Though there was a reduction in events in the medical management group, whether the use of dual antiplatelet therapy contributed significantly to the decreased event rate is unclear given that there was no single-platelet medical comparison group. The role for dual antiplatelet therapy for symptomatic intracranial stenosis thus remains uncertain.

Aspirin and clopidogrel for secondary prevention of early stroke recurrence

Data from the MATCH and FASTER trials raised the possibility that a short-term course of combination aspirin and clopidogrel may reduce recurrent ischaemic events in the immediate phase following stroke or TIA; the benefits of combination therapy in this context are currently under investigation in a number of randomized clinical trials (Table 15.3). In MATCH, the median time to enrolment after the index event was 15 days; in patients enrolled within 7 days there was a non-significant trend in favour of combination therapy. The FASTER trial randomized patients within 24 hours of stroke or TIA to aspirin versus aspirin/clopidogrel and simvastatin versus placebo in a 2×2 factorial design (23). The study, which was terminated prematurely due to poor recruitment, found a non-significant reduction in recurrent stroke in the combination antiplatelet group.

Data from the CHANCE trial suggest that, when initiated within 24 hours of stroke or TIA, stroke recurrence at 90 days is reduced by a short course (21 days) of combination aspirin/clopidogrel as compared with aspirin alone (24). Other ongoing prospective studies which are also investigating the role of short-term combination antiplatelet therapy in the acute phase after minor stroke and TIA, will determine if these findings will be replicated.

The CHANCE trial randomized 5170 Chinese patients and found that the hazard ratio at 90 days for the primary endpoint of ischaemic or haemorrhagic stroke was 0.68 (95% confidence interval (CI) 0.57–0.81, p <0.001) for the combination antiplatelet group (24, 25) The 90-day hazard ratio was 0.69 (95% CI 0.58–0.82, p <0.001) for the secondary endpoint of stroke, MI and vascular death. There was no difference in rates of haemorrhagic stroke (0.3% in each group) or moderate-to-severe extracranial haemorrhage (0.3% in each group). There was a non-significant increase in minor bleeding (1.2% vs 0.7%) in the combination group.

Implementation of other optimal secondary prevention strategies and post-stroke care in China and in the CHANCE population may differ from Western norms (26). Differences in proportions of stroke subtype, or other genetic, environmental, or undetermined factors may affect the benefit:risk ratio of combination antiplatelet therapy in other ongoing trials, thus whether results similar to that in CHANCE will be replicated has yet to be determined.

Secondary prevention of cardioembolic stroke

Cardioembolic stroke accounts for approximately one-fifth of all ischaemic stroke and is most commonly due to AF (27). With the exception of infective endocarditis, anticoagulation is the treatment of choice for secondary prevention of cardioembolic stroke from so-called 'major risk sources', which carry a substantial annual risk of embolization and high risk of recurrence (28). Choice of treatment is more controversial in the context of 'minor-risk' cardioembolic sources, which have the potential to cause stroke but do not have a high frequency of embolism or recurrence, and may be found incidentally.

Non-valvular atrial fibrillation

Non-valvular atrial fibrillation (NVAF) accounts for approximately 15% of all ischaemic stroke, and half of cardioembolic stroke. The embolic risks for paroxysmal and persistent AF are thought to be approximately equivalent (29). The attributable risk from AF increases with age: at age 50, 1.5% of ischaemic stroke is due to NVAF; at age 80, one-quarter is the result of AF (30). Both the prevalence of AF and the prevalence of associated stroke is expected to rise as the population ages; one US community survey found a 13% rise in the incidence of AF over the last two decades alone (31, 32). Furthermore, cardioembolic stroke in particular is associated with the highest burden of morbidity, mortality, and haemorrhagic transformation amongst ischaemic stroke subtypes. Therefore, an optimal secondary prevention in the context of NVAF is extremely important.

Unless a patient is known to have AF prior to or at the time of presentation with ischaemic stroke, detecting AF may be challenging. Sensitivity for detection of AF in an asymptomatic patient with conventional 24-hour Holter monitoring is approximately 5% (33). Detection of AF has been shown to improve with prolonged monitoring (34–36) and has been demonstrated to be superior to repeat Holter monitoring. The preliminary results of the EMBRACE trial, which randomized 572 patients over the age of 55 with recent cryptogenic stroke or TIA to a repeat Holter monitor versus 30-day event-triggered loop monitoring, found a 13% increase (3% vs 16%; 95% CI 9–18%, p <0.001) in detection of AF (37). However, devices for prolonged monitoring are not routinely available in the clinical setting.

Risk stratification for primary prevention of cardioembolic stroke due to AF is discussed elsewhere. The risk of recurrent stroke

Table 15.3 Ongoing and recently completed trials of short-term combination antiplatelet therapy for secondary prevention of acute ischaemic stroke and high-risk transient ischaemic attack

Trial	Intervention	Target enrolment, n	Time to enrolment	Primary outcome	Duration of follow-up
POINT (NCT00991029)	ASA ASA–C	4200	Within 12 hours	Vascular event rate	90 days
CHANCE[a] (NCT00979589)	ASA ASA–C	5100	Within 24 hours	Vascular event rate	3 months
COMPRESS[b] (NCT00814268)	ASA ASA–C	359	Within 48 hours	New DWI+ lesions on MRI	30 days
TARDIS (ISRCTN47823388)	ASA–DP–C ASA–DP	Start-up phase 350 Main phase 5000	Within 48 hours	Stroke severity at 90 days; recurrent stroke at 90 days is secondary outcome	90 days

ASA–C: aspirin plus clopidogrel; ASA–DP: aspirin plus dipyridamole; ASA–DP–C: aspirin plus dipyridamole plus clopidogrel.

[a] Completed; preliminary results announced February 2013.

[b] Recently completed.

is 6–10%/year after a cardioembolic stroke due to NVAF (38–40). A meta-analysis incorporating data from 29 randomized trials for primary and secondary prevention found that anticoagulation with dose-adjusted warfarin reduced the relative risk of stroke with NVAF by 64% (95% CI 49–74%) as compared with placebo/ no treatment or antiplatelet therapy (41). More recent trials have confirmed that combination antiplatelet therapy is also not a suitable option for secondary prevention in AF. The ACTIVE-W trial, which examined the use of combination aspirin–clopidogrel medication as an alternative to dose-adjusted warfarin in 6706 patients with AF, found a reduction in combined vascular endpoints (3.9%/ year vs 5.6%: relative risk (RR) 0.69; 95% CI 0.57–0.85) as well as stroke rates (2.39% vs 1.40%/year: RR=1.72; 95% CI 1.24–2.37, p=0.001) in the warfarin group. There was no significant difference in major bleeding (2.4% vs 2.2%) (42). The concurrent ACTIVE-A trial, which compared aspirin monotherapy versus combination aspirin–clopidogrel in 7554 patients unsuitable for warfarin, found an overall reduction of combined vascular events (6.8%/year vs 7.6%: RR 0.89; 95% 0.81–0.98, p=0.01) in the combination group, though the benefit of dual antiplatelet therapy for stroke prevention (2.4% vs 3.3%: RR 0.72; 95% CI 0.62–0.83) was marginal when rates of major bleeding were taken into account (2.0% vs 1.3% per year: RR 1.57; 95% CI 1.29–1.92) (43).

The challenges of maintaining safe and therapeutic levels of anticoagulation are well known, and even in the context of clinical trials, warfarin anticoagulation was only associated with an international normalized ratio (INR) in the target range of 2.0–3.0 approximately two-thirds of the time (44, 45). The efficacy of oral anticoagulation declines sharply when INR is subtherapeutic (46–48). In addition to exposing patients to potential risk of embolism when below target, INR above the therapeutic range is associated with an increased risk of serious or fatal haemorrhage. Intracranial haemorrhage accounts for approximately one-third of serious bleeding on warfarin therapy, but accounts for 90% of haemorrhage-associated deaths (49). Even with reversal, warfarin-associated intracranial haemorrhage, with a 75% risk of disability or death, has a higher rate of morbidity and mortality than spontaneous ICH (49–51). Risk of ICH is approximately doubled with an in-target INR and increases sharply thereafter, with a relative risk of haemorrhage of more than 8 with an INR greater than 4.0 (50, 52).

In recent years, several novel oral anticoagulants (NOACs) have been introduced for prevention of stroke and systemic embolism in NVAF. All available agents have been shown in large clinical trials to be equal, or, in the case of dabigatran 150 mg twice daily, superior to dose-adjusted warfarin for prevention of stroke and systemic embolism (43, 53–55). In addition, the rates of intracranial haemorrhage have been shown to be significantly lower with NOACs, though the mechanism by which this occurs has not yet been fully elucidated (Table 15.4; Figures 15.1 and 15.2). The proportion of participants with previous stroke, TIA, or systemic embolism varied markedly between studies (Table 15.4). In this subgroup, there was no significant benefit of NOACs over warfarin for prevention of recurrent stroke (AVERROES, which compared apixaban against aspirin, found a significant benefit in favour of apixaban for stroke prevention in the subgroup with a prior ischaemic event) (56) (Figure 15.3).

Given the improved safety, efficacy, and convenience associated with the NOACs over warfarin for NVAF, several guidelines now recommend that the NOACs be used for first-line primary and secondary prevention for stroke and systemic embolism in preference to (57, 58) or as an alternative to warfarin (59). However, challenges associated with these newer agents include increased cost, less established methods of coagulation monitoring, the lack of an effective antidote, partial renal clearance (with associated risk for accumulation in patients with severe renal insufficiency), and, in the case of dabigatran and apixaban, twice-daily dosing (60, 61). Furthermore, given that the NOACs have not been compared against one another in the context of a randomized trial, choice of agent is directed only by patient or physician preference and expert opinion.

Table 15.4 Trials demonstrating effectiveness of novel oral anticoagulants for stroke prevention in NVAF

Trial	Year	Comparison	Mechanism of NOAC	N	% with previous stroke/ TIA/systemic embolism	Design
RE-LY (43)	2009	Dabigatran 150 bid Dabigatran 110 bid Warfarin	Direct thrombin inhibitor	18113 AF + ≥1 RF	20.0%	Open-label (TTR 64%)
AVERROES (192)	2011	Apixaban 5 bid ASA 81 (64%)–325 od	Factor Xa inhibitor	5599 AF + ≥1 RF *Not suitable for warfarin*	13.6%	Double-blind
ROCKET-AF (53)	2011	Rivaroxaban 20 od Warfarin	Factor Xa inhibitor	14264 AF with 2–3 CHADS2 RF	54.7%	Double-blind (TTR 55%)
J-ROCKET-AF (55)	2012	Rivaroxaban 15 od Warfarin	Factor Xa inhibitor	1280 AF with ≥2 CHADS2 RF or LVEF ≥35%	63.5%	Double-blind (TTR 65%)
ARISTOTLE (54)	2011	Apixaban 5 bid Warfarin	Factor Xa inhibitor	18201 AF + ≥1 RF	19.4%	Double-blind (TTR 62%)

NOAC: novel oral anticoagulant; RF: risk factor for stroke or systemic embolism; TTR: time in therapeutic range for warfarin arm.

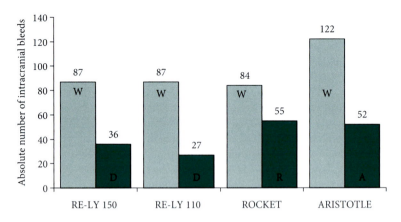

W = warfarin. D = dabigatran. R = rivaroxaban. A = apixaban

Fig. 15.1 Intracerebral bleeds in trials of warfarin versus NOAC in NVAF patients.

The role of surgical or endovascular therapy for AF is generally limited to those patients who cannot tolerate anticoagulation but are otherwise able to tolerate surgical or interventional therapy. Left atrial ligation has not been evaluated in large randomized trials. In the PROTECT-AF study, a non-inferiority trial, 707 patients with AF were randomized to percutaneous left atrial occlusion with a WATCHMAN device versus dose-adjusted warfarin. Patients in the endovascular group continued on warfarin for 45 days followed by combination aspirin–clopidogrel for 6 months. After a mean follow-up of 2.3 years, the endovascular group met non-inferiority criteria; the primary efficacy event, a composite of stroke, systemic embolism, and cardiovascular death occurred in 3.0% of the endo-vascular group and 4.3% in the control group (RR 0.71; 95% CI 0.44–1.30%/year) (62). The role for percutaneous occlusion for sec-ondary prevention, outside of clinical scenarios that preclude anti-coagulation for NVAF, has yet to be determined.

Mechanical valves

In older series, native valvular heart disease accounted for approxi-mately one-third of cardioembolic strokes (27), though most

patients now undergo surgical replacement with mechanical or bioprosthetic valves. Mechanical heart valves increase rate of thromboembolism through stasis inside the valve and by exposing the blood to the artificial valve surface (60).

A systematic review of observational studies incorporating 460 patients not on anticoagulants over 1225 patient-years of follow-up found a 1.8%/year risk of valve thrombosis, a 4.0% risk of major embolism, and 8.6%/year risk of any embolism, with a reduction of thromboembolic complication of approximately 75% in patients on dose-adjusted warfarin (63).

A meta-analysis of 11 trials including 2428 patients found that anti-platelet therapy in addition to dose-adjusted warfarin significantly reduced incidence of systemic embolism as compared to warfarin alone. Rates of minor bleeding, though not major bleeding or intra-cranial haemorrhage, were significantly increased (64). The American Heart Association (AHA)/American Stroke Association (ASA) recommends addition of aspirin 75–100 mg/day to dose-adjusted warfarin (target INR 2.5–3.5) for secondary prevention of stroke or systemic embolism in patients who have had an ischaemic stroke or systemic embolism in the context of therapeutic anticoagulation (28).

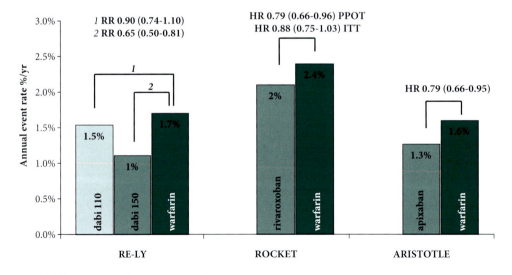

PPOT = per-protocol, on-treatment analysis
ITT = intention-to-treat analysis

Fig. 15.2 Stroke or systemic embolism in NVAF trials of NOAC versus warfarin.

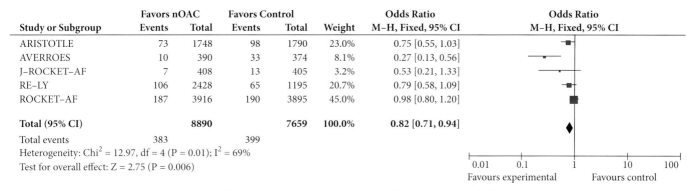

	Favors nOAC		Favors Control			Odds Ratio	Odds Ratio
Study or Subgroup	Events	Total	Events	Total	Weight	M–H, Fixed, 95% CI	M–H, Fixed, 95% CI
ARISTOTLE	73	1748	98	1790	23.0%	0.75 [0.55, 1.03]	
AVERROES	10	390	33	374	8.1%	0.27 [0.13, 0.56]	
J–ROCKET–AF	7	408	13	405	3.2%	0.53 [0.21, 1.33]	
RE–LY	106	2428	65	1195	20.7%	0.79 [0.58, 1.09]	
ROCKET–AF	187	3916	190	3895	45.0%	0.98 [0.80, 1.20]	
Total (95% CI)		**8890**		**7659**	**100.0%**	**0.82 [0.71, 0.94]**	
Total events	383		399				

Heterogeneity: Chi^2 = 12.97, df = 4 (P = 0.01); I^2 = 69%
Test for overall effect: Z = 2.75 (P = 0.006)

Fig. 15.3 Primary outcome in subgroup of patients with previous stroke, TIA, or systemic embolism in NVAF trials of NOAC.

Novel oral anticoagulants have not proven to be safe for prevention of stroke or systemic embolism in this group of patients. The randomized, open-label RE-ALIGN phase II trial, which compared dabigatran in doses ranging from 150–300 mg twice daily versus dose-adjusted warfarin in patients with mitral and/or aortic mechanical bileaflet valves, was halted early by the manufacturer due to an excess of thromboembolic events in participants and an increase in bleeding after surgery (65–67).

Acute myocardial infarction, cardiomyopathy, and left ventricular thrombus

Intracardiac thrombus may occur in one-third or more patients following a completed anterior MI, particularly if the infarct extends to the left ventricular (LV) apex (27, 68–71). Approximately 2.5% of patients overall and up to 10% with LV thrombus with acute MI experience stroke within 2–4 weeks of the event (68–71). The aggregate of available evidence examining both clinical and echocardiographic outcomes suggests that anticoagulation with warfarin or heparin reduces the risk of cerebral embolism and clot formation, although the optimal duration of therapy is unknown (69, 72–77). Current AHA/ASA guidelines recommend at least 3 months of oral anticoagulation with warfarin (target INR 2–3) for acute MI complicated by LV mural thrombus (28).

LV thrombus may also occur with chronic reduced LV ejection fraction. The annual rate of stroke in the context of congestive heart failure overall is approximately 2%, and risk for thromboembolism is proportional to the degree of LV systolic dysfunction and is markedly increased with concurrent AF (71, 78, 79). The indication for anticoagulation over antiplatelet therapy for stroke prevention in the context of depressed (≤35%) ejection fraction is unknown. The WATCH trial, which aimed to compare dose-adjusted warfarin with antiplatelet therapy for stroke prevention in heart failure, was terminated early due to lack of recruitment (80). The WARCEF trial, which randomized 2305 patients with LVEF 35% or lower (mean 25%±7.5) and sinus rhythm to aspirin 325 mg daily versus dose-adjusted warfarin (target INR 2.0–3.5) and followed for a mean of 3.5 years, found no significant difference between groups with regards to the primary outcome, a composite of ischaemic stroke, haemorrhage stroke, and death from any cause (7.47/100 patient years (pt-yr) vs 7.93: hazard ratio (HR) 0.93 (0.79–1.10)). Risk of ischaemic stroke was significantly decreased in the warfarin group (0.72/100 pt-yr vs 1.36: HR 0.52 (0.33–0.82), p=0.005) and there was no significant difference between groups with regards

to risk of ICH (0.12/100 pt-yr vs 0.05, HR 2.22 (0.43–11.66). The authors found no overall compelling indication for use of warfarin over aspirin in this patient group (62). The role, if any, for novel anticoagulants in this patient group has not yet been determined.

Patent foramen ovale

Approximately 25–30% of asymptomatic people have been shown to have a patent foramen ovale (PFO) in previous pathological series (81). Therefore, even if a PFO is found during investigations for the cause of stroke, there is a high probability that the defect is an incidental finding. Features on history or investigations that are thought to contribute to the likelihood of the PFO being implicated in stroke pathology include proximate or concurrent deep vein thrombosis/pulmonary embolism or venous hypercoagulable state, a history of Valsalva at the time of onset, and an associated atrial septal aneurysm (82).

In the PFO-ASA study, an observational study following 581 patients with cryptogenic stroke aged 18–55 for 4 years, 52% had no atrial septal defects and 37% had an isolated PFO. Of patients with stroke and PFO, 2.3% went on to have a recurrent event on aspirin 300 mg daily, as compared with 15.2% of patients with PFO and atrial septal aneurysm. In patients without any cardiac abnormalities, 4.2% experienced recurrence, while no patients with isolated atrial septal aneurysms experienced another event (83).

Available evidence from randomized trials suggests that there is no indication for routine percutaneous closure of PFO for secondary prevention. The CLOSURE I study, which randomized 909 patients aged 60 or under with cryptogenic stroke to percutaneous close with a STARFlex device versus medical therapy found no benefit in the closure group over 2 years of follow-up (primary end point of stroke, TIA, or systemic embolism 23 vs 29 events; 5.5% closure vs 6.8%: HR 0.78, 95% CI 0.45–1.35) and a higher rate of major vascular events and AF with device placement that was largely periprocedural (84). In the RESPECT trial, which randomized 980 patients to PFO closure versus medical therapy and followed patients for a mean of 2.5 years, there was a non-significant reduction in events in the procedural group (9 strokes vs 16: HR 0.49; 95% CI 0.22–1.11, p=0.08) (85). The PC Trial randomized 414 patients under the age of 60 with ischaemic stroke or TIA to PFO closure with an Amplatzer device versus medical therapy (either antiplatelet or anticoagulation at the investigator's discretion). There was a no significant reduction in the primary endpoint of death, non-fatal stroke, TIA, and peripheral embolism in the closure group (7 vs 11 events: HR 0.63; 95% CI 0.24–1.62). Mean follow-up was 4.1 years in the closure group and

Table 15.5 Trials of closure of patent foramen ovale versus medical therapy for cryptogenic stroke

Trial	Year	N, patient population	Comparison	Primary outcome	Follow-up	Annual stroke rate	Results
CLOSURE-I (84)	2012	909; Age 18–60 with cryptogenic stroke/TIA and PFO Mean age 45 y	PFO closure with STARFlex septal closure system vs medical therapy (warfarin INR 2.0–3.0, ASA 325, or both at discretion of site PI)	Stroke or TIA over 2 years, death from any cause over first 30 days, death from neurological cause from 31 days–2 years	2 years	**Closure:** 1.45% **Med:** 1.55%	*Primary endpoint:* 23 procedure vs 29 medical events (5.5% vs 6.8%), HR 0.78, 95% CI 0.45–1.35 *Stroke:* 3.1% vs 3.1%, (HR 0.94, 95% CI 0.43–2.07)
RESPECT (85)	2013	980; Age 18–60 with cryptogenic stroke/ TIA and PFO Mean age 45.9 y	PFO closure with Amplatzer PFO occluder vs medical therapy (ASA, warfarin, clopidogrel, ASA-dipyridamole at discretion of site PI)	Recurrent non-fatal or fatal ischaemic stroke or early death after randomization	2559 pts/yr mean 2.6 year (SD 2.0)	**Closure:** 0.65% **Med:** 1.34%	*Primary endpoint (all events were non-fatal ischaemic stroke):* 23 vs 29 events (1.8% vs 3.3% HR 0.49, 95% CI 0.22–1.11)
PC Trial (86)	2013	414; Age 18–60 with cryptogenic stroke/ TIA or peripheral embolism and PFO Mean age 44 y	PFO closure with Amplatzer PFO occluder vs medical therapy (ASA, thienopyridine, oral anticoagulation or no medication at discretion of PI)	Stroke or TIA over 2 years, death from any cause over first 30 days, death from neurologic cause from 31 days–2 years	1780 patient-years, mean 4.1 years in closure and 4.0 years in medical	**Closure:** 0.12% **Med:** 0.6%	*Primary endpoint:* 7 vs 12 events (3.4% vs 5.2%), HR 0.63, 95% CI 0.24–1.62) *Stroke:* 1 vs 5 (0.5% vs 2.4%, (HR 0.20, 95% CI 0.02–1.72)

PFO: patent foramen ovale.

4.0 years in the medical group (86) (Table 15.5). PFO closure for stroke of unknown cause remains controversial amongst clinicians (87), though given the existing data we do not advocate routine PFO closure over medical therapy for stroke of unknown cause at this time (Table 15.5; Figure 15.4).

Over 50% of atrial septal aneurysms may be associated with right-to-left shunt (88). In the PFO-ASA study, those with a PFO and associated septal aneurysm comprised approximately 10% of the study population and had a significantly higher rate of stroke recurrence than those with a PFO alone (83), though the evidence to guide decisions with regards to closure versus antiplatelet or anticoagulation therapy is lacking (84, 89) and is currently at the discretion of the patient and treating physician.

Blood pressure control

Hypertension is the most important modifiable risk factor for both ischaemic and haemorrhagic stroke, accounting for 35–50% of attributable risk (1, 90). Nearly 30% of the world adult population is hypertensive, and more than a third of modifiable stroke risk worldwide is attributable to elevated blood pressure in previous population-based series (1, 91).

There is a well-established log-linear relationship between both systolic and diastolic blood pressure and risk of primary cerebrovascular events (92). Meta-analyses have found that risk increases above 115 mmHg systolic and 75 mmHg diastolic though no clear 'safe' threshold has been established in the literature (90, 92). The association between systolic pressures and stroke risk is stronger than that of diastolic pressure (92–94). Hypertension is also more strongly associated with risk of haemorrhagic stroke than for ischaemic stroke, though it remains the most important modifiable risk factor for both stroke types.

Trials of blood pressure lowering have shown a similar association between reduction of systolic and diastolic pressure and risk of secondary cerebrovascular events after initial stroke or TIA (95–97). In a pooled analysis of seven randomized trials published before 2002 examining risk of recurrent vascular events with antihypertensive treatment in patients with previous ischaemic or haemorrhagic stroke or TIA, antihypertensive therapy was associated with collective risk reduction of recurrent stroke, MI, and all vascular events of 24% (OR 0.76; 95% CI 0.63–0.92), 21% (OR 0.79; 95% CI 0.63–0.98), and 21% (OR 0.79; CI 0.66–0.95) respectively. The benefits of antihypertensive treatment occurred in both hypertensive and normotensive subjects on subgroup analysis. Larger blood pressure reductions were associated with greater risk reduction for recurrent stroke (Table 15.6).

The association between degree of blood pressure reduction and risk reduction for secondary stroke was illustrated by the PROGRESS trial. The study randomized over 6000 patients (mean baseline blood pressure 147/86 mmHg) with previous stroke (ischaemic or haemorrhagic) or TIA to an antihypertensive regimen of perindopril 4 mg daily or placebo; indapamide 2.5 mg daily, a thiazide diuretic, was added as per the treating physician's discretion in the perindopril group as necessary. There was an overall blood pressure reduction of 9/4 mmHg in the treatment arm with a relative risk reduction (RRR) for fatal or non-fatal stroke of 28% (95% CI 17–38%). The benefits of therapy were most robust in the combination antihypertensive group with a blood pressure reduction of 12/5 mmHg and a RRR of 43% (95% CI 30–54%); the perindopril-only group had a lesser reduction (5/3 mmHg) and non-significant benefit on recurrent stroke (RRR 5%; 95% CI 19–23%). The significant associations of antihypertensive therapy with blood pressure reduction and risk reduction for stroke and all major vascular events were sustained in both hypertensive and normotensive participants (98).

A Primary outcome

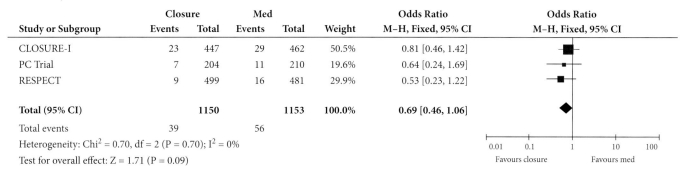

B Stroke outcome

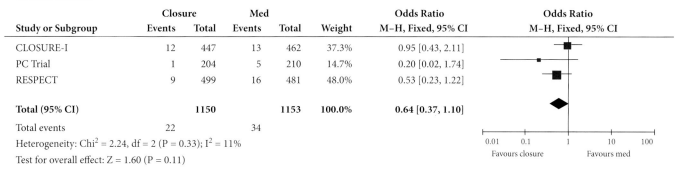

Fig. 15.4 Randomized trials of closure devices versus medical therapy in PFO patients. (A) Primary outcomes. (B) Stroke outcomes.

Table 15.6 Antihypertensive therapy trials for secondary stroke prevention comparing therapy to placebo (or no treatment)

Study	Year	N	Medication	Baseline blood pressure (mmHg)	Reduction in blood pressure (mmHg)	Results (95% CI)
HSCSG (193)	1974	452	Deserpine 1 mg daily + methylclothiazide 10 mg daily vs placebo	167/100	25.0/12.3	RR 0.78 (0.54–1.11)
Dutch TIA (194)	1993	1473	Atenolol 50 mg daily vs placebo	157/91	5.8/2.9	HR 0.82 (0.57–1.19)
TEST (195)	1995	720	Atenolol 50 mg daily vs placebo	161/88	4.0/3.0	RR 1.00 (0.75–1.35)
PROGRESS (98)	2001	6105 (1281 perindopril-only)	Perindopril 4 mg daily vs placebo	144/84	4.9/2.8	RRR 5% (−19%–23%)
PROGRESS (98)	2001	6105 (1770 combination)	Perindopril 4 mg daily + indapamide 2.5 mg daily vs double placebo	149/87	12.5/5.0	RRR 43% (30–54%)
HOPE (196)	2002	1013	Ramipril up to 10 mg daily	139/79	3.1/1.7	RRR 15% (−42%–30%)
FEVER (197)	2005	2368	Hydrochlorothiazide 12.5 md daily + (ER felodipine 5 mg daily vs placebo)	160/93	4.0/1.8	OR 0.81 (0.58–1.13)
SCOPE (198)	2005	194	Candesartan 8–16 mg daily vs placebo	166/90	3.6/1.6	RR 0.36 (0.18–0.73)
PRoFESS (99)	2008	20332	Telmisartan 80 mg daily vs placebo	144/84	3.8/2.0	HR 0.95 (0.86–1.04)
PATS (96)	2009	5665	Indapamide 2.5 mg daily	154/93	6.8/3.3	HR 0.69 (0.54–0.89)
SPS3	2013	3020	Blood pressure targets	145/80	138 & 127 (higher and lower target)	HR 0.81 (0.64–1.03)

[a] Thiazide diuretic, methyldopa, or bethanidine, guanthetidine, debrisoquine with or without adjunct methyldopa.

The PRoFESS trial demonstrated a similar non-significant benefit with a small blood pressure reduction in the treatment arm. The study randomized 20,332 patients (mean blood pressure 144/84 mmHg) with previous non-cardioembolic ischaemic stroke to telmisartan 80 mg daily or placebo. Blood pressure was lowered 4/2 mmHg in the telmisartan group; there was no significant reduction of recurrent stroke (HR 0.95; 95% CI 0.86–1.04) or major vascular events (HR 0.94; 95% CI 0.87–1.01). The authors attributed the lack of significant benefit in part to a lower mean blood pressure in the study group than in the PROGRESS trial and the modest reduction in blood pressure in the treatment arm. In addition, there was widespread use of other antihypertensive therapies in both the treatment and placebo groups (99).

A proportional risk-reduction per degree of systolic blood pressure lowering to similar that of the PROGRESS trial was sustained in a meta-regression analysis of the seven randomized antihypertensive trials published before 2002, where a 10 mmHg greater reduction in systolic blood pressure was associated with a reduction in risk of stroke of 31% ($R^2=0.71$) (90).

Though the benefits associated an approximate 10/5 mmHg reduction have been demonstrated, whether there is superior benefit of lowering blood pressure by a certain amount or to a particular absolute target is uncertain.

In addition, whether one particular class of antihypertensive medications or combination of medications confers superior protection against recurrent stroke is also uncertain as few trials have directly compared agents after stroke or TIA. The MOSES trial randomized 1405 hypertensive patients (mean office blood pressure 152/87 mmHg) with a history of ischaemic stroke, ICH, or TIA to receive 600 mg daily of eprosartan, an angiotensin receptor blocker, or 10 mg daily of nitrendipine, a calcium-channel blocker. The study included both multiple recurrent events and TIAs as primary end points in addition to ischaemic stroke and ICH. Blood pressure reduction was similar in both study groups with a reduction of 13/3 mmHg in the eprosartan group and 16/7 in the nitrendipine group. The study concluded that eprosartan conferred superior protection against secondary events (primary endpoints incidence density ratio (IDR) 0.79, 95% CI 0.66–0.96; cerebrovascular endpoint IDR 0.75; 95% CI 0.58–0.97), however, the difference in benefit was due mostly to a reduction in rate of TIA; there was no significant reduction in rates of recurrent ischaemic stroke. A significant proportion of participants in both groups were also taking additional antihypertensive medications during the course of the study (100).

Recently the results of The Secondary Prevention of Small Subcortical Strokes (SPS3) trial were presented. SPS3 examined the role of aggressive blood pressure in patients with symptomatic cerebral small vessel disease (101, 102). All 3020 patients were enrolled within 6 months of a symptomatic MRI-proven lacunar infarct and were randomized to less aggressive versus more aggressive blood pressure targets (systolic blood pressure 130–149 mmHg versus <130 mmHg); choice of antihypertensive agents was at the discretion of the site investigator. Approximately three-quarters of patients in the less aggressive arm and approximately two-thirds in the more aggressive arm achieved target blood pressure. Primary outcome was all recurrent stroke; mean follow-up was 3.7 years. There was almost a 20% non-significant reduction in all stroke in the lower target group (2.8%/year higher target vs 2.3%/year lower target: HR 0.81; 95% CI 0.64–1.03, p=0.08). When subdivided by stroke type, there was a two-third significant reduction in

haemorrhagic stroke (16 vs 6 events, 0.29%/year vs 0.11%/year: HR 0.37; 95% CI 0.15–0.95). Aggressive blood pressure treatment was well tolerated. There were 23 serious events related to hypotension (orthostatic syncope, stroke, MI, fall with injury, other) in the aggressively-treated group (0.40%/pt-year), half of which were syncopal events, and 15 (0.26% /pt-year) in the less aggressive group (HR 1.53; 95% CI 0.80–2.93, p=0.20). The results of the SPS3 BP target trial are best considered in the context of prior trials of long-term blood pressure lowering in patients with prior stroke and are congruent with their results (Table 15.6). For secondary prevention of lacunar stroke, we feel that a target blood pressure of <130 mmHg is overall achievable, safe, well tolerated, and reduces risk of recurrent stroke, haemorrhagic stroke in particular.

Current AHA/ASA and Scottish guidelines recommend the combination of a diuretic and an angiotensin-converting enzyme inhibitor on the basis of the PROGRESS trial as first-line antihypertensive therapy after stroke or TIA (Table 15.7).

Recent evidence suggests the variability of blood pressure—unprovoked high or low fluctuations independent of mean blood pressure—over weeks to months may also pose additional risk for both primary and recurrent stroke. A re-analysis of data from the UK-TIA secondary stroke prevention trial demonstrated elevated hazard ratios for cerebrovascular and cardiovascular events in patients with increased visit-to-visit blood pressure variability, as demonstrated by higher standard deviations and other measures of variability both dependent and independent of mean blood pressure (top-decile HR for SD systolic blood pressure over seven visits 6.22; 95% CI 4.16–9.29). Both variability and maximum systolic blood pressure were more predictive of risk of recurrent ischaemic events (103).

The same authors have hypothesized that additional protection against primary or secondary stroke may be conferred by certain antihypertensive drugs in part due to reducing blood pressure variability, though to date this conclusion is reached primarily from re-analysis of data from groups of participants (103–106) or primary prevention trials (103, 107) as opposed to individual patient data. Further prospective studies are required to further investigate the relationship between variability, risk of stroke, and the possible role of antihypertensive medication in mitigating risk.

To date, there is no specific prospective published data from large randomized trials to guide therapy for secondary prevention of other specific ischaemic stroke subtypes other than patients with small vessel disease. We exercise caution with regards to aggressive blood pressure reduction in the context of severe large artery disease, particularly in patients with poor collateralization on vascular imaging. A meta-analysis comparing risk of secondary ischaemic stroke on medical therapy in study cohorts with high (ECST and NASCET) versus low (UK-TIA) prevalence of carotid disease found that risk of stroke increased in both cohorts with increased blood pressure, but the association was less steep in the group with symptomatic carotid disease. In addition, an inverse relationship was seen in patients with at least 70% stenosis, but not unilateral carotid occlusion (95).

Blood pressure lowering after intracranial haemorrhage

Hypertension is the most important modifiable risk factor for spontaneous ICH. Highest rates of recurrence are amongst patients with lobar haemorrhages, thought to be more often associated with cerebral amyloid angiopathy than with hypertension. The risk of recurrence of lobar haemorrhage in previous series is two- to fourfold that

Table 15.7 Summary of current guidelines for blood pressure reduction for secondary stroke prevention

AHA/ASA	Canadian	Australian	ESO	SIGN
Ischaemic stroke BP reduction is recommended for both prevention of recurrent stroke and prevention of other vascular events in persons who have had an ischaemic stroke or TIA and are beyond the first 24 hours (*Class I; Level of Evidence A*) Because this benefit extends to persons with and without a documented history of hypertension, this recommendation is reasonable for all patients with ischaemic stroke or TIA who are considered appropriate for blood pressure reduction (*Class IIa; Level of Evidence B*). An absolute target blood pressure level and reduction are uncertain and should be individualized, but benefit has been associated with an average reduction of approximately 10/5 mmHg, and normal blood pressure levels have been defined as <120/80 mmHg by JNC 7 (*Class IIa; Level of Evidence B*). Several lifestyle modifications have been associated with blood pressure reduction and are a reasonable part of a comprehensive antihypertensive therapy (*Class IIa; Level of Evidence C*). These modifications include salt restriction; weight loss; consumption of a diet rich in fruits, vegetables, and low-fat dairy products; regular aerobic physical activity; and limited alcohol consumption. The optimal drug regimen to achieve the recommended level of reduction is uncertain because direct comparisons between regimens are limited. The available data indicate that diuretics or the combination of diuretics and an ACEI are useful (*Class I; Level of Evidence A*). The choice of specific drugs and targets should be individualized on the basis of pharmacological properties, mechanism of action, and consideration of specific patient characteristics for which specific agents are probably indicated (e.g. extracranial cerebrovascular occlusive disease, renal impairment, cardiac disease, and diabetes) (*Class IIa; Level of Evidence B*). *ICH* After the acute ICH period, absent medical contraindications, blood pressure should be well controlled, particularly for patients with ICH location typical of hypertensive vasculopathy (*Class I; Level of Evidence: A*). After the acute ICH period, a goal target of a normal blood pressure of <140/90 (<130/80 if diabetes or chronic kidney disease) is reasonable (*Class IIa; Level of Evidence: B*)	***All patients*** Patients with ischaemic stroke who are beyond the hyper-acute period should be prescribed antihypertensive treatment to target normal blood pressure. (*Evidence Level A*) Target blood pressure levels as per the Canadian Hypertension Education Program (CHEP) guidelines for prevention of stroke and other vascular events. —For the prevention of recurrent stroke in patients with diabetes or chronic kidney disease: <130 mmHg systolic and <80 mmHg diastolic. —Lowering blood pressure is recommended in patients with blood pressure <140/90 who have had a stroke	***All patients*** All stroke and TIA patients, whether normotensive or hypertensive, should receive blood pressure lowering therapy, unless contraindicated by symptomatic hypotension. (*Level A*) New blood pressure lowering therapy should commence before discharge for those with stroke or TIA, or soon after TIA if the patient is not admitted. (*Level B*)	*Ischaemic stroke* It is recommended that blood pressure be checked regularly. Blood pressure lowering is recommended after the acute phase, including in patients with normal blood pressure (*Class I, Level A*)	***All patients*** All patients with a previous stroke or TIA should be considered for treatment with an ACE inhibitor (e.g. perindopril) and thiazide (e.g. indapamide) regardless of blood pressure, unless contraindicated. (*Level A*) Patients with hypertension should be treated to <140/85 mmHg (<130/80 mmHg for patients with diabetes). (*Level D*)

of deep ICH in locations more typically associated with hypertensive haemorrhage (basal ganglia, thalamus, brainstem) (108, 109).

There are no dedicated trials examining blood pressure control in secondary prevention of spontaneous ICH and it is uncertain as to whether optimal targets for blood pressure reduction differ with respect to ischaemic versus haemorrhagic stroke. Patients with primary spontaneous ICH form a minority of subjects from secondary stroke prevention trials; data from the PROGRESS trial (ICH patients) found that patients in the combination therapy group had a significantly lower risk of first ICH (HR 0.44; 95% CI 0.28–0.69) and a non-significant reduction in recurrent ICH in the context of a small number of events with insufficient statistical power. There was a reduction in rates of both lobar and deep ICH (98).

Cholesterol

Epidemiological studies distinguishing ischaemic from haemorrhagic stroke have found an increased association between elevated lipid levels and ischaemic stroke, though the association is less robust than that between dyslipidaemia and ischaemic heart disease (IHD) (110). The weaker association with ischaemic stroke as compared to IHD may be due to heterogeneous stroke mechanisms; the available evidence suggests that large artery and small vessel stroke in particular are associated with elevated low-density lipoprotein (LDL) levels (111–113). Elevated total cholesterol, LDL, and triglycerides, and lower high-density lipoprotein (HDL) levels are associated with increased risk of ischaemic stroke (114–118). In addition to LDL, triglycerides have also been associated with large artery stroke in particular (119).

In a recent meta-analysis of 32 prospective studies (over 173,000 patients) on vascular risk and lipid levels, associated risk of coronary heart disease with low, intermediate, and very-low-density lipoprotein was fourfold that of ischaemic stroke, though there remained a modest association of ischaemic stroke with those atherogenic lipid fractions. Neither triglyceride nor HDL levels were independently associated with risk of stroke. There was no additional predictive value of apolipoprotein B or apoAI levels, and hazard ratios were not significantly affected by whether subjects had fasting lipid profiles or not (120). There was no association between lipid levels and haemorrhagic stroke, though several epidemiological studies have found, for unestablished reasons, an inverse association between haemorrhagic stroke and both serum cholesterol and LDL (114, 115, 121). Future studies examining individual stroke types will help to clarify this relationship.

The relationship between cholesterol-lowering drugs and stroke prevention is less than straightforward, as not all cholesterol-lowering medications are associated with modified risk of stroke. HMG-CoA reductase inhibitors (statins) are associated with both LDL reduction and with decreased risk of stroke as compared with placebo. Studies of statins for LDL reduction in primary and secondary prevention have shown a strong association between statin use and decreased risk of vascular events. A meta-analysis of all statin trials for primary and secondary vascular risk found a 21.1% relative risk reduction (95% CI 6.3%–33.5%) of stroke for every 1 mmol/L decrease in LDL cholesterol (122).

The SPARCL trial, which randomized 4731 patients with previous stroke or TIA (67% ischaemic stroke, 31% TIA, and 2% haemorrhagic) with 6 months of their event to atorvastatin 80 mg daily or placebo, found a decreased rate of recurrent fatal and non-fatal ischaemic stroke. There was a mean reduction on LDL of 1.4 mmol/L in the statin group. The atorvastatin arm had a significant reduction in fatal and non-fatal stroke (adjusted HR 0.84; 95% CI 0.71–0.99) and in all coronary events (HR 0.58; 95% CI 0.46–9.73), but not in overall mortality. A post hoc analysis found an increased risk of haemorrhagic stroke (HR 1.66; 95% CI 1.08–2.55) and decreased risk of ischaemic stroke (HR 0.78; 95% CI 0.66–0.94) with atorvastatin (123, 124). Haemorrhagic stroke was associated in univariate analysis with index haemorrhagic event (HR 5.65; 95% CI 2.82–11.30), male sex (HR 1.79; 95% CI 1.13–2.84), increased age (10-year increments, HR 1.42; 95% CI 1.16–1.74), and with stage 2 hypertension at the last study visit in multivariable analysis (HR 6.19; 95% CI 1.47–26.11). There was no association in the post hoc analysis between haemorrhagic risk and baseline LDL or cholesterol level, or recent LDL in treated patients (124). The authors suggested that the antithrombotic effect of statins may have contributed to the increased incidence of haemorrhage in the treatment arm (124).

The HPS study enrolled 3280 patients with a history of cerebrovascular disease (non-disabling ischaemic stroke, TIA or history of carotid intervention) no earlier than 6 months after their qualifying event, as well as 17,256 participants with other occlusive arterial disease or diabetes. Patients were randomized to receive simvastatin 40 mg daily or placebo. The treatment group had an average LDL reduction of 1 mmol/L and a significant reduction in first stroke as compared with placebo, though there was no significant reduction in rates of secondary stroke in the subset of participants with cerebrovascular disease. The results, which were unexpected, have been attributed to inclusion of heterogeneous stroke mechanisms, including haemorrhagic stroke, amongst the primary endpoints, as well as a significant time lapse (mean enrolment time 4.3 years post event) between index events and time to enrolment, beyond which the highest-risk period for a recurrent stroke had passed. There was a non-significant increase in haemorrhagic stroke (HR 1.91; 95% CI 0.92–3.96) in the treatment arm (125, 126).

Use of other LDL-lowering medications, however, including fibrates, resins, and dietary interventions, have not yielded similar risk reductions for stroke (127, 128). The protective mechanism of statins is thought to extend beyond cholesterol alone. The so-called pleiotropic effects of this class of medication are not entirely understood but they are thought to include anti-inflammatory, plaque-stabilizing, and antithrombotic effects, and improvement of endothelial function (126).

No studies in triglyceride reduction have been performed in a population with previous stroke. The VA-HIT trial found an association between gemfibrozil use and decreased risk of first stroke (RRR 31%; 95% CI 2–52%) in a population with IHD and low HDL. Plasma triglycerides were reduced 31% and HDL was increased by 10% in the treatment arm, though there was no significant effect on LDL levels (129).

Nicotinic acid, which increases HDL cholesterol and reduces LDL and triglycerides, is associated with a non-significant trend towards decreased risk of primary and secondary stroke and a significant decrease in carotid intima media thickness in meta-analysis (13). It is not well tolerated due to the side-effects of flushing, with a 55.4% discontinuation rate over 12 months in over 14,000 patients on extended release niacin (131).

Targets for LDL reduction for optimal secondary prevention of stroke are uncertain and are currently under investigation. In a post hoc analysis of the SPARCL trial, RRR for stroke was 28% for LDL concentrations of 1.8 mmol/L or lower as compared with higher than 2.6 mmol/L (132). Trials examining primary prevention of stroke amongst their endpoints have found that lower LDL levels are associated with decreased risk of stroke. In a meta-analysis of primary prevention trials using intensive versus standard statin therapy, there was a 13% (95% CI 4–22%) reduction in risk of risk of stroke and 16% (95% CI 8–24%) reduction in cardiovascular events in the intensive arm (122). In the Treating to New Targets trial, which randomized 10,001 patients with pre-existing coronary artery disease to high-dose (80 mg daily) or low-dose (10 mg) atorvastatin, there was a 25% reduction (HR 0.75; 95% CI 0.59–0.96) in risk of fatal and non-fatal stroke in the high-dose statin group (mean LDL 2.0 mmol/L) as compared to the low-dose group (mean LDL 2.6 mmol/L) over a 5-year follow-up period (118).

Though there is conflicting data from previous meta-analyses using primary prevention trials regarding the risk of haemorrhage with statin use, data from SPARCL suggest that patients with previous primary ICH are at increased risk for recurrent haemorrhage with statin therapy, particularly in the context of hypertension (124). Lowered LDL levels were not associated with haemorrhage risk in the SPARCL trial. We avoid use of statins in patients with previous primary ICH unless there are compelling indications from the perspective cardiovascular atherothrombotic risk and aim to ensure that blood pressure is well controlled in these patients. However, there is no general consensus regarding this practice.

Carotid surgery or stenting for symptomatic carotid disease

Carotid surgery

Carotid endarterectomy

Natural history data for stroke recurrence from symptomatic extracranial carotid stenosis is derived from older trials where

Table 15.8 Risk of ipsilateral stroke, perioperative stroke, and perioperative death by degree of stenosis in ECST, NASCET, and VACS (139)

Study	Year	Mean follow-up time	% stenosis	Ipsilateral ischaemic stroke and operative stroke or death (n/N)		Risk ratio (95% CI)
				Surgery	No surgery	
ECST	2003	**3** y	Near-occlusion	12/78	5/47	1.45 (0.54–3.85)
			70–99%	21/257	45/172	0.31 (0.19–0.51)
			50–69%	46/380	32/266	1.01 (0.66–1.54)
			30–49%	41/302	21/185	1.20 (0.73–1.96)
			<30%	84/783	37/538	1.56 (1.08–2.26)
NASCET	1998	**2.7** y	Near-occlusion	12/79	12/67	0.85 (0.41–1.76)
			70–99%	29/261	72/264	0.41 (0.27–0.61)
			50–69%	55/428	78/428	0.71 (0.51–0.97)
			30–49%	41/302	21/185	1.20 (0.73–1.96)
			<30%	27/212	28/213	0.97 (0.59–1.59)
VASCT	1991	**11.9** mo	70–99%	6/71	3/70	1.97 (0.51–7.58)
			50–69%	2/20	1/27	2.7 (0.26–27.74)

best medical optimization was most consistently comprised of only antiplatelet medications. In NASCET, 98% of patients were on antithrombotic therapy at the end of follow-up; 60% were taking antihypertensive medication and 15% lipid-lowering therapy at baseline (133). Current medical treatments, including antiplatelets, treatment of hypertension, glycaemic control, use of statins, and smoking cessation has led to lower risk of recurrent ischaemic stroke of all subtypes; statins in particular have been associated with decreased carotid plaque volume in human subjects and *in vitro* (134–136).

Data derived from the ECST trial and validated using the NASCET trial have been used to stratify risk of recurrent stroke based on patient age, sex, degree of carotid stenosis, presenting event (transient monocular blindness, hemispheric TIA, minor stroke, major stroke), time since last symptomatic event, and plaque characteristics (ulcerated versus smooth). So-called 'best medical therapy' from the non-surgical arms of the trial, from which recurrent stroke risk is calculated, does not uniformly include current best practices, including statin use (137).

The benefit of carotid endarterectomy (CEA) for symptomatic extracranial carotid stenosis has been established from three large randomized clinical trials (VACST, NASCET, ECST) and in pooled analysis (133, 138–142). A pooled analysis of the three trials by the Cochrane collaboration reanalysed the data using uniform criteria (NASCET criteria, which compared the lumen diameter at the site of maximal stenosis with maximal arterial lumen diameter distal to the occlusion). The study concluded that the benefit of endarterectomy is greatest in patients with stenosis greater than 70% and when performed within 2 weeks of the index event. The pooled analysis, which included data from 6092 patients and 35,000 patient-years of follow-up, found no benefit for endarterectomy in patients having less than 50% stenosis, a marginal benefit in patients with 50–69% stenosis (absolute risk reduction (ARR) 4.6%, p=0.04), and high benefit in patients with 70–99% stenosis without near occlusion

(collapse of the artery distal to the occlusion) (ARR 16.0%, p <0.001) (143) (Table 15.8).

The benefit of CEA in patients with 50–69% stenosis remains controversial. Subgroup analysis from NASCET and the pooled analysis suggest that only men benefit significantly from CEA with that degree of stenosis. It is hypothesized that smaller-calibre vessels in women may account for the sex differences with regards to perioperative and longer-term issues, including higher surgical and neurological morbidity and recurrent stenosis in women (144). Female patients, however, are generally underrepresented in the data and other analyses that demonstrate a clear gender difference in perioperative complications combine symptomatic and asymptomatic patients (28).

Optimal timing for endarterectomy also eludes consensus. In subgroup analysis, benefit of CEA was maximal in patients who were randomized within 2 weeks after their index event, with the benefit of the intervention progressively lost with successive delays (143). Though very early intervention is beneficial in patients with TIA or minor stroke, caution must be exercised in patients with larger strokes or haemorrhagic transformation due to the risks of hyperperfusion secondary to dysfunctional autoregulation in the context of damaged brain parenchyma with increased susceptibility for haemorrhage. Excellent results within 6 weeks of stroke have been reported in observational studies (145, 146); safety of endarterectomy in patients who have received tissue plasminogen activator has also been reported in small observational studies (147–149).

Extracranial–intracranial bypass

Extracranial–intracranial (EC–IC) bypass has not been shown to be of any benefit in patients with internal carotid narrowing or occlusion. This has been demonstrated in the EC–IC Bypass Study and in the most recent COSS study where positron emission tomography (PET) scan was used to select patients with evidence of haemodynamic ischemia due to inadequate collaterals (150).

Table 15.9 Major randomized trials comparing CAS to CEA for symptomatic[a] carotid stenosis

Study	Year	Mean follow-up time	Population	30-day outcome	Follow-up outcome
CAVATAS	2001	3 years	251 CAS 253 CEA	Disabling stroke or death: CAS 6.4% CEA 5.4%	Disabling stroke or death at 3 years: CAS 14.3% CEA 14.2% (HR 1.04, 95% CI 0.63–1.70)
SPACE	2006	24 months	605 CAS 595 CEA	Any stroke or death: CAS 6.84% CEA 6.34% (absolute risk difference 0.51%, 95% CI −1.89–2.91%)	Ipsilateral stroke, any periprocedural stroke or death: CAS 9.5% CEA 8.8% (HR 1.10, 95% CI 0.65–1.61)
EVA-3S	2008	4 years	260 CAS 257 CEA	Any stroke or death: CAS 9.6% CEA 3.9% (RR 2.5, 95% CI 1.2–5.1)	Any periprocedural stroke or death and any non-periprocedural ipsilateral stroke: CAS 11.1% CEA 6.2% (HR 1.97, 95% CI 1.06–3.67)
CREST	2010	2.5 years	1271 CAS 1251 CEA [a]47% of patients had asymptomatic stenosis	Death: CAS: 0.7% CEA: 0.3% P=0.18 Stroke: CAS: 4.1% CEA: 2.3% P=0.01 MI: CAS: 1.1% CEA: 2.3% P=0.03	Stroke, MI or death: CAS: 7.2% CEA: 6.8% (HR 1.11; 95% CI, 0.81 to 1.51; P=0.51)
ICSS	2010	120-day interim analysis (3-year planned follow up)	CAS: 855 CEA: 858	–	Stroke, death or periprocedural MI: CAS: 8.5% CEA: 5.2% (HR 1.69, 95% CI 1.16 to 2.45) Disabling stroke or death: CAS: 4.0% CEA: 3.2% (HR 1.28, 95% CI 0.77–2.11)

Carotid angioplasty and stenting

Carotid angioplasty and stenting (CAS) has emerged as a possible alternative to CEA. Four large randomized clinical trials (ICSS, SPACE, EVA-3S, and CREST) have compared stenting to endarterectomy for symptomatic carotid stenosis (Table 15.9). A recent meta-analysis of randomized trials comparing stenting with endarterectomy found that CEA was superior to CAS with regards to periprocedural stroke or death, particularly for symptomatic patients, but that CAS had a lower rate of periprocedural MI (151). Another meta-analysis combining data from ICSS, SPACE, and EVA-3S found that the difference between procedures with regards to periprocedural stroke and death was most marked within 7 days of the qualifying ischaemic event (2.8% CEA vs 9.4% CAS: RR 2.0; 95% CI 1.5–2.7), with the differences between groups progressively decreasing between 8 to 14 days (3.4% vs 8.1%) and 14 days or greater after the event (4.0% vs 7.3%) (152).

Currently, stenting is an option for patients with severe medical comorbidities that could contribute to an adverse surgical outcome, including patients with severe comorbidities (class III/IV CHF, class III/IV angina, left main coronary artery disease, LV ejection fraction less than 30%, recent MI, severe lung disease, or severe renal disease). Stenting is also an option for patients with unfavourable anatomical factors for carotid surgery, such as prior neck dissection or irradiation, postendarterectomy restenosis, surgically inaccessible lesions, contralateral carotid occlusion, contralateral vocal cord palsy, and tracheostomy (28).

The CAVATAS trial randomized 504 patients, 97% of whom had a symptomatic stenosis, and 93% of whom had experienced their event within the previous 6 months, to CEA or CAS. Rates of significant restenosis were significantly higher at 1 year in the CAS group (14% vs 4%, p <0.001). Stents were used in 26% of CAS patients and distal embolic protection devices were not employed. There was no significant difference in rates of stroke or death neither during the 30-day post-procedural period nor during the ensuing 3-year follow-up (153).

The SPACE trial, which had a non-inferiority design comparing CAS to CEA for symptomatic carotid stenosis, enrolled 1183 patients within 180 days of their event. The trial was stopped after its second interim analysis due to issues with funding and recruitment. There were no significant differences in rates of stroke or death at 30 days or at 2-year follow up, however, the trial was underpowered to detect non-inferiority. Rates of restenosis of greater than 70% were significantly higher in the CAS group (10.7 vs 4.6% by intention-to-treat). Though the trial has been criticized for its optional use of embolic protection devices (used for 27% of CAS cases), there was no significant difference in rates of stroke and death at 30 days between those patients treated with or without devices (154, 155).

EVA-3S, another non-inferiority trial comparing CAS to CEA, was stopped early due to higher rates in the CAS group of stroke and death 30 days post procedure (9.6 vs 3.9%: RR 2.5; 95% CI 1.2–5.1). Rates of ipsilateral stroke or death at 4 years were also higher in the CAS group, largely due to the high rate of periprocedural events (11.1 vs 6.2%: HR 1.97; 95% CI 1.06–3.67). The higher complication rate in the CAS group has been associated with heterogenous operator experience, and multiple types of stents and embolic protection devices. Use of embolic protection devices was optional early in the trial, and risk of stroke or death was significantly lower in those who were treated using such devices (156, 157).

The CREST trial enrolled 2502 patients with moderate to severe carotid stenosis, 53% of who were symptomatic within 180 days prior to enrolment. There was no significant difference between groups with regards to rate of stroke, MI or death in the periprocedural period or at estimated 4-year outcomes. Periprocedural rates for stroke were higher in the CAS group (4.1% CAS, 2.3% CEA); while periprocedural MI was significantly more frequent in the CEA cohort (1.1% CAS, 2.3% CEA). Patients over the age of 70 had significantly higher rates of the primary endpoint, which may be attributable to technical factors including vessel tortuosity and aortic arch calcification and atheroma (158).

The ICSS trial, which randomized 1713 patients with symptomatic stenosis 50% or greater within 12 months of their index event, found significantly higher rates of stroke, death, or periprocedural MI in the CAS group at the 120-day interim analysis. The higher rates of complications in the CAS group may have been attributable in part to two centres with particularly high complication rates. That dual antiplatelet therapy was recommended, but not mandatory in the stenting group may also have contributed to CAS adverse outcomes, though rates of combination therapy were not reported in the interim analysis (159).

We currently reserve stenting for patients with unfavourable anatomical factors or medical comorbidities. Evolution of stents and embolic protection devices and increased operator experience may eventually lead to better efficacy for stenting in comparison to endarterectomy.

Intracranial atherosclerotic disease

Atherosclerotic intracranial large-artery occlusive disease accounts for approximately 8–10% of ischaemic stroke in Caucasian populations; a higher prevalence has been found in black, Asian, and Hispanic patients (160). The commonest sites of symptomatic intracranial disease are the carotid siphon, middle cerebral artery, and intracranial vertebral and basilar arteries.

The recurrence rate of an ischaemic event from an intracranial large-artery source is high, even with current best medical therapy. In the WASID trial, which randomized patients to receive either ASA 1300 mg daily or dose-adjusted warfarin (target INR 2.0–3.0) the recurrence rate at 1 year for all recurrent ischaemic stroke was 15%. In the territory of the symptomatic artery, recurrence rate was 12% in the aspirin treatment arm and 11% in the warfarin arm, with more severe stenosis (≥70% as compared to <70%) associated with a higher risk of stroke in the territory of the narrowing (HR 2.03; 95% CI 1.9–3.22) (161). There was a 10% rate of recurrent stroke in the territory of the qualifying artery at 1 year in the SAMMPRIS trial, which assigned patients to angioplasty and stenting versus current best medical therapy for symptomatic severe stenosis (70–99%) of any major intracranial artery. Medical optimization included dual antiplatelet therapy, statin use, treatment of hypertension and a lifestyle modification programme targeting management of lipids, diabetes, smoking cessation, weight loss, and exercise (22) (Table 15.10).

In large randomized trials to date, neither anticoagulant nor revascularization therapies have proven more effective than medical management with antiplatelet medications and risk factor management with lipid and blood pressure control.

In the EC–IC Bypass trial, revascularization surgery was also shown to be ineffective as compared to antiplatelet therapy for preventing ischaemic events in patients with internal carotid or middle cerebral artery narrowing or occlusion (150). The COSS trial enrolled 195 recently symptomatic patients (<120 days after their index event) with atherosclerotic internal artery occlusion and haemodynamic compromise as determined by increased ipsilateral oxygen extraction on PET. Again, no benefit was found for EC–IC bypass as compared with best medical therapy, which included antithrombotic therapy and optimization of lipids, blood pressure, and blood glucose (162).

The SAMMPRIS trial, which compared stenting (Wingspan stent) to intensive medical therapy for intracranial stenosis, enrolled 451 patients with symptomatic stenosis of 70% or higher of a major intracranial artery within 30 days of their index event. Recruitment was terminated early due to an excess of stroke and death at 30 days in the stenting arm (14% stenting vs 5.8% medical). Follow-up at 1 year also found higher rates of stroke and death in the stenting group (20% vs 12.2%), mainly due to the excess of events during the periprocedural period (22).

Two large randomized trials failed to demonstrate dose-adjusted warfarin as superior to antiplatelet therapy for secondary prevention for intracranial atherosclerotic events. The WARSS trial compared randomized 2206 patients with non-cardioembolic ischaemic stroke to dose-adjusted warfarin (target INR 1.4–2.8) as compared versus aspirin 325 mg daily. There was no significant difference between groups with respect to rates of ischaemic stroke, death, or major haemorrhage. No additional benefit was seen for warfarin in a subgroup of 259 patients with symptomatic intracranial or extracranial large artery stenosis or occlusion (163). The WASID trial compared high-dose aspirin (1300 mg/day) to dose-adjusted warfarin (target INR 2.0–3.0) in 569 patients with symptomatic intracranial stenosis of 50% or higher. The risk of stroke in the territory of the stenotic artery was 19% at 1 year. Total risk of recurrent stroke over 1.8 years was 22% in both groups (HR 1.04; 95% CI 0.73–1.48), with a higher rate of adverse events in the warfarin group (161).

Randomized clinical trials have not demonstrated a benefit for warfarin anticoagulation for intracranial stenosis to date. There are not currently any data investigating newer antithrombotic agents

Table 15.10 Rates of recurrent stroke in the medical therapy arms in secondary stroke prevention trials for intracranial stenosis

Trial	Year	Number of patients assigned to medical therapy	Follow-up	Best medical therapy	Stroke rate
ECIC Bypass Study (150)	1985	189	44 months	ASA	Annualized rate: 9.5% all stroke 7.8% ipsilateral stroke
WASID (161)	2005	569	2 years	Warfarin (INR 2.0–3.0) or ASA 1300 mg daily	After the first year: 15% all stroke 12% ipsilateral stroke
GESICA (199) (observational study)	2006	102	23 months	At the treating physician's discretion	At end of follow-up: 13.7% all stroke (27% hemodynamic symptoms)
SAMMPRIS (22)	2011	227	11.9 months	ASA 325 mg daily and clopidogrel 75 mg daily, rosuvastatin, plus optimization of hypertension, lipids, diabetes, smoking cessation, weight loss and exercise planning	At end of follow-up: 14.1% all stroke 10.1% ipsilateral stroke
COSS (162)	2011	98	2 years	Antithrombotic therapy at physician's discretion, optimization of lipids, hypertension and blood glucose	At end of follow-up: 22.3% ipsilateral stroke (all stroke)

in intracranial stenosis. The optimal dose of aspirin in intracranial stenosis is uncertain, though in secondary prevention trials doses from 30–1300 mg have been shown to be effective, with higher doses associated with increased risk of gastrointestinal upset and gastrointestinal bleeding. In addition, there is no data directly comparing aspiring monotherapy versus combination antiplatelet therapy for intracranial stenosis.

No interventions to date have proven superior to antiplatelet therapy and optimization of blood pressure, serum cholesterol, blood glucose, and lifestyle modification. In a post hoc analysis of the WASID trial, patients with blood pressure higher than 140/90 and total cholesterol higher than 5.2 mmol/L had higher rates of recurrent ischaemic stroke (blood pressure HR 1.58; 95% CI 1.07–2.32; cholesterol HR 1.95; 1.29–2.97) (164).

In most instances, we recommend intensive medical management with antiplatelet therapy and risk factor modification. We caution against aggressive blood pressure reduction, particularly in the acute symptomatic phase, to avoid haemodynamic symptoms. There are compelling situations to consider stenting where medical management has failed, such as crescendo transient ischaemic attacks or recurrent and persistent haemodynamic symptoms, but there is no current evidence to support this from randomized controlled trials and the risk of periprocedural complications and in-stent restenosis must be weighed against the potential benefit. Whether other stents will prove superior to medical optimization in the future is uncertain. The VISSIT Intracranial Stent Study for Ischemic Therapy (clinical trials.gov NCT00816166), which is investigating a balloon-mounted stent versus best medical therapy, is currently underway.

Lifestyle modification

Blood glucose

Type 2 diabetes is associated with a two- to sixfold risk of first and recurrent ischaemic stroke and doubles the risk of stroke recurrence (165–169).

Three randomized controlled trials of intensive blood glucose control have failed to show a benefit for prevention of vascular events in patients with diabetes and history of vascular risk, cardiovascular events, or stroke. Patients with previous stroke comprised a small minority of the trial populations (170–172).

The PROactive study, which randomized patients with type 2 diabetes and macrovascular disease to pioglitazone or placebo, found no significant difference between groups overall for reduction of death or cardiovascular disease. In the subgroup of patients with stroke (19% of the study population) as their index vascular event, however, there was a 47% relative risk reduction in recurrent stroke (HR 0.53; 95% CI 0.34–0.85), and a 28% relative risk reduction in stroke, MI, or vascular death (HR 0.72; 95% CI 0.53–1.00) (173). These results have not yet been replicated in other randomized controlled trials. Rosiglitazone, another thiazolidinedione, has been associated with macrovascular risk (174). Future large randomized trials may clarify the role of this class of medications in stroke populations.

Recommendations from national guidelines with regards to glycaemic control for primary and secondary stroke prevention are summarized in Table 15.11.

Smoking cessation

There are no randomized controlled studies of smoking cessation for stroke prevention. Cigarette smoking is associated with a dose-response relationship for both ischaemic stroke and subarachnoid haemorrhage and is associated with increased risk of all stroke types (175–178). Second-hand and environmental tobacco smoke is also associated with increased risk of vascular events, including stroke (175, 179, 180). Observational studies have shown that the risk of stroke declines to that of non-smokers within 5 years of quitting smoking (181). Major national guidelines advocate smoking cessation for secondary prevention of stroke.

Table 15.11 Summary of current national guidelines for management of diabetes and glycaemic control for secondary stroke prevention

AHA/ASA	Canadian	Australian	ESO
Use of existing guidelines for glycaemic control and blood pressure targets in patients with diabetes is recommended for patients who have had a stroke or TIA (*Class I; Level of Evidence B*)	Glycaemic targets must be individualized; however, therapy in most patients with type 1 or type 2 diabetes should be targeted to achieve a glycated haemoglobin (HbA1c) level <7.0% in order to reduce the risk of microvascular complications [Evidence Level A] and, for individuals with type 1 diabetes, macrovascular complications. (*Evidence Level C*) To achieve an HbA1c <7.0%, patients with type 1 or type 2 diabetes should aim for a fasting plasma glucose or preprandial plasma glucose targets of 4.0–7.0 mmol/L (*Evidence Level B*)	Patients with glucose intolerance or diabetes should be managed in line with national guidelines for diabetes. (*Good practice point*)	It is recommended that blood glucose should be checked regularly. It is recommended that diabetes should be managed with lifestyle modification and individualized pharmacological therapy (*Class IV, GCP*). In patients with type 2 diabetes who do not need insulin, treatment with pioglitazone is recommended after stroke (*Class III, Level B*)

Vitamins

Hyperhomocysteinaemia has been associated with a twofold risk of stroke in epidemiological studies (182, 183). Studies to date have not shown that B-vitamins, which reduce total homocysteine, are effective in secondary stroke prevention. In the VITATOPS trial, 8164 patients with stroke or TIA were randomized within 7 months of their event to receive B vitamins (2 mg folic acid, 25 mg B_6, 0.5 mg B_{12} daily) versus placebo. There were no differences in rates of stroke, MI, or vascular death between groups (184). Another study comparing high-dose to low-dose B vitamins for secondary prevention of ischaemic stroke in 3680 patients found no difference in stroke recurrence between groups despite lowering total homocysteine by 2 mmol/L in the high-dose cohort (185).

In a meta-analysis of primary and secondary prevention trials, beta-carotene supplementation was associated with increased risk of cardiovascular death (RR 1.10; 95% CI 1.03–1.17) and vitamin E supplementation had no benefit for prevention of vascular events (186). Another meta-analysis of antioxidant use for primary and secondary prevention found a significantly increased risk of mortality with fat-soluble antioxidant supplementation (RR 1.05; 95% CI 1.02–1.08) (187).

There are no randomized controlled trials to support vitamin supplementation for secondary stroke prevention.

Exercise

There are no controlled studies to date examining the effects of physical activity on secondary stroke prevention. Data from primary prevention studies has shown that moderately and highly active adults have a reduced risk of stroke (188, 189), and a systematic review of fitness training after stroke did not demonstrate evidence of effect overall though individual studies found an increase in quality of life and reduction in level of impairment (190). Many major national guidelines advocate post-stroke exercise programmes.

References

1. O'Donnell MJ, Xavier D, Liu L, Zhang H, Chin SL, Rao-Melacini P, *et al.* Risk factors for ischaemic and intracerebral haemorrhagic stroke in 22 countries (the INTERSTROKE study): a case-control study. *Lancet.* 2010;376(9735):112–123.
2. Strong K, Mathers C, Bonita R. Preventing stroke: saving lives around the world. *Lancet Neurol.* 2007;6(2):182–187.
3. Pendlebury ST, Rothwell PM. Prevalence, incidence, and factors associated with pre-stroke and post-stroke dementia: a systematic review and meta-analysis. *Lancet Neurol.* 2009;8(11):1006–1018.
4. Rothwell PM, Algra A, Amarenco P. Medical treatment in acute and long-term secondary prevention after transient ischaemic attack and ischaemic stroke. *Lancet.* 2011;377(9778):1681–1692.
5. Hillen T, Coshall C, Tilling K, Rudd AG, McGovern R, Wolfe CD. Cause of stroke recurrence is multifactorial: patterns, risk factors, and outcomes of stroke recurrence in the South London Stroke Register. *Stroke.* 2003;34(6):1457–1463.
6. Sacco RL, Wolf PA, Kannel WB, McNamara PM. Survival and recurrence following stroke. The Framingham study. *Stroke.* 1982;13(3):290–295.
7. Rothwell PM, Coull AJ, Giles MF, Howard SC, Silver LE, Bull LM, *et al.* Change in stroke incidence, mortality, case-fatality, severity, and risk factors in Oxfordshire, UK from 1981 to 2004 (Oxford Vascular Study). *Lancet.* 2004;363(9425):1925–1933.
8. Baigent C, Blackwell L, Collins R, Emberson J, Godwin J, Peto R, *et al.* Aspirin in the primary and secondary prevention of vascular disease: collaborative meta-analysis of individual participant data from randomised trials. *Lancet.* 2009;373(9678):1849–1860.
9. A comparison of two doses of aspirin (30 mg vs 283 mg a day) in patients after a transient ischemic attack or minor ischemic stroke. The Dutch TIA Trial Study Group. *N Engl J Med.* 1991;325(18):1261–1266.
10. Swedish Aspirin Low-Dose Trial (SALT) of 75 mg aspirin as secondary prophylaxis after cerebrovascular ischaemic events. The SALT Collaborative Group. *Lancet.* 1991;338(8779):1345–1349.
11. Collaborative meta-analysis of randomised trials of antiplatelet therapy for prevention of death, myocardial infarction, and stroke in high risk patients. *BMJ.* 2002;324(7329):71–86.
12. Diener HC, Cunha L, Forbes C, Sivenius J, Smets P, Lowenthal A. European Stroke Prevention Study. 2. Dipyridamole and acetylsalicylic acid in the secondary prevention of stroke. *J Neurol Sci.* 1996;143(1–2):1–13.
13. Sze PC, Reitman D, Pincus MM, Sacks HS, Chalmers TC. Antiplatelet agents in the secondary prevention of stroke: meta-analysis of the randomized control trials. *Stroke.* 1988;19(4):436–442.
14. Halkes PH, van Gijn J, Kappelle LJ, Koudstaal PJ, Algra A. Aspirin plus dipyridamole versus aspirin alone after cerebral ischaemia of arterial origin (ESPRIT): randomised controlled trial. *Lancet.* 2006;367(9523):1665–1673.
15. A randomised, blinded, trial of clopidogrel versus aspirin in patients at risk of ischaemic events (CAPRIE). CAPRIE Steering Committee. *Lancet.* 1996;348(9038):1329–1339.
16. Sacco RL, Diener HC, Yusuf S, Cotton D, Ounpuu S, Lawton WA, *et al.* Aspirin and extended-release dipyridamole versus clopidogrel for recurrent stroke. *N Engl J Med.* 2008;359(12):1238–1251.

17. Diener HC, Bogousslavsky J, Brass LM, Cimminiello C, Csiba L, Kaste M, *et al*. Aspirin and clopidogrel compared with clopidogrel alone after recent ischaemic stroke or transient ischaemic attack in high-risk patients (MATCH): randomised, double-blind, placebo-controlled trial. *Lancet*. 2004;364(9431):331–337.

18. Bhatt DL, Fox KA, Hacke W, Berger PB, Black HR, Boden WE, *et al*. Clopidogrel and aspirin versus aspirin alone for the prevention of atherothrombotic events. *N Engl J Med*. 2006;354(16):1706–1717.

19. Benavente OR, Hart RG, McClure LA, Szychowski JM, Coffey CS, Pearce LA. Effects of clopidogrel added to aspirin in patients with recent lacunar stroke. *N Engl J Med*. 2012;367(9):817–825.

20. Markus HS, Droste DW, Kaps M, Larrue V, Lees KR, Siebler M, *et al*. Dual antiplatelet therapy with clopidogrel and aspirin in symptomatic carotid stenosis evaluated using Doppler embolic signal detection: the Clopidogrel and Aspirin for Reduction of Emboli in Symptomatic Carotid Stenosis (CARESS) trial. *Circulation*. 2005;111(17):2233–2240.

21. Wong KS, Chen C, Fu J, Chang HM, Suwanwela NC, Huang YN, *et al*. Clopidogrel plus aspirin versus aspirin alone for reducing embolisation in patients with acute symptomatic cerebral or carotid artery stenosis (CLAIR study): a randomised, open-label, blinded-endpoint trial. *Lancet Neurol*. 2010;9(5):489–497.

22. Chimowitz MI, Lynn MJ, Derdeyn CP, Turan TN, Fiorella D, Lane BF, *et al*. Stenting versus aggressive medical therapy for intracranial arterial stenosis. *N Engl J Med*. 2011;365(11):993–1003.

23. Kennedy J, Hill MD, Ryckborst KJ, Eliasziw M, Demchuk AM, Buchan AM. Fast assessment of stroke and transient ischaemic attack to prevent early recurrence (FASTER): a randomised controlled pilot trial. *Lancet Neurol*. 2007;6(11):961–969.

24. Wang Y, Wang Y, Zhao X, Liu L, Wang D, Wang C, *et al*. Clopidogrel and aspirin in Acute Minor Stroke or Transient Ischemic Attack (CHANCE). *N Engl J Med*. 2013(369):11–19.

25. Wang Y, Johnston SC. Rationale and design of a randomized, double-blind trial comparing the effects of a 3-month clopidogrel-aspirin regimen versus aspirin alone for the treatment of high-risk patients with acute nondisabling cerebrovascular event. *Am Heart J*. 2010;160(3):380–386 e1.

26. Liu L, Wang D, Wong KS, Wang Y. Stroke and stroke care in China: huge burden, significant workload, and a national priority. *Stroke*. 2011;42(12):3651–3654.

27. Cardiogenic brain embolism. The second report of the Cerebral Embolism Task Force. *Arch Neurol*. 1989;46(7):727–743.

28. Furie KL, Kasner SE, Adams RJ, Albers GW, Bush RL, Fagan SC, *et al*. Guidelines for the prevention of stroke in patients with stroke or transient ischemic attack: a guideline for healthcare professionals from the American Heart Association/American Stroke Association. *Stroke*. 2011;42(1):227–276.

29. Risk factors for stroke and efficacy of antithrombotic therapy in atrial fibrillation. Analysis of pooled data from five randomized controlled trials. *Arch Int Med*. 1994;154(13):1449–1457.

30. Ferro JM. Cardioembolic stroke: an update. *Lancet Neurol*. 2003;2(3):177–188.

31. Lip GY, Tse HF, Lane DA. Atrial fibrillation. *Lancet*. 2012;379(9816):648–661.

32. Miyasaka Y, Barnes ME, Gersh BJ, Cha SS, Bailey KR, Abhayaratna WP, *et al*. Secular trends in incidence of atrial fibrillation in Olmsted County, Minnesota, 1980 to 2000, and implications on the projections for future prevalence. *Circulation*. 2006;114(2):119–125.

33. Liao J, Khalid Z, Scallan C, Morillo C, O'Donnell M. Noninvasive cardiac monitoring for detecting paroxysmal atrial fibrillation or flutter after acute ischemic stroke: a systematic review. *Stroke*. 2007;38(11):2935–2940.

34. Hindricks G, Piorkowski C, Tanner H, Kobza R, Gerds-Li J-H, Carbucicchio C, *et al*. Perception of atrial fibrillation before and after radiofrequency catheter ablation: relevance of asymptomatic arrhythmia recurrence. *Circulation*. 2005;112(3):307–313.

35. Klemm HU, Ventura R, Rostock T, Brandstrup B, Risius T, Meinertz T, *et al*. Correlation of symptoms to ECG diagnosis following atrial fibrillation ablation. *J Cardiovasc Electrophysiol*. 2006;17(2):146–150.

36. Vasamreddy CR, Dalal D, Dong J, Cheng A, Spragg D, Lamiy SZ, *et al*. Symptomatic and asymptomatic atrial fibrillation in patients undergoing radiofrequency catheter ablation. *J Cardiovasc Electrophysiol*. 2006;17(2):134–139.

37. Gladstone D, The EMBRACE Trial Investigators. *Preliminary results of the Embrace Trial*. Late-Breaking Science Oral Abstracts, International Stroke Conference. 2013. <http://my.americanheart.org/idc/groups/ahamah-public/@wcm/@sop/@scon/documents/downloadable/ucm_449059.pdf>.

38. Independent predictors of stroke in patients with atrial fibrillation: a systematic review. *Neurology*. 2007;69(6):546–554.

39. Connolly SJ, Eikelboom J, Joyner C, Diener HC, Hart R, Golitsyn S, *et al*. Apixaban in patients with atrial fibrillation. *N Engl J Med*. 2011;364(9):806–817.

40. Connolly SJ, Pogue J, Hart RG, Hohnloser SH, Pfeffer M, Chrolavicius S, *et al*. Effect of clopidogrel added to aspirin in patients with atrial fibrillation. *N Engl J Med*. 2009;360(20):2066–2078.

41. Hart RG, Pearce LA, Aguilar MI. Meta-analysis: antithrombotic therapy to prevent stroke in patients who have nonvalvular atrial fibrillation. *Ann Intern Med*. 2007;146(12):857–867.

42. Connolly S, Pogue J, Hart R, Pfeffer M, Hohnloser S, Chrolavicius S, *et al*. Clopidogrel plus aspirin versus oral anticoagulation for atrial fibrillation in the Atrial fibrillation Clopidogrel Trial with Irbesartan for prevention of Vascular Events (ACTIVE W): a randomised controlled trial. *Lancet*. 2006;367(9526):1903–1912.

43. Connolly SJ, Ezekowitz MD, Yusuf S, Eikelboom J, Oldgren J, Parekh A, *et al*. Dabigatran versus warfarin in patients with atrial fibrillation. *N Engl J Med*. 2009;361(12):1139–1151.

44. Lader E, Martin N, Cohen G, Meyer M, Reiter P, Dimova A, *et al*. Warfarin therapeutic monitoring: is 70% time in the therapeutic range the best we can do? *J Clin Pharm Therapeut*. 2012;37(4):375–377.

45. Hylek EM. Vitamin K antagonists and time in the therapeutic range: implications, challenges, and strategies for improvement. *J Thromb Thrombolysis*. 2013 Apr;35(3):333–335.

46. Hylek EM, Skates SJ, Sheehan MA, Singer DE. An analysis of the lowest effective intensity of prophylactic anticoagulation for patients with nonrheumatic atrial fibrillation. *N Engl J Med*. 1996;335(8):540–546.

47. Secondary prevention in non-rheumatic atrial fibrillation after transient ischaemic attack or minor stroke. EAFT (European Atrial Fibrillation Trial) Study Group. *Lancet*. 1993;342(8882):1255–1262.

48. Adjusted-dose warfarin versus low-intensity, fixed-dose warfarin plus aspirin for high-risk patients with atrial fibrillation: Stroke Prevention in Atrial Fibrillation III randomised clinical trial. *Lancet*. 1996;348(9028):633–638.

49. Fang MC, Go AS, Chang Y, Hylek EM, Henault LE, Jensvold NG, *et al*. Death and disability from warfarin-associated intracranial and extracranial hemorrhages. *Am J Med*. 2007;120(8):700–705.

50. Rosand J, Eckman MH, Knudsen KA, Singer DE, Greenberg SM. The effect of warfarin and intensity of anticoagulation on outcome of intracerebral hemorrhage. *Arch Intern Med*. 2004;164(8):880–884.

51. Dowlatshahi D, Butcher KS, Asdaghi N, Nahirniak S, Bernbaum ML, Giulivi A, *et al*. Poor prognosis in warfarin-associated intracranial hemorrhage despite anticoagulation reversal. *Stroke*. 2012;43(7):1812–1817.

52. Hart RG, Tonarelli SB, Pearce LA. Avoiding central nervous system bleeding during antithrombotic therapy: recent data and ideas. *Stroke*. 2005;36(7):1588–1593.

53. Patel MR, Mahaffey KW, Garg J, Pan G, Singer DE, Hacke W, *et al*. Rivaroxaban versus warfarin in nonvalvular atrial fibrillation. *N Engl J Med*. 2011;365(10):883–891.

54. Granger CB, Alexander JH, McMurray JJ, Lopes RD, Hylek EM, Hanna M, *et al*. Apixaban versus warfarin in patients with atrial fibrillation. *N Engl J Med*. 2011;365(11):981–992.

55. Hori M, Matsumoto M, Tanahashi N, Momomura S, Uchiyama S, Goto S, *et al*. Rivaroxaban vs warfarin in Japanese patients with atrial fibrillation—the J-ROCKET AF study. *Circ J*. 2012;76(9):2104–2111.

56. Tanahashi N, Hori M, Matsumoto M, Momomura SI, Uchiyama S, Goto S, et al. Rivaroxaban versus Warfarin in Japanese Patients with Nonvalvular Atrial Fibrillation for the Secondary Prevention of Stroke: A Subgroup Analysis of J-ROCKET AF. *J Stroke Cerebrovasc Dis.* 2013;S1052–3057(12)00437-5.

57. You JJ, Singer DE, Howard PA, Lane DA, Eckman MH, Fang MC, et al. Antithrombotic therapy for atrial fibrillation: Antithrombotic Therapy and Prevention of Thrombosis, 9th ed: American College of Chest Physicians Evidence-Based Clinical Practice Guidelines. *Chest.* 2012;141(2 Suppl): e531S–75S.

58. Cairns JA, Connolly S, McMurtry S, Stephenson M, Talajic M. Canadian Cardiovascular Society atrial fibrillation guidelines 2010: prevention of stroke and systemic thromboembolism in atrial fibrillation and flutter. *Can J Cardiol.* 2011;27(1):74–90.

59. Furie KL, Goldstein LB, Albers GW, Khatri P, Neyens R, Turakhia MP, et al. Oral antithrombotic agents for the prevention of stroke in nonvalvular atrial fibrillation: a science advisory for healthcare professionals from the American Heart Association/American Stroke Association. *Stroke.* 2012;43(12):3442–3453.

60. Eikelboom JW, Hart RG. Antithrombotic therapy for stroke prevention in atrial fibrillation and mechanical heart valves. *Am J Hematol.* 2012;87 Suppl 1: S100–S107.

61. Ansell J. New oral anticoagulants should not be used as first-line agents to prevent thromboembolism in patients with atrial fibrillation. *Circulation.* 2012;125(1):165–170.

62. Homma S, Thompson JL, Pullicino PM, Levin B, Freudenberger RS, Teerlink JR, et al. Warfarin and aspirin in patients with heart failure and sinus rhythm. *N Engl J Med.* 2012;366(20):1859–1869.

63. Cannegieter SC, Rosendaal FR, Briet E. Thromboembolic and bleeding complications in patients with mechanical heart valve prostheses. *Circulation.* 2012;125:165–170.

64. Little SH, Massel DR. Antiplatelet and anticoagulation for patients with prosthetic heart valves. *Cochrane Database Syst Rev.* 2003;4:CD003464.

65. Van de Werf F, Brueckmann M, Connolly SJ, Friedman J, Granger CB, Hartter S, et al. A comparison of dabigatran etexilate with warfarin in patients with mechanical heart valves: the randomized, phase II study to evaluate the safety and pharmacokinetics of oral dabigatran etexilate in patients after heart valve replacement (RE-ALIGN). *Am Heart J.* 2012;163(6):931–937 e1.

66. O'Riordan M. *Study of dabigatran in mechanical heart valve patients halted.* <http://www.theheart.org>. 12 December 2012.

67. Food and Drug Administration. *FDA Drug Safety Communication: Pradaxa (dabigatran etexilate mesylate) should not be used in patients with mechanical prosthetic heart valves.* 2013 <http://www.fda.gov/Drugs/DrugSafety/ucm332912.htm> (accessed 28 April 2013).

68. Fuster V, Halperin JL. Left ventricular thrombi and cerebral embolism. *N Engl J Med.* 1989;320(6):392–394.

69. Natarajan D, Hotchandani RK, Nigam PD. Reduced incidence of left ventricular thrombi with intravenous streptokinase in acute anterior myocardial infarction: prospective evaluation by cross-sectional echocardiography. *Int J Cardiol.* 1988;20(2):201–207.

70. Sherman DG, Dyken ML, Fisher M, Harrison MJ, Hart RG. Cerebral embolism. *Chest.* 1986;89(2 Suppl):82S–98S.

71. Arboix A, Alio J. Acute cardioembolic cerebral infarction: answers to clinical questions. *Curr Cardiol Rev.* 2012;8(1):54–67.

72. Eigler N, Maurer G, Shah PK. Effect of early systemic thrombolytic therapy on left ventricular mural thrombus formation in acute anterior myocardial infarction. *Am J Cardiol.* 1984;54(3):261–263.

73. Held AC, Gore JM, Paraskos J, Pape LA, Ball SP, Corrao JM, et al. Impact of thrombolytic therapy on left ventricular mural thrombi in acute myocardial infarction. *Am J Cardiol.* 1988;62(4):310–311.

74. Nordrehaug JE, Johannessen KA, von der Lippe G. Usefulness of high-dose anticoagulants in preventing left ventricular thrombus in acute myocardial infarction. *Am J Cardiol.* 1985;55(13 Pt 1):1491–1493.

75. Davis MJ, Ireland MA. Effect of early anticoagulation on the frequency of left ventricular thrombi after anterior wall acute myocardial infarction. *Am J Cardiol.* 1986;57(15):1244–1247.

76. Gueret P, Dubourg O, Ferrier A, Farcot JC, Rigaud M, Bourdarias JP. Effects of full-dose heparin anticoagulation on the development of left ventricular thrombosis in acute transmural myocardial infarction. *J Am Coll Cardiol.* 1986;8(2):419–426.

77. Arvan S, Boscha K. Prophylactic anticoagulation for left ventricular thrombi after acute myocardial infarction: a prospective randomized trial. *Am Heart J.* 1987;113(3):688–693.

78. MacDougall NJ, Amarasinghe S, Muir KW. Secondary prevention of stroke. *Expert Rev Cardiovasc Ther.* 2009;7(9):1103–1115.

79. Cuadrado-Godia E, Ois A, Roquer J. Heart failure in acute ischemic stroke. *Curr Cardiol Rev.* 2010;6(3):202–213.

80. Massie BM, Krol WF, Ammon SE, Armstrong PW, Cleland JG, Collins JF, et al. The Warfarin and Antiplatelet Therapy in Heart Failure trial (WATCH): rationale, design, and baseline patient characteristics. *J Cardiac Fail.* 2004;10(2):101–112.

81. Hagen PT, Scholz DG, Edwards WD. Incidence and size of patent foramen ovale during the first 10 decades of life: an autopsy study of 965 normal hearts. *Mayo Clinic Proc.* 1984;59(1):17–20.

82. Caplan LR. *Caplan's Stroke: A Clinical Approach* (4th edn). Philadelphia, PA: Elsevier/Saunders; 2009.

83. Mas JL, Arquizan C, Lamy C, Zuber M, Cabanes L, Derumeaux G, et al. Recurrent cerebrovascular events associated with patent foramen ovale, atrial septal aneurysm, or both. *N Engl J Med.* 2001;345(24): 1740–1746.

84. Furlan AJ, Reisman M, Massaro J, Mauri L, Adams H, Albers GW, et al. Closure or medical therapy for cryptogenic stroke with patent foramen ovale. *N Engl J Med.* 2012;366(11):991–999.

85. Carroll JD, Saver JL, Thaler DE, Smalling RW, Berry S, MacDonald LA, et al. Closure of patent foramen ovale versus medical therapy after cryptogenic stroke. *N Engl J Med.* 2013;368(12):1092–1100.

86. Meier B, Kalesan B, Mattle HP, Khattab AA, Hildick-Smith D, Dudek D, et al. Percutaneous closure of patent foramen ovale in cryptogenic embolism. *N Engl J Med.* 2013;368(12):1083–1091.

87. Messe SR, Kent DM. Still no closure on the question of PFO closure. *N Engl J Med.* 2013;368(12):1152–1153.

88. Mugge A, Daniel WG, Angermann C, Spes C, Khandheria BK, Kronzon I, et al. Atrial septal aneurysm in adult patients. A multicenter study using transthoracic and transesophageal echocardiography. *Circulation.* 1995;91(11):2785–2792.

89. Homma S, Sacco RL, Di Tullio MR, Sciacca RR, Mohr JP. Effect of medical treatment in stroke patients with patent foramen ovale: patent foramen ovale in Cryptogenic Stroke Study. *Circulation.* 2002;105(22): 2625–2631.

90. Lawes CM, Bennett DA, Feigin VL, Rodgers A. Blood pressure and stroke: an overview of published reviews. *Stroke.* 2004;35(4):1024.

91. Mancia G, Ambrosioni E, Rosei EA, Leonetti G, Trimarco B, Volpe M. Blood pressure control and risk of stroke in untreated and treated hypertensive patients screened from clinical practice: results of the ForLife study. *J Hypertens.* 2005;23(8):1575–1581.

92. Lewington S, Clarke R, Qizilbash N, Peto R, Collins R. Age-specific relevance of usual blood pressure to vascular mortality: a meta-analysis of individual data for one million adults in 61 prospective studies. *Lancet.* 2002;360(9349):1903–1913.

93. Turnbull F, Neal B, Ninomiya T, Algert C, Arima H, Barzi F, et al. Effects of different regimens to lower blood pressure on major cardiovascular events in older and younger adults: meta-analysis of randomised trials. *BMJ.* 2008;336(7653):1121–1123.

94. Stamler J, Stamler R, Neaton JD. Blood pressure, systolic and diastolic, and cardiovascular risks. US population data. *Arch Intern Med.* 1993;153(5):598–615.

95. Rothwell PM, Howard SC, Spence JD. Relationship between blood pressure and stroke risk in patients with symptomatic carotid occlusive disease. *Stroke.* 2003;34(11):2583–2590.

96. Liu L, Wang Z, Gong L, Zhang Y, Thijs L, Staessen JA, et al. Blood pressure reduction for the secondary prevention of stroke: a Chinese trial and a systematic review of the literature. *Hypertens Res.* 2009;32(11):1032–1040.

97. Rashid P, Leonardi-Bee J, Bath P. Blood pressure reduction and secondary prevention of stroke and other vascular events: a systematic review. *Stroke*. 2003;34(11):2741–2748.

98. Randomised trial of a perindopril-based blood-pressure-lowering regimen among 6,105 individuals with previous stroke or transient ischaemic attack. *Lancet*. 2001;358(9287):1033–1041.

99. Yusuf S, Diener HC, Sacco RL, Cotton D, Ounpuu S, Lawton WA, et al. Telmisartan to prevent recurrent stroke and cardiovascular events. *N Engl J Med*. 2008;359(12):1225–1237.

100. Schrader J, Luders S, Kulschewski A, Hammersen F, Plate K, Berger J, et al. Morbidity and Mortality After Stroke, Eprosartan Compared with Nitrendipine for Secondary Prevention: principal results of a prospective randomized controlled study (MOSES). *Stroke*. 2005;36(6):1218–1226.

101. Benavente OR, White CL, Pearce L, Pergola P, Roldan A, Benavente MF, et al. The Secondary Prevention of Small Subcortical Strokes (SPS3) study. *Int J Stroke*. 2011;6(2):164–175.

102. SPS3 Study Group, Benavente OR, Coffey CS, Conwit R, Hart RG, McClure LA, et al. Blood-pressure targets in patients with recent lacunar stroke: the SPS3 randomised trial. *Lancet*. 2013;382:507–515

103. Rothwell PM, Howard SC, Dolan E, O'Brien E, Dobson JE, Dahlof B, et al. Effects of beta blockers and calcium-channel blockers on within-individual variability in blood pressure and risk of stroke. *Lancet Neurol*. 2010;9(5):469–480.

104. Webb AJ, Fischer U, Mehta Z, Rothwell PM. Effects of antihypertensive-drug class on interindividual variation in blood pressure and risk of stroke: a systematic review and meta-analysis. *Lancet*. 2010;375(9718):906–915.

105. Webb AJ, Fischer U, Rothwell PM. Effects of beta-blocker selectivity on blood pressure variability and stroke: a systematic review. *Neurology*. 2011;77(8):731–737.

106. Webb AJ, Rothwell PM. Effect of dose and combination of antihypertensives on interindividual blood pressure variability: a systematic review. *Stroke*. 2011;42(10):2860–2865.

107. Muntner P, Shimbo D, Tonelli M, Reynolds K, Arnett DK, Oparil S. The relationship between visit-to-visit variability in systolic blood pressure and all-cause mortality in the general population: findings from NHANES III, 1988 to 1994. *Hypertension*. 2011;57(2):160–166.

108. Passero S, Burgalassi L, D'Andrea P, Battistini N. Recurrence of bleeding in patients with primary intracerebral hemorrhage. *Stroke*. 1995;26(7):1189–1192.

109. Hill MD, Silver FL, Austin PC, Tu JV. Rate of stroke recurrence in patients with primary intracerebral hemorrhage. *Stroke*. 2000;31(1):123–127.

110. Lewington S, Whitlock G, Clarke R, Sherliker P, Emberson J, Halsey J, et al. Blood cholesterol and vascular mortality by age, sex, and blood pressure: a meta-analysis of individual data from 61 prospective studies with 55,000 vascular deaths. *Lancet*. 2007;370(9602):1829–1839.

111. Tirschwell DL, Smith NL, Heckbert SR, Lemaitre RN, Longstreth WT, Jr, Psaty BM. Association of cholesterol with stroke risk varies in stroke subtypes and patient subgroups. *Neurology*. 2004;63(10):1868–1875.

112. Imamura T, Doi Y, Arima H, Yonemoto K, Hata J, Kubo M, et al. LDL cholesterol and the development of stroke subtypes and coronary heart disease in a general Japanese population: the Hisayama study. *Stroke*. 2009;40(2):382–388.

113. Amarenco P, Labreuche J, Elbaz A, Touboul PJ, Driss F, Jaillard A, et al. Blood lipids in brain infarction subtypes. *Cerebrovasc Dis*. 2006;22(2-3):101–108.

114. Iso H, Jacobs DR, Jr, Wentworth D, Neaton JD, Cohen JD. Serum cholesterol levels and six-year mortality from stroke in 350,977 men screened for the multiple risk factor intervention trial. *N Engl J Med*. 1989;320(14):904–910.

115. Lindenstrom E, Boysen G, Nyboe J. Influence of total cholesterol, high density lipoprotein cholesterol, and triglycerides on risk of cerebrovascular disease: the Copenhagen City Heart Study. *BMJ*. 1994;309(6946):11–15.

116. Varbo A, Nordestgaard BG, Tybjaerg-Hansen A, Schnohr P, Jensen GB, Benn M. Nonfasting triglycerides, cholesterol, and ischemic stroke in the general population. *Ann Neurol*. 2011;69(4):628–634.

117. Bansal S, Buring JE, Rifai N, Mora S, Sacks FM, Ridker PM. Fasting compared with nonfasting triglycerides and risk of cardiovascular events in women. *JAMA*. 2007;298(3):309–316.

118. LaRosa JC, Grundy SM, Waters DD, Shear C, Barter P, Fruchart JC, et al. Intensive lipid lowering with atorvastatin in patients with stable coronary disease. *N Engl J Med*. 2005;352(14):1425–1435.

119. Bang OY, Saver JL, Liebeskind DS, Pineda S, Ovbiagele B. Association of serum lipid indices with large artery atherosclerotic stroke. *Neurology*. 2008;70(11):841–847.

120. Di Angelantonio E, Sarwar N, Perry P, Kaptoge S, Ray KK, Thompson A, et al. Major lipids, apolipoproteins, and risk of vascular disease. *JAMA*. 2009;302(18):1993–2000.

121. Goldstein LB. The complex relationship between cholesterol and brain hemorrhage. *Circulation*. 2009;119(16):2131–2133.

122. Amarenco P, Labreuche J. Lipid management in the prevention of stroke: review and updated meta-analysis of statins for stroke prevention. *Lancet Neurol*. 2009;8(5):453–463.

123. Amarenco P, Bogousslavsky J, Callahan A, 3rd, Goldstein LB, Hennerici M, Rudolph AE, et al. High-dose atorvastatin after stroke or transient ischemic attack. *N Engl J Med*. 2006;355(6):549–559.

124. Goldstein LB, Amarenco P, Szarek M, Callahan A, 3rd, Hennerici M, Sillesen H, et al. Hemorrhagic stroke in the Stroke Prevention by Aggressive Reduction in Cholesterol Levels study. *Neurology*. 2008;70(24 Pt 2):2364–2370.

125. Collins R, Armitage J, Parish S, Sleight P, Peto R. Effects of cholesterol-lowering with simvastatin on stroke and other major vascular events in 20536 people with cerebrovascular disease or other high-risk conditions. *Lancet*. 2004;363(9411):757–767.

126. Amarenco P, Labreuche J, Lavallee P, Touboul PJ. Statins in stroke prevention and carotid atherosclerosis: systematic review and up-to-date meta-analysis. *Stroke*. 2004;35(12):2902–2909.

127. Bucher HC, Griffith LE, Guyatt GH. Effect of HMGcoA reductase inhibitors on stroke. A meta-analysis of randomized, controlled trials. *Ann Int Med*. 1998;128(2):89–95.

128. Corvol JC, Bouzamondo A, Sirol M, Hulot JS, Sanchez P, Lechat P. Differential effects of lipid-lowering therapies on stroke prevention: a meta-analysis of randomized trials. *Arch Int Med*. 2003;163(6):669–676.

129. Bloomfield Rubins H, Davenport J, Babikian V, Brass LM, Collins D, Wexler L, et al. Reduction in stroke with gemfibrozil in men with coronary heart disease and low HDL cholesterol: The Veterans Affairs HDL Intervention Trial (VA-HIT). *Circulation*. 2001;103(23):2828–2833.

130. Bruckert E, Labreuche J, Amarenco P. Meta-analysis of the effect of nicotinic acid alone or in combination on cardiovascular events and atherosclerosis. *Atherosclerosis*. 2010;210(2):353–361.

131. Kamal-Bahl SJ, Burke T, Watson D, Wentworth C. Discontinuation of lipid modifying drugs among commercially insured United States patients in recent clinical practice. *Am J Cardiol*. 2007;99(4):530–534.

132. Amarenco P, Goldstein LB, Szarek M, Sillesen H, Rudolph AE, Callahan A, 3rd, et al. Effects of intense low-density lipoprotein cholesterol reduction in patients with stroke or transient ischemic attack: the Stroke Prevention by Aggressive Reduction in Cholesterol Levels (SPARCL) trial. *Stroke*. 2007;38(12):3198–3204.

133. Beneficial effect of carotid endarterectomy in symptomatic patients with high-grade carotid stenosis. North American Symptomatic Carotid Endarterectomy Trial Collaborators. *N Engl J Med*. 1991;325(7):445–453.

134. Migrino RQ, Bowers M, Harmann L, Prost R, LaDisa JF, Jr Carotid plaque regression following 6-month statin therapy assessed by 3T cardiovascular magnetic resonance: comparison with ultrasound intima media thickness. *J Cardiovasc Magn Reson*. 2011;13:37.

135. Abela GS, Vedre A, Janoudi A, Huang R, Durga S, Tamhane U. Effect of statins on cholesterol crystallization and atherosclerotic plaque stabilization. *Am J Ccardiol*. 2011;107(12):1710–1717.

136. Makris GC, Lavida A, Nicolaides AN, Geroulakos G. The effect of statins on carotid plaque morphology: a LDL-associated action or one more pleiotropic effect of statins? *Atherosclerosis*. 2010;213(1):8–20.

137. Rothwell PM, Mehta Z, Howard SC, Gutnikov SA, Warlow CP. Treating individuals 3: from subgroups to individuals: general principles and the example of carotid endarterectomy. *Lancet*. 2005;365(9455):256–265.

138. Mayberg MR, Wilson SE, Yatsu F, Weiss DG, Messina L, Hershey LA, et al. Carotid endarterectomy and prevention of cerebral ischemia in symptomatic carotid stenosis. Veterans Affairs Cooperative Studies Program 309 Trialist Group. *JAMA*. 1991;266(23):3289–3294.

139. Rerkasem K, Rothwell PM. Carotid endarterectomy for symptomatic carotid stenosis. *Cochrane Database Syst Rev*. 2011;4:CD001081.

140. Rothwell PM, Eliasziw M, Gutnikov SA, Fox AJ, Taylor DW, Mayberg MR, et al. Analysis of pooled data from the randomised controlled trials of endarterectomy for symptomatic carotid stenosis. *Lancet*. 2003;361(9352):107–116.

141. Randomised trial of endarterectomy for recently symptomatic carotid stenosis: final results of the MRC European Carotid Surgery Trial (ECST). *Lancet*. 1998;351(9113):1379–1387.

142. MRC European Carotid Surgery Trial: interim results for symptomatic patients with severe (70-99%) or with mild (0-29%) carotid stenosis. European Carotid Surgery Trialists' Collaborative Group. *Lancet*. 1991;337(8752):1235–1243.

143. Rothwell PM, Eliasziw M, Gutnikov SA, Warlow CP, Barnett HJ. Endarterectomy for symptomatic carotid stenosis in relation to clinical subgroups and timing of surgery. *Lancet*. 2004;363(9413):915–924.

144. Hugl B, Oldenburg WA, Neuhauser B, Hakaim AG. Effect of age and gender on restenosis after carotid endarterectomy. *Ann Vasc Surg*. 2006;20(5):602–608.

145. Eckstein HH, Ringleb P, Dorfler A, Klemm K, Muller BT, Zegelman M, et al. The Carotid Surgery for Ischemic Stroke trial: a prospective observational study on carotid endarterectomy in the early period after ischemic stroke. *J Vasc Surg*. 2002;36(5):997–1004.

146. Chaturvedi S, Bruno A, Feasby T, Holloway R, Benavente O, Cohen SN, et al. Carotid endarterectomy—an evidence-based review: report of the Therapeutics and Technology Assessment Subcommittee of the American Academy of Neurology. *Neurology*. 2005;65(6):794–801.

147. Crozier JE, Reid J, Welch GH, Muir KW, Stuart WP. Early carotid endarterectomy following thrombolysis in the hyperacute treatment of stroke. *Br J Surg*. 2011;98(2):235–238.

148. Bartoli MA, Squarcioni C, Nicoli F, Magnan PE, Malikov S, Berger L, et al. Early carotid endarterectomy after intravenous thrombolysis for acute ischaemic stroke. *Eur J Vasc Endovasc Surg*. 2009;37(5):512–518.

149. McPherson CM, Woo D, Cohen PL, Pancioli AM, Kissela BM, Carrozzella JA, et al. Early carotid endarterectomy for critical carotid artery stenosis after thrombolysis therapy in acute ischemic stroke in the middle cerebral artery. *Stroke*. 2001;32(9):2075–2080.

150. Failure of extracranial-intracranial arterial bypass to reduce the risk of ischemic stroke. Results of an international randomized trial. The EC/IC Bypass Study Group. *N Engl J Med*. 1985;313(19):1191–1200.

151. Liu ZJ, Fu WG, Guo ZY, Shen LG, Shi ZY, Li JH. Updated systematic review and meta-analysis of randomized clinical trials comparing carotid artery stenting and carotid endarterectomy in the treatment of carotid stenosis. *An Vasc Surg*. 2012;26(4):576–590.

152. Rantner B, Goebel G, Bonati LH, Ringleb PA, Mas JL, Fraedrich G. The risk of carotid artery stenting compared with carotid endarterectomy is greatest in patients treated within 7 days of symptoms. *J Vasc Surg*. 2013;57(3):619–626 e2.

153. Endovascular versus surgical treatment in patients with carotid stenosis in the Carotid and Vertebral Artery Transluminal Angioplasty Study (CAVATAS): a randomised trial. *Lancet*. 2001;357(9270):1729–1737.

154. Ringleb PA, Allenberg J, Bruckmann H, Eckstein HH, Fraedrich G, Hartmann M, et al. 30 day results from the SPACE trial of stent-protected angioplasty versus carotid endarterectomy in

symptomatic patients: a randomised non-inferiority trial. *Lancet*. 2006;368(9543):1239–1247.

155. Eckstein HH, Ringleb P, Allenberg JR, Berger J, Fraedrich G, Hacke W, et al. Results of the Stent-Protected Angioplasty versus Carotid Endarterectomy (SPACE) study to treat symptomatic stenoses at 2 years: a multinational, prospective, randomised trial. *Lancet Neurol*. 2008;7(10):893–902.

156. Mas JL, Chatellier G, Beyssen B, Branchereau A, Moulin T, Becquemin JP, et al. Endarterectomy versus stenting in patients with symptomatic severe carotid stenosis. *N Engl J Med*. 2006;355(16):1660–1671.

157. Mas JL, Trinquart L, Leys D, Albucher JF, Rousseau H, Viguier A, et al. Endarterectomy Versus Angioplasty in Patients with Symptomatic Severe Carotid Stenosis (EVA-3S) trial: results up to 4 years from a randomised, multicentre trial. *Lancet Neurol*. 2008;7(10):885–892.

158. Brott TG, Hobson RW, 2nd, Howard G, Roubin GS, Clark WM, Brooks W, et al. Stenting versus endarterectomy for treatment of carotid-artery stenosis. *N Engl J Med*. 2010;363(1):11–23.

159. Ederle J, Dobson J, Featherstone RL, Bonati LH, van der Worp HB, de Borst GJ, et al. Carotid artery stenting compared with endarterectomy in patients with symptomatic carotid stenosis (International Carotid Stenting Study): an interim analysis of a randomised controlled trial. *Lancet*. 2010;375(9719):985–997.

160. Arenillas JF. Intracranial atherosclerosis: current concepts. *Stroke*. 2011;42(1 Suppl): S20–3.

161. Chimowitz MI, Lynn MJ, Howlett-Smith H, Stern BJ, Hertzberg VS, Frankel MR, et al. Comparison of warfarin and aspirin for symptomatic intracranial arterial stenosis. *N Engl J Med*. 2005;352(13):1305–1316.

162. Powers WJ, Clarke WR, Grubb RL, Jr, Videen TO, Adams HP, Jr, Derdeyn CP. Extracranial-intracranial bypass surgery for stroke prevention in hemodynamic cerebral ischemia: the Carotid Occlusion Surgery Study randomized trial. *JAMA*. 2011;306(18):1983–1992.

163. Mohr JP, Thompson JL, Lazar RM, Levin B, Sacco RL, Furie KL, et al. A comparison of warfarin and aspirin for the prevention of recurrent ischemic stroke. *N Engl J Med*. 2001;345(20):1444–1451.

164. Chaturvedi S, Turan TN, Lynn MJ, Kasner SE, Romano J, Cotsonis G, et al. Risk factor status and vascular events in patients with symptomatic intracranial stenosis. *Neurology*. 2007;69(22):2063–2068.

165. Adachi H, Hirai Y, Tsuruta M, Fujiura Y, Imaizuml T. Is insulin resistance or diabetes mellitus associated with stroke? *Diabet Res Clin Pract*. 2001;51(3):215–223.

166. Dejong G, Vanraak L, Kessels F, Lodder J. Stroke subtype and mortality follow-up study in 998 patients with a first cerebral infarct. *J Clin Epidemiol*. 2003;56(3):262–268.

167. Harmsen P. Long-term risk factors for stroke: twenty-eight years of follow-up of 7457 middle-aged men in Goteborg, Sweden. *Stroke*. 2006;37(7):1663–1667.

168. Hart CL, Hole DJ, Smith GD. Risk factors and 20-year stroke mortality in men and women in the Renfrew/Paisley study in Scotland. *Stroke*. 1999;30(10):1999–2007.

169. Hu G, Jousilahti P, Sarti C, Antikainen R, Tuomilehto J. The effect of diabetes and stroke at baseline and during follow-up on stroke mortality. *Diabetologia*. 2006;49(10):2309–2316.

170. Duckworth W, Abraira C, Moritz T, Reda D, Emanuele N, Reaven PD, et al. Glucose control and vascular complications in veterans with type 2 diabetes. *N Engl J Med*. 2009;360(2):129–139.

171. Ismail-Beigi F, Craven T, Banerji MA, Basile J, Calles J, Cohen RM, et al. Effect of intensive treatment of hyperglycaemia on microvascular outcomes in type 2 diabetes: an analysis of the ACCORD randomised trial. *Lancet*. 2010;376(9739):419–430.

172. Patel A, MacMahon S, Chalmers J, Neal B, Billot L, Woodward M, et al. Intensive blood glucose control and vascular outcomes in patients with type 2 diabetes. *N Engl J Med*. 2008;358(24):2560–2572.

173. Dormandy JA, Charbonnel B, Eckland DJ, Erdmann E, Massi-Benedetti M, Moules IK, et al. Secondary prevention of macrovascular events in patients with type 2 diabetes in the PROactive Study (PROspective

pioglitAzone Clinical Trial In macroVascular Events): a randomised controlled trial. *Lancet*. 2005;366(9493):1279–1289.

174. Ajjan RA, Grant PJ. The cardiovascular safety of rosiglitazone. *Expert Opin Drug Saf*. 2008;7(4):367–376.

175. Kiechl S, Werner P, Egger G, Oberhollenzer F, Mayr M, Xu Q, *et al*. Active and passive smoking, chronic infections, and the risk of carotid atherosclerosis: prospective results from the Bruneck Study. *Stroke*. 2002;33(9):2170–2176.

176. Kurth T, Kase CS, Berger K, Gaziano JM, Cook NR, Buring JE. Smoking and risk of hemorrhagic stroke in women. *Stroke*. 2003;34(12):2792–2795.

177. Li C, Engstrom G, Hedblad B, Berglund G, Janzon L. Risk factors for stroke in subjects with normal blood pressure: a prospective cohort study. *Stroke*. 2005;36(2):234–238.

178. Wolf PA, D'Agostino RB, Kannel WB, Bonita R, Belanger AJ. Cigarette smoking as a risk factor for stroke. The Framingham Study. *JAMA*. 1988;259(7):1025–1029.

179. Bonita R, Duncan J, Truelsen T, Jackson RT, Beaglehole R. Passive smoking as well as active smoking increases the risk of acute stroke. *Tob Control*. 1999;8(2):156–160.

180. You RX, Thrift AG, McNeil JJ, Davis SM, Donnan GA. Ischemic stroke risk and passive exposure to spouses' cigarette smoking. Melbourne Stroke Risk Factor Study (MERFS) Group. *Am J Pub Health*. 1999;89(4):572–575.

181. Kawachi I, Colditz GA, Stampfer MJ, Willett WC, Manson JE, Rosner B, *et al*. Smoking cessation and decreased risk of stroke in women. *JAMA*. 1993;269(2):232–236.

182. Eikelboom JW, Hankey GJ, Anand SS, Lofthouse E, Staples N, Baker RI. Association between high homocyst(e)ine and ischemic stroke due to large- and small-artery disease but not other etiologic subtypes of ischemic stroke. *Stroke*. 2000;31(5):1069–1075.

183. Casas JP, Bautista LE, Smeeth L, Sharma P, Hingorani AD. Homocysteine and stroke: evidence on a causal link from mendelian randomisation. *Lancet*. 2005;365(9455):224–232.

184. B vitamins in patients with recent transient ischaemic attack or stroke in the VITAmins TO Prevent Stroke (VITATOPS) trial: a randomised, double-blind, parallel, placebo-controlled trial. *Lancet Neurol*. 2010;9(9):855–865.

185. Toole JF, Malinow MR, Chambless LE, Spence JD, Pettigrew LC, Howard VJ, *et al*. Lowering homocysteine in patients with ischemic stroke to prevent recurrent stroke, myocardial infarction, and death: the Vitamin Intervention for Stroke Prevention (VISP) randomized controlled trial. *JAMA*. 2004;291(5):565–575.

186. Vivekananthan DP, Penn MS, Sapp SK, Hsu A, Topol EJ. Use of antioxidant vitamins for the prevention of cardiovascular disease: meta-analysis of randomised trials. *Lancet*. 2003;361(9374):2017–2023.

187. Bjelakovic G, Nikolova D, Gluud LL, Simonetti RG, Gluud C. Mortality in randomized trials of antioxidant supplements for primary and secondary prevention: systematic review and meta-analysis. *JAMA*. 2007;297(8):842–857.

188. Lee CD, Folsom AR, Blair SN. Physical activity and stroke risk: a meta-analysis. *Stroke*. 2003;34(10):2475–2481.

189. Oczkowski W. Complexity of the relation between physical activity and stroke: a meta-analysis. *CJSM*. 2005;15(5):399.

190. Saunders DH, Greig CA, Mead GE, Young A. Physical fitness training for stroke patients. *Cochrane Database Syst Rev*. 2009;4:CD003316.

191. Field TS, Benavente OR. Current status of antiplatelet agents to prevent stroke. *Curr Neurol Neurosci Rep*. 2011;11(1):6–14.

192. Diener HC, Eikelboom J, Connolly SJ, Joyner CD, Hart RG, Lip GY, *et al*. Apixaban versus aspirin in patients with atrial fibrillation and previous stroke or transient ischaemic attack: a predefined subgroup analysis from AVERROES, a randomised trial. *Lancet Neurol*. 2012;11(3):225–231.

193. Effect of antihypertensive treatment on stroke recurrence. Hypertension-Stroke Cooperative Study Group. *JAMA*. 1974;229(4): 409–418.

194. Trial of secondary prevention with atenolol after transient ischemic attack or nondisabling ischemic stroke. The Dutch TIA Trial Study Group. *Stroke*. 1993;24(4):543–548.

195. Eriksson S, Olofsson B-O, Wester P-O. Atenolol in secondary prevention after stroke. *Cerebrovasc Dis*. 1995;5(1):21–25.

196. Yusuf S, Sleight P, Pogue J, Bosch J, Davies R, Dagenais G. Effects of an angiotensin-converting-enzyme inhibitor, ramipril, on cardiovascular events in high-risk patients. The Heart Outcomes Prevention Evaluation Study Investigators. *N Engl J Med*. 2000;342(3):145–153.

197. Liu L, Zhang Y, Liu G, Li W, Zhang X, Zanchetti A. The Felodipine Event Reduction (FEVER) Study: a randomized long-term placebo-controlled trial in Chinese hypertensive patients. *J Hypertension*. 2005;23(12):2157–2172.

198. Trenkwalder P, Elmfeldt D, Hofman A, Lithell H, Olofsson B, Papademetriou V, *et al*. The Study on COgnition and Prognosis in the Elderly (SCOPE)—major CV events and stroke in subgroups of patients. *Blood Pressure*. 2005;14(1):31–37.

199. Mazighi M, Tanasescu R, Ducrocq X, Vicaut E, Bracard S, Houdart E, *et al*. Prospective study of symptomatic atherothrombotic intracranial stenoses: the GESICA study. *Neurology*. 2006;66(8):1187–1191.

CHAPTER 16

Prognosis after stroke

Vincent Thijs

The science of prognostic studies

Determining the prognosis after stroke requires studies of excellent scientific quality (1–6). Biased studies provide incorrect information to the clinician and the patient and may impair the conduct of clinical trials. Biased studies may lead to overtreatment and abuse of resources when the prognosis of the patient is actually poor. Undertreatment may occur when patients are considered to have a poor prognosis, but actually will have a favourable outcome. For the patient and their family, being informed of a too optimistic or pessimistic outcome is obviously troubling. The consequences are severe when estimates of prognostic studies are used to send patients home from the emergency room after transient ischaemic attack (TIA) when they do actually have a high risk of recurrence. Similarly, biased estimates might lead to early discharge or withdrawal of care when care should actually be continued (7).

It is important to realize that prognostic studies offer probabilistic outcomes, rather than definite outcomes. As with any type of scientific study, prognostic studies suffer from drawbacks. Also, relying medical decision-making based on a single, published, high-quality study, may prove to be wrong, therefore validation in other independent studies and settings is required (3).

The inability to provide individual prognosis in most patients occurs because the results of prognostic studies derive from the average outcomes of a group of patients who are often different than the patient under consideration, because they are often performed in different healthcare settings, because treatment adherence and compliance is often not taken into account in prognostic models, and because not all prognostic variables may have been measured or were differently measured than in the patient under consideration. Therefore when prognosis is communicated to a patient or their family, it is wise to mention that a definite prognosis is difficult to make.

A few key principles of high-quality studies will be discussed here. The best estimates of outcome derive from population-based studies where no selection bias has occurred. Hospital-based studies may include patients that are different from the total population because of referral patterns or selection bias. Not all patients with stroke are admitted. Some patients die before they reach the hospital and many elderly patients that already reside in nursing homes may not be referred. Some general practitioners do not refer patients with very mild stroke. Sometimes hospital-based studies may be informative. For instance, in hospital-based studies accurate subtype classification is often more readily available or good imaging features are present.

In good prognostic studies, an inception cohort is used. Follow-up should start for all participants in about the same period

after stroke onset. Studies including patients recruited within a few hours after onset are optimal to catch early recurrent events. Before some seminal studies performed in the 1990s, prognosis after TIA was considered relatively benign, because most published studies did not consider very early recurrent events (8). Mixing patients that are recruited a few weeks or months after stroke onset, with patients that are recruited very early, as is often done in randomized clinical trials, provides biased estimates of prognosis. In acute stroke, deficits are often unstable in the very first hours after stroke onset and the effects of acute therapy like thrombolysis are sometimes not clear (9). Prognostic decision-making based on these hyperacute deficits is unwise and it is better to wait for at least 24 hours to gauge whether a deficit is permanent and communicate long-term prognosis.

The types of patients should be clearly defined. Mixing TIA patients with minor stroke patients may lead to a biased prognosis (9). Similarly, combining patients with anterior and posterior circulation lesions or ischaemic and haemorrhagic stroke may be erroneous.

Outcomes and prognostic parameters should be clearly defined and easily obtainable. All known prognostic factors should be measured at a defined time. The exact time depends on the purpose of the study. For hyperacute stroke, a prognostic tool should assess baseline parameters within a few hours, for long-term prognostication or for admittance to rehabilitation units an analysis after a few days is recommended. New prognostic models should incorporate already known prognostic factors before deciding on the value of a new tool. For prognosis of recovery, inclusion of age and initial impairment are quintessential. For recurrent stroke, stroke history is a powerful predictor of recurrent vascular events that is often omitted in prognostic studies. Similarly, if a prognostic tool is made an attempt should be made to compare it with the 'intuitive' prediction by the treating clinician.

The duration of follow-up and the number of recurrent events or rates of poor outcome should be adequate for statistical analyses. Loss to follow-up should be minimized and clearly mentioned by the authors. When loss to follow-up exceeds more than a few per cent of the patients the prognostic estimates become doubtful. Also, when using multivariable models to predict prognosis, a rule of thumb states that for each included prognostic variable about ten patients with a recurrent event or poor outcome should be included. For instance, at least 30 recurrent strokes should occur when one decides to study three prognostic variables, regardless of the number of patients that are included without recurrent stroke. In a study of prognosis after cryptogenic stroke, a high recurrence risk was found in patients with a combination of patent foramen ovale and atrial septal aneurysms; however, this was based on only 51 patients who suffered six endpoints (10).

A prognostic model should have a relatively high accuracy in predicting outcome. This is often measured by describing the area under the curve (AUC) or c-statistic of the prediction score (11, 12). The AUC is a value that estimates the capacity of a prognostic model to discriminate between a poor or a good prognosis or a high or low recurrence risk of stroke. To be meaningful in clinical practice AUC values or c-statistic values above 0.80 are recommended. A new measure, the net reclassification improvement (NRI) has been recommended to estimate the added value of a clinical score or prognostic model when multiple different models are available or when wants to test the addition of a new potential prognostic factor to an existing model. For instance in a model trying to improve the prediction of the development of malignant brain infarction, addition of emergent diffusion-weighted imaging (DWI) lesion volume led to correct classification in some patients previously thought not to develop malignant brain infarction, but also led to incorrect classification in some patients compared to the clinical model (13). Similarly, in patients not developing malignant brain infarction, addition of DWI lesion volume improved the prediction in some, but also worsened the prediction in others. The differences of the net changes in both groups are called the net improvement index. The model with imaging led to a net improvement index of 22%.

Independent validation by multiple studies in other healthcare settings adds to the robustness of the prediction score or prognostic model. Typically, AUC values in external validation cohorts will be less than the AUC obtained from the derivation cohort (3).

Finally, one has to realize that good and poor outcomes are defined differently from study to study and from outcome scale to outcome scale. Also, what doctors consider to be a poor prognosis, may be differently perceived by family or the patient. This is exemplified by the discussion of what is considered a good outcome after hemicraniectomy for malignant cerebral oedema or after severe intracerebral haemorrhage (14–16).

Recovery prediction after ischaemic stroke

In European population-based studies about 40% of patients who suffer a first ever stroke will be dead, dependent, or institutionalized 3 months later with some variation between healthcare systems (17).

When suffering a mild or disabling stroke, patients and their families are anxious to know whether their arm or leg weakness will recover, whether they will walk again or be able to communicate again, and care for themselves or survive. Most patients that will survive the initial stroke and do not suffer early recurrence or deterioration will have some degree of recovery (18, 19). Many studies have been performed to provide objective information about the outcome of this process. A few general principles are well accepted (19, 20). Recovery follows a non-linear logarithmic function over time with increased recovery speed in the first weeks after stroke followed by a subsequent flattening of the recovery curve and this irrespective of the initial stroke severity or affected neurological function (21, 22). Most studies indicate that at 6–12 months, functional outcome will not improve in a major way. This may be partly related to ceiling effects of most activities of daily living (ADL) scales (23–26). Age and the severity of initial clinical impairment are the most important prognostic markers (27). The younger the

patient, the more likely the patient will recover. Spectacular recoveries are often seen in patients suffering from stroke in their early twenties. In a study from the Austrian Stroke Registry, patients in their twenties had a 3.4-fold increase in good functional outcome, as compared with patients aged 55–65. As patients grow older and especially in the very old, good outcomes become less frequent, with a steep reduction in the proportion of good outcomes after age 75. The better outcome in young stroke survivors may result from increased support from family, more intensive rehabilitation, better adaptation systems, better-adapted neural recovery mechanisms or neuroplasticity, or collateral circulation. Elegant basic science studies have shown that the molecular programme executed after stroke supporting regeneration and neural function is quite different when stroke occurs in young compared to elderly rodents (28).

The initial impairment severity is, together with age, an important factor in recovery prediction. Mildly affected stroke patients generally have higher odds of recovery after stroke. A National Institutes of Health Stroke Scale (NIHSS) score below 5 is typically associated with a good outcome, with about 70% of good functional outcome (29). Be aware that the prognostic value of impairment scales, as measured in the very early minutes or hours after stroke onset, may not be that good (30). Recent studies, for instance, indicate that mild stroke patients often leave the hospital disabled. This is the reason why many stroke experts advocate thrombolytic treatment even when mild stroke is present. This practice is supported by subgroup analysis of the NINDS and ECASS 3 trials, although definitive data are lacking (31, 32).

Very severe neurological deficits within 24 hours after symptom onset, such as coma, complete paralysis, or very severe neurological impairment affecting multiple domains like global aphasia in combination with hemiplegia and eye deviation, is strongly indicative of a poor prognosis (33). Using neurological impairment scales, cut-offs indicative of poor recovery have been proposed, albeit with less than perfect discriminatory value (34, 35). NIHSS scores above 13 or 15 after a few days indicate permanent disability with a high likelihood (34). In the placebo arm of the NINDS study, patients with a NIHSS score higher than 17 plus atrial fibrillation almost invariably had a poor outcome (36).

Several models have been proposed to predict early recovery based on data obtained within the first hours after symptom onset (37–40). A model based on NIHSS and age in ischaemic stroke patients admitted within 6 hours, extensively validated with data from clinical trials, is able to predict mortality and functional outcome in approximately 70% of the patients, with an AUC of respectively 0.7 for mortality and 0.8 for functional independence. The model outperformed the impression of neurology residents regarding prognosis. The authors caution against the use of this model for individual prediction, but suggest its use in the inclusion criteria and design of clinical trials (37).

Another model, comprised of six easily obtainable variables has a similar predictive efficacy on independence and has been extensively validated in both haemorrhagic and ischaemic stroke, even in the first hours after stroke onset (41–43). The six variables are: (i) age, (ii) presence of dependency before stroke, (iii) whether the patient was living alone, and whether the patients is (iv) able to talk, (v) to walk without assistance, and (vi) capacity to lift their arms off the bed (41).

Both models are available as nomograms, but the authors advocate not using these models for individual prognosis.

These models do not incorporate other clinical features like stroke subtype or vascular risk factors. A model found that the presence of small vessel occlusion and diabetes influenced the prediction of excellent outcome in addition of age and baseline NIHSS, prestroke disability, and history of stroke (39, 40).

A model that was initially designed to predict in-hospital mortality after stroke (the iScore model) was recently shown to also predict very poor outcomes (death or institutionalization) after stroke within 30 days (44, 45). This model includes information about comorbidities like diabetes or the presence of cancer. The model was externally validated. The prognosis can be estimated using an online tool (46).

Table 16.1 compares the content of the four different prognostic scores.

As time passes, the prognostic value of impairment severity becomes clearer. If deficits do not subside or improve after a few days, prognostication becomes more accurate. The NIHSS is robust between days 2 and 9 to predict outcome as measured by the Barthel Index (BI) at 6 months or the modified Rankin scale (mRS) at 90 days (47, 48).

A simple, as yet unvalidated, model obtained 5 days after stroke using both NIHSS and age had AUC of 0.84 for predicting excellent outcome at 90 days (49). An analysis of patients enrolled in clinical trials showed that a combination of subcomponents from the NIHSS (such as the presence of dysarthria, facial palsy, or the motor score),

together with age and the number of vascular risk factors was predictive of good outcome (50). For instance, patients that were bedridden and needing constant care and supervision at 7 days (mRS score 5), being younger than 70 and having received tissue plasminogen activator, and having a NIHSS score at day 7 of lower than 17 (or no dysarthria with the NIHSS score and a leg strength <3) had a 60% chance of being able to walk independently at 3 months (mRS score 0–3).

The BI score obtained at day 5 (and day 9) is highly predictive of functional outcome at 90 days after stroke with an AUC of 0.83 (51).

Data from clinical trials in more than 6000 patients show that at 30 days, disability at 3 months can be almost exclusively determined from the mRS score with only 8% of patients improving or deteriorating more than 1 point on the scale (52).

Despite this flurry of studies, a systematic review of studies trying to predict the recovery of ADL found only a few studies of high scientific value (53). Age, baseline impairment severity as measured with a scale like the NIHSS or the Canadian Neurological Scale predicted poor ADL outcomes. The presence of only mild arm weakness predicted ADL recovery. Gender and the presence of atrial fibrillation did not seem to influence outcome per se.

When does stroke recovery end?

Most recovery occurs, on average, by 3–6 months after stroke (22). This recovery time varies by stroke severity: patients with mild

Table 16.1 Comparison of the content of four different prognostic scores

Predictive variables or characteristics	Essen model (37)	Six Simple Variables (5)	Acute Stroke Accurate Prediction model (7)	iScore (6)
Age	+	+	+	+
Time	<6 hours	Various	Day 1	Variable
Sex	–	–	–	+
Impairment scale	NIHSS	– [a]	NIHSS	CNS
Pre-stroke disability	–	Oxford handicap scale	+	+
Pre-stroke cognitive state	–	–	–	–
History of stroke	–	–	+	–
Family support	–	Living alone before stroke	–	–
Improvement between day 1 and day 5 as variable	–	–	–	–
Motor score upper limb	NIHSS	Able to lift arms	NIHSS subscale	CNS subscale
Motor score lower limb	NIHSS	Able to walk	NIHSS subscale	CNS subscale
Orientation and language	NIHSS	Glasgow Coma Scale verbal response	NIHSS subscale	CNS subscale
Stroke subtype	–	–	Small vessel occlusion versus no small vessel occlusion	TOAST
ADL assessment	–	–	–	–
Comorbid condition (diabetes, cancer, congestive heart failure, dialysis)	–	–	–	+
External validation	+	+	+	+
Mode of presentation	Nomogram	Nomogram	Nomogram	Website (46)

[a] Only the Oxfordshire Community Stroke project was used.

stroke typically recover within 2 months, patients with moderate stroke within 3 months, patients with severe stroke within 4 months, and patients with the most severe strokes have their functional recovery within 5 months from onset. Spectacular late recoveries have been reported (54).

Does the side of the lesion influence stroke prognosis?

The side of the ischaemic lesion does not seem to affect functional outcome (55). Care has to be taken to not underestimate the need of patients with low impairment scores and right hemispheric lesions as most neurological scales, like the NIHSSS, are more geared towards the recognition of left-sided hemisphere symptoms.

A magic number for recovery?

When patients have a mild to moderate motor deficit or aphasia 1–3 days after stroke onset, small studies have suggested that they will recover to about 70% of the maximum potential improvement (defined as the difference between the maximum score of the impairment and the initial impairment) at 90 days as measured with a motor scale or language battery that assessed naming and comprehension (56, 57) These findings were derived from small study populations and need validation in larger datasets.

Mortality prediction after ischaemic stroke

The 1-year mortality after ischaemic stroke is between 20% and 40% and the 30-day mortality is between 5% and 20% (58, 59). Prediction of short- and medium-term mortality is therefore highly relevant. There are, however, no scoring systems that are widely accepted.

Several risk scores were developed but not universally accepted because their sample size was small, stroke severity was not measured, the score was not easily usable by clinicians, the resulting AUCs were low, the models were not independently validated, or could not be transported to other healthcare settings (37, 40, 60–63)

In the framework of the Get With The Guidelines (GWTG) programme, a risk score for in-hospital mortality was developed in 274,988 ischaemic stroke patients from more than 1000 hospitals in the United States (64). A model with the NIHSS alone, was almost as good as a model that incorporated NIHSS with other characteristics (age, arrival via ambulance, history of atrial fibrillation, previous stroke, previous myocardial infarction, carotid stenosis, diabetes mellitus, peripheral vascular disease, hypertension, history of dyslipidaemia, current smoking, and weekend or night admission). This model was in turn superior to a model that did not include the NIHSS. A nomogram was provided for the models with and without NIHSS. These data are routinely collected within the GWTG programme and can easily be implemented in the GWTG web tool. It is unclear whether this model is useful in other healthcare settings, as the hospitalization duration was relatively short and mortality low.

The iSCORE mentioned earlier was developed specifically to predict mortality in inpatients with ischaemic stroke. It incorporates clinical, prestroke disability and relevant comorbidities (diabetes, atrial fibrillation, congestive heart failure, cancer, dialysis) (44). It was developed in Canada in a derivation sample of 8223 patients

with internal validation in 4039 and external validation in 3270 patients. There was quite close agreement between observed and predicted mortality. Further studies will need to study the transportability of this score to other healthcare settings before becoming widely accepted.

Recovery of specific neurological deficits commonly found in stroke patients

Motor recovery

The prognosis of arm motor recovery in hemiplegic stroke patients is poor with good functional outcome in only 5–20% (65–67). The severity of early motor impairment is the biggest predictor of outcome, regardless of which test is used (68). Dependent on the severity of stroke, major upper extremity recovery beyond 11 weeks is very unlikely (67). If some arm grip is present within the first weeks, outcome is not as bad, whereas the absence of a hand grip within a month is indicative of very poor motor outcome (65). The function of the leg matters too. If motor function in the leg returns in the first week, the chance of regaining dexterity of the arm is much higher (69). Conversely, absence of return of motor function in the leg within 2 weeks is associated with poor functional arm outcome. In one study of 102 patients with a flaccid arm due to middle cerebral artery infarction studied serially only 10.6% recovered manual dexterity after 6 months (69). The optimal time for outcome prediction of the arm was at 4 weeks: a Fugl–Meyer score of more than 18 had a 94% chance of functional arm recovery, but only 0.09% if this level was not achieved.

Recently, early indicators of functional recovery of the arm have been proposed: the presence of finger extension and shoulder abduction within 72 hours had a very high probability of regaining functional arm recovery at 6 months (70). This finding could however not be replicated in another study, which tested wrist and shoulder extension within 48 hours (71). The differences might be related to the cut-offs as to what is considered functional arm recovery.

Hemianopia

Few studies have systematically evaluated recovery factors and the time to recovery in patients with hemianopia due to stroke (72–74). The available prospective studies suggest that total recovery of hemianopia is possible, but that partial recovery is more frequent and occurs in up to 72%. The recovery process is mostly complete at 6 months (72). Quadrantanopia has a better prognosis than hemianopia. Better recovery is present when the striate cortex is spared (72, 73) and when the lower visual field is affected (74). The recovery process occurs mostly in the periphery of the visual field (72, 73).

Neglect and anosognosia

The neglect syndrome is a constellation of impairments related to attention to self and the outside world occurring in lesions in the contralateral hemisphere (75). Neglect is typically a multidimensional syndrome, comprising subsyndromes like anosognosia for hemiplegia, asomatognosia, extinction, motor neglect, visuospatial neglect which individually may have different severities and may influence prognosis differently. There is also no universally accepted, standardized scale for assessing neglect. In the Copenhagen Stroke Study, a large community based stroke study with 600 patients measured within the first week after stroke, anosognosia for motor deficit and visual field cuts, but not neglect (as assessed by a cancellation test and by asking the patient to reach for the affected arm) per se, had an independent negative effect on prognosis regarding to ADL, discharge to home or rehabilitation length (76). Other studies, often mixing anosognosia and hemineglect, found a deleterious effect on rehabilitation efforts and poorer prognosis (77, 78).

Again, the time of assessment and the scale used is important (79). Acute recovery of some aspects of neglect is frequently seen even in severely affected patients within a few days after stroke (77). Neglect persisting at admission into a rehabilitation facility is probably a factor that has a negative influence on global outcome. Though symptoms of neglect may gradually wane, a long-lasting effect on postural control and gait impairment has been described (80).

Dysphagia

Dysphagia may show a different recovery pattern after stroke than hemiparesis with dysphagia showing an apparent high rate of good outcome (81–84). This may, however, be a false assumption as studies show the persistence of subclinical deficits in many patients. In one study of 91 dysphagic patients studied within 5 days after stroke about three-quarters of stroke patients had taken up their pre-stroke diet by 3 months, but at least 10% had persistent dysphagia after 3 months with half of the patients requiring enteral feeding.

Few studies have examined whether the dysphagia completely resolved using imaging techniques like videofluoroscopy. One large study showed a high rate of aspiration on videofluoroscopy at 6 months, despite an 87% rate of resumption of the normal diet. Persistent clinical swallowing abnormalities were also frequent (85).

In a study of patients who underwent videofluoroscopy because of dysphagia at 40 days after stroke, factors strongly related to persistent dysphagia were inadequate or no tongue-to-palate contact, reduced laryngeal elevation, the presence of pyriform sinus residue, coating of the pharyngeal wall, and aspiration (86).

Walking

Being able to walk independently is a major goal for stroke patients and the rehabilitation team. The following predictors are predictive of resuming walking within 30 days in a recent systematic review: lower age, milder severity of paresis, less reduced leg power, absence of hemianopia, smaller size of brain lesion, and type of stroke (87). In a large prospective study, recovery of walking function occurred in 95% of the patients within the first 11 weeks after stroke, with more rapid recovery and stabilization in mild to moderate leg weakness (88, 89). When paresis is initially very severe, no further improvement was seen after 11 weeks in about 95% of the patients. Patients who did not regain some strength in the leg within the first week after stroke were not able to walk at 3 months (89). Later recovery of walking ability, up to 1 year, has, however, been described in selected patients with initially flaccid paralysis of the lower limb, undergoing delayed outpatient rehabilitation (90).

Aphasia

Language deficits are common following left hemisphere stroke. About 60% of patients with aphasia had permanent language impairments after stroke, based on the Western Aphasia battery. The best time to predict language outcome was at 2–4 weeks after stroke onset. Improvement compared to initial baseline occurred in most patients. Auditory comprehension appears to be the function that improves most in patients with large lesions compared to verbal and written expression. The outcome after aphasia is quite variable and depends mostly on the severity of initial aphasia, the general severity of the stroke, and the location and size of the lesions. The impact of age and intelligence on aphasia recovery is unclear. Education and gender do not influence the recovery pattern in a major way. Similarly, handedness has not been shown to influence the recovery in a significant way. More extensive lesions affecting language areas like Broca's or Wernicke's regions impair recovery of the disrupted language function. Global aphasia often evolves to Broca-type aphasia. Fluent aphasias rarely evolve into non-fluent types.

Sensory abnormalities

Somatosensory impairment defined as either impaired tactile sensation, impaired stereognosis, or proprioception is common after stroke. Few studies have systematically evaluated the recovery of sensory impairment after stroke. This is a difficult area to study objectively as there are different ways to estimate sensory impairments going from questionnaires, clinical, and electrophysiological tools. As in other types of impairment, recovery over time is observed, mainly dependent on the initial severity of somatosensory impairment and general stroke severity (57).

Ataxia

Few studies have examined recovery after cerebellar stroke. Recovery after ataxia can be spectacular as evidenced by the absence of any neurological impairment after decompression or cerebellectomy for space-occupying cerebellar infarcts. A retrospective study in a rehabilitation setting showed large functional improvements after cerebellar infarction (91). Recovery is less good when there is additional brainstem involvement and when the stroke-related disability is severe.

Mortality and disability after intubation

A study reviewed the outcomes after intubation of patients with severe ischaemic or haemorrhagic stroke due to neurological or respiratory reasons (92). The mortality was 58% (range 46–75%) at 30 days and 68% (range 59–80%) at 1–2 years. Still, despite this poor outcome, one-third of the survivors had a good clinical outcome.

Recovery and mortality prediction after intracerebral haemorrhage

Intracerebral haemorrhage (ICH) accounts for about 15% of all strokes (93). Prognosis after ICH is worse with a higher rate of death and less complete recovery than ischaemic stroke. However, this might just reflect the fact that ICH lesion volumes are generally larger than the ischaemic lesion volumes. In fact the outcome seems comparable between the two groups when correction for initial stroke severity is applied (94). Improvement in functional outcome was observed in one-third of the patients who survived the ICH between hospital discharge and 12 months (95). The mortality after intracerebral haemorrhage is about 35–52% within 30 days after stroke onset, with many patients dying within 48 hours after stroke onset, purportedly related to early withdrawal of care in many patients (95–98).

A multitude of prognostic models have been developed for ICH (99–101). However, none of the prognostic algorithms has gained widespread acceptance, like coma prediction models after cardiac arrest (102). Relevant models include in addition to age and the severity of consciousness impairment (e.g. Glasgow Coma Scale or NIHSS), the volume of the ICH, the presence of intraventricular extension and midline shift as relevant parameters for predicting outcome. A comparison of the prognostic systems is shown in Table 16.2.

However, many of the developed models have several flaws (100). Data for deriving the models were obtained retrospectively, the cohorts were small, the validation was lacking or incomplete, the data definitions were not provided, and some patients underwent surgical treatment. Death was often the only outcome that was

considered. In most of the models in whom an AUC was calculated it was above 0.8, indicating quite good prognostic performance. However, the proportion of patients in whom outcome was predicted as universally poor was often limited, casting doubt on the relevance of the models in clinical practice, especially when deciding whether intensive treatment is warranted. Few models assessed recovery as the outcome parameter. Only one study assessed whether a prognostic score performed better than the clinician's judgement. The Essen ICH score performed better than the admitting physician's estimation (103).

Another issue that is heavily debated is the bias induced by do not resuscitate (DNR) orders and early withdrawal of care in the prognostic capacity of these models. A report showed that commonly used models overestimate mortality rates in patients who do not receive early DNR orders and underestimate mortality rates when patients receive early DNR orders (7, 104). When both

Table 16.2 Comparison of prognostic scores used in intracerebral haemorrhage

	Stroke data bank score (101)	Cincinatti (99)	ICH score (95, 107)	Functional score (108)	Essen ICH score (103)
Outcome	Mortality and poor outcome	30-day mortality and Glasgow Outcome Scale score	30-day mortality and modified Rankin Scale score	Functional independence at 90 days (Glasgow Outcome Scale ≥4)	Functional independence Barthel Index score >95 at 90 days
Location	Supratentorial	Supra-and infratentorial	Supra-and infratentorial	Supra-and infratentorial	Supra-and infratentorial
Predictors	GCS score <8, ICH volume >72 mL, IVH presence, pulse pressure >85 mmHg	GCS score (≤8, 9–15) and ICH volume in three categories (<30 mL, 30–60 mL, >60 mL)	GCS score, ICH volume, IVH presence, infratentorial location, age (maximum score is 5)	ICH volume, lobar, deep or infratentorial, age, GCS score, pre-ICH cognitive impairment	Age Total NIHSS LOC (as in NIHSS)
Scoring system	NA	NA	GCS score 3–4: 2 5–12: 1 13–15: 0 ICH ≥30 mL: 1 Infratentorial ICH: 1 IVH: 1 Age ≥80: 1 0–6 points	ICH <30 mL: 4 ICH 30–60 mL: 2 Age <70: 2 70–79: 1 I CH Lobar: 2 ICH Deep: 1 GCS ≥9: 2 Pre-ICH cognitive impairment absent: 1	Age: 60–69: 1 70–79: 2 80 or more: 3 NIH 0–5: 0 6–10: 1 11–15: 2 16–20: 3 20 or more/coma: 4 NIH LOC Drowsy: 1 Stupor: 2 Coma: 3
Scoring range			0–6 (lower is better)	0–11 (higher is better)	0–11 (lower is better)
	Both features present:93% 30-day mortality, 94% poor 1-year outcome, both absent 3% mortality, 17% poor 1 year outcome	GCS score ≤8 and ICH volume >60 mL predicted mortality in 91% of patients	All patients with scores of 5 died	ICH volume (<30 mL), ICH location (lobar) presence, GCS score >8, age <70, no cognitive impairment: 82% good functional outcome (91% if no DNR orders), if none of these features present and age >80, no good outcomes were observed	Score of >3 had a 94.5% NPV for good functional outcome, score of 7 had a PPV of 86% for mortality
Tested in other study population	Yes	Yes	Yes	No	Yes
Influence of early DNR	Yes	Yes	Yes	No	Uncertain

groups of patients are combined, the differences cancel out and the perception of good accuracy is created. Early DNR orders may be a surrogate for pre-existing disability, comorbidity, or the perception that prognosis is dire based on the clinician's intuition or reflect a general attitude or hospital culture of hopelessness in the care of patients with acute ICH. There is an association between hospitals that frequently institute early (within 24 hours after stroke onset) DNR orders (here seen as a surrogate for the aggressiveness of therapy), and mortality from ICH, after correction from case-mix differences between hospitals (105).

Another related problem is that if the prognostic scores are based on variables that are already in common clinical use to withdraw care, this may lead to a self-fulfilling prophecy on the efficacy of the prognostic score to predict death, but even more dangerously withdrawal of care in some patients who might have survived or recovered reasonably well (106). On the other hand, if care is not withdrawn in any patients carrying a poor prognosis, this might avoid disability in a few patients but at the expense of many more patients surviving with severe disability, a situation that many elderly people consider worse than death.

Conclusion

Providing a prognosis after stroke is a difficult decision. Over the past years, strides have been made in overcoming the limitations of prognostic decision-making in stroke. Headway has been made in creating prognostic scores that are clinically relevant and useful. Finding a universally accepted prognostic tool currently remains a dream. As with any result of scientific study in medicine, common sense is required when making decisions using prognostic scores. Their value lies in opening up the discussion with patients and family about outcome, and in clinical trials where they can be used to better design the target population for the intervention.

References

1. Laupacis A, Wells G, Richardson WS, Tugwell P. Users' guides to the medical literature. V. How to use an article about prognosis. Evidence-Based Medicine Working Group. *JAMA.* 1994;272(3):234–237.
2. Moons KG, Altman DG, Vergouwe Y, Royston P. Prognosis and prognostic research: application and impact of prognostic models in clinical practice. *BMJ.* 2009;338:b606.
3. Altman DG, Vergouwe Y, Royston P, Moons KG. Prognosis and prognostic research: validating a prognostic model. *BMJ.* 2009;338:b605.
4. Counsell C, Dennis M. Systematic review of prognostic models in patients with acute stroke. *Cerebrovasc Dis.* 2001;12(3):159–170.
5. Moons KG, Royston P, Vergouwe Y, Grobbee DE, Altman DG. Prognosis and prognostic research: what, why, and how? *BMJ.* 2009;338:b375.
6. Rothwell PM. Prognostic models. *Pract Neurol.* 2008;8(4):242–253.
7. Zahuranec DB, Morgenstern LB, Sanchez BN, Resnicow K, White DB, Hemphill JC, 3rd. Do-not-resuscitate orders and predictive models after intracerebral hemorrhage. *Neurology.* 2010;75(7):626–633.
8. Johnston SC, Gress DR, Browner WS, Sidney S. Short-term prognosis after emergency department diagnosis of TIA. *JAMA.* 2000;284(22):2901–2906.
9. Johnston SC, Easton JD. Are patients with acutely recovered cerebral ischemia more unstable? *Stroke.* 2003;34(10):2446–2450.
10. Mas JL, Arquizan C, Lamy C, Zuber M, Cabanes L, Derumeaux G, *et al.* Recurrent cerebrovascular events associated with patent foramen ovale, atrial septal aneurysm, or both. *N Engl J Med.* 2001;345(24):1740–1746.
11. Steyerberg EW, Vickers AJ, Cook NR, Gerds T, Gonen M, Obuchowski N, *et al.* Assessing the performance of prediction models: a framework for traditional and novel measures. *Epidemiology.* 2010;21(1):128–138.
12. Pencina MJ, D'Agostino RB, Sr., D'Agostino RB, Jr, Vasan RS. Evaluating the added predictive ability of a new marker: from area under the ROC curve to reclassification and beyond. *Stat Med.* 2008;27(2):157–172; discussion 207–112.
13. Thomalla G, Hartmann F, Juettler E, Singer OC, Lehnhardt FG, Kohrmann M, *et al.* Prediction of malignant middle cerebral artery infarction by magnetic resonance imaging within 6 hours of symptom onset: a prospective multicenter observational study. *Ann Neurol.* 2010;68(4):435–445.
14. Weil AG, Rahme R, Moumdjian R, Bouthillier A, Bojanowski MW. Quality of life following hemicraniectomy for malignant MCA territory infarction. *Can J Neurol Sci.* 2011;38(3):434–438.
15. Kelly AG, Holloway RG. Health state preferences and decision-making after malignant middle cerebral artery infarctions. *Neurology.* 2010;75(8):682–687.
16. Rabinstein AA, Diringer MN. Withholding care in intracerebral hemorrhage: realistic compassion or self-fulfilling prophecy? *Neurology.* 2007;68(20):1647–1648.
17. Heuschmann PU, Wiedmann S, Wellwood I, Rudd A, Di Carlo A, Bejot Y, *et al.* Three-month stroke outcome: the European Registers of Stroke (EROS) investigators. *Neurology.* 2011;76(2):159–165.
18. Kwakkel G, Kollen B, Lindeman E. Understanding the pattern of functional recovery after stroke: facts and theories. *Restor Neurol Neurosci.* 2004;22(3-5):281–299.
19. Jongbloed L. Prediction of function after stroke: a critical review. *Stroke.* 1986;17(4):765–776.
20. Kwakkel G, Wagenaar RC, Kollen BJ, Lankhorst GJ. Predicting disability in stroke—a critical review of the literature. *Age Ageing.* 1996;25(6):479–489.
21. Jorgensen HS, Nakayama H, Raaschou HO, Vive-Larsen J, Stoier M, Olsen TS. Outcome and time course of recovery in stroke. Part I: Outcome. The Copenhagen Stroke Study. *Arch Phys Med Rehabil.* 1995;76(5):399–405.
22. Jorgensen HS, Nakayama H, Raaschou HO, Vive-Larsen J, Stoier M, Olsen TS. Outcome and time course of recovery in stroke. Part II: time course of recovery. The Copenhagen Stroke Study. *Arch Phys Med Rehabil.* 1995;76(5):406–412.
23. Kwon S, Hartzema AG, Duncan PW, Min-Lai S. Disability measures in stroke: relationship among the Barthel Index, the Functional Independence Measure, and the Modified Rankin Scale. *Stroke.* 2004;35(4):918–923.
24. Weimar C, Kurth T, Kraywinkel K, Wagner M, Busse O, Haberl RL, *et al.* Assessment of functioning and disability after ischemic stroke. *Stroke.* 2002;33(8):2053–2059.
25. Kasner SE. Clinical interpretation and use of stroke scales. *Lancet Neurol.* 2006;5(7):603–612.
26. Horgan NF, O'Regan M, Cunningham CJ, Finn AM. Recovery after stroke: a 1-year profile. *Disabil Rehabil.* 2009;31(10):831–839.
27. Knoflach M, Matosevic B, Rucker M, Furtner M, Mair A, Wille G, *et al.* Functional recovery after ischemic stroke—a matter of age: data from the Austrian Stroke Unit Registry. *Neurology.* 2012;78(4):279–285.
28. Popa-Wagner A, Carmichael ST, Kokaia Z, Kessler C, Walker LC. The response of the aged brain to stroke: too much, too soon? *Curr Neurovasc Res.* 2007;4(3):216–227.
29. Khatri P, Conaway MR, Johnston KC. Ninety-day outcome rates of a prospective cohort of consecutive patients with mild ischemic stroke. *Stroke.* 2012;43(2):560–562.
30. Smith EE, Abdullah AR, Petkovska I, Rosenthal E, Koroshetz WJ, Schwamm LH. Poor outcomes in patients who do not receive intravenous tissue plasminogen activator because of mild or improving ischemic stroke. *Stroke.* 2005;36(11):2497–2499.
31. Bluhmki E, Chamorro A, Davalos A, Machnig T, Sauce C, Wahlgren N, *et al.* Stroke treatment with alteplase given 3.0-4.5 h after onset of acute ischaemic stroke (ECASS III): additional outcomes and subgroup analysis of a randomised controlled trial. *Lancet Neurol.* 2009;8(12):1095–1102.
32. Recombinant tissue plasminogen activator for minor strokes: the National Institute of Neurological Disorders and Stroke rt-PA Stroke Study experience. *Ann Emerg Med.* 2005;46(3):243–252.

33. Bamford J, Sandercock P, Dennis M, Burn J, Warlow C. Classification and natural history of clinically identifiable subtypes of cerebral infarction. *Lancet.* 1991;337(8756):1521–1526.

34. Muir KW, Weir CJ, Murray GD, Povey C, Lees KR. Comparison of neurological scales and scoring systems for acute stroke prognosis. *Stroke.* 1996;27(10):1817–1820.

35. Adams HP, Jr, Davis PH, Leira EC, Chang KC, Bendixen BH, Clarke WR, et al. Baseline NIH Stroke Scale score strongly predicts outcome after stroke: a report of the Trial of Org 10172 in Acute Stroke Treatment (TOAST). *Neurology.* 1999;53(1):126–131.

36. Frankel MR, Morgenstern LB, Kwiatkowski T, Lu M, Tilley BC, Broderick JP, et al. Predicting prognosis after stroke: a placebo group analysis from the National Institute of Neurological Disorders and Stroke rt-PA Stroke Trial. *Neurology.* 2000;55(7):952–959.

37. Weimar C, Konig IR, Kraywinkel K, Ziegler A, Diener HC. Age and National Institutes of Health Stroke Scale Score within 6 hours after onset are accurate predictors of outcome after cerebral ischemia: development and external validation of prognostic models. *Stroke.* 2004;35(1):158–162.

38. Johnston KC, Connors AF, Jr, Wagner DP, Haley EC, Jr Predicting outcome in ischemic stroke: external validation of predictive risk models. *Stroke.* 2003;34(1):200–202.

39. Johnston KC, Wagner DP, Wang XQ, Newman GC, Thijs V, Sen S, et al. Validation of an acute ischemic stroke model: does diffusion-weighted imaging lesion volume offer a clinically significant improvement in prediction of outcome? *Stroke.* 2007;38(6):1820–1825.

40. Johnston KC, Connors AF, Jr, Wagner DP, Knaus WA, Wang X, Haley EC, Jr A predictive risk model for outcomes of ischemic stroke. *Stroke.* 2000;31(2):448–455.

41. Counsell C, Dennis M, McDowall M, Warlow C. Predicting outcome after acute and subacute stroke: development and validation of new prognostic models. *Stroke.* 2002;33(4):1041–1047.

42. Counsell C, Dennis M, McDowall M. Predicting functional outcome in acute stroke: comparison of a simple six variable model with other predictive systems and informal clinical prediction. *J Neurol Neurosurg Psychiatry.* 2004;75(3):401–405.

43. Teale EA, Forster A, Munyombwe T, Young JB. A systematic review of case-mix adjustment models for stroke. *Clin Rehabil.* 2012;26(9):771–786

44. Saposnik G, Kapral MK, Liu Y, Hall R, O'Donnell M, Raptis S, et al. IScore: a risk score to predict death early after hospitalization for an acute ischemic stroke. *Circulation.* 2011;123(7):739–749.

45. Saposnik G, Raptis S, Kapral MK, Liu Y, Tu JV, Mamdani M, et al. The iScore predicts poor functional outcomes early after hospitalization for an acute ischemic stroke. *Stroke.* 2011;42(12):3421–3428.

46. Saposnik G. iSCORE online tool. <http://www.sorcan.ca/iscore/> (accessed 6 March 2012).

47. Kwakkel G, Veerbeek JM, van Wegen EE, Nijland R, Harmeling-van der Wel BC, Dippel DW, et al. Predictive value of the NIHSS for ADL outcome after ischemic hemispheric stroke: does timing of early assessment matter? *J Neurol Sci.* 2010;294(1–2):57–61.

48. Kerr DM, Fulton RL, Lees KR, for the VC. Seven-Day NIHSS is a sensitive outcome measure for exploratory clinical trials in acute stroke: evidence from the Virtual International Stroke Trials Archive. *Stroke.* 2012 May;43(5):1401–1403.

49. Johnston KC, Barrett KM, Ding YH, Wagner DP. Acute stroke accurate prediction I. Clinical and imaging data at 5 days as a surrogate for 90-day outcome in ischemic stroke. *Stroke.* 2009;40(4):1332–1333.

50. Hallevi H, Albright KC, Martin-Schild SB, Barreto AD, Morales MM, Bornstein N, et al. Recovery after ischemic stroke: criteria for good outcome by level of disability at day 7. *Cerebrovasc Dis.* 2009;28(4):341–348.

51. Kwakkel G, Veerbeek JM, Harmeling-van der Wel BC, van Wegen E, Kollen BJ, Early prediction of functional outcome after stroke I. Diagnostic accuracy of the Barthel Index for measuring activities of daily living outcome after ischemic hemispheric stroke: does early poststroke timing of assessment matter? *Stroke.* 2011;42(2):342–346.

52. Ovbiagele B, Lyden PD, Saver JL, Collaborators V. Disability status at 1 month is a reliable proxy for final ischemic stroke outcome. *Neurology.* 2010;75(8):688–692.

53. Veerbeek JM, Kwakkel G, van Wegen EE, Ket JC, Heymans MW. Early prediction of outcome of activities of daily living after stroke: a systematic review. *Stroke.* 2011;42(5):1482–1488.

54. Smania N, Gandolfi M, Aglioti SM, Girardi P, Fiaschi A, Girardi F. How long is the recovery of global aphasia? Twenty-five years of follow-up in a patient with left hemisphere stroke. *Neurorehabil Neural Repair.* 2010;24(9):871–875.

55. Fink JN, Frampton CM, Lyden P, Lees KR, Virtual International Stroke Trials Archive I. Does hemispheric lateralization influence functional and cardiovascular outcomes after stroke?: an analysis of placebo-treated patients from prospective acute stroke trials. *Stroke.* 2008;39(12):3335–3340.

56. Lazar RM, Minzer B, Antoniello D, Festa JR, Krakauer JW, Marshall RS. Improvement in aphasia scores after stroke is well predicted by initial severity. *Stroke.* 2010;41(7):1485–1488.

57. Prabhakaran S, Zarahn E, Riley C, Speizer A, Chong JY, Lazar RM, et al. Inter-individual variability in the capacity for motor recovery after ischemic stroke. *Neurorehabil Neural Repair.* 2008;22(1):64–71.

58. Appelros P, Nydevik I, Viitanen M. Poor outcome after first-ever stroke: predictors for death, dependency, and recurrent stroke within the first year. *Stroke.* 2003;34(1):122–126.

59. Hankey GJ, Jamrozik K, Broadhurst RJ, Forbes S, Burvill PW, Anderson CS, et al. Five-year survival after first-ever stroke and related prognostic factors in the Perth Community Stroke Study. *Stroke.* 2000;31(9):2080–2086.

60. Konig IR, Ziegler A, Bluhmki E, Hacke W, Bath PM, Sacco RL, et al. Predicting long-term outcome after acute ischemic stroke: a simple index works in patients from controlled clinical trials. *Stroke.* 2008;39(6):1821–1826.

61. Solberg OG, Dahl M, Mowinckel P, Stavem K. Derivation and validation of a simple risk score for predicting 1-year mortality in stroke. *J Neurol.* 2007;254(10):1376–1383.

62. Wang Y, Lim LL, Heller RF, Fisher J, Levi CR. A prediction model of 1-year mortality for acute ischemic stroke patients. *Arch Phys Med Rehabil.* 2003;84(7):1006–1011.

63. Wang Y, Lim LL, Levi C, Heller RF, Fischer J. A prognostic index for 30-day mortality after stroke. *J Clin Epidemiol.* 2001;54(8):766–773.

64. Smith EE, Shobha N, Dai D, Olson DM, Reeves MJ, Saver JL, et al. Risk score for in-hospital ischemic stroke mortality derived and validated within the Get With the Guidelines-Stroke Program. *Circulation.* 2010;122(15):1496–1504.

65. Heller A, Wade DT, Wood VA, Sunderland A, Hewer RL, Ward E. Arm function after stroke: measurement and recovery over the first three months. *J Neurol Neurosurg Psychiatry.* 1987;50(6):714–719.

66. Wade DT, Langton-Hewer R, Wood VA, Skilbeck CE, Ismail HM. The hemiplegic arm after stroke: measurement and recovery. *J Neurol Neurosurg Psychiatry.* 1983;46(6):521–524.

67. Nakayama H, Jorgensen HS, Raaschou HO, Olsen TS. Recovery of upper extremity function in stroke patients: the Copenhagen Stroke Study. *Arch Phys Med Rehabil.* 1994;75(4):394–398.

68. Coupar F, Pollock A, Rowe P, Weir C, Langhorne P. Predictors of upper limb recovery after stroke: a systematic review and meta-analysis. *Clin Rehabil.* 2012. Apr;26(4):291–313.

69. Kwakkel G, Kollen BJ, van der Grond J, Prevo AJ. Probability of regaining dexterity in the flaccid upper limb: impact of severity of paresis and time since onset in acute stroke. *Stroke.* 2003;34(9):2181–2186.

70. Nijland RH, van Wegen EE, Harmeling-van der Wel BC, Kwakkel G. Presence of finger extension and shoulder abduction within 72 hours after stroke predicts functional recovery: early prediction of functional outcome after stroke: the EPOS cohort study. *Stroke.* 2010;41(4):745–750.

71. Prager EM, Lang CE. Predictive ability of 2-day measurement of active range of motion on 3-mo upper-extremity motor function in people with poststroke hemiparesis. *Am J Occup Ther.* 2012;66(1):35–41.

72. Messing B, Ganshirt H. Follow-up of visual field defects with vascular damage of the geniculostriate visual pathway. *Neuro-Ophthalmology.* 1987;7(4):231–242.

73. Celebisoy M, Celebisoy N, Bayam E, Kose T. Recovery of visual-field defects after occipital lobe infarction: a perimetric study. *J Neurol Neurosurg Psychiatry.* 2011;82(6):695–702.

74. Tiel K, Kölmel H. Patterns of recovery from homonymous hemianopia subsequent to infarction in the distribution of the posterior cerebral artery. *Neuro-Ophthalmology.* 1991;11:33–39.

75. Heilman KM, Valenstein E, Watson RT. Neglect and related disorders. *Semin Neurol.* 2000;20(4):463–470.

76. Pedersen PM, Jorgensen HS, Nakayama H, Raaschou HO, Olsen TS. Hemineglect in acute stroke—incidence and prognostic implications. The Copenhagen Stroke Study. *Am J Phys Med Rehabil.* 1997;76(2):122–127.

77. Jehkonen M, Ahonen JP, Dastidar P, Koivisto AM, Laippala P, Vilkki J, et al. Visual neglect as a predictor of functional outcome one year after stroke. *Acta Neurol Scand.* 2000;101(3):195–201.

78. Jehkonen M, Laihosalo M, Kettunen JE. Impact of neglect on functional outcome after stroke: a review of methodological issues and recent research findings. *Restor Neurol Neurosci.* 2006;24(4-6):209–215.

79. Bowen A, McKenna K, Tallis RC. Reasons for variability in the reported rate of occurrence of unilateral spatial neglect after stroke. *Stroke.* 1999;30(6):1196–1202.

80. van Nes IJ, van Kessel ME, Schils F, Fasotti L, Geurts AC, Kwakkel G. Is visuospatial hemineglect longitudinally associated with postural imbalance in the postacute phase of stroke? *Neurorehabil Neural Repair.* 2009;23(8):819–824.

81. Smithard D, O'Neill P, England R, Park C, Wyatt R, Martin D, et al. The natural history of dysphagia following a stroke. *Dysphagia.* 1997;12(4):188–193.

82. Gordon C, Hewer RL, Wade DT. Dysphagia in acute stroke. *Br Med J (Clin Res Ed).* 1987;295(6595):411–414.

83. Barer DH. The natural history and functional consequences of dysphagia after hemispheric stroke. *J Neurol Neurosurg Psychiatry.* 1989;52(2):236–241.

84. Kidd D, Lawson J, Nesbitt R, MacMahon J. The natural history and clinical consequences of aspiration in acute stroke. *QJM.* 1995;88(6):409–413.

85. Mann G, Hankey GJ, Cameron D. Swallowing function after stroke: prognosis and prognostic factors at 6 months. *Stroke.* 1999;30(4):744–748.

86. Han T, Paik N, Park J, Kwon B. The prediction of persistent dysphagia beyond six months after stroke. *Dysphagia.* 1998;23(1):59–64.

87. Craig LE, Wu O, Bernhardt J, Langhorne P. Predictors of poststroke mobility: systematic review. *Int J Stroke.* 2011;6(4):321–327.

88. Jorgensen HS, Nakayama H, Raaschou HO, Olsen TS. Recovery of walking function in stroke patients: the Copenhagen Stroke Study. *Arch Phys Med Rehabil.* 1995;76(1):27–32.

89. Wandel A, Jorgensen HS, Nakayama H, Raaschou HO, Olsen TS. Prediction of walking function in stroke patients with initial lower extremity paralysis: the Copenhagen Stroke Study. *Arch Phys Med Rehabil.* 2000;81(6):736–738.

90. Dam M, Tonin P, Casson S, Ermani M, Pizzolato G, Iaia V, et al. The effects of long-term rehabilitation therapy on poststroke hemiplegic patients. *Stroke.* 1993;24(8):1186–1191.

91. Kelly PJ, Stein J, Shafqat S, Eskey C, Doherty D, Chang Y, et al. Functional recovery after rehabilitation for cerebellar stroke. *Stroke.* 2001;32(2):530–534.

92. Holloway RG, Benesch CG, Burgin WS, Zentner JB. Prognosis and decision making in severe stroke. *JAMA.* 2005;294(6):725–733.

93. Roger VL, Go AS, Lloyd-Jones DM, Benjamin EJ, Berry JD, Borden WB, et al. Executive summary: heart disease and stroke statistics—2012 update: a report from the American Heart Association. *Circulation.* 2012;125(1):188–197.

94. Chiu D, Peterson L, Elkind MS, Rosand J, Gerber LM, Silverstein MD. Comparison of outcomes after intracerebral hemorrhage and ischemic stroke. *J Stroke Cerebrovasc Dis.* 2010;19(3):225–229.

95. Hemphill JC, 3rd, Farrant M, Neill TA, Jr Prospective validation of the ICH Score for 12-month functional outcome. *Neurology.* 2009;73(14):1088–1094.

96. Broderick J, Connolly S, Feldmann E, Hanley D, Kase C, Krieger D, et al. Guidelines for the management of spontaneous intracerebral hemorrhage in adults: 2007 update: a guideline from the American Heart Association/American Stroke Association Stroke Council, High Blood Pressure Research Council, and the Quality of Care and Outcomes in Research Interdisciplinary Working Group. *Stroke.* 2007;38(6):2001–2023.

97. Zurasky JA, Aiyagari V, Zazulia AR, Shackelford A, Diringer MN. Early mortality following spontaneous intracerebral hemorrhage. *Neurology.* 2005;64(4):725–727.

98. Naidech AM, Bernstein RA, Bassin SL, Garg RK, Liebling S, Bendok BR, et al. How patients die after intracerebral hemorrhage. *Neurocrit Care.* 2009;11(1):45–49.

99. Broderick JP, Brott TG, Duldner JE, Tomsick T, Huster G. Volume of intracerebral hemorrhage. A powerful and easy-to-use predictor of 30-day mortality. *Stroke.* 1993;24(7):987–993.

100. Ariesen MJ, Algra A, van der Worp HB, Rinkel GJ. Applicability and relevance of models that predict short term outcome after intracerebral haemorrhage. *J Neurol Neurosurg Psychiatry.* 2005;76(6):839–844.

101. Tuhrim S, Dambrosia JM, Price TR, Mohr JP, Wolf PA, Hier DB, et al. Intracerebral hemorrhage: external validation and extension of a model for prediction of 30-day survival. *Ann Neurol.* 1991;29(6):658–663.

102. Wijdicks EF, Hijdra A, Young GB, Bassetti CL, Wiebe S. Practice parameter: prediction of outcome in comatose survivors after cardiopulmonary resuscitation (an evidence-based review): report of the Quality Standards Subcommittee of the American Academy of Neurology. *Neurology.* 2006;67(2):203–210.

103. Weimar C, Benemann J, Diener HC. Development and validation of the Essen Intracerebral Haemorrhage Score. *J Neurol Neurosurg Psychiatry.* 2006;77(5):601–605.

104. Creutzfeldt CJ, Becker KJ, Weinstein JR, Khot SP, McPharlin TO, Ton TG, et al. Do-not-attempt-resuscitation orders and prognostic models for intraparenchymal hemorrhage. *Crit Care Med.* 2011;39(1):158–162.

105. Hemphill JC, 3rd, Newman J, Zhao S, Johnston SC. Hospital usage of early do-not-resuscitate orders and outcome after intracerebral hemorrhage. *Stroke.* 2004;35(5):1130–1134.

106. Becker KJ, Baxter AB, Cohen WA, Bybee HM, Tirschwell DL, Newell DW, et al. Withdrawal of support in intracerebral hemorrhage may lead to self-fulfilling prophecies. *Neurology.* 2001;56(6):766–772.

107. Hemphill JC, 3rd, Bonovich DC, Besmertis L, Manley GT, Johnston SC. The ICH score: a simple, reliable grading scale for intracerebral hemorrhage. *Stroke.* 2001;32(4):891–897.

108. Rost NS, Smith EE, Chang Y, Snider RW, Chanderraj R, Schwab K, et al. Prediction of functional outcome in patients with primary intracerebral hemorrhage: the FUNC score. *Stroke.* 2008;39(8):2304–2309.

CHAPTER 17

Silent cerebral infarcts and microbleeds

Bo Norrving

Introduction

The existence of clinically silent cerebrovascular lesions was reported by neuropathologists decades ago (1–4). However, the full extent of silent lesions was not recognized until the introduction of modern neuroimaging techniques, which allowed identification of subclinical cerebrovascular disease during life. Initial studies focused on silent cerebral infarcts (SCIs) detected by computed tomography (CT) in patients with acute stroke. During the 1990s and onwards, studies were extended to cohorts from the healthy general population, and CT was replaced by magnetic resonance imaging (MRI), a much more sensitive technique to detect small vascular lesions in the brain. Several longitudinal clinical and neuroimaging studies have subsequently been performed to study the progression and prognostic impact of SCI. The 'discovery' of cerebral microbleeds (CMBs) is more recent (5, 6) and concurs with the introduction of MRI imaging protocols that are sensitive to detect haemosiderin.

Studies on SCIs and CMBs have drastically changed the perspective of relative proportions between silent and symptomatic cerebrovascular disease. Silent vascular brain lesions far outnumber symptomatic cerebrovascular disease presenting as transient ischaemic attack (TIA) and stroke: based on a provisional estimate silent cerebrovascular lesions are 15 times more common than lesions causing clinically apparent stroke (7). The clinical implications of silent cerebrovascular disease in influencing prognosis for vascular events, cognitive impairment, and stroke recovery, and in interfering with brain function have been increasingly recognized. Furthermore, SCIs and CMBs frequently coexist with neurodegenerative disease and may act synergistically in increasing cognitive deficits, disabilities, and other symptoms.

Definitions and terminology

In the upcoming revision of the International Classification of Diseases (ICD) from ICD-10 to ICD-11 by the World Health Organization (WHO), SCIs and silent cerebral microbleeds (SCMs) will appear under the block of 'Cerebrovascular Diseases' in the chapter 'Diseases of the Nervous System', and under the heading 'Cerebrovascular disease with no acute cerebral symptom'. SCI is defined as a brain infarct that has not caused acute focal dysfunction of the brain, and SMB is defined analogously. These definitions will replace some older terms like 'unrecognized' or 'covert' cerebral infarcts. Furthermore, the term 'cerebral' will be used rather than 'brain'. It is emphasized that SCB and SMB should not be labelled 'stroke'—the latter term is reserved for cerebrovascular disorders that cause acute neurological dysfunction. The definition of SCI and SMB is well compatible with the knowledge that incidentally detected lesions in the brain are not innocent but important determinants for cognitive impairment, dementia, micturition dysfunction, and gait disorders—SCI and SMBs are *silent* only in the aspect that they have not caused *acute* cerebral dysfunction.

Silent cerebral infarcts

Clinical and neuroimaging diagnostic issues

Diagnosing a visualized infarct as 'silent' is challenging, and several potential sources of error should be recognized. A careful history is needed since well-documented previous clinical symptoms and even hospital admissions resulting in a diagnosis of TIA or stroke, may not be adequately recalled by a patient self-report (8). Careful questioning may reveal that symptoms possibly related to the location of a SCI were actually present but ignored due to lack of awareness of stroke-like symptoms in the elderly and in their families (9). Furthermore clinical symptoms may fail to be recognized as TIA or stroke even when brought to medical attention. There is a long list of 'stroke chameleons', i.e. uncommon presentations of stroke that may be missed (10), see Chapters 4 and 7–9. Indirect data also support the concept that a proportion of cerebral ischaemic events may escape clinical recognition: in a large German cohort with TIA and stroke patients, left hemispheric symptoms were significantly more common than those from the right hemisphere, and the side asymmetry increased with decreasing severity of symptoms (11). Presumably, left hemispheric ischaemic lesions may more often be symptomatic due to clinical recognition of speech abnormalities whereas right hemispheric ischaemia may more often be unrecognized due to non-eloquent localization or neglect. If one assumes that ischaemic lesions should be symmetrical between hemispheres, one may recalculate that one in eight ischaemic strokes and one in fur TIAs may be clinically missed.

However, the majority of infarcts judged as silent have probably not been associated with unrecognized or forgotten acute focal neurological symptoms. Localization and size are important determinants if a brain lesion will cause clinical symptoms or be asymptomatic: silent infarcts can obviously go undetected if they occur in clinically ineloquent regions of the brain. A recent systematic review of pathology of lacunar ischaemic stroke in humans found that the pathology of infarcts causing acute stroke symptoms or not was largely similar (12).

The neuroimaging diagnostic criteria for silent cerebral infarcts have been variable across studies (13–15), hampering comparisons of findings. Recently, a report on neuroimaging standards for research into small vessel disease and its contribution to ageing and neurodegeneration has been published (16). The report proposes that for deep SCIs only lesions that cavitate should be regarded as silent cerebral infarcts. Studies have shown that not all (symptomatic) acute, small, deep infarcts cavitate with time: some appear as white matter hyperintensities whereas some are not visualized at all with time. As a consequence, the distinction between silent brain infarcts and white matter hyperintensities of presumed vascular origin is less sharp than previously recognized, or reported in scientific studies. Estimates of the proportion of acute, small, deep infarcts that cavitate are variable and range from 28–94% (17, 18). Cavitation may be related to time and size of the lesion, but also to neuroimaging methods such as MRI sequences (19). It should be recognized that a very small proportion of cavitated lesions appearing as a SCI may have been caused by a previous small bleeding. The variable fates of small vessel disease-related lesions and convergence of aetiologically different lesions to result in similar late appearances on MRI is illustrated in Figure 17.1.

Presumed silent cerebral infarcts need to be carefully separated from prominent perivascular spaces (Virchow-Robin Spaces), a distinction which may have been overseen in early reports. Perivascular spaces are fluid-filled spaces that follow a typical course of a vessel penetrating/transversing the brain through grey or white matter (16). They will appear linear when imaged parallel to the course of the vessel, and round or ovoid (with a diameter less than 2 mm) when imaged perpendicular to the course of the vessel. Characteristics and distinguishing features of MRI findings of lacunes, perivascular space, white matter hyperintensities and other imaging findings are given in Figure 17.2.

In patients with symptoms of TIA or stroke and multiple lesions on CT or conventional MRI, it may be difficult to determine whether a visualized infarct is recent and symptomatic, or old and clinically silent (20, 21). This issue may be solved by diffusion-weighted MRI, if it was performed in the acute phase. However, even MRI is not perfectly sensible to detect small acute ischaemic lesions: in patients with lacunar syndromes up to 30% of cases may be MRI negative (22).

A recent addition to the spectrum of silent brain infarcts is cerebral microinfarcts, very small (<1 mm) often cortical infarcts, that are not detected on conventional structural MRI (23). Cerebral microinfarcts may be up to 15 times more frequent than 'conventional' SCIs. Their role in contributing to clinical features and prognosis is currently unclear and merits further study.

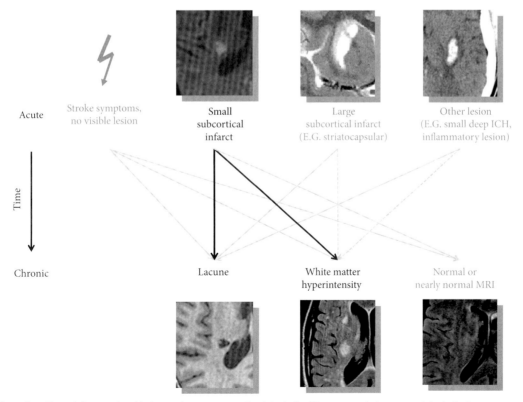

Fig. 17.1 Variable fates of small vessel disease-related lesions and convergence of aetiologically different acute lesions to result in similar late appearances on MRI: arrows indicate possible late fates of acute imaging findings; black arrows indicate common fates of recent small subcortical infarcts; solid grey arrows indicate less common and grey dashed arrows indicate least common late fates, according to best available current knowledge. Lancet Neurology 2013;12:in press (16) (with permission).

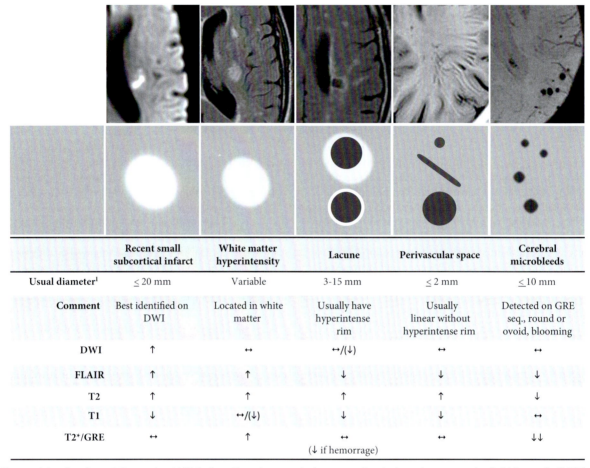

	Recent small subcortical infarct	White matter hyperintensity	Lacune	Perivascular space	Cerebral microbleeds
Usual diameter[1]	≤ 20 mm	Variable	3-15 mm	≤ 2 mm	≤ 10 mm
Comment	Best identified on DWI	Located in white matter	Usually have hyperintense rim	Usually linear without hyperintense rim	Detected on GRE seq., round or ovoid, blooming
DWI	↑	↔	↔/(↓)	↔	↔
FLAIR	↑	↑	↓	↓	↓
T2	↑	↑	↑	↑	↓
T1	↓	↔/(↓)	↓	↓	↔
T2*/GRE	↔	↑	↔ (↓ if hemorrage)	↔	↓↓

Fig. 17.2 Characteristics of small vessel disease-related MRI findings: illustrative examples (upper panel) and schematic representation (middle panel) of MRI features of different small vessel disease-related changes on typical scans are shown together with a summary of imaging characteristics (lower panel) for individual lesions. h: increased signal; i: decreased signal; n: isointense signal. (Lancet Neurology 2013;12:in press (16) (with permission).)

Silent infarcts in patients without prior transient ischaemic attack and stroke

Prevalence, risk factors, and imaging characteristics

Several studies have shown that SCI are often seen in healthy elderly in the general population. Findings in six population-based studies are summarized in Figure 17.3 (24).

The Cardiovascular Health Study (CHS) (25, 26) of 3660 subjects older than 65 years of age, found a prevalence of 28% among those without known prior stroke. Similar age-specific prevalences were reported from the Atherosclerosis Risk in Communities (ARIC) study of 1737 persons (27, 28).

In the Rotterdam Scan Study (29) 1077 persons 60–90 years of age were examined with cerebral MRI. For 259 participants (24%) one or more infarcts on MRI were seen: 217 patients had only SCIs and 42 had symptomatic infarcts. Thus, SCIs were five times as prevalent as symptomatic brain infarcts. Prevalence of SCIs increased with age, from 8% in the 60–64-year-old patients to 35% among those aged 85–90 years old, and were more frequent in women (age-adjusted odds ratio (OR) 1.4; 95% confidence interval (CI) 1.0–1.8).

In the Framingham Heart Study (30), a population-based cohort of 2081 subjects across a wide range of ages (34–97 years), the overall prevalence was 12.3%, nearly identical for both genders. As in previous reports, SCIs were common after age 50 and increased linearly with age. A similar pattern of SCIs was observed in the Framingham Offspring Study (31).

SCIs are also common in patients with other types of vascular disease. In the SMART Study (32) on patients with a mean age of 58 years with coronary heart disease, peripheral arterial disease, or abdominal aortic aneurysm the prevalence of SCI on MRI was 17%, comparable to the prevalence seen in population-based studies of healthy elderly in the age group 65–69 years. In persons with asymptomatic carotid stenosis, proportions of 15% and 30% were reported based on CT scan (33, 34).

With respect to morphological characteristics of SCI, findings from the different studies are quite consistent (29). SCIs are usually small, with 60–93% being less than 1.5 cm in diameter, and about three-quarters are single. The majority (70–94%) are localized to basal ganglia or subcortical matter, whereas less than 15% are cortical. SCIs are localized to the pons or cerebellum in up to 15% of cases. Thus, the majority of SCIs share imaging characteristics of lacunar infarcts caused by subcortical penetrating artery disease (see Chapter 4), and pathological studies show that the morphology and pathophysiological features between symptomatic and silent small deep infarcts were similar (35).

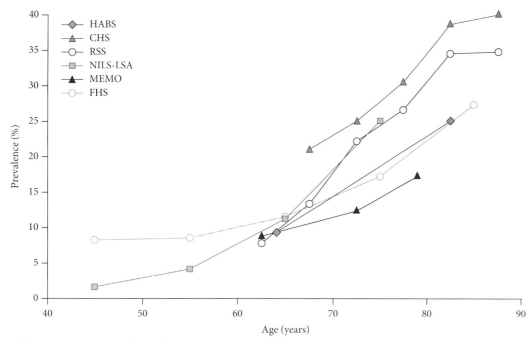

Fig. 17.3 Prevalence of silent versus symptomatic brain infarcts with increasing age, as reported in six population-based studies. (From: Vermeer SE, Longstreth WT, Koudstaal PJ. Silent brain infarcts: a systematic review. Lancet Neurology 2007;6:611–19, (with permission).)

Silent brain infarcts are closely linked to ischaemic white matter lesions (WMLs). WMLs are even more prevalent in the elderly than SCIs (36–38), and the two conditions share most risk factors and show a high degree of covariance (30, 39). As discussed earlier, the distinction between the two conditions may be less sharp than previously thought.

Risk factors

Besides the steep increase in prevalence of SCIs with age, a strong association with hypertension, with ORs between 2 and 3, is also a general finding across studies (24). Besides systolic, diastolic and pulse pressure, several studies have noted an association between SCI and various other indices of blood pressure dysregulation, including nocturnal non-dipping (40, 41), ambulatory blood pressure and blood pressure variability (42, 43), and exaggerated blood pressure response to mental stressors (44).

Findings for other traditional vascular risk factors, such as diabetes, smoking, and homocysteinaemia, are more variable between studies (24). Many studies show magnitudes of risk factor estimates comparable with symptomatic stroke, but non-significant results with large confidence intervals. The lack of consistent findings is likely due to small sample size, and possibly imprecise determinations of risk factors. As acute symptomatic and silent cerebral infarcts share similar pathologies, it is most likely that the underlying risk factors should be largely similar.

Gender effects also differ between studies. Whereas a 30–40% increased risk was observed in the Rotterdam study (29) and in the lacunar infarct substudy of the CHS (45), no difference was observed in other studies (27, 30, 46).

Effects and prognostic implication of silent cerebral infarcts

The increasing recognition that SCIs are associated with cognitive decline, depressed mood, and increased risk for stroke represents a scientific advance of major importance for public health.

Several cross-sectional studies have shown that SCI are related to decreased cognitive functioning (26, 45, 47, 48). Similar associations with cognitive decline as for SCIs have been reported for periventricular and subcortical WMLs (36, 49, 50). Coexisting high-degree WMHs and silent infarcts appear to have independent, additive effects (50). The cognitive effects of SCIs and WMLs presumably result from disruption and degradation of white matter pathways connecting functionally related cortical (particularly frontal) and subcortical structures. Further aspects on silent cerebrovascular disease and cognition/dementia are described in Chapter 19.

Depression in the elderly appears also to be part of the spectrum of cognitive effects linked to SCI: high prevalences (51–94%) of SCI have been reported in patients with pre-senile or senile major depression (51) and such findings have been associated with poor short-term response to antidepressant treatment (52). In the CHS (53) depressive symptoms were not only correlated with silent cerebral infarcts at baseline, but also persistence of depressive symptoms during follow-up (54). A role for silent cerebral infarcts as a potential cause of depression in the elderly was also recently reported in a prospective study by Saavedra Perez et al. (55). SCIs are also linked to subtle neurological abnormalities and gait disturbances in the elderly, and appear to have a synergistic effect with white matter ischaemic lesions (56).

SCIs commonly progress, and in longitudinal studies new SCIs are severalfold more common than clinically apparent stroke (8). In the CHS (57), 17.7% of the 1433 participants developed incident SCIs over 5 years on follow-up MRI; over the same period only 2.7% of the participants experienced a clinically apparent stroke. Severity of WMLs on initial MRI was the strongest predictor of new SCIs. The presence of SCIs, periventricular WMLs, and generalized brain atrophy at baseline, as well as their progression, are associated with a steeper cognitive decline on follow-up, in particular affecting information processing speed and executive function (57–63). In the Rotterdam Scan Study the risk of dementia more than doubled in persons with SCIs at baseline; this decline was restricted to people who had new SCIs during follow-up (64).

SCI is also an important and independent risk factor for future stroke. Among patients with SCIs, the CHS study reported a 7.3% incidence of stroke during 4 years, representing a twofold increased risk compared to persons without SCIs (65). An even higher risk was found in the Rotterdam Study (11.7% during 4.2 years among persons with SCIs at baseline), representing a fourfold increase in risk after adjustment for other risk factors. Also for this outcome SCIs and WMLs appear to additively increase the risk (39, 66).

Therapy of silent cerebral infarcts in persons without prior transient ischaemic attack or stroke

The vast majority of SCIs are small and deep and reflect penetrating artery disease, a pathogenesis shared with lacunar infarcts (see Chapter 4). SCIs are associated with cognitive effects and increased rates of stroke, which appear to be intermediate between those seen in the general population and among patients with a clinically apparent lacunar infarct (see Chapter 4).

Should then the same principles as in secondary stroke prevention also be applied in persons found to have a SCI?

As yet, there is very little solid evidence to guide clinical practice on preventive measures in persons found to have a SCI. A comprehensive risk factor screen and adaptation of principles for vascular disease prevention in general appears justified, given the associations with risk factors and SCIs. Among the modifiable risk factors, careful blood pressure control likely plays a major role in the long term. Physical activity may also have a protective role in the development of SCIs, as suggested by the Northern Manhattan Study (67). Unless there is another clear indication present, SCI per se is not currently regarded as an indication for an antiplatelet agent. The low prevalence of carotid artery disease and cardioembolic sources associated with SCIs appears not to warrant the broad use of screening with ultrasound or echocardiography in the absence of physical signs at examination.

Further research will have to show if preventive measures of people with SCI free from stroke and TIA should be more aggressive than the general principles for primary vascular prevention currently most widely used.

Silent cerebral infarcts in patients with symptomatic cerebral ischaemia

Prevalence, risk factors, and imaging characteristics

Several studies have documented that SCIs are prevalent in patients admitted with a first TIA or stroke. Early studies using first-generation CT equipment reported relatively low proportions (11–13%), whereas later studies (68–73) reported prevalences ranging from 23–38%. SCIs are more prevalent in patients with lacunar infarction than in those with atherothrombotic or cardioembolic infarcts (70, 72, 73). Most SCIs (up to 85%) are small and deep, whereas cortical infarcts account for 10–24% (69, 70, 74). The latter localization may more often involve the right hemisphere or the posterior cerebral artery territory than other cortical areas, and may more often be linked to a cardioembolic cause (75, 76).

Risk factors for SCIs in patients with TIA and stroke appear similar to findings in the general population, with strong and consistent associations with age and hypertension, whereas associations with

several other traditional risk factors have been reported in single or few reports. The design of trials examining these issues is quite heterogeneous, and several studies have low statistical power.

Recent studies have also shown that SCIs are highly prevalent in patients with young stroke. In the SIFAP study (77) silent infarcts on MRI were seen in 20% of patients with a first-ever stroke, and in 11.4% of patients with TIA and no history of a previous cerebrovascular event. Similar findings were reported in the Helsinki Young Stroke Study (78).

Clinical effects of silent cerebral infarcts in patients with transient ischaemic attack or stroke

Whereas several studies have reported that mortality and morbidity is not influenced by the presence of SCIs in cohorts of patients with stroke or TIA (68–70, 72, 75), relatively crude outcome measures and short times of follow-up have been used in these studies. However, the Dutch TIA Study reported that residual symptoms of any kind were more common in patients with SCIs than in those without (74), and both SCI and WML were associated with an increased risk of recurrent stroke (79, 80). Two studies (72, 76) have reported that SCIs at baseline incurred a higher risk of recurrent stroke and vascular events.

A consistent association with SCI and prognosis has been found in patients with lacunar infarcts (81, 82). In four studies (83–86) SCI, hypertension, diabetes, and presence of any cardioembolic source were independent predictors of future stroke risk, and presence of SCI may also affect long-term survival (85). Presence of SCIs and WMLs have also been found to be independent predictors of worse functional outcome (85, 87), in line with a general perception that more advanced small-artery disease at the time of the index ischaemic event may limit the possibility of functional recovery of the brain.

SCI is also an important risk factor for mild cognitive impairment and dementia after stroke, as further discussed in Chapter 19.

New silent infarcts after stroke

Early occurrence of silent cerebral infarcts may be quite common although the issue has been addressed in only a few reports. In an unselected ischaemic stroke population, the rate of new lesions seen on diffusion-weighted MRI at 1 week was 34% (88); most of these events were clinically silent whereas only 2% were accompanied by clinical symptoms of recurrent ischaemia. Another recent study found a 10% rate of new lesions on diffusion-weighted MRI 1 month after TIA or minor stroke and half of these new lesions were asymptomatic (89). Progression of SCI over a longer timeframe has mainly been investigated in patients with lacunar infarcts, in whom new silent infarcts develop at a rate of at least twice that of new symptomatic lacunae (for review, see (81)). After about 3 years, almost half of all patients had developed silent infarcts as well as progression of leucoaraiosis (90). The clinical effects of new SCIs have not been well studied.

Therapy

There are few clinical trial and observational data on therapeutic issues with respect to SCI in patients with TIA and stroke. Whereas more aggressive secondary preventive approaches may be appealing if there is evidence of widespread SCIs and WMLs at baseline, benefits of combining antithrombotic regimens may well be offset by increased adverse effects, as illustrated by the MATCH and SPS3 trials (91, 92).

Careful control of blood pressure is a cornerstone in secondary stroke prevention, but the effect of progression of SCIs is uncertain. A CT substudy of the PROGRESS trial on blood pressure lowering therapy in patients with stroke found no significant effect on therapy on the rate on silent brain infarcts over 3.9 years (93). However, a MRI substudy showed that the blood pressure-lowering regimen stopped or delayed the progression of WMLs (94). With respect to carotid surgery there are no data to support that the presence of SCIs should affect the decisions whether to operate or not.

Cerebral microbleeds

CMBs are small (2–5 mm) hypointense lesions on paramagnetic sensitive MRI sequences such as T2*-weighted gradient-echo (GRE) or susceptibility-weighted sequences. They are most often located in the cortico-subcortical junction, deep grey or white matter in the cerebral hemispheres, brainstem, and cerebellum. The common occurrence of CMBs has only been recognized since the mid 1990s (5, 6), as CMBs are generally not visualized on CT or fluid attenuated inversion recovery (FLAIR), T1- or T2-weighted MRI sequences. There has been substantial progress in the understanding of CMBs during recent years (recently summarized in a comprehensive monograph (95)), but there are several areas in need of further study.

Neuroimaging characteristics

GRE or T2*-weighted MRI is a highly sensitive technique in the detection of old and recent cerebral haemorrhage. Haemosiderin remains permanently stored at sites of previous bleedings so MRI findings of CMBs represent the cumulative burden of such lesions during life. Autopsy studies have confirmed that the small hypointense foci on GRE MRI correspond to perivascular haemosiderin-laden macrophages and ischaemic necrosis, and are residues of vascular leakage of blood cells in vessels smaller than 200 μm (96, 97). Neuroimaging criteria are available to separate CMBs from flow voids of vessels, calcium or iron deposits in the basal ganglia, and cerebral cavernous malformations (95, 98, 99).

Recent studies have highlighted the importance of imaging techniques in the sensitivity to detect CMBs. Use of MRI with higher magnetic field strengths increases the sensitivity of CMB detection substantially (up to twofold) (6, 95), which needs to be recognized in interpreting reported prevalences of CMBs in different patient cohorts and across studies. Standardized visual rating scales for CMBs have been recently developed (100, 101). Neuroimaging standards for CMBs are included in the recent COEN report on imaging standards for small vessel disease (16).

Prevalence of cerebral microbleeds in different populations

The first studies on prevalence of CMBs in the general population indicated that the prevalence was quite low, for example, 6.4% in the Austrian Stroke Prevention Study (102) and 4.7% in the Framingham study (103). Both of these studies included mainly quite young age groups. In a later population-based study, the AGES-Reykjavik study (104) 11.1% were reported in a cohort with a mean age of 76 years. In the more recent Rotterdam Scan Study (105) a rate of 23.5% was reported, using more sensitive MRI techniques. Thus, the proportions of persons with CMBs approach those of SCIs in the general population.

In cohorts of patients with ischaemic stroke the average prevalence of CNBs is 40%, with highest rates (up to 65%) in patients with ischaemic cerebral small-vessel disease (SCI and WMLs) (95). Chronic hypertension has appeared as a risk factor in several, but not all studies. Other frequently reported risk factors include diabetes, cholesterol, and antithrombotic drug use. CMBs appear to be more prevalent among subjects of Asian origin compared with Caucasians, but this finding may be linked with differences in patient selection criteria.

The prevalence of CMBs is particularly high among patients with intracerebral haemorrhage (ICH), ranging from 47–97% (mean 68%). CMB is also associated with cerebral amyloid angiopathy, which is the dominating cause for primary lobar ICH in the elderly. The presence of multiple, strictly lobar haemorrhages, including CMBs, has been shown to be highly specific for severe cerebral amyloid angiopathy in elderly patients with no other definitive cause of the ICH (95, 99, 106), and is an important prerequisite to establish the diagnosis of cerebral amyloid angiopathy in life (106–108). In contrast, ICH related to high blood pressure is associated with CMBs characteristically localized to the deep hemispheric regions, brainstem, and cerebellum. However, substantial overlap between the two patterns certainly exists.

CMBs are also a characteristic imaging feature of cerebral autosomal dominant arteriopathy with subcortical infarcts and leucoencephalopathy (CADASIL) (see Chapter 14). CMBs are also seen in about a quarter of patients with Alzheimer disease (98), presumably related to coincidence with cerebral amyloid angiopathy.

Clinical significance and prognostic implications

Initially thought to have no effect on cerebral function, there is now increasing evidence that CMBs may affect cognition, as further discussed in Chapter 19. The issue is methodologically complex because CMBs often coexist with SCIs and WMLs, which are known to cause cognitive impairment. However, a study that matched for presence of SCI and WML found that CMBs were associated with cognitive impairment, mainly executive dysfunction (109). Hypothetically, CMBs may affect cognition through tissue loss in the frontal lobes and basal ganglia disrupting frontal-basal ganglia connections, but the precise mechanisms are still unknown.

The prognostic implications of CMBs are currently evolving. Since CMBs may be viewed as a potential marker of a bleeding-prone microangiopathy, there are a large number of associations in which CMBs may play a role for prognosis and therapy, such as the safety of antithrombotic drugs and thrombolytic therapy, the risk of ICH, and clinical deterioration.

Studies have shown that CMB may increase the risk of ICH and possibly also ischaemic stroke (110). In patients with ICH, the presence of lobar CMBs is associated with an increased risk of recurrent ICH (95, 111).

With respect to CMBs and the risk of haemorrhagic complications of thrombolytic therapy, it appears that in patients with a small number of CMBs the risk of thrombolysis-related ICH may be slightly greater than in patients without CMBs, but it is unlikely that any small increased risk should overweight the benefit of thrombolytic therapy.

In a cross-sectional study CMBs were more common in antithrombotic drug users, and aspirin use was related to the lobal association of CMBs (112). Furthermore, patients with CMBs have been reported to have a higher risk of ICH during warfarin therapy (113), but this finding is not consistent (114). The role of CMBs in promoting anticoagulant-related ICHs is currently being studied in a large randomized trial. A key question is whether the increased risk for ICH associated with cerebral amyloid angiopathy-related CMBs is sufficient to tip treating physicians away from prescribing antiplatelet and anticoagulant therapy for patients with appropriate indications.

At present, the detection of CMBs does not influence choice of therapy after TIA and stroke. However, this issue is currently a major research field. Until these questions are answered, caution must be used in basing treatment decisions on limited observational data.

References

1. Fisher CM. Lacunes: small deep cerebral infarcts. *Neurology*. 1965;15: 774–784.
2. Fisher CM. The arterial lesions underlying lacunes. *Acta Neuropathologica (Berlin)*. 1969;12:1–15.
3. De Reuck J, Sieben G, De Coster W, vander Ecken H. Stroke pattern and topography of cerebral infarcts: a clinicopathological study. *Eur Neurol*. 1981;20:411–415.
4. Fisher CM. Lacunar infarcts: a review. *Cerebrovasc Dis*. 1991;1:311–20.
5. Offerbacher H, Fazekas F, Schmidt R, Koch M, Fazekas G, Kapeller P. MR of cerebral abnormalities concomitant with primary intracerebral hematomas. *AJNR Am J Neuroradiol*. 1996;17:573–78.
6. Greenberg SM, Vernooij MW, Cordonnier C, Viswanathan A, Al-Shahi Salman R, Warach S, *et al.* for the Microbleed Study Group. Cerebral microbleeds: a guide to detection and interpretation. *Lancet Neurol*. 2009;8:165–74.
7. Leary MC and Saver JL. Annual incidence of first silent stroke in the United States: a preliminary estimate. *Cerebrovasc Dis*. 2003;16:280–285.
8. Vermeer SE, den Heijer T, Koudstaal PJ, Oudkerk M, Hofman A, Breteler MM. Incidence and risk factors of silent brain infarcts in the population-based Rotterdam Scan Study. *Stroke*. 2003;34:392–396.
9. Saini M, Ikram K, Hilal S, Qiu A, Venketasubramanian N, Chen C. Silent stroke: not listened to rather than silent. *Stroke*. 2012;11:3102–3104.
10. Edlow JA, Selim MH. Atypical presentations of acute cerebrovascular syndromes. *Lancet Neurol*. 2011;10:550–560.
11. Foerch C, Misselwitz B, Sitzer M, Berger K, Steinmetz H, Neuman-Haefelin T, Arbetitsgruppe Schlaganfall Hessen. Difference in recognition of right and left hemisphereic stroke. *Lancet*. 2005;366:392–393.
12. Potter GM, Doubal FN, Jackson CA, Chappell FM, Sudlow CL, Dennis MS, *et al.* Counting cavitating lacunes underestimates the burden of lacunar infarction. *Stroke*. 2010;41:267–272.
13. Zhu YC, Tzourio C, Soumare A, Azoyer B, Dufouil C, Chabriat H. Severity of dilated Virchow-Robin spaces is associated with age, blood pressure, and MRI markers of small vessel disease: a population-based study. *Stroke*. 2010;41:2483–2490.
14. Zhu YC, Dufouil C, Tzourio C, Chabriat H. Silent brain infarcts: a review of MRI diagnostic criteria. *Stroke*. 2011;42:1140–1145.
15. Potter GM, Marlborough FJ, Wardlaw JM. Wide variation in definition, detection, and description of lacunar lesions on imaging. *Stroke*. 2010;42:359–366.
16. The Centers of Excellence in Neurodegeneration Vascular Imaging Standards Working Group. Neuroimaging standards for research into small vessel disease and its contribution to ageing and neurodegeneration: a united approach. *Lancet Neurol*. 2013;12:822–838.
17. Potter G, Doubal F, Jackson C, Sudlow C, Dennis M, Wardlaw J. Associations of clinical stroke misclassification ('clinical-imaging dissociation') in acute ischemic stroke. *Cerebrovasc Dis*. 2010;29:395–402.
18. Moreau F, Patel S, Lauzon ML, McCreary CR, Goyal M, Frayne R, *et al.* Cavitation after acute symptomatic lacunar stroke depends on time, location, and MRI sequence. *Stroke*. 2012;43:1837–1842.
19. Bokura H, Kobayashi S, Yamaguchi S. Distinguishing silent lacunar infarction from enlarged Virshow-Robin spaces: a magnetic resonance imaging and pathological study. *J Neurol*. 1998;245:116–122.
20. Kang D, Charlela JA, Ezzeddine MA, Warach S. Association of ischemic lesion patterns on early diffusion-weighted imaging with TOAST stroke subtypes. *Arch Neurol*. 2003;60:1730–1734.
21. Schulz UG, Briley D, Meagher T, Molyneux A, Rothwell PM. Diffusion-weighted MRI in 300 patients presenting late with subacute transient ischemic attack or minor stroke. *Stroke*. 2004;35:2459–2465.
22. Doubal FN, Dennis MS, Wardlaw JM. Characteristics of patients with minor ischaemic strokes and negative MRI: a cross sectional study. *J Neurol Neurosurg Psychiatry*. 2011;82:540–542.
23. Smith EE, Schneider JA, Wardlaw JM, Greenberg SM. Cerebral microinfarcts: the invisible lesions. *Lancet Neurol*. 2012;11:272–282.
24. Vermeer SE, Longstreth WT, Koudstaal PJ. Silent brain infarcts: a systematic review. *Lancet Neurology*. 2007;6:611–619.
25. Bryan RN, Wells SW, Miller TJ, Elster AD, Jungreis CA, Poirier VC, *et al.* Infarctlike lesions in the brain: prevalence and anatomic characteristics at MR imaging of the elderly—data from The Cardiovascular Health Study. *Radiology*. 1997;202:47–54.
26. Price TR, Manolio TA, Kronmal RA, Kittner SJ, Yue NC, Robbins J, *et al.* Silent brain infarction on magnetic resonance imaging and neurological abnormalities in community-dwelling older adults. The Cardiovascular Health Study CHS Collaborative Research Group. *Stroke* 1997;28:1158–1164.
27. Howard G, Wagenknecht LE, Cai J, Cooper L, Kraut MA, Toole JF. Cigarette smoking and other risk factors for silent cerebral infarction in the general population. *Stroke*. 1998;29:913–917.
28. Bryan RN, Caj J, Burke G, Hutchinson RG, Liao D, Toole JF, *et al.* Prevalence and anatomic characteristics of infarct-like lesions on MR images of middle-aged adults: the atherosclerosis risk in communities study. *AJNR Am J Neuroradiol*. 1999;20:1273–1280.
29. Vermeer SE, Koudstaal PJ, Oudkerk M, Hofman A, Breteler MMB. Prevalence and risk-factors of silent brain infarcts in the population-based Rotterdam Scan Study. *Stroke*. 2002;33:21–25.
30. DeCarli C, Massaro J, Harvey D, Hald J, Tullberg M, Au R, *et al.* Measures of brain morphology and infarction in the Framingham Heart Study: establishing what is normal. *Neurobiol Aging*. 2005;26: 491–510.
31. Das RR, Seshadri S, Beiser AS, Kelly-Hayes M, Au R, Himali JJ, *et al.* Prevalence and correlates of silent cerebral infarcts in the Framingham offspring study. *Stroke*. 2008;39:2929–2935.
32. Giele JLP, Witkamp TD, Mali WPTM, van der Graaf Y, for the SMART Study Group. Silent brain infarcts in patients with manifest vascular disease. *Stroke*. 2004;35:742–746.
33. Norris JW, Zhu CZ. Silent stroke and carotid stenosis. *Stroke*. 1992;23:483–485.
34. Brott T, Tomsick T, Feinberg W, Johnson C, Biller J, Broderisk J, *et al.* Baseline silent cerebral infarction in the Asymptomatic Carotid Atherosclerosis Study. *Stroke*. 1994;25:1122–1129.
35. Bailey EL, Smith C, Sudlow CLM, Wardlaw JM. Pthology of lacunar ischeaemic stroke in humans—a systematic review. *Brain Pathol*. 2012;22:583–591.
36. Longstreth WT Jr, Manolio TA, Arnold A, Burke GL, Bryan N, Jungreis CA, *et al.* Clinical correlates of white matter findings on cranial magnetic resonance imaging of 3301 elderly people. The Cardiovascular Health Study. *Stroke*. 1996;27:1274–1282.
37. Liao D, Cooper L, Cai J, Toole JF, Bryan NR, Hutschinson RG, *et al.* Presence and severity of white matter lesions and hypertension, its treatment, and its control. The ARIC Study. Atherosclerosis risk in communities study. *Stroke*. 1996;27:2262–2270.
38. De Leeuw F-E, de Groot JC, Achten E, Oudkerk M, Ramos LMP, Heijboer R, *et al.* Prevalence of cerebral white matter lesions in elderly people: a

population based magnetic resonance imaging study. The Rotterdam Scan Study. *J Neurol Neurosurg Psychiatry.* 2001;70:9–14.

39. Kuller LH, Longstreth WT Jr, Arnold AM, Bernick C, Bryan RN, Beauchamp NJ Jr. White matter hyperintensity on cranial magnetic resonance imaging: a predictor of stroke. *Stroke.* 2004;35:1821–1825.

40. Kairo K, Matsuo T, Kobayashi H, Imiya M, Matsuo M, Shimada K. Elation between nocturnal fall of blood pressure and silent cerebrovascular damage in elderly hypertensives: advanced silent cerebrovascular damage in extreme dippers. *Hypertension.* 1996;27:130–135.

41. Kairo K, Motai K, Mitsuhashi T, Suzuki T, Nakagawa Y, Ikeda U, *et al.* Autonomic nervous system dysfunction in elderly hypertensive patients with abnormal blood pressure variation. Relation to silent cerebrovascular disease. *Hypertension.* 1997;30:1504–1510.

42. Shimada K, Kawamoto A, Matsubayashi K, Ozawa T. Silent cerebrovascular disease in the elderly. Correlation with ambulatory pressure. *Hypertension.* 1990;16:692–699.

43. Goldstein IB, Bartzokis G, Hance DB, Shapiro D. Relationship between blood pressure and subcortical lesions in healthy elderly people. *Stroke.* 1998;29:765–772.

44. Waldstein SR, Siegel EL, Lefkowitz D, Maier KJ, Brown JR, Obuchowski AM, *et al.* Stress-induced blood pressure reactivity and silent cerebrovascular disease. *Stroke.* 2004;35:1294–1298.

45. Longstreth WT Jr, Bernick C, Manolio TA, Bryan N, Jungreis CA, Price TR. Lacunar infarcts defined by magnetic resonance imaging of 3600 elderly people: the Cardiovascular Health Study. *Arch Neurol.* 1998;55:1217–1225.

46. Kobayashi S, Okada K, Koide H, Bokura H, Yamaguchi S. Subcortical silent brain infarction as a risk factor for clinical stroke. *Stroke.* 1997;28:1932–1939.

47. Matsui T, Arai H, Yuzuriha T, Yao H, Miura M, Hashimoto S, *et al.* Elevated plasma homocysteine levels and risk of silent brain infarcts in elderly people. *Stroke.* 2001;32:1116–1119.

48. Maeshima S, Moriwaki H, Ozaki F, Okita R, Yamaga H, Ueyoshi A. Silent cerebral infarction and cognitive function in middle-aged neurologically healthy subjects. *Acta Neurol Scand.* 2002;105:179–184.

49. De Groot JC, de Leeuw FE, Oudkerk M, van Gijn J, Hofman A, Jolles J, *et al.* Cerebral white matter lesions and cognitive function: The Rotterdam Scan Study. *Ann Neurol* 2000;47: 145–151.

50. Mosley TH, Knopman DS, Catellier DJ, Bryan N, Hutchinson RG, Grothues CA, *et al.* Cerebral MRI findings and cognitive functioning. The Atherosclerosis Risk in Communities Study. *Neurology.* 2005;64:2056–2062.

51. Fujikawa T, Yamawaki S, Youhounda Y. Incidence of silent cerebral infarction in patients with major depression. *Stroke.* 1993;24:1631–1634.

52. Fujikawa T, Yokota N, Muraoka M, Yamawaki S. Response of patients with major depression and silent cerebral infarction to antidepressant drug therapy, with emphasis on central nervous system adverse reactions. *Stroke.* 1996;27:2040–2042.

53. Steffens DC, Helms MJ, Krishnan KR, Burke GL. Cardiovascular disease and depression symptoms in the Cardiovascular Health Study. *Stroke.* 1999;30:2159–2166.

54. Steffens DC, Krishnan RR, Crump C, Burke GL. Cerebrovascular disease and evolution of depressive symptoms in the Cardiovascular Health Study. *Stroke.* 2002;30:1636–1644.

55. Saavedra Perez HC, Direk N, Hofman A, Vernoij MW, Tiemeier H, Ikram MA. Silent brain infarcts: a cause of depression in the elderly? *Psychiatry Res.* 2013;211:180–182.

56. Van der Flier WM, van Straaten ECW, Barkhof F, Verdelho A, Madureira S, Pantoni L, *et al.* Small vessel disease and general cognitive function in non-disabled elderly: the LADIS study. *Stroke.* 2005;36:2116–2120.

57. Longstreth WT Jr, Dulberg C, Manolio TA, Lewis MR, Beauchamp NJ Jr, O'Leary D, *et al.* Incidence, manifestations and predictors of brain infarcts defined by serial cranial magnetic resonance imaging in the elderly. The Cardiovascular Health Study. *Stroke.* 2002;33:2376–2382.

58. De Groot JC, de Leeuw FE, Oudkerk M, van Gijn J, Hoffman A, Jolles J, *et al.* Periventricular cerebral white matter lesions predict rate of cognitive decline. *Ann Neurol.* 2002;52:335–341.

59. Kuller LH, Lopez OL, Jagust WJ, Becker JT, DeKosky ST, Lyketsos C, *et al.* Determinants of vascular dementia in the Cardiovascular Health Study. *Neurology.* 2005;64:1548–1552.

60. Longstreth WT Jr, Arnold AM, Beauchamp NJ, Manolio TA, Lefkowitz D, Jungreis C, *et al.* Incidence, manifestations, and predictors of worsening white matter on serial cranial magnetic resonance imaging in the elderly. The Cardiovascular Health Study. *Stroke.* 2005;36:56–61.

61. Prins ND, van Dijk EJ, den Heijer T, Vermeer SE, Jolles J, Koudstaal PJ, *et al.* Cerebral small-vessel disease and decline in information processing speed, executive function and memory. *Brain.* 2005;128:2034–2041.

62. Schmidt R, Ropele S, Enzinger C, Petrovic K, Smith S, Schmidt H, *et al.* White matter lesion progression, brain atrophy, and cognitive decline: the Austrian Stroke Prevention Study. *Ann Neurol.* 2005;58:610–616.

63. Gouw AA, van der Flier WM, Fazekas F, van Straaten EC, Pantoni L, Poggesi A, *et al.* LADIS Study Group. Progression of white matter hyperintensities and incidence of new lacunes over a 3-year period: the Leukoaraiosis and Disability study. *Stroke.* 2008;39:1414–1420.

64. Vermeer SE, Prins ND, den Heijer T, Hofman A, Koudstaal PJ, Breteler MM. Silent brain infarcts and the risk of dementia and cognitive decline. *N Engl J Med.* 2003;348:1215–1222.

65. Bernick C, Kuller L, Dulberg C, Longstreth WT Jr, Manolio TA, Beauchamp N, *et al.* Silent MRI infarcts and the risk of future stroke: the Cardiovascular Health Study. *Neurology.* 2001;57:1222–1229.

66. Vermeer SE, Hollander M, van Dijk EJ, Hofman A, Koudstaal PJ, Breteler MMB. Silent brain infarcts and white matter lesions increase stroke risk in the general population. The Rotterdam Scan Study. *Stroke.* 2003;34:1126–1129.

67. Willey JZ, Moon YP, Paik MC, Yoshita M, DeCarli C, Sacco RL, *et al.* Lower prevalence of silent brain infarcts in the physically active. The Northern Manhattan Study. *Neurology.* 2011;76:2112–2118.

68. Ricci S, Celani MG, La Rosa F, Righetti E, Duca E, Caputo N. Silent brain infarctions in patients with first-ever stroke. *Stroke.* 1993;24:647–651.

69. Jörgensen HS, Nakayama H, Raaschou HO, Olsen GJ. Silent infarction in acute stroke patients. Prevalence, risk factors, and clinical significance: the Copenhagen Stroke Study. *Stroke.* 1994;25:97–104.

70. Boon A, Lodder J, Heuts-van Raak I, Kessels F. Silent brain infarcts in 755 consecutive patients with a first-ever supratentorial ischemic stroke. *Stroke.* 1994;25:2384–2390.

71. Davis PH, Clarke WR, Bendixen BH, Adams HP Jr, Woolson RF, Culebras A. Silent cerebral infarction in patients enrolled in the TOAST Study. *Neurology.* 1996;46:942–48.

72. Corea F, Henon H, Pasquier F, Leys D. Silent infarcts in stroke patients: patient characteristics and effects on 2-year outcome. *J Neurol.* 2001;248:271–278.

73. Adachi T, Kobayashi S, Yamaguchi S. Frequency and pathogenesis of silent subcortical brain infarction in acute first-ever ischemic stroke. *Intern Med.* 2002;41:103–108.

74. Herderschee D, Hijdra A, Algra A, Koudstaal PJ, Kappelle LJ, van Gijn J, for the Dutch TIA Trial Study Group. Silent stroke in patients with transient ischemic attack or minor ischemic stroke. *Stroke.* 1992;23:1220–1224.

75. Chodosh EH, Foulkes MA, Kase CS, Wolf PA, Mohr JP, Hier DB, *et al.* Silent stroke in the NINCDS stroke data bank. *Neurology.* 1988;38:1674–1679.

76. EAFT Study Group. Silent brain infarction in nonrheumatic atrial fibrillation: EAFT Study Group European Atrial Fibrillation Trial. *Neurology.* 1996;46:159–165.

77. Rolfs A, Fazekas F, Grittner U, Dichgans M, Martus P, Holzhausen M, *et al.* Stroke in Young Fabry Patients (SIFAP) Investigators. Acute cerebrovascular disease in the young: the Stroke in Young Fabry Patients study. *Stroke.* 2013;44:340–349.

78. Putaala J, Kurkinen M, Tarvos V, Salonen O, Kaste M, Tatlisumak T. Silent brain infarcts and leukoaraiosis in young adults with first-ever ischemic stroke. *Neurology.* 2009;72:1823–1829.

79. Van Swieten JC, Kappelle LJ, Algra A, van Latum JC, Koudstaal PJ, van Gijn J. Hypodensity of the cerebral white matter in patients with transient ischemic attack or minor stroke: influence on the rate of subsequent stroke: Dutch TIA Trial Study Group. *Ann Neurol.* 1992;32:177–183.

80. The Dutch TIA Trial Study Group. Predictors of major vascular events in patients with transient ischemic attack or nondisabling stroke. *Stroke.* 1993;24:527–531.

81. Norrving B. Long-term prognosis after lacunar infarction. *Lancet Neurology.* 2003;2:238–245.

82. Norrving B. Lacunar infarcts: no black holes in the brain are benign. *Pract Neurol.* 2008;8:222–228.

83. Staaf G, Lindgren A, Norrving B. Pure motor stroke from presumed lacunar infarct: long-term prognosis for survival and risk of recurrent stroke. *Stroke.* 2001;32:2592–2596.

84. Kazui S, Levi CR, Jones EF, Quang L, Calafiore P, Donnan GA. Lacunar stroke: transoesophageal echocardiographic factors influencing long-term prognosis. *Cerebrovasc Dis.* 2001;12:325–330.

85. De Jong G, Kessels F, Lodder J. Two types of lacunar infarcts. Further arguments from a study on prognosis. *Stroke.* 2002;33:2072–2076.

86. Yamamoto Y, Akiguchi I, Oiwa K, Hayashi M, Kasai T, Ozasa K. Twenty-four-hour blood pressure and MRI as predictive factors for different outcomes in patients with lacunar infarct. *Stroke.* 2002;33:297–305.

87. Samuelsson M, Söderfelt B, Olsson GB. Functional outcome in patients with lacunar infarction. *Stroke.* 1996;27:842–846.

88. Kang DW, Latour LL, Chalela JA, Dambrosia J, Warach S. Early ischemic lesion recurrence within a week after acute ischemic stroke. *Ann Neurol.* 2003;54:66–74.

89. Coutts SB, Hill MD, Simon JE, Sohn C-H, Scott JN, Demchuk AM, for the VISION Study Group. Silent ischemia in minor stroke and TIA patients identified on MR imaging. *Neurology.* 2005;65:513–517.

90. Van Zagten M, Boiten J, Kessels F, Lodder J. Significant progression of white matter lesions and small deep (lacunar) infarcts in patients with stroke. *Arch Neurol.* 1996;53:650–655.

91. Diener HC, Bogousslavsky J, Brass LM, Cimminiello C, Csiba L, Kaste M, *et al.* MATCH investigators. Aspirin and clopidogrel compared with clopidogrel alone after recent ischaemic stroke or transient ischaemic attack in high-risk patients (MATCH): randomised, double-blind, placebo-controlled trial. *Lancet.* 2004;364:331–337.

92. SPS3 Investigators, Benavente OR, Hart RG, McClure LA, Szychowski JM, Coffey CS, *et al.* Effects of clopidogrel added to aspirin in patients with recent lacunar stroke. *N Engl J Med.* 2012;367:817–825.

93. Hasegawa Y, Yamaguchi T, Omae T, Woodward M, Chalmers J. PROGRESS CT Substudy Investigators. Effects of perindopril-based blood pressure lowering and of patient characteristics on the progression of silent brain infarcts: the Perindopril Protection against Recurrent Stroke Study (PROGRESS) CT Substudy in Japan. *Hypertens Res.* 2004;27:147–156.

94. Dufouil C, Chalmers J, Coskun O, Besancon V, Bousser MG, Guillon P, *et al.* Effects of blood pressure lowering on cerebral white matter hyperintensities in patients with stroke: the PROGRESS (perindopril protection against recurrent stroke study) magnetic resonance substudy. *Circulation.* 2005;112:1644–1650.

95. Werring DJ (ed). *Cerebral Microbleeds. Pathophysiology to Clinical Practice.* Cambridge: Cambridge University Press; 2011.

96. Fazekas F, Kleinert R, Robb G, Kleinert G, Kapeller P, Schmidt R, *et al.* Histopathologic analysis of foci of signal loss on gradient-echo T2*-weighted MR images in patients with spontaneous intracerebral hemorrhage: evidence of microangiopathy-related microbleeds. *Am J Neuroradiol.* 1999;20:637–642.

97. Tanaka A, Ueno Y, Nakayama Y, Takano K, Takebayashi S. Small chronic hemorrhages and ischemic lesions in association with spontaneous intracerebral hematomas. *Stroke.* 1999;30:1637–1642.

98. Koennecke H-C. Cerebral microbleeds on MRI. Prevalence, associations, and potential clinical implications. *Neurology.* 2006;66:165–171.

99. Viswanathan A and Chabriat H. Cerebral microhemorrhage. *Stroke.* 2006;37:550–555.

100. Gregoire SM, Chaudhary UJ, Brown MM, Yousry TA, Kallis C, Jäger HR, *et al.* The Microbleed Anatomical Rating Scale (MARS): reliability of a tool to map brain microbleeds. *Neurology.* 2009;73:1759–1766.

101. Cordonnier C, Potter GM, Jackson CA, Doubal F, Keir S, Sudlow CL, *et al.* Improving interrater agreement about brain microbleeds: development of the Brain Observer MicroBleed Scale (BOMBS). *Stroke.* 2009;40:94–99.

102. Robb G, Schmidt R, Kapeller P, Lechner A, Hartung HP, Fazekas F. MRI evidence of past cerebral microbleeds in a healthy elderly population. *Neurology.* 1999;52:991–994.

103. Jeerakathil T, Wolf PA, Beiser A, Hald JK, Au R, Kase CS, *et al.* Cerebral microbleeds: prevalence and associations with cardiovascular risk factors in the Framingham Study. *Stroke.* 2004;35:1831–1835.

104. Sveinbjornsdottir S, Sigurdsson S, Aspelund T, Kjartansson O, Eiriksdottir G, Valtysdottir B, *et al.* Cerebral microbleeds in the population based AGES-Reykjavik study: prevalence and location. *J Neurol Neurosurg Psychiatry.* 2008;79:1002–1006.

105. Vernooij MW, van der Lugt A, Ikram MA, Wielopolski PA, Niessen WJ, Hofman A, *et al.* Prevalence and risk factors of cerebral microbleeds: The Rotterdam Scan Study. *Neurology.* 2008;70:1208–1214.

106. Knudsen KA; Rosand J, Karluk D, Greenberg SM. Clinical diagnosis of cerebral amyloid angiopathy: validation of the Boston criteria. *Neurology.* 2001;56:537–539.

107. Greenberg SM, Finkelstein SP, Schaefer PW. Petechial hemorrhages accompanying lobar hemorrhage: detection by gradient-echo MRI. *Neurology.* 1996;46:1751–1754.

108. Rosand J, Mizukansky A, Kumar A, Wisco JJ, Smith EE, Betensky RA, *et al.* Spatial clustering of hemorrhages in probable cerebral amyloid angiopathy. *Ann Neurol.* 2005;58:459–462.

109. Werring DJ, Frazer DW, Coward LJ, Losseff NA, Watt H, Cipolotti L, *et al.* Cognitive dysfunction in patients with cerebral microbleeds on T2*-weighted gradient-echo MRI. *Brain.* 2004;127:2265–2275.

110. Fan YH, Zhang L, Lam WW, Mok VC, Wong KS. Cerebral microbleeds as a risk factor for subsequent intracerebral hemorrhage among patients with acute ischemic stroke. *Stroke.* 2003;34:2459–2462.

111. Greenberg SM, Eng JA, Ning M, Smith EE, Rosand J. Hemorrhage burden predicts recurrent intracerebral hemorrhage after lobar hemorrhage. *Stroke.* 2004;35:1415–1420.

112. Vernooij MW, Haag MD, van der Lugt A, Hofman A, Krestin GP, Stricker BH, *et al.* Use of antithrombotic drugs and the presence of cerebral microbleeds: the Rotterdam Scan Study. *Arch Neurol.* 2009;66: 714–720

113. Lee SH, Ryu WS, Roh JK. Cerebral microbleeds are a risk factor for warfarin-related intracerebral haemorrhage. *Neurology.* 2009;72:171–176.

114. Orken DN, Kenengil G, Uysal E, Forta H. Cerebral microbleeds in ischemic stroke patients on warfarin treatment. *Stroke.* 2009;40:3638–3640.

CHAPTER 18

Complications after stroke

Hanne Christensen, Elsebeth Glipstrup,
Nis Høst, Jens Nørbæk, and Susanne Zielke

Introduction

Complications are frequent in stroke, especially in severe stroke. Hardly any patient with severe stroke goes through stroke unit treatment without any complications as complications including infections, falls, deterioration, pain, ischaemic heart disease, and others occur in more than 60% of patients. Focus should be on prevention and early detection of complications. Often the patients cannot give a clear history due to the stroke. It is therefore necessary to look for complications during patient care and rounds in a systematic way, otherwise severe complications may be overlooked. There are few data to guide the management of complications in stroke (1, 2) and treatment remains guided by best practice and clinical experience, which also forms the primary basis for major parts of this chapter. This chapter aims to give a concise and practically oriented summary of complications after stroke for the clinician. Some of the issues are also covered from other perspectives in Chapter 10.

Infections

Frequencies and causes of infections

Infections are frequent in patients with stroke and are often related to the clinical severity of the stroke and the subsequent immobilization (3). Post-stroke immunosuppression is likely to result from the sympathico-adrenal activation seen predominantly after severe stroke, and this may further contribute to the susceptibility of stroke patients to infections (4). By far the most frequent infections are urinary tract infections and pneumonia. Infections are reported to occur in up to half of patients in stroke units. Infections are most frequent in patients with severe stroke and significant comorbidities and may contribute further to poor outcome. The number of infections may be reduced by early mobilization and specific preventive measures, e.g. prevention of aspiration by systematic dysphagia screening.

When to suspect?

Infections are to be suspected based on specific symptoms, such as productive coughing but often the more diffuse systemic symptoms including a confused state are predominant.

Clinical presentations

Patients often present with a slight increase in body temperature (37.5–37.9°C), subtle neurological deterioration, mental confusion, and/or increasing C-reactive protein (CRP) and white blood cell (WBC) counts. Pre-disposing conditions such as dysphagia—increasing the risk of aspiration—or urinary tract infection (UTI) call for special attention. Infections may be an important differential diagnosis to recurrent stroke in especially frail elderly people in whom it may cause an apparent progression in an existing hemiparesis. After severe stroke infections tend to present most commonly on day 2 or 3 as a specific pattern but may present at any time during stroke care.

How to investigate?

If the clinical picture is dominated by systemic symptoms a general workup including blood samples for CRP, WBC, blood culture, urinary dip test—followed by urinary culture in case of positive findings—lung stethoscopy, and chest x-ray is recommended. Spinal tap is only indicated based on clinical signs of a neuroinfection as in other infectious patients.

Urinary tract infections

Bacteriuria with no clinical symptoms and no increase in WBC or CRP is not an UTI; this is, however, a frequent finding in a stroke population. Male patients often have concomitant prostate hyperplasia and female patients may have chronic urinary incontinence for various reasons: both conditions are related to residual urine and bacteriuria. UTIs are reported in 10% of patients in the first month following stroke (2).

Diagnosis

Urine dip test followed by a urine culture if dip test positive and supplemented by WBC count, CRP level, and blood culture in patients with septic symptoms. Routine urine dip test may be performed on admission. *Escherichia coli* infection of some severity has a specific foetor.

Treatment

Treatment is based on oral antibiotics in minor cases and systemic therapy in cases with septic symptoms or dysphagia and no other indication for gastric tube. Rational use of antibiotics follows local resistance patterns and therefore regional/hospital guidelines.

Further measures include avoidance of permanent urinary catheter as well as use of bedpans and increasing use of intermittent catheterization and most importantly reinstituting usual voiding positions as soon as possible in order to achieve regular complete bladder emptying.

Pneumonia

Specific pulmonary symptoms may be subtle in patients recovering from severe stroke, however fulminant lobar pneumonia may also occur. Most often basal bronchopneumonias related to immobilization and reduced basal ventilation are observed (Figures 18.1

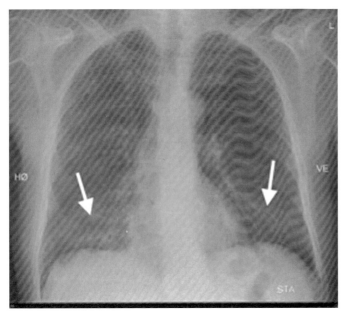

Fig. 18.1 Chest x-ray showing bronchopneumonia with basal infiltrations.

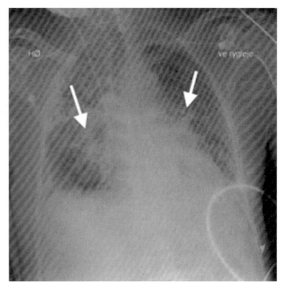

Fig. 18.3 Chest x-ray showing signs of aspiration pneumonia with affection of upper lobes.

and 18.2). In patients with dysphagia, aspiration pneumonias, which are most commonly observed in the upper lobes, are observed (Figure 18.3). Classic lobar pneumonia is rarely seen; patients with chronic obstructive lung disease often present with exacerbations during subacute stroke. Pneumonia is reported to occur in 10% of patients with stroke (2).

Diagnosis

In straightforward cases, a reliable clinical diagnosis can be made based on symptoms including coughing and expectoration, fever, increased respiratory rate, and asymmetric crepitation on lung stethoscopy, often accompanied by pain or discomfort at the back of the thorax.

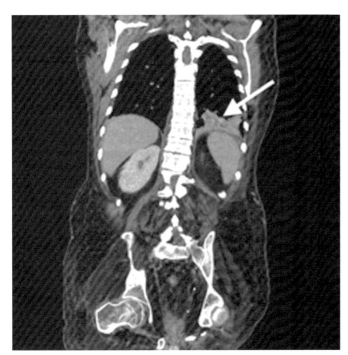

Fig. 18.2 CT scan showing bronchopneumonia with basal left infiltration.

Diagnosis is confirmed by chest x-ray or CT. A tracheal suctioning sample for culture before treatment is recommended together with CRP and WBC supplemented by blood culture as well as arterial gases in more severe cases. Further observation of the patient includes monitoring of respiratory rate and oxygen saturation, e.g. every second hour or continuously.

General treatment

Pneumonia is treated with antibiotics and supplemented with lung physiotherapy (continuous positive airway pressure) in patients with no pleural effusion. Rational use of antibiotics follows local resistance patterns and therefore regional/hospital guidelines.

Oxygen supplementation (2–4 L/min) is generally considered to palliate and stabilize the oxygen saturation, however oxygen must be used with caution in patients with COPD or other chronic conditions characterized with continued increased arterial blood gas carbon dioxide, as oxygen supplementation may suppress the respiratory impulse. Structured changing in positioning in order to obtain air-shift in all pulmonary regions is mandatory in the immobilized patient. Follow-up of vital values and blood tests are necessary to monitor the treatment response.

Antibiotic treatment

Specific recommendations depend on local resistance patterns and consequently local antibiotics protocols should be followed. Culture and determination of resistance patterns are mandatory.

Prophylactic antibiotics do not improve outcome after stroke. This approach has been tested in the context of post-stroke immunosuppression and the high risk of infections after stroke. In clear-cut cases it is justified to start antibiotics based on clinical findings before having all test results as in our clinical experience this reduces the total morbidity due to the infection in patients after stroke.

Prevention by dysphagia screening

A number of approaches to dysphagia testing have been described ranging from a simple water-drinking test to filming the actual swallowing process. No doubt the more refined methods will reveal more cases; however, in our clinical experience it is very important to ensure that all patients are tested on admission, even by a simpler method. The set-up for a GUSS test is illustrated in Figure 18.4.

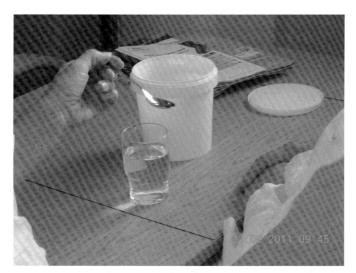

Fig. 18.4 Gugging Swallowing Screen (GUSS). Material: water, teaspoon, food thickener (direct swallowing test).

Venous thromboembolism (deep venous thromboembolism and pulmonary embolism)

Frequencies and causes of venous thromboembolism

Deep venous thromboembolism (DVT) is reported to occur in 10–15% of patients after stroke and pulmonary embolism (PE) in up to 3–4% of patients. A number of factors increase the risk of venous thromboembolism (VTE): most importantly immobilization. Also comorbidity, including neoplastic conditions, as well as genetic predisposition for VTE increases the risk.

When to suspect?

Pain in the calf of a lower paretic extremity should raise the suspicion of DVT. In the majority of patients not only is motor activity reduced on the affected side after stroke but also sensory function and neurological symptoms such as neglect may further obscure the patient's subjective symptoms. It is therefore reasonable to do DVT detection workup based on clinical findings, even without complaints from the patient.

It is recommended to inspect the lower extremities of an immobilized stroke patient during rounds at regular intervals (daily or every other day) focusing on signs of DVT as well as possible lesions from unregistered trauma and pressure sores.

Clinical presentations

The onset of DVT is most commonly subacute with increasing symptoms from venous stasis including pain, oedema, and reddening of the leg. Symptoms may start at the level of the ankle and ascend up above the knee. The patient with stroke may, due to stroke-related symptoms, not be aware of or able to localize the discomfort.

If PEs occur, most commonly a sudden severe deterioration is observed. The patient typically becomes circulatory unstable with tachycardia and decreasing blood pressure and increasing respiratory rate. Sudden death may be the sole clinical presentation. Arterial blood gas will show decreasing tensions of both oxygen and carbon dioxide. Less severe presentations of PE remain a differential diagnosis to pneumonia.

How to investigate

If DVT is suspected based on clinical findings, a blood sample for analysis of D-dimer is recommended as first-line workup. In case this is elevated, further workup is needed—D-dimer is a phase reactant and does not represent a specific diagnosis of VTE; in case of a normal D-dimer differential diagnosis should primarily be explored.

Unnoticed trauma on the paretic side may give rise to clinical suspicion of DVT, especially in patients with neglect.

In suspicion of PE both a D-dimer and an arterial blood gas should be obtained and analysed acutely. If D-dimer is increased and the arterial blood gas shows decreasing tensions of oxygen and carbon dioxide, further workup should be attempted acutely. With confirmation of PE considerations as to anticoagulant therapy and/or thrombolysis should be weighed against the risk of haemorrhagic transformation. As a general rule anticoagulation carries an acceptable risk of cerebral bleeding complications, while thrombolysis is expected to carry an unacceptable risk. Therapy of PE in the stroke patient will often require assistance from a cardiologist.

Diagnosis

DVT is confirmed by Doppler ultrasound (Figure 18.5) of the lower extremity. Doppler ultrasound has a high diagnostic sensitivity and specificity if thrombosis is visualized above the knee; however, in cases with strong clinical signs visualization of thrombosis even at a more distal location will be considered diagnostic by most clinicians.

Phlebography (Figure 18.6) is time-consuming and painful for the patient, and is only rarely used.

In circulatory unstable patients with PE, echocardiography will typically demonstrate right ventricular dilatation and signs of increased pulmonary pressure. Rarely, a central pulmonary clot can be directly visualized.

High-resolution CT of the chest (Figure 18.7) is now a routine test that is available 24/7 in many hospitals or at least on a next-day basis and will visualize even smaller PEs. Ventilation–perfusion scintigraphy remains an option in some centres and has a high sensitivity and specificity for PE but remains a daytime examination.

Treatment

Primary treatment is anticoagulation initiated by therapeutic doses of low-molecular-weight heparin (LMWH) and followed by 3–6 months of oral anticoagulation. In some cases, transferral to a specialized unit for thrombectomy or local thrombolysis may improve outcome, and such specialized centres should be consulted regarding deteriorating patients.

Prevention

First-line prevention of VTE is mobilization; a simple clinical rule is to get the patient out of bed for at least 6 hours a day; however, when looking at the total risk of an individual patient concurrent diseases with increased risk of VTE such as cancer must be taken into account. The risk of VTE in immobilized patients is reduced by LMWH in preventive doses (5), which can also be used in cerebral haemorrhage after the first 24–48 hours (6). LMWH is effective in preventive doses and is indicated in actively treated patients that cannot yet be sufficiently mobilized. Compression stockings do not prevent VTE in patients after stroke (7, 8); however, pneumatic compression has recently shown a clinically relevant reduction in the risk of VTE (9).

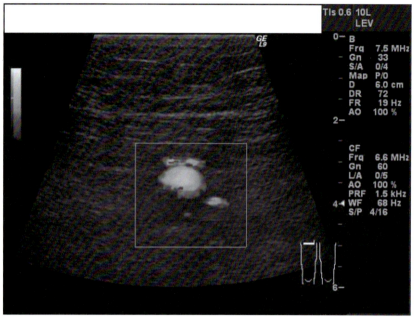

Fig. 18.5 Doppler ultrasound of DVT. Also see figure in colour plate section

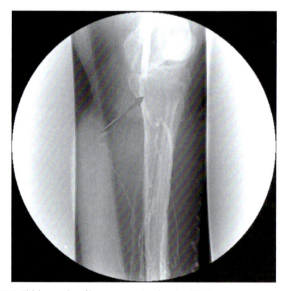

Fig. 18.6 Phlebography of lower extremity showing DVT.

Cardiac complications

Cardiac complications are common after stroke, especially in the acute phase, and care should be taken in assessing whether the cardiac manifestations are linked causally to the stroke, or are merely new-onset manifestations of the shared risk factors and pathophysiology of vascular disease (10).

Cardiac complications accompanying or ensuing stroke include arrhythmia, predominantly in the form of atrial fibrillation, ischaemic heart disease, and congestive heart failure (Box 18.1).

Arrhythmia and electrocardiography in general

Atrial fibrillation is the most common cardiac arrhythmia in general and in the stroke patient in particular, where as a general rule

it presents an indication for oral anticoagulation (11). Initiation of anticoagulant therapy is typically postponed for 2–3 weeks after major stroke in order to avoid increasing the risk of haemorrhagic transformation.

Atrial fibrillation often exists without specific symptoms, especially in the elderly. It is diagnosed from an electrocardiogram (ECG) with irregular R–R intervals without visual P-waves, and with varying degrees of tachycardia (Figure 18.8). Typical symptoms include palpitations, shortness of breath, oppression, light-headedness, and fainting. Prolonged, rapid atrial fibrillation may induce cardiomyopathy with overt heart failure.

ECG changes in general are quite common after stroke, and may represent signs of pre-existing heart disease, may be due to new-onset manifest cardiac complications, or may arise as a referred consequence of the intracerebral event.

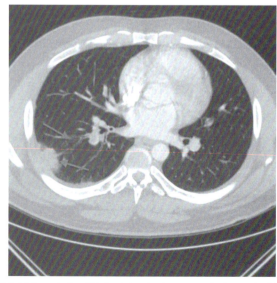

Fig. 18.7 High-resolution CT of peripheral pulmonary embolism and infiltration.

Box 18.1 Cardiac complications

Cardiac complications after stroke are common and include:

◆ Arrhythmia, especially atrial fibrillation

◆ Ischaemic heart disease

◆ Heart failure.

Care should be taken in detecting and addressing these aspects of the stroke patient phenotype, preferably through close collaboration between neurologist and cardiologist

Box 18.2 Digoxin loading

Oral loading (preferred choice):

◆ Total 10–15 mcg/kg

◆ 25% of dose immediately

◆ 25% of dose after 2–4 hours

◆ 25% after 8 hours

◆ Last 25% after 8 hours.

Intravenous loading:

◆ Total dose is reduced with 20–25%

◆ 50% immediately

◆ 25% after 8 hours

◆ Last 25% after 8 hours

◆ Always ensure that creatinine and potassium are in the normal range before treatment—if not consult a specialist

◆ Remember to plan continued oral treatment.

Side effects are dose dependent and include conduction block: telemetry makes monitoring easier.

Apart from considering anticoagulant therapy, the issue of antiarrhythmic therapy including the need for immediate rate regulation, possible specific heart failure therapy, and long-term strategy as to returning to, and maintaining, sinus rhythm should be addressed with the help of a cardiologist. Rapid ventricular action with heart rate higher than 130 beats/minute and resulting decrease in blood pressure are frequently observed in patients with acute, severe stroke and/or concurrent infections. Initial rate control can be obtained by digoxin loading orally or intravenously (Box 18.2). If not urgent, it may be preferable to start the patient on maintenance dose according to age, weight, and creatinine. When the patient is mobilized additional rate reduction therapy is often needed, a beta-blocker or a calcium channel blocker being the common choice.

Excess of ventricular ectopic beats and ventricular tachycardia can also occur with increased incidence after stroke and may lead to haemodynamic instability and even death.

An ECG should always be part of the initial workup of the stroke patient allowing not only for abnormalities to be detected but also

as a basis for later comparison. In either case ECG changes signify a poorer prognosis for the stroke patient, and measures should be taken to ameliorate the consequences whenever possible.

On-site telemetry in the neurology department is helpful in detecting and monitoring arrhythmias including paroxysmal atrial fibrillation in the acute stroke patients. Seven-day Holter

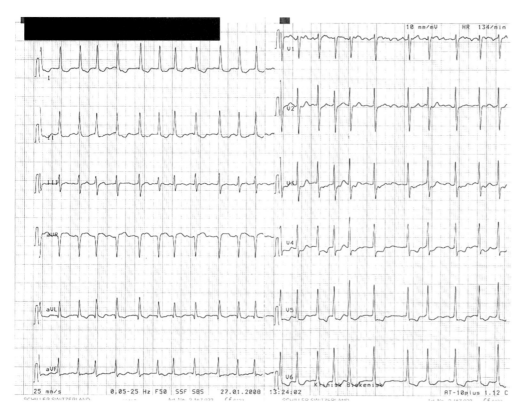

Fig. 18.8 ECG from a 66-year-old woman with hypercholesterolemia, hypertension, and recently diagnosed paroxysmal atrial fibrillation.

monitoring is regarded as the gold standard for detecting atrial fibrillation but remains very time consuming. Use of a number of more easily applicable methods including nurse pulse assessment, bipolar ECG, finger probes, modified blood pressure monitor, serial ECG, mobile cardiac outpatient telemetry, and event loop recorders have been reported after stroke, however, direct comparison of the methods is still lacking. At the moment the choice is best guided by local availability and the rule of thumbs that the length of the monitoring reflects the sensitivity for paroxysmal atrial fibrillation. Use of high-cost methods such as implanted loop recorders is only rarely warranted after stroke and repeated manual pulse assessment may represent a relevant approach.

Ischaemic heart disease

The risk of myocardial infarction is significantly increased after stroke, both acutely and at long-term follow-up, and coronary heart disease has been found to be highly prevalent at autopsy in stroke patients (12). Stroke ranges as a coronary heart disease risk equivalent in secondary prevention of cardiovascular events.

Increased concentration of serological markers of myocardial damage, such as troponins, is a common finding following ischaemic stroke, even in the absence of specific symptoms of myocardial ischaemia, and often gives rise to considerations such as the need for further examinations and therapy focused on coronary heart disease (13). However, the need for coronary catheterization resulting possibly in percutaneous coronary intervention and need for prolonged antithrombotic therapy may interfere with bleeding risk during stroke evolvement, and the strategy must be carefully individualized in close collaboration between neurologist and cardiologist (11).

Heart failure

Congestive heart failure (CHF) may be a consequence of pre-existing ischaemic heart disease or prolonged tachycardia with acute hypertension and/or fluid overload as potential precipitating factors. The incidence of CHF after acute stroke is not precisely known, however, CHF has a profound negative impact on prognosis of the stroke patient (Figure 18.9).

An ECG with signs of arrhythmia and/or extensive myocardial infarction in patients presenting clinically with dyspnoea and,

depending upon degree of decompensation, tachycardia and stethoscopic rales, should always elicit a fast-track cardiological workup. This will include echocardiography, plans for invasive examination, directions for specific medical therapy, and considerations as to possible device therapy with implantable cardioverter-defibrillator and/or CRT (cardiac resynchronization therapy).

Pending cardiological evaluation and specific examinations as outlined earlier, the neurologist's hypothesis of CHF may be corroborated serologically by increased levels of natriuretic peptides (e.g. pro-BNP) and radiologically by chest x-ray showing cardiomegaly and excess interstitial pulmonary fluid.

A special form of cardiomyopathy, stress-induced apical ballooning syndrome, or Takotsubo cardiomyopathy (named after the resemblance of the left ventricle during systole to the shape of a Japanese octopus trap), is receiving increased attention as a possible feature of stroke. Takotsubo cardiomyopathy seems to occur in as much as 1–2% of patients with ischaemic stroke, with the patient presenting features of acute coronary syndrome and heart failure. Specific examinations addressing the suspicion of Takotsubo cardiomyopathy include echocardiography and coronary angiography (which will rule out coronary artery disease) and therapy is focused on the transient heart failure, which signifies the syndrome.

Falls

Frequencies and causes of falls

Patients with stroke are at high risk of falls, and fall rates have been reported to range from 14–65% while in hospitals. Older age, infections, cognitive impairment, neglect, depression, continence problems, visual problems, balance problems, leg weakness, sensory loss, and foot problems may increase the risk of falls. Falls are the most frequent complication to stroke.

Prevention of falls

There is very little high-quality evidence on successful approaches to reducing falls. Strength and balance training, vitamin D supplementation, and strategies targeting falls risk factors may reduce falls episodes and reduce harm. Falls precautions may also include use of alarm systems, use of special equipment (e.g. enclosure beds), or

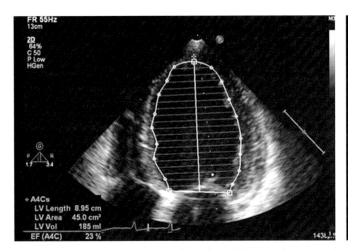
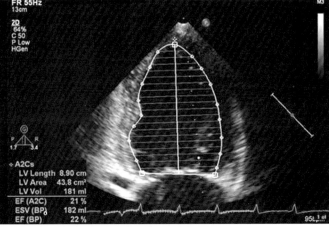

Fig. 18.9 Stills from transthoracic echocardiography with biplane volume-estimation of left ventricular ejection fraction (LVEF).

placing the call buttons and the patient's belongings very close to the patient, aiming at reducing the need to get up. In some cases, it may be necessary to have a sitter with the patient for limited periods to ensure patient safety (14).

Pressure ulcer and skin care

Frequencies and clinical presentation

The frequency of pressure ulcers after stroke depends on both care and stroke severity. Reported frequencies therefore range from 0.6–25%. Known consequences of stroke, like poor mobility and incontinence, increase the risk of skin breaks and pressure ulcers occur more often in severe stroke. The sacrum, buttocks, and heels are the usual predilection sites for pressure ulcers.

Best practice to prevent pressure ulcer

◆ The patient should be examined for skin breakdown when repositioned and after sitting.

◆ Use of the Braden Scale (<http://www.bradenscale.com/images/bradenscale.pdf>) in nursing practice can assist the prediction of stroke patients at high risk of developing pressure ulcers (15).

◆ Frequent turning should be ensured in bedridden patients.

Lower urinary symptoms

Frequencies and causes of lower urinary symptoms

Up to 94% of stroke patients report at least one symptom of lower urinary tract symptoms (LUTS) 1 month after stroke onset. The exact causative mechanism of LUTS following a stroke is unknown. The pathophysiology in an individual patient remains mostly multifactorial.

When to suspect?

Paresis in the legs and symptoms of UTI on admission is associated with and increases the severity of LUTS following stroke. Medical conditions such as UTI, dehydration, mental confusion, depression, constipation, urinary retention, and symptoms induced by drugs such as diuretics, sedatives, anticholinergics, and antihypertensives contribute to transient urinary incontinence.

Clinical presentations

Most frequent symptoms of LUTS among stroke patients are nocturia, urgency, increased daytime frequency, and urinary incontinence.

How to investigate?

◆ LUTS is best evaluated by a 3-day voiding diary recording the times of micturition, day and night, incontinence episodes, pad usage, and fluid intake.

◆ The optimal method to evaluate the burden of LUTS is by a validated questionnaire, e.g. The Danish Prostate Symptom Score (DAN-PSS) (validated in stroke patients) (16, 17).

How and when to treat?

◆ Reduce number of factors that contribute to LUTS (18).

◆ LUTS must be addressed if symptoms bother the patient and if addressing LUTS can be included in the patient's rehabilitation programme.

◆ LUTS training requires adequate cognitive function to adhere to an active training programme.

Best practice to treat LUTS is:

◆ Bladder training programme: timed voiding regimen with gradually progressive voiding intervals with an ideal interval of 3–4 hours or/and

◆ Pelvic muscle training: intensive with training sessions 3–4 times per week repeating 8–10 sustained contraction each time.

In patients with cognitive impairment, LUTS treatment includes:

◆ Timed voiding with fixed time interval.

◆ Habit voiding with toileting according to patient's natural voiding pattern

◆ Prompted voiding: teaching to initiate toileting is a technique in which the patient is instructed or reminded to urinate according to a predetermined schedule, usually beginning at intervals as often as one hour.

Bladder ultrasound-scanning is an easy nurse- or nurse-assistant-provided examination that can also be performed on the sitting patient: it is not required to transfer the patient back to bed in order to perform a bladder scan. Figure 18.10 illustrates a bladder scan on a sitting person.

Constipation

When to suspect?

Constipation is a common complication in acute stroke; up to 55% of patients develop new-onset constipation within 4 weeks after stroke, and it is already frequent on the third day after stroke. Its occurrence is associated with dependence and use of bedpan for defecation.

Clinical presentation and diagnosis

Constipation is identified according to ROME criteria and a stool diary (Box 18.3).

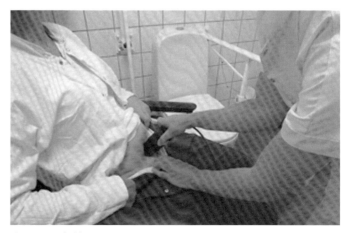

Fig. 18.10 Bladder scan in a sitting person.

Box 18.3 Rome criteria for constipation

1. Straining in >25% defecations

2. Lumpy or hard stools in >25% defecations

3. Sensation of incomplete evacuation in >25% defecations

4. Sensation of anorectal obstruction/blockade in >25% defecations

5. Manual manoeuvres to facilitate >2% defecations

6. ≤3 defecations/ week.

If the patient fulfilled two or more of the diagnostic criteria in a consecutive 7-day stool diary, constipation is diagnosed.

How and when to treat?

Best practice to treat and prevent constipation is (19):

♦ To offer all patients already on admission a structured assessment, with subsequent interventions (Box 18.4).

♦ During admission, daily registration in the patient's stool-diary and follow-up on interventions.

♦ To ensure a stool pattern with more than three stools per week:

• Planned toileting according to the patient daily habits

• Sufficient fluid intake

• Medication (stool softeners, laxatives and enemas) if bowel movements three times or fewer per week.

Acute/subacute organic delirium

Incidence

Organic delirium occurs in all neurological patients, but also constitutes a frequent complication to strokes with an incidence rate of 15–45% (20). Delirium requires a fairly long inpatient stay, together with a permanently reduced level of functioning and an increased mortality rate (21) (Box 18.5).

Patients at risk

Left-sided cerebral lesions, advanced age, male gender, cerebral illnesses such as dementia, previous apoplexy, schizophrenia, sensory defects, multiple morbidity/polypharmacy, a poor nutritional state, a low level of functioning, alcohol, and drug abuse similarly predispose an individual to the illness (22, 23).

Symptoms

Typical presentations may include reduced attention, confusion of thought, disorientation, and memory problems, disturbance of circadian rhythm, muscular activity, language, perception, and

---

Box 18.4 Assessment for constipation

♦ Physical function history

♦ Digital rectal examination

♦ Bowel symptom history

♦ Education (targeted verbal information with provision of booklet).

Box 18.5 Definition of organic delirium

ICD 10: 'Organic delirium (WHO DF05.x) is a neuropsychiatric syndrome reflecting a disturbance of normal neuronal communication. It invariably involves reduced awareness and clarity of consciousness, which typically fluctuate throughout the day. Delirium is characterized by a sudden onset, taking place from hours to days, disturbance of circadian rhythm and changes in muscular activity.'

---

emotion (depressive symptoms). Delusions and hallucinations (auditory and visual) occur frequently. Delirium may be characterized exclusively by hyperactivity or hypoactivity (10%), but most often a mixture of the two is seen (24, 25).

Investigation

Delirium often results from multiple factors.

In the patient history focus should be on: premorbid physical and mental level of functioning, all drugs taken including over-the-counter drugs, start of symptoms and their development, previous episodes of confusion, sensory impairment, aids (hearing aids, glasses, etc.), social conditions, chronic illnesses (24).

Recommended tests: haemoglobin, WBC count (including differential count), CRP level, calcium, electrolytes, creatinine and carbamide, liver tests, glucose, thyroid stimulating hormone (TSH), and urine dipstick. If indications appear: run ECG, urine and blood cultures.

When necessary the following examinations may further supplement: chest x-ray, coronary enzymes, envenomation tests, arterial puncture, supplementary cultivation (expectorate, skin), lumbar puncture, EEG, vitamin B_{12}, and folate.

Prevention and screening (26, 27)

Primary

♦ Ensure sufficient intake of food and drink

♦ early mobilization.

♦ Avoid moving the patient between departments and between wards/rooms.

♦ Calendar and clock in the ward.

♦ Avoid hypoxia and hypotension.

♦ Observe circadian rhythm with special focus on night rest and day sleep.

♦ Permanent nursing staff (possibly a permanent presence in the room).

♦ Prevent constipation and urine retention.

♦ Drugs review (avoid, if possible, drugs with anticholinergic effect).

♦ Muted lights at night.

♦ Help patient to gain self-control and greater understanding of the situation.

♦ Involvement of the patient's own network or family.

Secondary

♦ Early identification of the condition.

♦ Attention directed towards prodromal symptoms:

• Problems with falling asleep/fretful sleep with nightmares, form for recording sleep

- Symptoms of anxiety and depression
- Problems with concentration
- Tiredness with a tendency to doze off in the course of the day
- Sensitivity to light and sound.

◆ Introduction of CAM (Confusion Assessment Method), e.g. CAM-ICU, as the delirium-monitoring instrument.

Treatment

Treatment of delirium is first and foremost a non-pharmacological nursing effort. Nursing care should be directed as described in the 'Primary prophylaxis' section.

Identification and correction of underlying cause(s)

Optimization of the somatic condition: supply of oxygen at arterial oxygen saturation lower than 93%, blood transfusion in case of anaemia, normalize glucose, fluid, and electrolyte balance, avoid constipation and urine retention (frequent bladder scans), prevent and treat pain, ensure adequate nutrition.

Do not interrupt administration of vital medication.

Pharmacological treatment

Haloperidol is the drug of choice (28). Haloperidol can be taken as a tablet, as a liquid formulation, and by injection. Haloperidol is a potent antipsychotic agent and, in addition to this, has a powerful unspecified sedative effect, which is advantageous in that it normalizes the circadian rhythm and eases the sometimes violent psychomotor agitation in the delirious patient. The cerebral sensitivity to haloperidol increases with age. A younger patient needs a larger dose in order to obtain the desired sedation. The doses in Table 18.1 are meant as a guide only. In strong psychomotor agitation the dosage level needs to increase (also the 'as needed' (PRN) administration) and often it is practical with parenteral administration.

This dosage suggestion is based on parenteral administration. Haloperidol should be given regularly for the night. PRN prescription is given for lack of sleep and for psychomotor agitation. If PRN medication is administered in order for the patient to obtain sleep this is added to the regular prescription for the next day.

Haloperidol is titrated until night rest has been obtained in at least two succeeding nights. After that the dose may be halved. If night time sleep is unchanged on subsequent nights, haloperidol may be discontinued. For susceptible patients *prophylactic treatment* with haloperidol 0.5–2.5 mg at night may be considered.

Since haloperidol metabolizes hepatically the dosage should be reduced if the patient has reduced liver function. Patients with basal ganglia dysfunction (Parkinson disease and atypical Parkinson disease/dementia with Lewy bodies) are at an increased risk of side effects. Another important side effect is orthostatism with its risk of falling and fractures. Extrapyramidal side effects are rarely seen in the case of a temporary treatment. ECG should be available before

the start of medical treatment, and this ought to be repeated daily in the first 3 days after the start of treatment, in that haloperidol may result in a prolonged QTC interval.

Benzodiazepines should be avoided in the case of delirium. Electroconvulsive therapy may be considered if there is a lack of effect of the medical treatment.

Further suggested reading includes the NICE guidelines (29) and the European Delirium Association website (<http://www.europeandeliriumassociation.com>).

Depression

Incidence of depression

Post-stroke depression occurs in a third of stroke survivors in comparison to approximately 10% of population controls. This may be a conservative estimate as patients with communicative deficits have been excluded from the majority of studies. Post-stroke depression has repeatedly been associated with poorer recovery and rehabilitation as well as reduced quality of life and functional status. Depression is also very frequent in patients with other neurological conditions such as Parkinson disease or epilepsy, and in patients with other medical conditions.

Symptoms and diagnosis

Symptoms of depression may be obscured by communicative disorders or other cognitive deficits and often the use of standard diagnostic scales such as, e.g. the Hamilton Scale, does not appear meaningful in this patient population. Often therapists or nurses notice that the patient is losing motivation and appetite and no longer foresees a good outcome. Most often the clinical presentation is dominated by loss of hope and enjoyment of everyday pleasures, together with new or increased sleeping difficulty; the patient often feel that he or she is to blame for the situation and just wants to be left alone. Diagnostic tools such as the Geriatric Depression Scale (30) (see Figure 18.11) may be very useful in patients without severe language disorder; sometimes the diagnosis may be based on the clinical presentation alone.

Treatment

The use of antidepressants significantly reduces the burden of depressive symptoms in patients with neurological disorders and medical conditions; few data are available on the effect on quality of life and functional outcome (31, 32). In our clinical experience, patients with symptoms of post-stroke depression and, e.g. reduced motivation for rehabilitation, appear to benefit from antidepressive treatment as they are enabled to take up the training programme again.

Pharmaceutical treatment

The patient's age and comorbidities must be taken into account when starting treatment and low doses and slow increases in dosing is generally recommended. A selective serotonin re-uptake inhibitor (SSRI) is first line, tricyclic antidepressants have cardiac side effects, a noradrenaline-selective reuptake inhibitor may be useful if sleeping difficulties or anxiety is dominating problems. Dryness of the mouth is the most common side effect in low doses but may cause caries. Citalopram 10 mg × 1 (morning) or mirtazapine 15 mg × 1 (night) are first-line treatments. After at least

Table 18.1 Haloperidol dosing in different age groups: benzodiazepines should be avoided!

<50 years old	60–70 years old	70–80 years old	>80 years old
5 mg every night	2.5–5 mg every night	1–2.5– mg every night	0.5–1 mg every night
+2.5 mg PRN	+1–2 mg PRN	+1–2 mg PRN	+0.5–1 mg PRN

6 months of treatment, the indication must be revised aiming at withdrawal.

Emotionalism
Incidence and clinical presentation of emotionalism

Emotionalism occurs in 20–25% of stroke patients most often weeks after stroke onset and may persist in some. Emotionalism is uncontrolled busts of crying or laughter—bar far most often crying in patents after stroke—that does not have a basis in the patient's actual feelings. Emotionalism is related to depression but often the patient has no significant signs of depression. The condition is socially disabling due to stress and embarrassment.

Treatment of emotionalism

Only a few trials exist in this field, and none that compares pharmaceutical interventions to psychological interventions.

Geriatric Depression Scale (Short Form)

Patient's Name: _____   Date: _____

Instructions: Choose the best answer for how you felt over the past week.

No.	Question	Answer	Score
1.	Are you basically satisfied with your life?	YES/NO	
2.	Have you dropped many of your activites and interests?	YES/NO	
3.	Do you feel that life is empty?	YES/NO	
4.	Do you offen get bored?	YES/NO	
5.	Are you in good spirits most of the time?	YES/NO	
6.	Are you afraid that something bad is going to happen to you?	YES/NO	
7.	Do you feel happy most of the time?	YES/NO	
8.	Do you often feel helpless?	YES/NO	
9.	Do you prefer to stay at home, rather than going our and doing new things?	YES/NO	
10.	Do you feel you have more problems with memory than most?	YES/NO	
11.	Do you think it is wonderful be alive?	YES/NO	
12.	Do you feel pretty worthless the way you are now?	YES/NO	
13.	Do you feel full of energy?	YES/NO	
14.	Do you feel that your situation is hopeless?	YES/NO	
15.	Do you think at most people are better off than you are?	YES/NO	
		TOTAL	

Scoring:
Assign one point for each of these answers:

1. NO	4. YES	7. NO	10. YES	13. NO
2. YES	5. NO	8. YES	11. NO	14. YES
3. YES	6. YES	9. YES	12. YES	15. YES

A score of 0 to 5 is normal. A score above 5 suggests depression.

Source:
- Yesavage J.A., Brink T.L., Rose T.L et al. Development and validation of a geriatric depression screening scale: a preliminary report. J. Psychiatr. Res. 1983; 17:37-49.

Fig. 18.11 The Geriatric Depression Scale.

Antidepressants of any class appear to be effective in a systematic review (33). In clinical experience SSRIs in low dose, e.g. citalopram 10 mg × 1, is very effective and with an almost immediate onset of effect in comparison to the effect in depression.

Seizures

Less than 5% of patients present with generalized seizures within 24 hours of stroke onset, however 11% later develop post-stroke seizures within 5 years (34). Only a cortical location and possibly severe stroke predict later occurrence of seizures (35).

As seizures most commonly have onset after discharge, this issue will generally be dealt with by the general practitioner or during an acute readmission.

Clinical presentation

Generalized tonic–clonic seizures are most common, however, primary partial seizures possibly with secondary generalization are observed. Movement disorders including dystonia may in rare cases result from stroke and present differential diagnosis.

Investigation

EEG may be helpful to confirm diagnosis especially during the seizure; however, focal activity is more the rule than the exception after stroke, which may complicate interpretation. It is generally recommended to perform imaging, in most cases a non-contrast CT to rule out new events or other causal pathology including subdural haematoma.

Diagnosis

Single seizures especially in the acute phase of stroke are not epilepsy and do not require treatment. Only repeated seizures are epilepsy and need treatment.

Treatment

Status epilepticus is extremely rare in post-stroke seizures and therefore loading or aggressive acute treatment with benzodiazepines are hardly ever needed but may result in respiratory insufficiency. First-line treatment is lamotrigine starting with 25 mg × 2 and increased to 100 mg × 2 during 3 weeks. Carbamazepine and oxcarbamazepine are efficient but may cause unacceptable changes in salt and liver enzymes in an elderly population. Valproic acid is another option; however, this may cause encephalopathy in the elderly as well as increasing liver enzymes.

Pain

Pain is frequent after stroke and is reported in up to 75% of all patients, most frequently as a painful shoulder (36). In the first week headache is common (37), also in patients with smaller lesions such as lacunar infarcts, and most often located ipsilateral to the cerebral lesion. In the chronic phase musculoskeletal pain is common and often related to permanent loss of motor function. Central pain does not occur until weeks or months after stroke onset and therefore mostly after discharge. All lesions that involve the ascending sensory tracts may cause central pain; however, this probably occurs most frequently after thalamic stroke and Wallenberg syndrome. Overall frequencies of 3–9% are reported (38).

Table 18.2 Pharmacological treatment for neuropathic pain

Drug	Starting dose	Maximum dose
Amitriptyline (TCA)	10–25 mg	75 (150) mg
Pregabalin	(25–) 75–150 mg	600 mg
Lamotrigine	25 mg	200–400 mg

Clinical presentation

Patients often do not report pain spontaneously so they need to be asked in a systematic way in order to allow for more than one coexisting pain type. A late presentation, with pain from an area with sensory deficits, points towards a central pain syndrome. In nociceptive pain, the pain is often related to a joint (commonly shoulder or hip) or presents as lower back pain and relate to physical activity.

Diagnosis and treatment

Diagnosis is primarily clinical but may involve imaging of joints or other musculoskeletal structures.

Nociceptive pain is treated in stroke patients as in other patients; however, frail elderly patients are generally susceptible to side effects from drugs. Non-pharmacological measures aiming at reducing the load on the painful joint and towards better positioning at night are first-line treatment. Pharmacological treatment is often needed and paracetamol 1 g four times daily or given as a retarded formulation if available is often sufficient.

Central pain management remains often more complicated. Cutaneous administration (ointments/gel) with local anaesthetics may reduce the need of other medication. Otherwise antidepressants or antiepileptics reduce pain (see Table 18.2).

Post-stroke fatigue

Post-stroke fatigue is extremely common after stroke and may be the main cause of reduced quality of life and prolonged sick leave in minor stroke and TIA. There are so far no evidence-based interventions for post-stroke fatigue (39). In clinical practice, information and counselling appears to be helpful; it is generally accepted that the fatigue is relieved spontaneously at least 3–6 months after stroke and that taking breaks during the day together with physical decreases the degree of fatigue experienced by the patient.

References

1. Indredavik B, Rohweder G, Naalsund E, Lydersen S. Medical complications after stroke. *Stroke*. 2008;39:414–420.
2. Kumar S, Selim MH, Caplan LR. Medical complications after stroke. *Lancet Neurol*. 2010;9:105–118.
3. Westendorp WF, Nederkoorn PJ, Vermeij J-D, Dijkgraaf MG, van de Beek D. Post-stroke infection: a systematic review and metanalysis. *BMC Neurol*. 2011;11:1–10.
4. Harms H, Reimnitz P, Bohner G, Werich T, Klingebiel R, Meisel C, et al. Influence of stroke localization on autonomic activation, immunodepression, and post-stroke infection. *Cerebrovasc Dis*. 2011;32:552–560.
5. Shorr AF, Jackson WL, Sherner JH, Moores LK. Difference between low-molecular-weight heparin and unfractionated heparin for venous thromboembolism prevention following ischemic stroke: a metaanalysis. *Chest*. 2008;1:149–155.

6. Paciaroni M, Agnelli G, Venti M, Alberti A, Acciarresi M, Caso V. Efficacy and safety of anticoagulants in the prevention of venous thromboembolism in patients with acute cerebral hemorrhage: a metaanalysis of controlled studies. *J Thromb Haemost.* 2011;9:893–898.

7. CLOTS Trial Collaboration, Dennis M, Sandercock PA, Reid J, Graham G, Venables G, Rudd A, Bowler G. Effectiveness of thigh-length graduated compression stockings to reduce the risk of deep vein thrombosis after stroke (CLOTS trial 1): a multicentre, randomised controlled trial. *Lancet.* 2009;373:1958–1965.

8. CLOTS (Clots in Legs or sTockings after Stroke) Trial Collaboration. Thigh-length versus below-knee stockings for deep venous thrombosis prophylaxis after stroke: a randomized controlled trial. *Ann Intern Med.* 2010;153:553–562.

9. Effectiveness of intermittent pneumatic compression in reduction of risk of deep vein thrombosis in patients who have had a stroke (CLOTS 3): a multicentre randomised controlled trial. CLOTS (Clots in Legs Or sTockings after Stroke) Trials Collaboration. *Lancet,* 2012;382:516–524.

10. Prosser J, Macgregor L, Lees KR, Diener H-C, Hacke, Davis S. Predictors of early cardiac morbidity and mortality after ischemic stroke. *Stroke.* 2007;38:2295–2302.

11. European Heart Rhythm Association; European Association for Cardio-Thoracic Surgery, Camm AJ, Kirchhof P, Lip GY, Schotten U, et al. Guidelines for the management of atrial fibrillation: the Task Force for the Management of Atrial Fibrillation of the European Society of Cardiology (ESC). *Eur Heart J.* 2010;31:2369–2429. <http://www.escardio.org/guidelines-surveys/esc-guidelines/GuidelinesDocuments/guidelines-afib-FT.pdf>.

12. Touzé E, Varenne O, Chatellier G, Peyrar S, Rothwell PM, Mas J-L Risk of myocardial infarction and vascular death after transient ischemic attack and ischemic stroke. A systematic review and meta-analysis. *Stroke.* 2005;36:2748–2755.

13. Jensen J, Atar D, Mickley H Mechanism of troponin elevation in patients with acute ischemic stroke. *Am J Cardiol.* 2007;99:867–870.

14. Batchelor F, Hill K, Mackintosh S, Said C. What works in falls prevention after stroke? A systematic review and meta-analysis. *Stroke.* 2010;41:1715–1722.

15. Comfort EH. Reducing pressure ulcer incidence through Braden Scale Risk Assesment and support surface use. *Adv Skin Care.* 2008;21:330–334.

16. Hansen BJ, Flyger H, Brasso K, Schou J, Nordling J, Thorup Andersen J, et al. Validation of the self-administered Danish Prostatic Symptom Score (DAN-PSS-1) system for use in benign prostatic hyperplasia. *Br J Urol.* 1995;76:451–458.

17. Tibaek S, Dehlendorff C. Validity of the Danish Prostate Symptom Score questionnaire in stroke. *Acta Neurol Scand.* 2009 Dec;120(6):411–417.

18. Thomas LH, Cross S Barrett J, French B, Leathley M, Sutton CJ, Watkins C. Treatment of urinary incontinence after stroke in adults. 2009. [Update of *Cochrane Database Syst* Rev 2005;3:CD004462; PMID: 16034933]. *Cochrane Database Syst Rev.* 1:CD004462.

19. Harari D, Norton C, Lockwood, Cameron S. Treatment of constipation and fecal incontinence in stroke patients. Randomized controlled trial. *Stroke.* 2004;2349–2555.

20. Oldenbeuving AW, de Kort PL, Jansen BP, Algra A, Kappelle LJ, Roks G. Delirium in the acute phase after stroke: incidence, risk factors, and outcome. *Neurology.* 2011;76:993–999.

21. Melkas S, Laurila JV, Vataja R, Oksala N, Jokinen H, Pohjasvaara T, et al. Post-stroke delirium in relation to dementia and long-term mortality. *Int J Geriatr Psychiatry.* 2012;27:401–408.

22. Dahl MH, Ronning OM, Thommessen B. Delirium in acute stroke – prevalence and risk factors. *Acta Neurol Scand Suppl.* 2010:39–43.

23. McManus J, Pathansali R, Hassan H, Ouldred E, Cooper D, Stewart R, et al. The course of delirium in acute stroke. *Age Ageing.* 2009;38:385–389.

24. Trzepacz PT, Baker RW, Greenhouse J. A symptom rating scale for delirium. *Psychiatry Res.* 1988;23:89–97.

25. McManus J, Pathansali R, Stewart R, Macdonald A, Jackson S. Delirium post-stroke. *Age Ageing.* 2007;36:613–618.

26. Inouye SK, Bogardus ST, Jr., Charpentier PA, Leo-Summers L, Acampora D, Holford TR, et al. A multicomponent intervention to prevent delirium in hospitalized older patients. *N Engl J Med.* 1999;340:669–676.

27. Inouye SK, van Dyck CH, Alessi CA, Balkin S, Siegal AP, Horwitz RI. Clarifying confusion: the confusion assessment method. A new method for detection of delirium. *Ann Intern Med.* 1990;113:941–948.

28. Lonergan E, Britton AM, Luxenberg J, Wyller T. Antipsychotics for delirium. *Cochrane Database Syst Rev.* 2007;2:CD005594.

29. National Institute for Health and Clinical Excellence. *CG103: Delirium.* London: NICE. <http://guidance.nice.org.uk/CG103/Guidance>.

30. Yesavage JA, Brink TL, Rose TL, Lum O, Huang V, Adey M, Leirer VO. Development and validation of a geriatric depression screening scale: a preliminary report. *J Psychiatr Res.* 1982–1983;17(1):37–49.

31. Price A, Rayner L, Okon-Rocha E, Evans A, Valsrai K, Higginson IJ, Hotopf M. Antidepressants for the treatment of depression in neurological disorders: a systematic review and meta-analysis of randomized controlled trials. *J Neurol Neurosurg Psychiatry.* 2011;82:914–923.

32. Rayner L, Price A, Evans A, Valsraj K, Higginson IJ, Hotopf M. Antidepressants for depression in physically ill people. *Cochrane Database Syst Rev.* 2010;3:CD007503.

33. Hackett ML, Yang M, Anderson CS, Horrocks JA, House A. Pharmaceutical interventions for emotionalism after stroke. *Cochrane Database Syst Rev.* 2010;2:CD003690.

34. Burn J, Dennis M, Bamford J, Sandercock P, Wade D, Warlow C. Epileptic seizures after a first stroke: the Oxfordshire community stroke project. *BMJ.*1997;315:1582–1587.

35. Bladin CF, Alexandrov AV, Bellavance A, Bornstein N, Chambers B, Coté R, et al. for the Seizures After Stroke Study Group. *Arch Neurol.* 2000;57:1617–1622.

36. Lindgren I, Jönsson A-C, Norrving B, Lindgren A. Shoulder pain after stroke. A prospective population-based study. *Stroke.* 2007;38:343–348.

37. Vestergaard K, Andersen G, MI Nielsen, Jensen TS. Headache in stroke. *Stroke.* 1993;24:1621–1624.

38. Klit H, Finneruo NB, Jensen TS. Central post-stroke pain: clinical characteristics, pathophysiology, and management. *Lancet Neurol.* 2009;8:857–868.

39. McGeough E, Pollock A, Smith LN, Dennis M, Sharpe M, Lewis S, Mead GE. Interventions for post-stroke fatigue. *Cochrane Database Syst Rev.* 2009; 3:CD007030.

CHAPTER 19

Vascular cognitive impairment and dementia

Didier Leys, Kei Murao, and Florence Pasquier

Introduction

Stroke and dementia are frequent and often associated in the same patient. Their association can be encountered either in the diagnostic workup of patients attending a memory clinic, or during the follow-up of stroke patients (1). The term 'vascular dementia' (VaD) is used to describe a dementia syndrome likely to be the direct consequence of stroke lesions (2, 3), while the term post-stroke dementia (PSD) is a more general term that includes all types of dementia occurring after a stroke, irrespective of the presumed cause (4). Therefore, VaD accounts for only a part of PSD, while it may sometimes occur without any clinical history of stroke (4) and be the consequence of so-called 'silent' lesions of the brain of vascular origin. VaD is the second most common cause of dementia after Alzheimer disease (AD): it accounts for 10–50% of all cases of dementia, depending on regional variations and criteria used (1, 5, 6). Both ischaemic and haemorrhagic strokes lead to a high risk of cognitive impairment and dementia (1, 5, 7). About one in ten patients is demented before having a first-ever stroke, one in ten develops new-onset dementia after a first-ever stroke, and more than one in three develops dementia after a recurrent stroke (5). A vascular origin of cognitive impairment is frequent, and often preventable: therefore, patients could benefit from early detection and therapy. An accurate diagnosis of vascular cognitive impairment or VaD is necessary (8, 9). Dementia is probably the tip of the iceberg, accounting for a small part of the cognitive consequences of stroke, as most of these consequences are represented by cognitive-impairment without dementia (8, 9), and are due to the coexistence of vascular and degenerative lesions of the brain (4, 10, 11).

Epidemiology

Vascular cognitive impairment (VCI) and VaD can occur in patients with or without clinical evidence of stroke.

Post-stroke cognitive impairment and dementia

Prevalence

The prevalence of PSD varies largely according to various factors such as selection criteria of cohorts, setting, and delay of cognitive assessment after stroke (1). The pooled prevalence of PSD 1 year after stroke ranges from a lowest value of 7.4% in population-based studies conducted in first-ever strokes and excluding patients with pre-existing dementia, and a highest value of 41.3% in hospital-based studies including recurrent strokes and patients with pre-existing dementia (5). In all case–control studies, the prevalence of dementia was higher in stroke survivors than in matched controls (12, 13). Some patients with PSD were, however, already demented before stroke: the prevalence of pre-existing dementia is 14.4% in all patients with stroke in hospital-based studies, 9.1% in all patients with history of stroke in community-based studies, and 8.5% in stroke patients reaching the follow-up in hospital-based studies (5).

Incidence

The incidence of new-onset PSD varies also largely between population- and hospital-based studies. In population-based studies it increases from 5% 1 year after stroke, up to 12% after 5 years (1.7% per year: 95% confidence interval (CI) 1.4–2.0%), while in hospital-based studies it increases from 18% after 3 months up to 35% after 5 years (3.0% per year: 95% CI 1.3–4.7%) (5). Stroke patients have a ninefold increased risk of new-onset dementia after 1 year, compared to controls without stroke (5). A population-based study showed that the relative risk of being demented in stroke survivors was 8.8 after 1 year, and decreased to 2.0 after 25 years (14). The incidence of AD is also doubled 25 years after stroke (14), but we should bear in mind that any study conducted 25 years after a stroke has limitations due to the low quality of the baseline assessment performed in the 1980s, and the highly selected profile of patients who survive 25 years, who are usually younger, had less severe strokes, and are not representative of the general population of stroke patients.

Risk factors

From a systematic review of available literature published before 1 May 2009, risk factors for PSD were demographic factors (female gender, increasing age, and non-white ethnicity), vascular risk factors (high blood pressure, diabetes mellitus, atrial fibrillation), stroke features (haemorrhagic origin, dysphasia, left hemisphere location, recurrent stroke, multiple strokes), stroke complications (hypoxic-ischaemic episodes, incontinence, confusion, early seizures), and structural brain changes (leucoaraiosis, cortical atrophy, medial temporal lobe atrophy) (5).

When dementia was already present before stroke, factors associated with dementia are factors associated with both VaD (diabetes mellitus, atrial fibrillation, ischaemic heart disease, previous transient ischaemic attacks of strokes, arterial hypertension, smoking, multiple strokes, silent strokes, white matter changes), and AD (female gender, low education, family history of dementia, medial temporal lobe atrophy) (5), suggesting a heterogeneity of PSD.

Influence of post-stroke dementia on stroke outcome

Stroke patients with PSD have a higher mortality rate after stroke (15, 16): in the New York cohort, the cumulative proportion of survivors at 5 years after stroke was 39% for stroke patients with dementia and 75% for non-demented stroke patients (15). Dementia diagnosed 3 months after stroke is also associated with an increased risk of recurrence (17). A possible explanation is that dementia may be a surrogate marker for multiple vascular risk factors that may increase the risk of recurrence (17), but less intensive management of stroke patients with cognitive impairment, and lack of compliance, may also play a role (17). Patients with dementia are also more likely to develop delirium at the acute stage (18), depressive symptoms (19), and seizures (20).

Vascular cognitive impairment and vascular dementia without clinical evidence of stroke

Comparisons between epidemiological studies are impeded by methodological differences. One of the major difficulties is to decide whether or not patients with AD associated with vascular lesions (ADv) should be counted as AD patients, VaD patients, or in a specific group of ill-defined ADv patients.

Prevalence

An old European Community Concerted Action reanalysed all information available on the prevalence of VaD in Europe before 1990(21): of 23 surveys, only 5 met the following criteria: (i) dementia defined according to the DSM-III criteria or equivalent, (ii) case finding through direct individual examination, (iii) at least 300 subjects over 65 years, and (iv) inclusion of institutionalized persons. The sex-specific prevalence of VaD/AD over the age of 60 was 2.6% for men and 2.1% for women. It increased with age and remained generally higher in men, ranging from 3.2–4.8% (2.2–2.9% in women) between 70 and 79 years and from 3.5–16.3% (2.8–9.2% for women) between 80 and 89 years. The prevalence of AD was twice higher than that of VaD (21). In Japan, VaD accounts for more than 50% of dementias after 65 years (22). Several consistent findings can be identified: (i) age-dependence, (ii) sex difference, and (iii) ethnic differences.

At autopsy, cases of pure VaD are very uncommon (23). The association of AD and stroke lesions is frequent (24).

Incidence

Because of an excess in mortality due to vascular death in patients with VaD, cross-sectional studies may underestimate their frequency. In the few available data, substantial variations in the incidence rates have been observed. Over 75 years, the annual incidence rates of VaD are 900/100,000 in men and 1200/100,00 in women (25). In Japan, the VaD:AD ratio shifted from 1.8:1 to 1.1:1 (26); the prevalence of VaD decreased more in men than in women and matched an overall decline in stroke incidence (26). These findings suggest that stroke prevention may decrease the risk of VaD.

Mortality

The mortality rate is higher in VaD than in AD (15).

How to diagnose vascular cognitive impairment and dementia?

The cornerstone in the evaluation of a patient with dementia is to record a detailed clinical and neurological history and examination, including an interview of an informant. The assessment of social functions, daily living activities, psychiatric symptoms, and behavioural changes, are part of the routine evaluation. Besides, a proof of stroke lesions is needed and is provided by imaging or autopsy.

Mental status examination

The bedside mental status examination includes the Mini Mental State Examination (MMSE) (27). Its main limitation in stroke patients is that it emphasizes language, does not include timed elements, is not sensitive to mild deficits, and is influenced by education and age. However, this test is so popular and widely used across different cultures, that it is always part of the evaluation. The Montreal Cognitive Assessment (MoCA) was developed as another a global cognitive screening test that is more adapted to stroke patients (28). It can be downloaded for free in 34 different languages, at <http://www.mocatest.org>. It picks up more cognitive abnormalities than the MMSE (29). All patients with a score of 30/30 at the MoCA have 30/30 at the MMSE, while many patients with 30 at the MMSE have scores between 20 and 29 at the MoCA test (29, 30). Its higher sensitivity is in part due to the inclusion of tests for executive functions, especially useful in stroke patients. Other screening instruments for VaD include a four- to ten-word memory test with delayed recall, cube drawing test for copy verbal fluency test (number of animals named in 1 minute), Luria's alternating hand sequence or finger rings and one-letter cancellation test (3). Usually more detailed neuropsychological assessments are needed to cover memory functions (short- and long-term memory), abstract thinking, judgement, aphasia, apraxia, agnosia, orientation, attention executive functions, and speed of information processing (6, 31, 32).

Brain imaging

Brain imaging is crucial to identify the most likely cause of dementia. Magnetic resonance imaging (MRI) has a higher sensitivity than computed tomography (CT) to detect brain lesions, medial temporal lobe atrophy, white matter changes, and microbleeds. Positron emission tomography with the Pittsburg compound B (PIB) may help identifying the presence of cerebral amyloid angiopathy because of its capacity to detect cerebrovascular beta-amyloid in during life (33).

Diagnostic criteria for vascular dementia

The two key elements for a diagnosis of VaD are the definition of dementia (6), and the definition of the vascular disorder (34, 35).

All currently available criteria are consensus criteria, summarized in Tables 19.1–19.4. They were not derived from prospective community-based studies on vascular factors affecting cognition, and they are not based on detailed natural histories (2) (3, 6, 35, 36). They are mainly or exclusively based on the infarct concept and were designed to have a high specificity, i.e. to diagnoses cases of VaD as pure as possible. Moreover, they have been poorly implemented and validated (6, 36).

Table 19.1 DSM-IV criteria for diagnosis of vascular dementia (53)

Require focal neurological signs and symptoms or laboratory evidence of focal neurological damage clinically judged to be related to the disturbance
Time course specified by sudden cognitive and functional losses
Brain imaging requirements: not detailed
Reasonably broad but lack detailed clinical and radiological guidelines

Table 19.2 ICD-10 criteria for diagnosis of vascular dementia (34, 54)

Require unequal distribution of cognitive deficits, focal signs as evidence of focal brain damage, and significant cerebrovascular disease judged to be aetiologically related to the dementia
Brain imaging requirements: not detailed
Specify altogether six subtypes of VaD
Highly selective
Lack of detailed guidelines, e.g. unequal cognitive deficits and neuroimaging, aetiological cues, and heterogeneity

Table 19.3 ADDTC criteria for diagnosis of vascular dementia (2)

Exclusively criteria for ischaemic VaD (IVaD)
Require (i) evidence of two or more ischaemic strokes by history neurological signs or neuroimaging studies, or (ii) in case of a single stroke a clearly documented temporal relationship (not detailed), and always a neuroradiological evidence of at least one infarct outside the cerebellum
Ischaemic white matter changes on CT or MRI do not qualify as brain imaging evidence of probable IVaD, but may support the diagnosis
Includes a list of features supporting or casting doubt on a diagnosis of probable IVaD

Variations in defining the dementia syndrome (6, 13), and the vascular cause (34, 37), has led to a critical consequence: different definitions give different point prevalence estimates, identify different groups of subjects, and further identify different types and distribution of lesions.

The current criteria for VaD are not interchangeable; they identify different numbers and cluster of patients labelled as VaD. The DSM-IV criteria are less restrictive compared to the ICD-10, the ADDTC and the NINDS–AIREN criteria (34, 38). The clinical criteria for VaD of older origin (38) do not specify brain imaging requirements for the diagnosis in detail. The ADDTC requires one CT or T1-weighted MRI infarct outside cerebellum, but white matter lesions do not qualify for support of probable IVD. The NINDS–AIREN criteria require multiple infarcts (more than one cortico-subcortical or lacunar) or extensive white matter lesions (CT or T1-weighted MRI), but accept also a clinically 'strategic' single infarct as an

Table 19.4 NINDS–AIREN criteria for diagnosis of vascular dementia (3, 120)

Include dementia syndrome, cerebrovascular disease, and a relationship between dementia and cerebrovascular disorders
Cerebrovascular disease defined by the presence of focal neurological signs and detailed brain imaging evidence of ischaemic changes in the brain
Relationship between dementia and cerebrovascular disorder based on the onset of dementia within 3 months following a recognized stroke, or on abrupt deterioration in cognitive functions or fluctuating, stepwise progression of cognitive deficits
Include a list of features consistent with the diagnosis, or making the diagnosis uncertain or unlikely
Different levels of certainty of the clinical diagnosis (probable, possible, definite) are included
Inter-rater reliability from moderate to substantial (kappa 0.46 to 0.72)

evidence of 'relevant cerebrovascular disease'. As evaluated neuropathologically the ADDTC criteria seem to be more sensitive and the NINDS-AIREN criteria more specific, but neither is perfect (39). In a neuropathological series sensitivity of the NINDS–AIREN criteria was 58% and specificity 80% (39). The criteria successfully excluded AD in 91% of cases, and the proportion of combined cases misclassified as probable VaD was 29% (39). Compared to the ADDTC criteria, the NINDS–AIREN criteria were more specific and they better excluded combined cases (54% vs 29%) (39).

Clinical patterns of vascular cognitive impairment and vascular dementia

The cognitive syndrome

The cognitive syndrome of VaD is characterized by the coexistence of:

1. A memory deficit, less severe than in AD, consisting of impaired recall, relative preservation of recognition, and better benefit from cues (40).

2. A dysexecutive syndrome, including impairment in goal formulation, initiation, planning, organizing, sequencing, executing, set-sifting, and set-maintenance, as well as in abstracting (40–42). It relates to lesions affecting the prefrontal subcortical circuit including prefrontal cortex, caudate, pallidum, thalamus, and the thalamo-cortical circuit (genu anterior limb of the internal capsule, anterior centrum semiovale, and anterior corona radiata) (43).

3. Slowed information processing.

4. Mood and personality changes.

These features are typical for cases with subcortical lesions. Patients with cortical lesions often have in addition a combination of different cortical neuropsychological syndromes (41). Features that make the diagnosis of VaD uncertain or unlikely include early onset and progressive worsening of memory deficit or some other cognitive cortical deficit in the absence of corresponding focal lesions on brain imaging (3).

Associated neurological features

Clinical neurological findings are frequent and indicate the presence of focal brain lesions that occur early in the time-course of VaD. They include mild motor and sensory deficits, decreased coordination, brisk tendon reflexes, Babinski sign, field cut, bulbar signs including dysarthria and dysphagia, extrapyramidal signs (mainly rigidity and akinesia), gait disorder (hemiplegic, apractic-atactic, or small-stepped), unsteadiness and unprovoked falls, as well as urinary frequency and urgency (3, 44–47). In cortical VaD, typical clinical features are sensorimotor changes and abrupt onset of cognitive impairment and aphasia, and in subcortical VaD pure motor hemiparesis, bulbar signs, and dysarthria (46).

Associated behavioural features

Depression, anxiety, emotional lability and incontinence, and other psychiatric symptoms are frequent in VaD (44). Depression, apathy, emotional incontinence, and psychomotor retardation are frequent in subcortical VaD (41, 42).

Heterogeneity of vascular cognitive impairment and dementia

VaD may be classified in several categories based upon: (i) the underlying vascular pathology, (ii) the type of brain lesions, (iii) the location of brain lesions, (iv) the clinical syndrome. The subtypes of VaD that are included in current classifications are the cortical type (or multi-infarct dementia), the subcortical type (or small-vessel dementia), and the strategic infarct type (3, 42, 46, 48–51). Other classifications also include hypoperfusion dementia (3, 42, 49, 52), haemorrhagic dementia, hereditary VaD, and combined AD with cerebrovascular disease.

None of the current clinical criteria for VaD include detailed criteria for their subtypes. The DSM-IV (53) did not specify subtypes. The ICD-10 (54) included six subtypes with superficial descriptions (acute onset, multi-infarct, subcortical, mixed cortical and subcortical, other, and unspecified). The ADDTC (2) criteria do not specify detailed subtypes, but highlight that classification of ischaemic VaD for research purposes should specify features of the infarcts that may differentiate of the disorder, such as location (cortical, white matter, periventricular, basal ganglia, thalamus), size (volume), distribution (large, small, or microvessel), severity (chronic ischaemia versus infarction), aetiology (embolism, atherosclerosis, arteriosclerosis, cerebral amyloid angiopathy hypoperfusion). The NINDS–AIREN criteria (3) include without detailed description cortical VaD, subcortical VaD, Binswanger's disease, and thalamic dementia.

Cortical vascular dementia

Cortical VaD relates to large-vessel disease, cardiac emboli, and hypoperfusion. It shows prominently cortical and cortico-subcortical arterial territorial and distal field infarcts (Figure 19.1). Typical clinical features are lateralized sensorimotor changes and abrupt onset of cognitive impairment and aphasia (55). Some combination of cortical neuropsychological

syndromes has been suggested to be present in cortical VaD (41). The occurrence of dementia depends on two factors: the total volume of brain loss because of infarcts and haemorrhages (56), and the location of these lesions (57). It has also been suggested that it may depend on the presence and volume of perifocal ischaemic damage (58). There is no clear cut-off point on the volume of infarction resulting in dementia. This group is heterogeneous in terms of aetiologies, vascular mechanisms, brain changes, and clinical presentation.

Strategic infarct vascular dementia

Focal, often small, ischaemic lesions involving specific sites critical for higher cortical functions have been classified separately. This group shows most heterogeneity. Isolated brain infarcts or haemorrhages may lead to dementia. In such cases, dementia is due to the location of the lesion, rather than the volume of brain loss. The following cortical locations have been associated with dementia: left angular gyrus infarcts (59), right hemisphere angular gyrus infarcts, inferomesial temporal infarcts (60, 61), and mesial frontal infarcts (62, 63). Isolated subcortical vascular lesions consist of lacunar infarcts, deep territorial infarcts, and deep haemorrhages, disrupting specific subcortical–cortical functional loops crucial for the maintenance of cognitive status (64). Dementia has been reported in thalamic (65) (Figure 19.2), left-sided capsular genu (66), and caudate nuclei infarcts (67–69). However, the concept of strategic infarct was introduced in the era of CT scans, and has not been revised since MRI has become the standard for stroke care. 'Strategic' locations have been described in single cases or in small series; however, in case reports with first generations of computed tomographic CT scans, another vascular lesion of the brain cannot be excluded and may interfere with the neuropsychological profile (70, 71). We cannot completely exclude that, in a few cases, there was another lesion that was not seen on CT scan. Moreover, in elderly patients without follow-up after stroke, the contribution of Alzheimer lesions to the neuropsychological profile cannot be excluded (4, 7, 72). The concept of strategic stroke should, therefore, be revisited with modern imaging techniques and a longer follow-up.

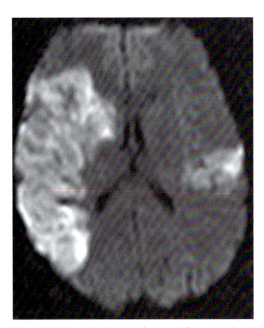

Fig. 19.1 Bilateral middle cerebral artery infarct on diffusion-weighted imaging at the acute stage.

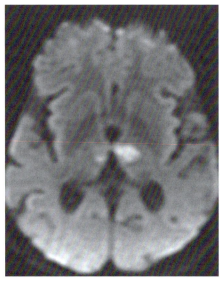

Fig. 19.2 Bithalamic infarct on diffusion-weighted imaging at the acute stage.

Subcortical vascular dementia

Subcortical VaD includes small-vessel disease as primary vascular cause, lacunar infarcts, white matter lesions, and microbleeds as primary types of brain lesions, and subcortical location as the primary location of lesions. Ischaemic lesions in VaD affect especially the prefrontal subcortical circuit that includes prefrontal cortex, caudate, pallidum, and the thalamo-cortical circuit (genu or anterior limb of the internal capsule, anterior centrum semiovale, and anterior corona radiata) (43).

The most prominent symptoms are of subcortical type. Lacunar infarcts appear as small miliary softening, mostly located in the putamen, thalamus, or pons, or in the deep white matter (57). They are small (5–15 mm) cavitations filled by a fine network of astrocytic processes, macrophages, and siderophages, surrounded by fibrillary and protoplasmic astrocytes and sometimes also by haemosiderin pigments. They are the consequence of the occlusion of one single, deep perforating artery (73). Multiple lacunes, in association with diffuse white matter changes, have been reported as the anatomical substrate of progressive cognitive decline in some patients who were clinically diagnosed as having AD, in the absence of a history of stroke and of a stepwise course of dementia (74). In demented patients with similarly progressive decline and absence of clinical strokes, diffuse white matter changes without lacunes have been described at autopsy (75). These cases were, however, clinically diagnosed as VaD. Such small-vessel diseases are usually due to chronic arterial hypertension (73). Small-vessel disease is the consequence of the occlusion of one single, deep perforating artery, caused by segmental fibrinoid degeneration with lipohyalinosis (73). Many perforating branches have multiple stenosis and poststenotic dilatations, suggesting that some haemodynamic events might also play a role, rather than local thrombosis (76). Stroke patients with lacunes are more likely to have white matter changes (77, 78) and to develop dementia (79) than patients with other stroke subtypes.

Subcortical VaD is characterized by an abrupt onset (days to weeks), a stepwise deterioration with episodes of recovery after worsening, and a fluctuating course. Sometimes, cognitive symptoms evolve relatively insidiously and can even be slowly progressive (2, 3, 44, 45, 55). The survival is lower than that of the general population or of AD (37). Detailed studies on the natural history of subcortical VaD are lacking.

The cognitive syndrome of subcortical VaD is characterized by: (i) mild memory deficits consisting of impaired recall, relative intact recognition, less severe forgetting, and better benefit from cues than in AD (40); (ii) a dysexecutive syndrome including impairment in goal formulation, initiation, planning, organizing, sequencing, executing, set-sifting and self-maintenance, as well as in abstracting (40–42); and behavioural changes including depression, personality change, emotional lability and incontinence, inertia, emotional bluntness, and psychomotor retardation (41, 42).

The clinical neurological findings especially early in the course of subcortical VaD include episodes of mild upper motor neuron signs (drift, reflex asymmetry in coordination), gait disorder (apractic-atactic or small-stepped), imbalance and falls, urinary frequency and incontinence, dysarthria, dysphagia, extrapyramidal signs (hyperkinesias, rigidity), and depression (80–84). However, often these focal neurological signs are subtle (85).

Small deep infarcts in the basal ganglia, centrum semiovale, or brainstem, are often associated with leucoencephalopathy (77, 78).

Dementia is not always present in patients with a lacunar state. So-called Binswanger disease may be considered in patients with pathological evidence of the underlying vasculopathy lacunes and leucoencephalopathy (Figure 19.3). Pathological examination of cases of Binswanger disease show diffuse or patchy rarefaction of myelin predominating in the periventricular and occipital regions of the centrum semiovale and associated with gliosis and spongiosis (57). The U fibres, internal capsules, and cerebral cortex are usually spared (45). White matter changes are associated with multiple lacunes in the white matter and basal ganglia (45). Binswanger's encephalopathy may represent the end-stage pathology of lacunar state (57). However, the existence of Binswanger disease as a specific type of VaD remains controversial (86). Dementia may occur after several strokes, when patients have dysarthria, dysphagia, 'Marche à petits pas', incontinence, spasmodic laughing or crying, and parkinsonism. In other cases, multiple brain infarcts are recognized on brain imaging, in patients with dementia and no clear clinical evidence of stroke. Multiple lacunes in association with diffuse cerebral white matter changes have been reported as the anatomical substrate of progressive cognitive decline in some patients who were clinically diagnosed as having AD, in the absence of a history of stroke and a stepwise course of dementia (74).

Most cases of multiple lacunar infarcts with leucoencephalopathy are due to lipohyalinosis of the deep perforating arteries, which is the favoured chronic arterial hypertension (73). However, other causes may be associated with a higher risk of dementia in stroke patients. Cerebral autosomal dominant arteriopathy with subcortical infarcts and leucoencephalopathy (CADASIL) is an autosomal dominant arteriopathy due to a mutation in the *NOTCH3* gene (87) on chromosome 19. Usually lacunar infarcts occur between 40 and 50 years of age, and dementia occurs in one-third of patients with lacunes, and is almost always present before death (88). Mild cognitive impairment, of subcortical type, is probably present years before occurrence of dementia, but dementia occurs in a stepwise fashion in a setting of several strokes, and is rarely progressive. MRI is always abnormal in symptomatic subjects: it shows confluent hyperintensities in the white matter and lacunar infarcts (89).

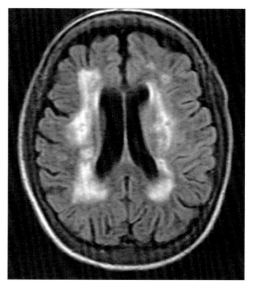

Fig. 19.3 Severe white matter changes on fluid attenuated inversion recovery sequences.

Other rare arteriolopathies leading to multiple lacunar infarcts and dementia have been recognized. Their origin remains unknown, but genetic studies might help to classify them: non-CADASIL Binswanger-like syndromes without arterial hypertension.

Vascular cognitive impairment and dementia without detectable stroke lesions

Role of white matter changes in post-stroke dementia

One-third to one-half of patients with pathological evidence of VaD lack a history of clinically recognized stroke (90). The question remains whether chronic ischaemia plays an important role in VaD. The role of haemodynamic factors and hypoxemia in the pathogenesis of PSD has already been mentioned (91). Several authors have found no evidence of chronic ischaemic states in VaD, studied by means of positron emission tomography (PET) (92, 93). However, presence of arterial borderzones in the deep white matter and the high susceptibility of oligodendroglial cells to ischaemia, along with the findings of widespread, histopathologically verified non-infarct damage in patients with VaD, suggest that chronic ischaemic leucoencephalopathies leading to VaD do exist (94).

Chronic ischaemia without infarction in the carotid territory might be an exceptional cause of dementia, attributed to a 'misery perfusion' with PET studies (64). This type of dementia might be reversible after correcting correction of the haemodynamic deficit (64). The term 'incomplete white matter infarction', has been suggested (95) to describe a rarefaction of the deep white matter, with diffuse partial loss of myelin sheets, axons and oligodendroglial cells, and mild astrocytic and macrophagic reactions in association with a central small-vessel disorder. It correlates to the frequent finding of white matter changes on CT and MRI scans in elderly patients (95). The brain damage may be more severe, and affect several of the most sensitive structures of the brain, leading to laminar necrosis of the neocortex, hippocampal degeneration, Purkinje cell loss of the cerebellar cortex, and deep cerebral white matter demyelination.

White matter changes may be associated with subtle cognitive and behavioural changes (96, 97). The functions which are the most sensitive to white matter changes are memory, attention, and frontal lobe function (96, 97).

Role of microbleeds in post-stroke dementia

Brain microbleeds are small dot-like lesions appearing as hypo signal on gradient echo T2*-weighted MRI sequences (98) (see Figure 19.4). They represent microscopic areas of old haemosiderin deposits (99). They are frequent in the setting of symptomatic cerebrovascular disease and also in older healthy people, suggesting a link with cerebral amyloid angiopathy (98). Their use as diagnostic or prognostic biomarkers remains uncertain (98). More recently, they have been highlighted as a potential key factor in the pathogenesis of Alzheimer's disease (100), connecting the main pathological contributors of amyloid accumulation and cerebrovascular damage. The question of whether they contribute to the cognitive syndrome remains uncertain, but it has been shown that AD patients with brain microbleeds decline more rapidly (101), and are more severe (102).

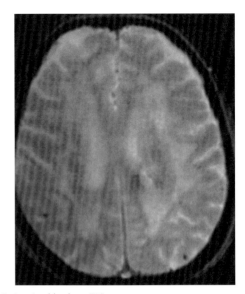

Fig. 19.4 Brain microbleeds on T2* sequences.

Role of Alzheimer pathology

Medial temporal lobe atrophy, known to be associated with an increased risk for AD (103), is more frequent in stroke patients who have pre-existing dementia (104), and is associated with an increased risk of new-onset PSD (105), leading to the hypothesis that many cases of PSD may be due to AD (7, 104). Alzheimer and vascular lesions of the brain are frequently associated at autopsy (24, 106). The links between PSD and AD are probably closer than expected (4). Shared risk factors of the two clinical entities may be responsible for their co-occurrence. Besides advancing age, one of them might be the epsilon 4 allele of the apolipoprotein E gene.

It has been shown that the basis of the interaction between vascular risk factors and Alzheimer pathology is at the level of the neurovascular unit, where perivascular and vascular cells, glia, and neurons are in close contact (107). Both the structure and the function of the neurovascular unit are modified under the effect of amyloid beta peptide in patients with AD lesions, and ischaemia in ischaemic stroke (107). Ischaemia is a powerful modulator of cerebral amyloidogenesis, while amyloid beta peptide has potent cerebrovascular effects (107). These structural and functional changes will contribute to cognitive impairment (Figure 19.5).

The multifactorial origin of vascular cognitive impairment

From a clinical point of view, dementia is probably due to stroke alone in the following circumstances: (i) in young stroke patients who become demented after one or several strokes; (ii) when the clinician has a high level of certainty that the cognitive functioning of the patient was normal before stroke, impaired immediately after, and does not worsen over time or even slightly improve; (iii) when the lesions are located in strategic areas; and (iv) when a specific vascular condition known to cause dementia is proven by pathological data or a specific marker (e.g. CADASIL).

Many cases of dementia occurring in stroke patients are probably the consequence of the cumulative effect of the cerebrovascular lesions, Alzheimer pathology, and white matter changes. Even when these changes do not lead to dementia by

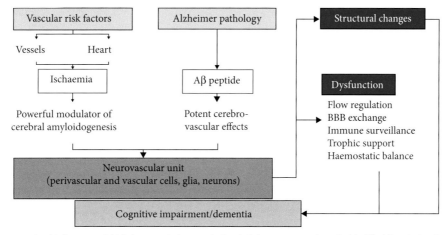

Fig. 19.5 Interaction between vascular risk factors and Alzheimer pathology at the level of the neurovascular unit. Modified from Iadecola, C., The overlap between neurodegenerative and vascular factors in the pathogenesis of dementia. (Modified from Iadecola, C., The overlap between neurodegenerative and vascular factors in the pathogenesis of dementia. Acta Neuropathol, 120(3), 287–96.)

themselves, their cumulative effect may reach the threshold of lesions required to produce dementia (4). When stroke, white matter changes, or both, occur in a patient with asymptomatic Alzheimer pathology the period of preclinical AD may be shortened (4) (72).

Management of patients with vascular cognitive impairment and dementia

Stroke prevention

Patients with dementia after stroke are significantly less frequently treated with aspirin or warfarin than non-demented patients (17). However, trials of secondary prevention of stroke usually exclude patients with obvious dementia. As a consequence, optimal secondary prevention of stroke in patients with dementia remains speculative. Anticoagulation is not recommended in dementia, and carotid endarterectomy is thought to be associated with increased risk of the therapeutic procedure. However, this has never been evaluated. Therefore, stroke prevention trials should include dementia as a secondary end-point.

Acute stroke management

Stroke patients with pre-existing cognitive impairment often have an underlying brain pathology which could be associated with an increased bleeding risk, such as brain microbleeds (100), usually associated with cerebral amyloid angiopathy in Alzheimer's disease (AD) (108), hypertensive micro-angiopathy in vascular dementia (109), or both. Besides this possible increased bleeding risk, patients with cognitive impairment are also less likely to recover because of the presence of brain lesions, impaired brain plasticity, and possibly higher sensitivity to the neurotoxic effects on brain cells of recombinant tissue plasminogen activator (rtPA) (110). For these reasons, patients with cognitive impairment may have a worse outcome after intravenous thrombolytic therapy than matched patients without cognitive impairment. In practice, demented patients are less frequently treated with intravenous rtPA, even in the absence of contraindication (111), but there is no evidence that this self-limitation is appropriate. There is no randomized controlled trial conducted in patients with dementia or

cognitive impairment, but some indirect evidence that the presence of cognitive impairment should not prevent to treat patients with rtPA if otherwise appropriate (112, 113).

Symptomatic treatment

No drug has so far been approved for the treatment of VaD. Nevertheless, approved anti-Alzheimer drugs have been tested in VaD and in AD with coexistent vascular lesions. Cholinesterase inhibitors (114– 117) and memantine (118) have some effect but the magnitude is small and there is heterogeneity between studies (119). The benefit can be either due to the effect on coexisting AD, or a non-specific effect on the pathways interrupted by the vascular lesions of the brain. Besides, treatments of anxiety and depression may provide some benefit in eligible patients.

References

1. Leys D, Henon H, Mackowiak-Cordoliani MA, Pasquier F. Post-stroke dementia. *Lancet Neurol.* 2005;4(11):752–759.
2. Chui HC, Victoroff JI, Margolin D, Jagust W, Shankle R, Katzman R. Criteria for the diagnosis of ischemic vascular dementia proposed by the State of California Alzheimer's Disease Diagnostic and Treatment Centers. *Neurology.* 1992;42(3 Pt 1):473–480.
3. Roman GC, Tatemichi TK, Erkinjuntti T, Cummings JL, Masdeu JC, Garcia JH, *et al.* Vascular dementia: diagnostic criteria for research studies. Report of the NINDS-AIREN International Workshop. *Neurology.* 1993;43(2):250–260.
4. Pasquier F, Leys D. Why are stroke patients prone to develop dementia? *J Neurol.* 1997;244(3):135–142.
5. Pendlebury ST, Rothwell PM. Prevalence, incidence, and factors associated with pre-stroke and post-stroke dementia: a systematic review and meta-analysis. *Lancet Neurol.* 2009;8(11):1006–1018.
6. Erkinjuntti T, Ostbye T, Steenhuis R, Hachinski V. The effect of different diagnostic criteria on the prevalence of dementia. *N Engl J Med.* 1997;337(23):1667–1674.
7. Cordonnier C, Leys D, Dumont F, Deramecourt V, Bordet R, Pasquier F, *et al.* What are the causes of pre-existing dementia in patients with intracerebral haemorrhages? *Brain.* 2010;133(11):3281–3289.
8. Hachinski V. The 2005 Thomas Willis Lecture: stroke and vascular cognitive impairment: a transdisciplinary, translational and transactional approach. *Stroke.* 2007;38(4):1396–1396.
9. Hachinski V, Donnan GA, Gorelick PB, Hacke W, Cramer SC, Kaste M, *et al.* Stroke: working toward a prioritized world agenda. *Stroke.* 2010;41(6):1084–1099.

10. Iadecola C. Neurovascular regulation in the normal brain and in Alzheimer's disease. *Nat Rev Neurosci.* 2004;5(5):347–360.

11. Iadecola C, Gorelick PB. Converging pathogenic mechanisms in vascular and neurodegenerative dementia. *Stroke.* 2003;34(2):335–337.

12. Censori B, Manara O, Agostinis C, Camerlingo M, Casto L, Galavotti B, et al. Dementia after first stroke. *Stroke.* 1996;27(7):1205–1210.

13. Pohjasvaara T, Erkinjuntti T, Vataja R, Kaste M. Dementia three months after stroke. Baseline frequency and effect of different definitions of dementia in the Helsinki Stroke Aging Memory Study (SAM) cohort. *Stroke.* 1997;28(4):785–792.

14. Kokmen E, Whisnant JP, O'Fallon WM, Chu CP, Beard CM. Dementia after ischemic stroke: a population-based study in Rochester, Minnesota (1960-1984). *Neurology.* 1996;46(1):154–159.

15. Tatemichi TK, Paik M, Bagiella E, Desmond DW, Pirro M, Hanzawa LK. Dementia after stroke is a predictor of long-term survival. *Stroke.* 1994;25(10):1915–1919.

16. Henon H, Durieu I, Lebert F, Pasquier F, Leys D. Influence of prestroke dementia on early and delayed mortality in stroke patients. *J Neurol.* 2003;250(1):10–16.

17. Moroney JT, Bagiella E, Tatemichi TK, Paik MC, Stern Y, Desmond DW. Dementia after stroke increases the risk of long-term stroke recurrence. *Neurology.* 1997;48(5):1317–1325.

18. Henon H, Lebert F, Durieu I, Godefroy O, Lucas C, Pasquier F, et al. Confusional state in stroke: relation to preexisting dementia, patient characteristics, and outcome. *Stroke.* 1999;30(4):773–779.

19. Verdelho A, Henon H, Lebert F, Pasquier F, Leys D. Depressive symptoms after stroke and relationship with dementia: a three-year follow-up study. *Neurology.* 2004;62(6):905–911.

20. Cordonnier C, Henon H, Derambure P, Pasquier F, Leys D. Influence of pre-existing dementia on the risk of post-stroke epileptic seizures. *J Neurol Neurosurg Psychiatry.* 2005;76(12):1649–1653.

21. Rocca WA, Hofman A, Brayne C, Breteler MM, Clarke M, Copeland JR, et al. The prevalence of vascular dementia in Europe: facts and fragments from 1980-1990 studies. EURODEM-Prevalence Research Group. *Ann Neurol.* 1991;30(6):817–824.

22. Ueda K, Kawano H, Hasuo Y, Fujishima M. Prevalence and etiology of dementia in a Japanese community. *Stroke.* 1992;23(6):798–803.

23. Hulette C, Nochlin D, McKeel D, Morris JC, Mirra SS, Sumi SM, et al. Clinical-neuropathologic findings in multi-infarct dementia: a report of six autopsied cases. *Neurology.* 1997;48(3):668–672.

24. Victoroff J, Mack WJ, Lyness SA, Chui HC. Multicenter clinicopathological correlation in dementia. *Am J Psychiatry.* 1995;152(10):1476–1484.

25. Aronson MK, Ooi WL, Morgenstern H, Hafner A, Masur D, Crystal H, et al. Women, myocardial infarction, and dementia in the very old. *Neurology.* 1990;40(7):1102–1106.

26. Kiyohara Y, Yoshitake T, Kato I, Ohmura T, Kawano H, Ueda K, et al. Changing patterns in the prevalence of dementia in a Japanese community: the Hisayama study. *Gerontology.* 1994;40(Suppl 2):29–35.

27. Folstein MF, Folstein SE, McHugh PR. "Mini-mental state". A practical method for grading the cognitive state of patients for the clinician. *J Psychiatr Res.* 1975;12(3):189–198.

28. Nasreddine ZS, Phillips NA, Bedirian V, Charbonneau S, Whitehead V, Collin I, et al. The Montreal Cognitive Assessment, MoCA: a brief screening tool for mild cognitive impairment. *J Am Geriatr Soc.* 2005;53(4):695–699.

29. Pendlebury ST, Cuthbertson FC, Welch SJ, Mehta Z, Rothwell PM. Underestimation of cognitive impairment by mini-mental state examination versus the Montreal cognitive assessment in patients with transient ischemic attack and stroke: a population-based study. *Stroke.* 2010;41(6):1290–1293.

30. Dong Y, Sharma VK, Chan BP, Venketasubramanian N, Teoh HL, Seet RC, et al. The Montreal Cognitive Assessment (MoCA) is superior to the Mini-Mental State Examination (MMSE) for the detection of vascular cognitive impairment after acute stroke. *J Neurol Sci.* 2010;299(1-2):15–18.

31. Pohjasvaara T, Erkinjuntti T, Ylikoski R, Hietanen M, Vataja R, Kaste M. Clinical determinants of post-stroke dementia. *Stroke.* 1998;29(1):75–81.

32. Hachinski V, Iadecola C, Petersen RC, Breteler MM, Nyenhuis DL, Black SE, et al. National Institute of Neurological Disorders and Stroke-Canadian Stroke Network vascular cognitive impairment harmonization standards. *Stroke.* 2006;37(9):2220–2241.

33. Johnson KA, Gregas M, Becker JA, Kinnecom C, Salat DH, Moran EK, et al. Imaging of amyloid burden and distribution in cerebral amyloid angiopathy. *Ann Neurol.* 2007;62(3):229–234.

34. Wetterling T, Kanitz RD, Borgis KJ. Comparison of different diagnostic criteria for vascular dementia (ADDTC, DSM-IV, ICD-10, NINDS-AIREN). *Stroke.* 1996;27(1):30–36.

35. Erkinjuntti T. Clinical criteria for vascular dementia: the NINDS-AIREN criteria. *Dementia.* 1994;5(3-4):189–192.

36. Rockwood K, Parhad I, Hachinski V, Erkinjuntti T, Rewcastle B, Kertesz A, et al. Diagnosis of vascular dementia: Consortium of Canadian Centres for Clinical Cognitive Research concensus statement. *Can J Neurol Sci.* 1994;21(4):358–364.

37. Skoog I, Nilsson L, Palmertz B, Andreasson LA, Svanborg A. A population-based study of dementia in 85-year-olds. *N Engl J Med.* 1993;328(3):153–158.

38. Verhey FR, Lodder J, Rozendaal N, Jolles J. Comparison of seven sets of criteria used for the diagnosis of vascular dementia. *Neuroepidemiology.* 1996;15(3):166–172.

39. Gold G, Giannakopoulos P, Montes-Paixao Junior C, Herrmann FR, Mulligan R, Michel JP, et al. Sensitivity and specificity of newly proposed clinical criteria for possible vascular dementia. *Neurology.* 1997;49(3):690–694.

40. Desmond DW, Erkinjuntti T, Sano M, Cummings JL, Bowler JV, Pasquier F, et al. The cognitive syndrome of vascular dementia: implications for clinical trials. *Alzheimer Dis Assoc Disord.* 1999;13 Suppl 3:S21–S29.

41. Mahler ME, Cummings JL. Behavioral neurology of multi-infarct dementia. *Alzheimer Dis Assoc Disord.* 1991;5(2):122–130.

42. Cummings JL. Vascular subcortical dementias: clinical aspects. *Dementia.* 1994;5(3-4):177–180.

43. Cummings JL. Frontal-subcortical circuits and human behavior. *Arch Neurol.* 1993;50(8):873–880.

44. Roman GC. Senile dementia of the Binswanger type. A vascular form of dementia in the elderly. *JAMA.* 1987;258(13):1782–1788.

45. Babikian V, Ropper AH. Binswanger's disease: a review. *Stroke.* 1987;18(1):2–12.

46. Erkinjuntti T, Ketonen L, Sulkava R, Sipponen J, Vuorialho M, Iivanainen M. Do white matter changes on MRI and CT differentiate vascular dementia from Alzheimer's disease? *J Neurol Neurosurg Psychiatry.* 1987;50(1):37–42.

47. Ishii N, Nishihara Y, Imamura T. Why do frontal lobe symptoms predominate in vascular dementia with lacunes? *Neurology.* 1986;36(3):340–345.

48. Wallin A, Blennow K. The clinical diagnosis of vascular dementia. *Dementia.* 1994;5(3-4):181–184.

49. Brun A. Pathology and pathophysiology of cerebrovascular dementia: pure subgroups of obstructive and hypoperfusive etiology. *Dementia.* 1994;5(3–4):145–147.

50. Loeb C, Meyer JS. Vascular dementia: still a debatable entity? *J Neurol Sci.* 1996;143(1-2):31–40.

51. Konno S, Meyer JS, Terayama Y, Margishvili GM, Mortel KF. Classification, diagnosis and treatment of vascular dementia. *Drugs Aging.* 1997;11(5):361–373.

52. Sulkava R, Erkinjuntti T. Vascular dementia due to cardiac arrhythmias and systemic hypotension. *Acta Neurol Scand.* 1987;76(2):123–128.

53. American Psychiatric Association. *Diagnostic and Statistical Manual of Mental Disorders (DSM-IV).* Washington, DC: American Psychiatric Association; 1994.

54. World Health Organization. *The ICD-10 Classification of Mental and Behavioural Disorders. Diagnostic criteria for research.* Geneva: World Health Organization; 1993.

55. Erkinjuntti T. Types of multi-infarct dementia. *Acta Neurol Scand.* 1987;75(6):391–399.

56. Erkinjuntti T, Haltia M, Palo J, Sulkava R, Paetau A. Accuracy of the clinical diagnosis of vascular dementia: a prospective clinical and post-mortem neuropathological study. *J Neurol Neurosurg Psychiatry.* 1988;51(8):1037–1044.

57. De Reuck J, Crevits L, De Coster W, Sieben G, vander Eecken H. Pathogenesis of Binswanger chronic progressive subcortical encephalopathy. *Neurology.* 1980;30(9):920–928.

58. Brun A, Englund E. Neuropathological brain mapping. *Dement Geriatr Cogn Disord.* 1997;8(2):123–127.

59. Benson DF, Cummings JL. Angular gyrus syndrome simulating Alzheimer's disease. *Arch Neurol.* 1982;39(10):616–620.

60. Ott BR, Saver JL. Unilateral amnesic stroke. Six new cases and a review of the literature. *Stroke.* 1993;24(7):1033–1042.

61. Caplan LR, Hedley-Whyte T. Cuing and memory dysfunction in alexia without agraphia. A case report. *Brain.* 1974;97(2):251–262.

62. Alexander MP, Freedman M. Amnesia after anterior communicating artery aneurysm rupture. *Neurology.* 1984;34(6):752–757.

63. Damasio AR, Graff-Radford NR, Eslinger PJ, Damasio H, Kassell N. Amnesia following basal forebrain lesions. *Arch Neurol.* 1985;42(3):263–271.

64. Baron JC, Bousser MG, Rey A, Guillard A, Comar D, Castaigne P. Reversal of focal "misery-perfusion syndrome" by extra-intracranial arterial bypass in hemodynamic cerebral ischemia. A case study with 15O positron emission tomography. *Stroke.* 1981;12(4):454–459.

65. Graff-Radford NR, Tranel D, Van Hoesen GW, Brandt JP. Diencephalic amnesia. *Brain.* 1990;113(Pt 1):1–25.

66. Tatemichi TK, Desmond DW, Prohovnik I. Strategic infarcts in vascular dementia. A clinical and brain imaging experience. *Arzneimittelforschung.* 1995;45(3A):371–385.

67. Bhatia KP, Marsden CD. The behavioural and motor consequences of focal lesions of the basal ganglia in man. *Brain.* 1994;117(Pt 4):859–876.

68. Caplan LR, Schmahmann JD, Kase CS, Feldmann E, Baquis G, Greenberg JP, et al. Caudate infarcts. *Arch Neurol.* 1990;47(2):133–143.

69. Mendez MF, Adams NL, Lewandowski KS. Neurobehavioral changes associated with caudate lesions. *Neurology.* 1989;39(3):349–354.

70. Godefroy O, Rousseaux M, Leys D, Destee A, Scheltens P, Pruvo JP. Frontal lobe dysfunction in unilateral lenticulostriate infarcts. Prominent role of cortical lesions. *Arch Neurol.* 1992;49(12):1285–1289.

71. Godefroy O, Rousseaux M, Pruvo JP, Cabaret M, Leys D. Neuropsychological changes related to unilateral lenticulostriate infarcts. *J Neurol Neurosurg Psychiatry.* 1994;57(4):480–485.

72. Snowdon DA, Greiner LH, Mortimer JA, Riley KP, Greiner PA, Markesbery WR. Brain infarction and the clinical expression of Alzheimer disease. The Nun Study. *JAMA.* 1997;277(10):813–817.

73. Fisher CM. Lacunes: Small, Deep Cerebral Infarcts. *Neurology.* 1965;15:774–784.

74. Pantoni L, Garcia JH, Brown GG. Vascular pathology in three cases of progressive cognitive deterioration. *J Neurol Sci.* 1996;135(2):131–139.

75. Englund E, Brun A, Alling C. White matter changes in dementia of Alzheimer's type. Biochemical and neuropathological correlates. *Brain.* 1988;111(Pt 6):1425–1439.

76. De Reuck J, Vander Eecken H. The arterial angioarchitecture in lacunar state. *Acta Neurol Belg.* 1976;76(3):142–149.

77. Hijdra A, Verbeeten B, Jr, Verhulst JA. Relation of leukoaraiosis to lesion type in stroke patients. *Stroke.* 1990;21(6):890–894.

78. Leys D, Pruvo J, Scheltens P, Rondepierre P, Godefroy O, Leclerc X, et al. Leuko-araiosis: relationship with the types of focal lesions occuring in acute cerebrovascular disorders. *Cerebrovasc Dis.* 1992;2:169–176.

79. Henon H, Vroylandt P, Durieu I, Pasquier F, Leys D. Leukoaraiosis more than dementia is a predictor of stroke recurrence. *Stroke.* 2003;34(12):2935–2940.

80. Baezner H, Blahak C, Poggesi A, Pantoni L, Inzitari D, Chabriat H, et al. Association of gait and balance disorders with age-related white matter changes: the LADIS study. *Neurology.* 2008;70(12):935–942.

81. Firbank MJ, O'Brien JT, Pakrasi S, Pantoni L, Simoni M, Erkinjuntti T, et al. White matter hyperintensities and depression—preliminary results from the LADIS study. *Int J Geriatr Psychiatry.* 2005;20(7):674–679.

82. O'Brien JT, Firbank MJ, Krishnan MS, van Straaten EC, van der Flier WM, Petrovic K, et al. White matter hyperintensities rather than lacunar infarcts are associated with depressive symptoms in older people: the LADIS study. *Am J Geriatr Psychiatry.* 2006;14(10):834–841.

83. Poggesi A, Pracucci G, Chabriat H, Erkinjuntti T, Fazekas F, Verdelho A, et al. Urinary complaints in nondisabled elderly people with age-related white matter changes: the Leukoaraiosis And DISability (LADIS) Study. *J Am Geriatr Soc.* 2008;56(9):1638–1643.

84. van Straaten EC, Fazekas F, Rostrup E, Scheltens P, Schmidt R, Pantoni L, et al. Impact of white matter hyperintensities scoring method on correlations with clinical data: the LADIS study. *Stroke.* 2006;37(3):836–840.

85. Skoog I. The relationship between blood pressure and dementia: a review. *Biomed Pharmacother.* 1997;51(9):367–375.

86. Pantoni L, Garcia JH. The significance of cerebral white matter abnormalities 100 years after Binswanger's report. A review. *Stroke.* 1995;26(7):1293–1301.

87. Joutel A, Corpechot C, Ducros A, Vahedi K, Chabriat H, Mouton P, et al. Notch3 mutations in CADASIL, a hereditary adult-onset condition causing stroke and dementia. *Nature.* 1996;383(6602):707–710.

88. Chabriat H, Vahedi K, Iba-Zizen MT, Joutel A, Nibbio A, Nagy TG, et al. Clinical spectrum of CADASIL: a study of 7 families. Cerebral autosomal dominant arteriopathy with subcortical infarcts and leukoencephalopathy. *Lancet.* 1995;346(8980):934–939.

89. Chabriat H, Bousser MG, Pappata S. Cerebral autosomal dominant arteriopathy with subcortical infarcts and leukoencephalopathy: a positron emission tomography study in two affected family members. *Stroke.* 1995;26(9):1729–1730.

90. Yoshitake T, Kiyohara Y, Kato I, Ohmura T, Iwamoto H, Nakayama K, et al. Incidence and risk factors of vascular dementia and Alzheimer's disease in a defined elderly Japanese population: the Hisayama Study. *Neurology.* 1995;45(6):1161–1168.

91. Moroney JT, Bagiella E, Desmond DW, Paik MC, Stern Y, Tatemichi TK. Risk factors for incident dementia after stroke. Role of hypoxic and ischemic disorders. *Stroke.* 1996;27(8):1283–1289.

92. Frackowiak RS, Pozzilli C, Legg NJ, Du Boulay GH, Marshall J, Lenzi GL, et al. Regional cerebral oxygen supply and utilization in dementia. A clinical and physiological study with oxygen-15 and positron tomography. *Brain.* 1981;104(Pt 4):753–778.

93. Brown WD, Frackowiak RS. Cerebral blood flow and metabolism studies in multi-infarct dementia. *Alzheimer Dis Assoc Disord.* 1991;5(2):131–143.

94. Englund E. Neuropathology of white matter lesions in vascular cognitive impairment. *Cerebrovasc Dis.* 2002;13Suppl 2:11–15.

95. Brun A, Englund E. A white matter disorder in dementia of the Alzheimer type: a pathoanatomical study. *Ann Neurol.* 1986;19(3):253–262.

96. Tarvonen-Schroder S, Raiha I, Kurki T, Rajala T, Sourander L. Clinical characteristics of rapidly progressive leuko-araiosis. *Acta Neurol Scand.* 1995;91(5):399–404.

97. Tarvonen-Schroder S, Roytta M, Raiha I, Kurki T, Rajala T, Sourander L. Clinical features of leuko-araiosis. *J Neurol Neurosurg Psychiatry.* 1996;60(4):431–436.

98. Cordonnier C, Al-Shahi Salman R, Wardlaw J. Spontaneous brain microbleeds: systematic review, subgroup analyses and standards for study design and reporting. *Brain.* 2007;130(Pt 8):1988–2003.

99. Fazekas F, Kleinert R, Roob G, Kleinert G, Kapeller P, Schmidt R, *et al.* Histopathologic analysis of foci of signal loss on gradient-echo T2*-weighted MR images in patients with spontaneous intracerebral hemorrhage: evidence of microangiopathy-related microbleeds. *AJNR Am J Neuroradiol.* 1999;20(4):637–642.

100. Cordonnier C, van der Flier WM, Sluimer JD, Leys D, Barkhof F, Scheltens P. Prevalence and severity of microbleeds in a memory clinic setting. *Neurology.* 2006;66(9):1356–1360.

101. Henneman WJ, Sluimer JD, Cordonnier C, Baak MM, Scheltens P, Barkhof F, *et al.* MRI biomarkers of vascular damage and atrophy predicting mortality in a memory clinic population. *Stroke.* 2009;40(2):492–498.

102. Tang WK, Chen YK, Lu JY, Chu WC, Mok VC, Ungvari GS, *et al.* Cerebral microbleeds and symptom severity of post-stroke depression: a magnetic resonance imaging study. *J Affect Disord.* 2011;129(1-3):354-8

103. Jobst KA, Smith AD, Barker CS, Wear A, King EM, Smith A, *et al.* Association of atrophy of the medial temporal lobe with reduced blood flow in the posterior parietotemporal cortex in patients with a clinical and pathological diagnosis of Alzheimer's disease. *J Neurol Neurosurg Psychiatry.* 1992;55(3):190–194.

104. Henon H, Pasquier F, Durieu I, Pruvo JP, Leys D. Medial temporal lobe atrophy in stroke patients: relation to pre-existing dementia. *J Neurol Neurosurg Psychiatry.* 1998;65(5):641–647.

105. Cordoliani-Mackowiak MA, Henon H, Pruvo JP, Pasquier F, Leys D. Post-stroke dementia: influence of hippocampal atrophy. *Arch Neurol.* 2003;60(4):585–590.

106. Jellinger KA, Attems J. Prevalence and pathogenic role of cerebrovascular lesions in Alzheimer disease. *J Neurol Sci.* 2005;229–230:37–41.

107. Iadecola C. The overlap between neurodegenerative and vascular factors in the pathogenesis of dementia. *Acta Neuropathol.* 2010;120(3):287–296.

108. Ellis RJ, Olichney JM, Thal LJ, Mirra SS, Morris JC, Beekly D, *et al.* Cerebral amyloid angiopathy in the brains of patients with Alzheimer's disease: the CERAD experience, Part XV. *Neurology.* 1996;46(6):1592–1596.

109. Jellinger KA. The pathology of ischemic-vascular dementia: an update. *J Neurol Sci.* 2002;203–204:153–157.

110. Querfurth HW, LaFerla FM. Alzheimer's disease. *N Engl J Med.* 2010;362(4):329–344.

111. Saposnik G, Cote R, Rochon PA, Mamdani M, Liu Y, Raptis S, *et al.* Care and outcomes in patients with ischemic stroke with and without preexisting dementia. *Neurology.* 2011;77(18):1664–1673.

112. Alshekhlee A, Li C, Chuang S, Vora N, Edgell R, Kitchener J, *et al.* Does dementia increase risk of thrombolysis? A case-control study. *Neurology.* 2011;76:1575–1580.

113. Saposnik G, Kapral MK, Cote R, Rochon PA, Wang J, Raptis S, *et al.* Is pre-existing dementia an independent predictor of outcome after stroke? A propensity score-matched analysis. *J Neurol.* 2012;259(11):2366–2375.

114. Meyer JS, Chowdhury MH, Xu G, Li YS, Quach M. Donepezil treatment of vascular dementia. *Ann N Y Acad Sci.* 2002;977:482–486.

115. Auchus AP, Brashear HR, Salloway S, Korczyn AD, De Deyn PP, Gassmann-Mayer C. Galantamine treatment of vascular dementia: a randomized trial. *Neurology.* 2007;69(5):448–458.

116. Moretti R, Torre P, Antonello RM, Cazzato G. Rivastigmine in subcortical vascular dementia: a comparison trial on efficacy and tolerability for 12 months follow-up. *Eur J Neurol.* 2001;8(4):361–362.

117. Dichgans M, Markus HS, Salloway S, Verkkoniemi A, Moline M, Wang Q, *et al.* Donepezil in patients with subcortical vascular cognitive impairment: a randomised double-blind trial in CADASIL. *Lancet Neurol.* 2008;7(4):310–318.

118. Orgogozo JM, Rigaud AS, Stoffler A, Mobius HJ, Forette F. Efficacy and safety of memantine in patients with mild to moderate vascular dementia: a randomized, placebo-controlled trial (MMM 300). *Stroke.* 2002;33(7):1834–1839.

119. Kavirajan H, Schneider LS. Efficacy and adverse effects of cholinesterase inhibitors and memantine in vascular dementia: a meta-analysis of randomised controlled trials. *Lancet Neurol.* 2007;6(9):782–792.

120. Lopez OL, Larumbe MR, Becker JT, Rezek D, Rosen J, Klunk W, *et al.* Reliability of NINDS-AIREN clinical criteria for the diagnosis of vascular dementia. *Neurology.* 1994;44(7):1240–1245.

CHAPTER 20

Brain repair after stroke

Steven C. Cramer

Brain repair—a definition

Brain repair refers to restoration of brain structure or function after an insult such as stroke. This repair can be spontaneous or therapeutically induced. Repair contrasts with therapeutic strategies that aim to prevent cerebrovascular disease, and with approaches that aim to limit extent of injury from a new stroke, such as neuroprotection or reperfusion. Instead, repair is focused on regrowth, repair, restoration, rewiring, and rehabilitation.

Current therapies for a new stroke reduce disability in only a subset of patients. The only drug approved to treat acute stroke is tissue plasminogen activator (tPA) (1, 2). A limited fraction of patients receive this medicine (3), in large part due to the narrow time window for safe drug administration. Despite recent data supporting administration of intravenous tPA up to 4.5 hours after ischaemic stroke onset, it continues to be true that only a minority of acute stroke patients receive this drug, with recent estimates being that approximately 5% of stroke patients receive this medication (4). Moreover, of those so treated, half or more have significant long-term disability (1, 2). Because most repair-based approaches have a time window measured in days rather than hours, any repair-based approach that achieves regulatory approval will likely have the potential to help a large proportion of patients affected by stroke.

Spontaneous recovery from stroke

Animal models and preclinical studies have characterized the neurobiology of spontaneous stroke recovery. After an experimental infarct, brain regions become excitable, in some cases showing gamma-aminobutyric acid (GABA) receptor downregulation and increased N-methyl-D-aspartate (NMDA) receptor binding. Expression changes for a number of genes, for example, resulting in increased levels of several growth factors. Angiogenesis is accompanied by structural changes in axons, dendrites, and synapses, and thus in both white matter and grey matter. These changes are often preferentially seen in the area surrounding an infarct, and in areas with network connections to injured zones. In many cases, parallels exist with normal development and with learning. Preclinical studies provide mechanistic insights, and also suggest therapeutic targets for improving recovery (5–10).

Direct cellular and molecular measures are difficult to obtain in human subjects. Non-invasive neuroimaging studies have provided insights in human subjects, and in general have been concordant with findings in animals. A number of methods have been found useful to study human brain function, structure, physiology, and metabolism in this context, including transcranial magnetic stimulation, electroencephalography, magnetoencephalography, functional magnetic resonance imaging, positron emission tomography, and near infrared spectroscopy (11, 12). Overall, results indicate that a focal injury such as stroke not only reduces local tissue function, but also has distant effects on activity in a number of brain areas connected within a distributed network, with recent studies emphasizing the importance of network interactions after stroke (13–15). Thus after a single unilateral suptratentorial stroke, multiple changes can be seen within multiple brain areas of the affected hemisphere. Such changes have been described with subcortical strokes and with cortical strokes. Diaschisis refers to a depression in activity seen in areas that are not injured but which share a connection with injured zones (16). Over time, resolution of diaschisis can be followed by overactivation of network nodes, a pattern reminiscent of the brain during increased effort in healthy subjects. Changes in cortical map representations are also seen in relation to behavioural recovery, with numerous patterns having been described (5, 8, 17–20).

Changes in the function of brain networks can also be seen within the contralesional hemisphere. In general, the contribution of the contralesional hemisphere to spontaneous behavioural recovery after stroke seems largest in subjects with the greatest injury and deficits (21–23), a fact that might also have significant bearing in the therapeutic arena (24). Attention has therefore been paid to laterality of activity as a measure of altered brain function (25, 26). Changes in laterality are related to stroke-induced changes in interhemispheric interactions (27), a finding that suggests that improved function of ipsilesional brain regions might in part be facilitated by normalizing interhemispheric interactions (28).

Therapies to promote brain repair

Many categories of restorative therapy are under study in relation to promoting brain repair (10, 29–31). Many have reached the point of human study, though in general most are in early phase trials. The current emphasis is on the study of single agents, a key step to understanding therapeutic efficacy. Over time, it is likely that combinations of therapy will be examined as well. Some restorative therapies are started in the early days after stroke onset, aiming to amplify innate repair mechanisms. Other restorative therapies are initiated months after stroke onset, at a time when most spontaneous behavioural recovery has occurred, and so have as the goal induction of new neural plasticity.

The restorative therapeutic effect has been evaluated for a number of growth factors in preclinical stroke studies. Many have shown a significant effect on behavioural outcome when initiated 24 hours post stroke or longer. Growth factors are appealing as a restorative agent because of their established role in normal development, and in some cases because years of experience (outside of stroke indications) have provided insights into their effects in humans. Most human stroke studies to date have examined the haematopoietic growth factors, such as granulocyte colony-stimulating factor (32) or erythropoietin (33, 34). Growth factors are generally large proteins, for which central nervous system (CNS) ingress is limited. A number of strategies have been proposed to overcome this, such as helping growth factors to cross the blood–brain barrier via conjugation to a molecular Trojan horse (35). Another strategy has been to transfect an exogenous stem cell with a gene encoding for a growth factor, as has been studied for fibroblast growth factor-2 (36), glial cell line-derived neurotrophic factor (37), brain-derived neurotrophic factor (38), vascular endothelial growth factor (39), placenta growth factor (40), or hepatocyte growth factor (41).

The post-stroke restorative effect of other large molecules is also under study. One approach in this context focuses on neutralizing factors that inhibit growth in the adult CNS, with the overall model being that neural repair after stroke after CNS injury is limited by the lack of a permissive growth environment. Three major inhibitors that contribute to this environment have been described: myelin-associated glycoprotein, oligo-myelin glycoprotein, and Nogo-A. Blockade of these inhibitors, such as with a monoclonal antibody, promotes axonal growth (42, 43) and is being examined in human studies as a means to improve outcomes.

Numerous small molecules have also been examined to improve outcome after stroke. In many cases, these represent drugs that have already been approved for other indications and are now being examined for effects on stroke recovery. Some of these drugs, such as amphetamine, levodopa, ropinirole, and escitalopram, target specific neurotransmitter systems, while this is less true for other drugs such as inosine, sildenafil, and niacin. There have been some noteworthy positive studies in this category, such as the FLAME study of 118 patients, which found that fluoxetine started within 10 days of stroke had a favourable effect on long-term motor outcome as compared to placebo (44). Other examples include the study by Jorge et al., which found that escitalopram started within 3 months of stroke onset improved cognitive outcomes at 1 year in 129 patients (45); and the study by Scheidtmann et al., which found that levodopa started within 6 months of stroke onset improved motor function in 53 patients (46).

Cell-based therapies are receiving increased attention, with numerous cell types under consideration (47, 48). One therapeutic strategy is to administer pharmacological compounds that target endogenous neural stem cells. The most common cell-based therapy is to directly administer exogenous stem cells, examples of which include transformed tumour cells, adult stem cells such as marrow stromal cells, stem cells with modified genes or a bioscaffold, umbilical cord cells, placental cells, fetal stem cells, and embryonic stem cells. Such exogenous cells can be autologous, allogeneic, or xenografts. Promising results in human subjects with stroke have been reported with the administration of intravenous marrow stromal cells (49, 50). Cellular therapies hold great promise but can introduce complexities not always encountered with other restorative therapies, such stability of therapy during manufacturing and delivery, the long-term fate of the administered cells, ethical concerns raised in procurement of some cells, and the potential effects introduced by concomitant immunosuppressive drugs if required.

A number of intensive activity-based therapy regimens have been studied. A key example is constraint-induced therapy, an approach that trains the affected limb while restraining the non-affected limb, in order to overcome learned disuse of the affected limb. In the EXCITE trial, constraint-induced therapy was associated with significant gains in motor outcome in 222 patients enrolled 3–9 months after stroke onset (51), with these effects enduring for years (52). The constraint induced approach is also being studied in non-motor domains, such as aphasia (53). The timing of such intensive therapies may be as important as the content. The VECTORS trial examined arm motor constraint induced therapy early after stroke and found that in 52 patients enrolled within 1 month of stroke onset, higher intensity of therapy was associated with poorer behavioural outcome at day 90 (54)—too much too soon can be harmful. The LEAPS trial compared two therapies focused on gait in 408 patients within 2 months of stroke, and found that treadmill training with body-weight support did not differ from progressive exercise at home managed by a physical therapist in effects on walking ability 1 year after stroke (55). While effects of these therapeutic approaches did not differ, the LEAPS trial did find that a majority of patients with stroke can experience significant behavioural gains when therapy is initiated weeks after stroke onset, with 52% of treated patients showing improved gait velocity 1 year after stroke onset. An intervention started on the first day post stroke that improved gait velocity in a majority of patients 12 months post stroke would garner great praise; this should be no less true when the therapy is initiated weeks after stroke onset.

Important questions remain for activity-based regimens focused on intensive therapy, such as the optimal timing and amount of training, how to design the content of training in order to maximize generalizability of therapy effects across real-life challenges, adjusting content of training in relation to time after stroke, and the potential to maximize treatment effects by combining with pharmacological therapies.

The effect of therapy delivered by robotic devices has also been examined. Numerous robotic devices are under study (56–59). Robotic devices offer potential advantages, such as consistent and long-lasting output, programmability, utility for virtual reality applications, high precision, great potential for telerehabilitation and so reaching underserved regions, and the potential for an improved therapist:patient ratio (60). However, challenges remain. Lo et al., in 127 patients who were in the chronic phase of stroke, found that robot-assisted therapy did not significantly improve motor function after 12 weeks, as compared with usual care or intensive therapy, though in secondary analyses, robot-assisted therapy improved outcomes over 36 weeks as compared with usual care but not with intensive therapy (61). Factors that might represent avenues for improving the impact of robotic therapy include more fully defining the relationship between robotic therapy and traditional physiotherapy and matching the right patients with the right robotic devices and protocols.

The brain is an electrical organ, suggesting the potential for brain stimulation to promote brain repair and thereby improve outcomes after stroke. Many forms of brain stimulation have been examined, including repetitive transcranial magnetic stimulation, theta burst stimulation, epidural cortical stimulation, transcranial direct current stimulation, and stimulation via a laser-based device. There is precedence for a focus on brain stimulation, as the gold standard therapy for major depression remains a form of brain stimulation, electroconvulsive therapy. Some results have been favourable (62, 63) while others have not (64, 65). Some brain stimulation therapies can have bidirectional effects and so, for example, can be set to reduce activity, such as in brain areas that might be interfering with recovery or set to increase activity, such as in dormant brain areas where increased activity is desired. The maximum impact of stimulation-based approaches to brain repair might be seen when protocols take fullest advantage of the potential of this approach to differentially stimulate different brain areas, with high temporal resolution.

Humans are cognitive creatures and so the potential exists to enhance outcomes with approaches focused on cognitive skills. Athletes who envision successful performances in their minds can improve their scores. Building on the neurobiology of mirror neuron systems, therapies have been devised that incorporate motor imagery and motor observation (66). Other cognitive strategies include those that incorporate music (67), and those focused on overcoming neglect and hemi-inattention (68).

Principles of brain repair after stroke

Brain repair after stroke is not a one-size-fits-all undertaking. Instead, the effectiveness of restorative therapies can be maximized with attention to certain principles (69). The evidence for several of these is considered here.

First, brain repair is time-sensitive. Treating stroke recovery is a four-dimensional issue. The cellular and biochemical underpinnings of recovery, many of which are potential therapeutic targets, evolve over time (8, 70, 71). Some biological targets are only relevant to repair during a specific time period after stroke. Furthermore, some therapies can have different effects on stroke depending on timing. For example, long-term effects of a GABA agonist or NMDA receptor blocker can be favourable if administered in the early hours after stroke (72, 73) but deleterious if initiated days later (74–76), and the reverse may be true for matrix metalloproteinases (77).

These time windows might vary across therapies and across species. Ren et al. found that the neurotrophic factor Osteogenic protein-1 enhanced sensorimotor recovery in rats when initiated at 1 day after stroke or at 3 days after stroke, but not later (78). Biernaskie et al. compared 5 weeks of enriched rehabilitation to a control intervention in rats with experimental stroke and found improved behavioural outcomes when enriched rehabilitation was started 5 days after stroke, smaller gains when therapy was started 14 days after stroke, and no such gains when therapy was started 30 days after stroke (79). The LEAPS study of human subjects found that an activity-based intervention initiated 6 months after stroke provided the same long-term behavioural gains as when therapy was initiated 2 months after stroke (55), though effects of therapy initiated at earlier timepoints after stroke were not studied.

Second, brain repair is experience-dependent. Since the classic study by Feeney et al. (80), which showed that a stimulant promoted improved motor outcome after experimental stroke in rodents only when the drug was paired with training, increasing evidence suggests that a restorative therapy needs reinforcement and shaping through experience to produce best behavioural results. A number of subsequent studies support this conclusion (81–85). As pharmacological and cellular therapies gain traction, increased attention will be needed to patient experiences that occur concomitant with the therapy of interest, as these experiences can influence therapeutic efficacy. Issues of interest might include the timing, content, and intensity of such experiences.

Third, patient stratification is likely important to studies of post-stroke brain repair. Numerous variables have been found to be potential predictors of stroke outcome, including location and size of injury (86, 87), genotype (88, 89), measures of brain function (90), and affective disorders (91, 92). Such measures may be of pivotal value in defining the population most likely to benefit from a given therapy (see Figure 20.1), as stroke is a very heterogeneous condition. This point is further considered later in the discussion of biomarkers.

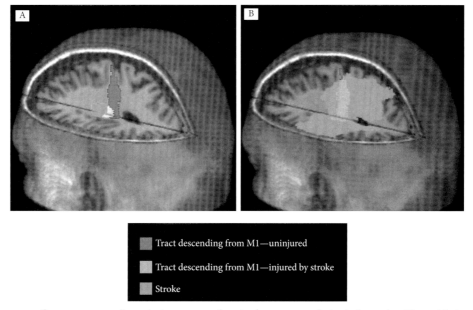

Tract descending from M1—uninjured
Tract descending from M1—injured by stroke
Stroke

Fig. 20.1 Extent of injury to a specific motor tract predicts gains in arm motor function from a course of robotic therapy in subjects with chronic stroke (87). Two examples of stroke injury to the corticospinal tract descending from primary motor cortex are provided. The subject in (A) had only 37.5% of this tract injured by stroke and had a gain of 11 points on the Fugl–Meyer scale, while the subject in (B) had 93.4% of this tract injured by stroke and had a gain of only 1 point. In this study, tract-specific injury was stronger than infarct volume or baseline clinical status at predicting gains. Such findings might be incorporated into clinical trials, for example, as an entry criterion, for identifying subjects with sufficient biological substrate to improve from therapy. Also see figure in colour plate section.

Fourth, modality-specific measures might be useful to measure treatment effects when the target is brain repair (93). The reasons for this approach revolve around the fact that restorative therapies achieve their effect by improving the function of specific neural systems. Improvement is seen in neural systems where surviving substrate is amenable to repair: a behaviour for which the underlying brain regions are destroyed by stroke is less likely to improve than a behaviour for which the underlying brain regions are accessible to a restorative therapy. For example, a patient whose stroke partially spares the motor system but utterly destroys the language system may show gains in strength but not aphasia in response to a restorative therapy. Furthermore, this patient may or may not show gains in global stroke outcome measures such as the modified Rankin Scale score. Such motor gains might be considered worthwhile by many patients and so important to measure in clinical trials. Modality-specific endpoints are aligned with this strategy, akin to their utility for understanding spontaneous stroke recovery, where the rate and degree of gains often vary widely across behavioural modalities (94–96). Improvement in global clinical status is of course a goal of paramount importance, but a treatment that provides gains by promoting neuroplasticity might demonstrate maximum effect in brain networks that have subtotal injury, underscoring the complementary value of endpoints that measure these modality-specific treatment effects. A number of modality-specific endpoints have been successfully incorporated into clinical trials and indeed have been the basis for regulatory approval (97).

Fifth, the nature of brain organization *prior* to stroke influences *post-stroke* brain plasticity. For example, in healthy subjects, some behaviours such as language or hand movement tend to be highly lateralized (i.e. generation of the behaviour involves mainly one hemisphere), and other behaviours such as bulbar and facial movement tend to be less lateralized (i.e. generation of the behaviour involves both hemispheres). These differences remain apparent after stroke. Cramer and Crafton (98) found that face movement is more bilaterally organized than is shoulder or arm movement in healthy subjects (i.e. before any stroke), and that this remains true after stroke. Such a difference could have functional implications. Hamdy et al. found that the cortical representation for swallowing is normally bilaterally organized (99). Not surprisingly, therefore, dysphagic patients who recovered after stroke showed an increase in their cortical pharyngeal map size within the contralesional hemisphere, whereas patients who remained dysphagic did not show this change (100). For reorganization of brain maps after stroke, the pattern of brain reorganization can influence behavioural status, and this pattern is at times constrained by features of normal brain organization.

Implications for clinical trials of brain repair after stroke

The rapidly expanding knowledge base about brain repair and its application to humans, as already discussed, inform the design of restorative trials, a topic that has been reviewed in detail (101).

In the design of restorative stroke clinical trials, some points can be gleaned from lessons learned in the setting of acute stroke trials (102–106). Topics include methodological quality of preclinical programmatic development (106, 107), choice of entry criteria (108), and choice of outcome measures (109). The value of modality-specific endpoints for studies of restorative agents has

been discussed earlier in this chapter. Dose–response relationships are important to define, and might change with increasing time after stroke.

Another point learned from acute stroke trials useful to repair-based trials is the need to align anatomical and physiological features of patient enrolees with those present in preclinical models. Concern over this issue was raised in relation to translation of epidural motor cortex stimulation, where rodent and primate studies showing efficacy of this intervention required preserved motor-evoked responses (110–113) but a phase III human trial (64) did not. In a post hoc analysis, Nouri and Cramer found that human patients receiving stimulation and who had a preserved motor evoked response were 2.5 times more likely to achieve the primary efficacy endpoint (67% vs 27%, p <0.05) than human patients receiving stimulation who did not have a preserved motor evoked response, possibly due to differences in sensorimotor cortex grey matter volumes (114).

In contrast with the neuroprotective and reperfusion therapies examined in many acute stroke trials, repair-based therapies are influenced by experience, training, and environment. Acute stroke therapies such as tPA generally exert their effect rapidly, around the time of therapy administration, while for a repair-based trial, many of the biological events that improve final behavioural outcome occur over the days to weeks that follow therapy initiation. As already mentioned, a subject's experiences, concomitant training, and environment can each interact with a repair-based therapy in defining the final therapy effects. Issues such as caregiver status (115, 116), affective state (91, 117, 118), and socioeconomic factors (119) might also significantly influence restorative therapy effects. Both the quantity and the quality of such influences can affect brain repair and behavioural outcome (120–127). Genetic factors might also be an important consideration to studies aiming to therapeutically induce brain plasticity from stroke (88, 89, 128–132). Also, certain medications are can *adversely* influence brain plasticity, repair, and recovery from stroke (80, 133–137), and so are covariates of interest to a restorative stroke trial.

Influences that arise between the time that a repair-based therapy is initiated and the time of final clinical trial outcome assessment thus require substantial consideration in a repair-based trial because they can interact with repair-based therapy and modify its effects. There are multiple ways that study design might address these issues. In some cases, these influences can be precisely controlled, such as via entry criteria or by carefully controlling the details of any study-administered concomitant therapy such as physiotherapy or speech therapy. When external influences cannot be controlled, study design can insure that they are at least measured. Such an approach provided useful insights in one recent repair-based stroke clinical trial, where the amount of outside physiotherapy (i.e. physiotherapy occurring in parallel with trial participation, but prescribed by private physicians, outside of trial jurisdiction), was found to differ significantly between active and placebo treatment arms (138). Such measures can then be treated as planned covariates of interest in statistical analyses.

Repair-based therapies have the potential to examine within-subject treatment effects, as a baseline behavioural measure can be obtained prior to initiating therapy. Even when a restorative therapy is introduced early after stroke, the time window is generally at least 24 hours. Measuring within-subject behavioural change offers potential statistical advantages over cross-sectional outcome assessments, and so is a consideration in the design of restorative stroke trials (139).

Biomarkers have the potential to strengthen clinical trials of brain repair after stroke. A biomarker can be defined as a measure that provides insight into a tissue state or disease state, and in a clinical trial context would provide information beyond that available from bedside exam. Biomarkers have the potential to identify patients most likely to respond to a treatment (Figure 20.1), and so might reduce variance and increase study power (140–142). A biomarker might also provide insight into a treatment's mechanism of action (143–145), which can provide useful insights at the stage of protocol development, or to refine the target patient population, for example, as suggested by hippocampal size in distinguishing responders from non-responders to Donepezil for improving cognitive outcome after stroke (146). There are important caveats in the selection of any biomarker (147), for example, the utility of a biomarker is highest when its relationships with the disease process and with the therapy are well understood (148, 149).

A number of specific measures are potentially available to serve as biomarkers in the context of a restorative stroke trial. Simple measures derived from blood testing have been proposed (150, 151). Imaging-based methods can provide anatomical measures of injury (87, 152), tissue status such as cortical thickness (153), white matter tract integrity (62, 86, 87, 154, 155), regional brain function (90, 156, 157), network interactions (15), or chemical state (158, 159). Physiological assessments might also be useful (160) and indeed complementary (86, 114). Measures of injury to a predefined functional brain region, such as the extent of insult to the hand region of primary motor cortex (161), white matter cholinergic projections (162), or left temporal language areas (163), might provide useful insights into the likelihood that a particular therapy will be able to promote repair in a specific target region.

Concluding comments

Preclinical and human studies are providing increased insight into the neurobiology of spontaneous recovery after stroke. This information is opening the door to a number of potential restorative therapies, many of which are in human clinical trials. When applied according to selected neurobiological principles, these therapies have the potential to improve outcome for many patients after stroke.

References

1. Hacke W, Kaste M, Bluhmki E, Brozman M, Davalos A, Guidetti D, et al. Thrombolysis with alteplase 3 to 4.5 hours after acute ischemic stroke. *N Engl J Med.* 2008 Sep 25;359(13):1317–1329.

2. Tissue plasminogen activator for acute ischemic stroke. The National Institute of Neurological Disorders and Stroke rt-PA Stroke Study Group. *N Engl J Med.* 1995 Dec 14;333(24):1581–1587.

3. Reed S, Cramer S, Blough D, Meyer K, Jarvik J. Treatment with tissue plasminogen activator and inpatient mortality rates for patients with ischemic stroke treated in community hospitals. *Stroke.* 2001;32(8):1832–1840.

4. Adeoye O, Hornung R, Khatri P, Kleindorfer D. Recombinant tissue-type plasminogen activator use for ischemic stroke in the United States: a doubling of treatment rates over the course of 5 years. *Stroke.* 2011 Jul;42(7):1952–1955.

5. Cramer S, Chopp M. Recovery recapitulates ontogeny. *Trends Neurosci.* 2000;23(6):265–271.

6. Wieloch T, Nikolich K. Mechanisms of neural plasticity following brain injury. *Curr Opin Neurobiol.* 2006 Jun;16(3):258–264.

7. Nudo RJ. Neural bases of recovery after brain injury. *J Commun Disord.* 2011 Sep–Oct;44(5):515–520.

8. Li S, Carmichael ST. Growth-associated gene and protein expression in the region of axonal sprouting in the aged brain after stroke. *Neurobiol Dis.* 2006 Aug;23(2):362–373.

9. Arai K, Lo EH. Experimental models for analysis of oligodendrocyte pathophysiology in stroke. *Exp Transl Stroke Med.* 2009;1:6.

10. Zhang ZG, Chopp M. Neurorestorative therapies for stroke: underlying mechanisms and translation to the clinic. *Lancet Neurol.* 2009 May;8(5):491–500.

11. Cramer SC, Riley JD. Neuroplasticity and brain repair after stroke. *Curr Opin Neurol.* 2008 Feb;21(1):76–82.

12. Ward NS. Human brain mapping of the motor system after stroke. In Cramer SC, Nudo RJ (eds) *Brain Repair After Stroke* (pp. 113–123). Cambridge: Cambridge University Press; 2010.

13. Sharma N, Baron JC, Rowe JB. Motor imagery after stroke: relating outcome to motor network connectivity. *Ann Neurol.* 2009 Nov;66(5):604–616.

14. Grefkes C, Nowak DA, Eickhoff SB, Dafotakis M, Kust J, Karbe H, et al. Cortical connectivity after subcortical stroke assessed with functional magnetic resonance imaging. *Ann Neurol.* 2008 Feb;63(2):236–246.

15. Carter AR, Astafiev SV, Lang CE, Connor LT, Rengachary J, Strube MJ, et al. Resting interhemispheric functional magnetic resonance imaging connectivity predicts performance after stroke. *Ann Neurol.* 2010 Mar;67(3):365–375.

16. von Monakow C. *Diaschisis*, 1914. In Pribram K (ed) *Brain and Behavior 1: Mood, States and Mind (pp. 26–34).* Baltimore, MD: Penguin Books; 1969.

17. Nudo R. Recovery after damage to motor cortical areas. *Curr Opin Neurobiol.* 1999;9(6):740–747.

18. Ward NS, Cohen LG. Mechanisms underlying recovery of motor function after stroke. *Arch Neurol.* 2004 Dec;61(12):1844–1848.

19. Yozbatiran N, Cramer SC. Imaging motor recovery after stroke. *NeuroRx.* 2006 Oct;3(4):482–488.

20. Wieloch T, Nikolich K. Mechanisms of neural plasticity following brain injury. *Curr Opin Neurobiol.* 2006 Jun;16(3):258–264.

21. Netz J, Lammers T, Homberg V. Reorganization of motor output in the non-affected hemisphere after stroke. *Brain.* 1997;120:1579–1586.

22. Turton A, Wroe S, Trepte N, Fraser C, Lemon R. Contralateral and ipsilateral EMG responses to transcranial magnetic stimulation during recovery of arm and hand function after stroke. *Electroencephalogr Clin Neurophysiol.* 1996;101:316–328.

23. Heiss WD, Thiel A. A proposed regional hierarchy in recovery of post-stroke aphasia. *Brain Lang.* 2006 Jul;98(1):118–123.

24. Bradnam LV, Stinear CM, Barber PA, Byblow WD. Contralesional hemisphere control of the proximal paretic upper limb following stroke. *Cereb Cortex.* 2012 Nov;22(11):2662–2671.

25. Cramer S, Nelles G, Benson R, Kaplan J, Parker R, Kwong K, et al. A functional MRI study of subjects recovered from hemiparetic stroke. *Stroke.* 1997;28(12):2518–2527.

26. Calautti C, Naccarato M, Jones PS, Sharma N, Day DD, Carpenter AT, et al. The relationship between motor deficit and hemisphere activation balance after stroke: A 3T fMRI study. *NeuroImage.* 2007 Jan 1;34(1):322–331.

27. Murase N, Duque J, Mazzocchio R, Cohen L. Influence of interhemispheric interactions on motor function in chronic stroke. *Ann Neurol.* 2004 Mar;55(3):400–409.

28. Floel A, Cohen LG. Recovery of function in humans: cortical stimulation and pharmacological treatments after stroke. *Neurobiol Dis.* 2010 Feb;37(2):243–251.

29. Cramer SC. Repairing the human brain after stroke. II. Restorative therapies. *Ann Neurol.* 2008 May 14;63(5):549–560.

30. Cheeran B, Cohen L, Dobkin B, Ford G, Greenwood R, Howard D, et al. The future of restorative neurosciences in stroke: driving the

translational research pipeline from basic science to rehabilitation of people after stroke. *Neurorehabil Neural Repair.* 2009 Feb;23(2):97–107.

31. Knecht S, Hesse S, Oster P. Rehabilitation after stroke. *Dtsch Arztebl Int.* 2011 Sep;108(36):600–606.

32. Schabitz WR, Laage R, Vogt G, Koch W, Kollmar R, Schwab S, et al. AXIS: a trial of intravenous granulocyte colony-stimulating factor in acute ischemic stroke. *Stroke.* 2010 Nov;41(11):2545–2551.

33. Wang L, Zhang Z, Wang Y, Zhang R, Chopp M. Treatment of stroke with erythropoietin enhances neurogenesis and angiogenesis and improves neurological function in rats. *Stroke.* 2004 Jul;35(7):1732–1737.

34. Cramer SC, Fitzpatrick C, Warren M, Hill MD, Brown D, Whitaker L, *et al.* The beta-hCG+erythropoietin in acute stroke (BETAS) study: a 3-center, single-dose, open-label, noncontrolled, phase IIa safety trial. *Stroke.* 2010 May;41(5):927–931.

35. Zhang Y, Pardridge WM. Blood-brain barrier targeting of BDNF improves motor function in rats with middle cerebral artery occlusion. *Brain Res.* 2006 Sep 21;1111(1):227–229.

36. Kim BO, Tian H, Prasongsukarn K, Wu J, Angoulvant D, Wnendt S, *et al.* Cell transplantation improves ventricular function after a myocardial infarction: a preclinical study of human unrestricted somatic stem cells in a porcine model. *Circulation.* 2005 Aug 30;112(9 Suppl):I96–104.

37. Horita Y, Honmou O, Harada K, Houkin K, Hamada H, Kocsis JD. Intravenous administration of glial cell line-derived neurotrophic factor gene-modified human mesenchymal stem cells protects against injury in a cerebral ischemia model in the adult rat. *J Neurosci Res.* 2006 Nov 15;84(7):1495–1504.

38. Zhao L-X, Zhang J, Cao F, Meng L, Wang D-M, Li Y-H, *et al.* Modification of the brain-derived neurotrophic factor gene: a portal to transform mesenchymal stem cells into advantageous engineering cells for neuroregeneration and neuroprotection. *Exp Neurol.* 2004;190(2):396–406.

39. Iwase T, Nagaya N, Fujii T, Itoh T, Murakami S, Matsumoto T, *et al.* Comparison of angiogenic potency between mesenchymal stem cells and mononuclear cells in a rat model of hindlimb ischemia. *Cardiovasc Res.* 2005 Jun 1;66(3):543–551.

40. Liu H, Honmou O, Harada K, Nakamura K, Houkin K, Hamada H, *et al.* Neuroprotection by PlGF gene-modified human mesenchymal stem cells after cerebral ischaemia. *Brain.* 2006 Oct;129(Pt 10):2734–2745.

41. Zhao MZ, Nonoguchi N, Ikeda N, Watanabe T, Furutama D, Miyazawa D, *et al.* Novel therapeutic strategy for stroke in rats by bone marrow stromal cells and ex vivo HGF gene transfer with HSV-1 vector. *J Cereb Blood Flow Metab.* 2006 Sep;26(9):1176–1188.

42. Domeniconi M, Filbin MT. Overcoming inhibitors in myelin to promote axonal regeneration. *J Neurol Sci.* 2005 Jun 15;233(1-2):43–47.

43. Buchli AD, Schwab ME. Inhibition of Nogo: a key strategy to increase regeneration, plasticity and functional recovery of the lesioned central nervous system. *Ann Med.* 2005;37(8):556–567.

44. Chollet F, Tardy J, Albucher JF, Thalamas C, Berard E, Lamy C, *et al.* Fluoxetine for motor recovery after acute ischaemic stroke (FLAME): a randomised placebo-controlled trial. *Lancet Neurol.* 2011 Feb;10(2):123–130.

45. Jorge RE, Acion L, Moser D, Adams HP, Jr, Robinson RG. Escitalopram and enhancement of cognitive recovery following stroke. *Arch Gen Psychiatry.* 2010 Feb;67(2):187–196.

46. Scheidtmann K, Fries W, Muller F, Koenig E. Effect of levodopa in combination with physiotherapy on functional motor recovery after stroke: a prospective, randomised, double-blind study. *Lancet.* 2001;358:787–790.

47. Lindvall O, Kokaia Z. Stem cell research in stroke: how far from the clinic? *Stroke.* 2011 Aug;42(8):2369–2375.

48. Savitz SI, Chopp M, Deans R, Carmichael ST, Phinney D, Wechsler L. Stem Cell Therapy as an Emerging Paradigm for Stroke (STEPS) II. *Stroke.* 2011 Mar;42(3):825–829.

49. Bang OY, Lee JS, Lee PH, Lee G. Autologous mesenchymal stem cell transplantation in stroke patients. *Ann Neurol.* 2005 Jun;57(6):874–882.

50. Honmou O, Houkin K, Matsunaga T, Niitsu Y, Ishiai S, Onodera R, *et al.* Intravenous administration of auto serum-expanded autologous mesenchymal stem cells in stroke. *Brain.* 2011 June;134(6):1790–1807.

51. Wolf SL, Winstein CJ, Miller JP, Taub E, Uswatte G, Morris D, *et al.* Effect of constraint-induced movement therapy on upper extremity function 3 to 9 months after stroke: the EXCITE randomized clinical trial. *JAMA.* 2006 Nov 1;296(17):2095–2104.

52. Wolf SL, Winstein CJ, Miller JP, Thompson PA, Taub E, Uswatte G, *et al.* Retention of upper limb function in stroke survivors who have received constraint-induced movement therapy: the EXCITE randomised trial. *Lancet Neurol.* 2008 Jan;7(1):33–40.

53. Berthier ML, Pulvermuller F. Neuroscience insights improve neurorehabilitation of poststroke aphasia. *Nat Rev Neurol.* 2011 Feb;7(2):86–97.

54. Dromerick A, Lang C, Powers W, Wagner J, Sahrmann S, Videen T, *et al.* Very Early Constraint-Induced Movement Therapy (VECTORS): Phase II trial results. *Stroke.* 2007;38:465.

55. Duncan PW, Sullivan KJ, Behrman AL, Azen SP, Wu SS, Nadeau SE, *et al.* Body-weight-supported treadmill rehabilitation after stroke. *N Engl J Med.* 2011 May 26;364(21):2026–2036.

56. Brewer BR, McDowell SK, Worthen-Chaudhari LC. Poststroke upper extremity rehabilitation: a review of robotic systems and clinical results. *Topics Stroke Rehabil.* 2007 Nov–Dec;14(6):22–44.

57. Volpe BT, Huerta PT, Zipse JL, Rykman A, Edwards D, Dipietro L, *et al.* Robotic devices as therapeutic and diagnostic tools for stroke recovery. *Arch Neurol.* 2009 Sep;66(9):1086–1090.

58. Reinkensmeyer D, Emken J, Cramer S. Robotics, motor learning, and neurologic recovery. *Annu Rev Biomed Eng.* 2004 Aug;6:497–525.

59. Balasubramanian S, Klein J, Burdet E. Robot-assisted rehabilitation of hand function. *Curr Opin Neurol.* 2010 Dec;23(6):661–670.

60. Cramer SC. Brain repair after stroke. *N Engl J Med.* 2010 May 13;362(19):1827–1829.

61. Lo AC, Guarino PD, Richards LG, Haselkorn JK, Wittenberg GF, Federman DG, *et al.* Robot-assisted therapy for long-term upper-limb impairment after stroke. *N Engl J Med.* 2010 May 13;362(19):1772–1783.

62. Lindenberg R, Zhu LL, Ruber T, Schlaug G. Predicting functional motor potential in chronic stroke patients using diffusion tensor imaging. *Hum Brain Mapp.* 2012 May;33(5):1040–1051.

63. Ackerley SJ, Stinear CM, Barber PA, Byblow WD. Combining theta burst stimulation with training after subcortical stroke. *Stroke.* 2010 Jul;41(7):1568–1572.

64. Levy R, Benson R, Winstein C, for the Everest Study Investigators (eds). *Cortical stimulation for upper-extremity hemiparesis from ischemic stroke: Everest Study Primary Endpoint Results.* International Stroke Conference; 2008; New Orleans, LA.

65. Pomeroy VM, Cloud G, Tallis RC, Donaldson C, Nayak V, Miller S. Transcranial magnetic stimulation and muscle contraction to enhance stroke recovery: a randomized proof-of-principle and feasibility investigation. *Neurorehabil Neural Repair.* 2007 Nov–Dec;21(6):509–517.

66. Small SL, Buccino G, Solodkin A. The mirror neuron system and treatment of stroke. *Dev Psychobiol.* 2012;54(3):293–310.

67. Sarkamo T, Tervaniemi M, Laitinen S, Forsblom A, Soinila S, Mikkonen M, *et al.* Music listening enhances cognitive recovery and mood after middle cerebral artery stroke. *Brain.* 2008 Mar;131(Pt 3):866–876.

68. Ramachandran VS, Altschuler EL. The use of visual feedback, in particular mirror visual feedback, in restoring brain function. *Brain.* 2009 Jul;132(Pt 7):1693–1710.

69. Cramer SC, Sur M, Dobkin BH, O'Brien C, Sanger TD, Trojanowski JQ, *et al.* Harnessing neuroplasticity for clinical applications. *Brain.* 2011 Jun;134(Pt 6):1591–1609.

70. Stroemer R, Kent T, Hulsebosch C. Enhanced neocortical neural sprouting, synaptogenesis, and behavioral recovery with D-amphetamine therapy after neocortical infarction in rats. *Stroke.* 1998;29(11):2381–2395.

71. Jones T, Schallert T. Overgrowth and pruning of dendrites in adult rats recovering from neocortical damage. *Brain Res.* 1992;581:156–160.

72. Green AR, Hainsworth AH, Jackson DM. GABA potentiation: a logical pharmacological approach for the treatment of acute ischaemic stroke. *Neuropharmacology.* 2000 Jul 10;39(9):1483–1494.

73. Ovbiagele B, Kidwell CS, Starkman S, Saver JL. Neuroprotective agents for the treatment of acute ischemic stroke. *Curr Neurol Neurosci Rep.* 2003 Jan;3(1):9–20.

74. Kozlowski D, Jones T, Schallert T. Pruning of dendrites and restoration of function after brain damage: Role of the NMDA receptor. *Restor Neurol Neurosci.* 1994;7:119–126.

75. Wahlgren N, Martinsson L. New concepts for drug therapy after stroke. Can we enhance recovery? *Cerebrovasc Dis.* 1998;8 Suppl 5:33–38.

76. Barth T, Hoane M, Barbay S, Saponjic R. Effects of glutamate antagonists on the recovery and maintenance of behavioral function after brain injury. In Goldstein L (ed) *Restorative Neurology: Advances in Pharmacotherapy for Recovery After Stroke* (pp. 91–120). Armonk, NY: Futura Publishing Co., Inc.; 1998.

77. Zhao BQ, Tejima E, Lo EH. Neurovascular proteases in brain injury, hemorrhage and remodeling after stroke. *Stroke.* 2007 Feb;38(2 Suppl):748–752.

78. Ren J, Kaplan P, Charette M, Speller H, Finklestein S. Time window of intracisternal osteogenic protein-1 in enhancing functional recovery after stroke. *Neuropharmacology.* 2000;39(5):860–865.

79. Biernaskie J, Chernenko G, Corbett D. Efficacy of rehabilitative experience declines with time after focal ischemic brain injury. *J Neurosci.* 2004 Feb 4;24(5):1245–1254.

80. Feeney D, Gonzalez A, Law W. Amphetamine, Halperidol, and experience interact to affect the rate of recovery after motor cortex injury. *Science.* 1982;217:855–857.

81. Garcia-Alias G, Barkhuysen S, Buckle M, Fawcett JW. Chondroitinase ABC treatment opens a window of opportunity for task-specific rehabilitation. *Nat Neurosci.* 2009 Sep;12(9):1145–1151.

82. Fang PC, Barbay S, Plautz EJ, Hoover E, Strittmatter SM, Nudo RJ. Combination of NEP 1-40 treatment and motor training enhances behavioral recovery after a focal cortical infarct in rats. *Stroke.* 2010 Mar;41(3):544–549.

83. Starkey ML, Schwab ME. Anti-Nogo-A and training: Can one plus one equal three? *Exp Neurol.* 2012 May;235(1):53–61.

84. Hovda D, Feeney D. Amphetamine with experience promotes recovery of locomotor function after unilateral frontal cortex injury in the cat. *Brain Res.* 1984;298:358–361.

85. Adkins DL, Hsu JE, Jones TA. Motor cortical stimulation promotes synaptic plasticity and behavioral improvements following sensorimotor cortex lesions. *Exp Neurol.* 2008 Jul;212(1):14–28.

86. Stinear CM, Barber PA, Smale PR, Coxon JP, Fleming MK, Byblow WD. Functional potential in chronic stroke patients depends on corticospinal tract integrity. *Brain.* 2007 Jan;130(Pt 1):170–180.

87. Riley JD, Le V, Der-Yeghiaian L, See J, Newton JM, Ward NS, et al. Anatomy of stroke injury predicts gains from therapy. *Stroke.* 2011 Feb;42(2):421–426.

88. Siironen J, Juvela S, Kanarek K, Vilkki J, Hernesniemi J, Lappalainen J. The Met allele of the BDNF Val66Met polymorphism predicts poor outcome among survivors of aneurysmal subarachnoid hemorrhage. *Stroke.* 2007 Oct;38(10):2858–2860.

89. Cramer SC, Procaccio V. Correlation between genetic polymorphisms and stroke recovery. Analysis of the GAIN Americas and GAIN International Studies. *Eur J Neurol.* 2012 May;19(5):718–724.

90. Cramer SC, Parrish TB, Levy RM, Stebbins GT, Ruland SD, Lowry DW, et al. Predicting functional gains in a stroke trial. *Stroke.* 2007 Jul;38(7):2108–2114.

91. Lai SM, Duncan PW, Keighley J, Johnson D. Depressive symptoms and independence in BADL and IADL. *J Rehabil Res Dev.* 2002 Sep–Oct;39(5):589–596.

92. Gillen R, Tennen H, McKee TE, Gernert-Dott P, Affleck G. Depressive symptoms and history of depression predict rehabilitation efficiency in stroke patients. *Arch Phys Med Rehabil.* 2001 Dec;82(12):1645–1649.

93. Cramer SC, Koroshetz WJ, Finklestein SP. The case for modality-specific outcome measures in clinical trials of stroke recovery-promoting agents. *Stroke.* 2007 Apr;38(4):1393–1395.

94. Hier D, Mondlock J, Caplan L. Recovery of behavioral abnormalities after right hemisphere stroke. *Neurology.* 1983;33:345–350.

95. Marshall R, Perera G, Lazar R, Krakauer J, Constantine R, DeLaPaz R. Evolution of cortical activation during recovery from corticospinal tract infarction. *Stroke.* 2000;31(3):656–661.

96. Markgraf C, Green E, Hurwitz B, Morikawa E, Dietrich W, McCabe P, et al. Sensorimotor and cognitive consequences of middle cerebral artery occlusion in rats. *Brain Res.* 1992;575(2):238–246.

97. Goodman AD, Brown TR, Edwards KR, Krupp LB, Schapiro RT, Cohen R, et al. A phase 3 trial of extended release oral dalfampridine in multiple sclerosis. *Ann Neurol.* 2010 Oct;68(4):494–502.

98. Cramer SC, Crafton KR. Somatotopy and movement representation sites following cortical stroke. *Exp Brain Res.* 2006 Jan;168(1–2):25–32.

99. Hamdy S, Aziz Q, Rothwell JC, Singh KD, Barlow J, Hughes DG, et al. The cortical topography of human swallowing musculature in health and disease. *Nature Med.* 1996 Nov;2(11):1217–1224.

100. Hamdy S, Aziz Q, Rothwell J, Power M, Singh K, Nicholson D, et al. Recovery of swallowing after dysphagic stroke relates to functional reorganization in the intact motor cortex. *Gastroenterology.* 1998;115(5):1104–1112.

101. Cramer SC. Issues in clinical trial methodology for brain repair after stroke. In Cramer SC, Nudo RJ (eds) *Brain Repair After Stroke* (pp. 172–182). Cambridge: Cambridge University Press; 2010.

102. Grotta J, Bratina P. Subjective experiences of 24 patients dramatically recovering from stroke. *Stroke.* 1995 Jul;26(7):1285–1288.

103. Fisher M, Ratan R. New perspectives on developing acute stroke therapy. *Ann Neurol.* 2003 Jan;53(1):10–20.

104. Gladstone D, Black S, Hakim A. Toward wisdom from failure: lessons from neuroprotective stroke trials and new therapeutic directions. *Stroke.* 2002 Aug;33(8):2123–2136.

105. Fisher M, Feuerstein G, Howells DW, Hurn PD, Kent TA, Savitz SI, et al. Update of the Stroke Therapy Academic Industry Roundtable Preclinical Recommendations. *Stroke.* 2009 Jun;40(6):2244–2250.

106. Philip M, Benatar M, Fisher M, Savitz SI. Methodological quality of animal studies of neuroprotective agents currently in phase II/III acute ischemic stroke trials. *Stroke.* 2009 Feb;40(2):577–581.

107. Savitz SI, Fisher M. Future of neuroprotection for acute stroke: in the aftermath of the SAINT trials. *Ann Neurol.* 2007 May;61(5):396–402.

108. Uchino K, Billheimer D, Cramer S. Entry criteria and baseline characteristics predict outcome in acute stroke trials. *Stroke.* 2001;32(4):909–16.

109. Duncan P, Jorgensen H, Wade D. Outcome measures in acute stroke trials: a systematic review and some recommendations to improve practice. *Stroke.* 2000;31(6):1429–1438.

110. Adkins-Muir D, Jones T. Cortical electrical stimulation combined with rehabilitative training: enhanced functional recovery and dendritic plasticity following focal cortical ischemia in rats. *Neurol Res.* 2003 Dec;25(8):780–788.

111. Kleim J, Bruneau R, VandenBerg P, MacDonald E, Mulrooney R, Pocock D. Motor cortex stimulation enhances motor recovery and reduces peri-infarct dysfunction following ischemic insult. *Neurol Res.* 2003 Dec;25(8):789–793.

112. Plautz E, Barbay S, Frost S, Friel K, Dancause N, Zoubina E, et al. Post-infarct cortical plasticity and behavioral recovery using concurrent cortical stimulation and rehabilitative training: a feasibility study in primates. *Neurol Res.* 2003 Dec;25(8):801–810.

113. Teskey G, Flynn C, Goertzen C, Monfils M, Young N. Cortical stimulation improves skilled forelimb use following a focal ischemic infarct in the rat. *Neurol Res.* 2003 Dec;25(8):794–800.

114. Nouri S, Cramer SC. Anatomy and physiology predict response to motor cortex stimulation after stroke. *Neurology*. 2011 Sep;77(11):1076–1083.

115. Smith J, Forster A, Young J. Cochrane review: information provision for stroke patients and their caregivers. *Clin Rehabil*. 2009 Mar;23(3):195–206.

116. Glass TA, Matchar DB, Belyea M, Feussner JR. Impact of social support on outcome in first stroke. *Stroke*. 1993 Jan;24(1):64–70.

117. Jonsson AC, Lindgren I, Hallstrom B, Norrving B, Lindgren A. Determinants of quality of life in stroke survivors and their informal caregivers. *Stroke*. 2005 Apr;36(4):803–808.

118. Mukherjee D, Levin RL, Heller W. The cognitive, emotional, and social sequelae of stroke: psychological and ethical concerns in post-stroke adaptation. *Topics Stroke Rehabil*. 2006 Fall;13(4):26–35.

119. McFadden E, Luben R, Wareham N, Bingham S, Khaw KT. Social class, risk factors, and stroke incidence in men and women: a prospective study in the European prospective investigation into cancer in Norfolk cohort. *Stroke*. 2009 Apr;40(4):1070–1077.

120. Kwakkel G. Impact of intensity of practice after stroke: issues for consideration. *Disabil Rehabil*. 2006 Jul 15–30;28(13–14):823–830.

121. Kwakkel G, Wagenaar R, Twisk J, Lankhorst G, Koetsier J. Intensity of leg and arm training after primary middle-cerebral-artery stroke: a randomised trial. *Lancet*. 1999 Jul 17;354(9174):191–196.

122. Dobkin B. *The Clinical Science of Neurologic Rehabilitation*. New York: Oxford University Press; 2003.

123. Van Peppen RP, Kwakkel G, Wood-Dauphinee S, Hendriks HJ, Van der Wees PJ, Dekker J. The impact of physical therapy on functional outcomes after stroke: what's the evidence? *Clin Rehabil*. 2004 Dec;18(8):833–862.

124. Cicerone KD, Dahlberg C, Malec JF, Langenbahn DM, Felicetti T, Kneipp S, et al. Evidence-based cognitive rehabilitation: updated review of the literature from 1998 through 2002. *Arch Phys Med Rehabil*. 2005 Aug;86(8):1681–1692.

125. Bhogal S, Teasell R, Speechley M. Intensity of aphasia therapy, impact on recovery. *Stroke*. 2003 Apr;34(4):987–993.

126. Jones T, Chu C, Grande L, Gregory A. Motor skills training enhances lesion-induced structural plasticity in the motor cortex of adult rats. *J Neurosci*. 1999;19(22):10153–10163.

127. Johansson B. Brain plasticity and stroke rehabilitation. The Willis lecture. *Stroke*. 2000 Jan;31(1):223–230.

128. Kleim JA, Chan S, Pringle E, Schallert K, Procaccio V, Jimenez R, et al. BDNF val66met polymorphism is associated with modified experience-dependent plasticity in human motor cortex. *Nat Neurosci*. 2006 Jun;9(6):735–737.

129. Alberts MJ, Graffagnino C, McClenny C, DeLong D, Strittmatter W, Saunders AM, et al. ApoE genotype and survival from intracerebral haemorrhage. *Lancet*. 1995 Aug 26;346(8974):575.

130. Niskakangas T, Ohman J, Niemela M, Ilveskoski E, Kunnas TA, Karhunen PJ. Association of apolipoprotein E polymorphism with outcome after aneurysmal subarachnoid hemorrhage: a preliminary study. *Stroke*. 2001 May;32(5):1181–1184.

131. Cramer SC, Procaccio V. Correlation between genetic polymorphisms and stroke recovery. Analysis of the GAIN Americas and GAIN International Studies. *Eur J Neurol*. 2012 May;19(5):718–724.

132. Pearson-Fuhrhop KM, Cramer SC. Genetic influences on neural plasticity. *PMR*. 2010 Dec;2(12 Suppl 2):S227–S240.

133. Butefisch C, Davis B, Wise S, Sawaki L, Kopylev L, Classen J, et al. Mechanisms of use-dependent plasticity in the human motor cortex. *Proc Natl Acad Sci U S A*. 2000 Mar 28;97(7):3661–3665.

134. Goldstein L, Sygen in Acute Stroke Study Investigators. Common drugs may influence motor recovery after stroke. *Neurology*. 1995;45:865–871.

135. Troisi E, Paolucci S, Silvestrini M, Matteis M, Vernieri F, Grasso MG, et al. Prognostic factors in stroke rehabilitation: the possible role of pharmacological treatment. *Acta Neurol Scand*. 2002 Feb;105(2):100–106.

136. Conroy B, Zorowitz R, Horn SD, Ryser DK, Teraoka J, Smout RJ. An exploration of central nervous system medication use and outcomes in stroke rehabilitation. *Arch Phys Med Rehabil*. 2005 Dec;86(12 Suppl 2):S73–S81.

137. Lazar R, Fitzsimmons B, Marshall R, Berman M, Bustillo M, Young W, et al. Reemergence of stroke deficits with midazolam challenge. *Stroke*. 2002 Jan;33(1):283–285.

138. Cramer S, Dobkin B, Noser E, Rodriguez R, Enney L. A randomized, placebo-controlled, double-blind study of ropinirole in chronic stroke. *Stroke*. 2009 Sep;40(9):3034–3038.

139. Calautti C, Baron J. Functional neuroimaging studies of motor recovery after stroke in adults: a review. *Stroke*. 2003 Jun;34(6):1553–1566.

140. Toth G, Albers GW. Use of MRI to estimate the therapeutic window in acute stroke: is perfusion-weighted imaging/diffusion-weighted imaging mismatch an EPITHET for salvageable ischemic brain tissue? *Stroke*. 2009 Jan;40(1):333–335.

141. Donnan GA, Baron JC, Ma H, Davis SM. Penumbral selection of patients for trials of acute stroke therapy. *Lancet Neurol*. 2009 Mar;8(3):261–269.

142. Feuerstein GZ, Zaleska MM, Krams M, Wang X, Day M, Rutkowski JL, et al. Missing steps in the STAIR case: a Translational Medicine perspective on the development of NXY-059 for treatment of acute ischemic stroke. *J Cereb Blood Flow Metab*. 2008 Jan;28(1):217–219.

143. Carey J, Kimberley T, Lewis S, Auerbach E, Dorsey L, Rundquist P, et al. Analysis of fMRI and finger tracking training in subjects with chronic stroke. *Brain*. 2002 Apr;125(Pt 4):773–788.

144. Johansen-Berg H, Dawes H, Guy C, Smith S, Wade D, Matthews P. Correlation between motor improvements and altered fMRI activity after rehabilitative therapy. *Brain*. 2002 Dec;125(Pt 12):2731–2742.

145. Koski L, Mernar T, Dobkin B. Immediate and long-term changes in corticomotor output in response to rehabilitation: correlation with functional improvements in chronic stroke. *Neurorehabil Neural Repair*. 2004 Dec;18(4):230–249.

146. Roman GC, Salloway S, Black SE, Royall DR, Decarli C, Weiner MW, et al. Randomized, placebo-controlled, clinical trial of donepezil in vascular dementia: differential effects by hippocampal size. *Stroke*. 2010 Jun;41(6):1213–1221.

147. Milot MH, Cramer SC. Biomarkers of recovery after stroke. *Current Opin Neurol*. 2008 Dec;21(6):654–659.

148. Fleming T, DeMets D. Surrogate end points in clinical trials: are we being misled? *Ann Intern Med*. 1996;125(7):605–613.

149. Bucher H, Guyatt G, Cook D, Holbrook A, McAlister F. Users' guides to the medical literature: XIX. Applying clinical trial results. A. How to use an article measuring the effect of an intervention on surrogate end points. Evidence-Based Medicine Working Group. *JAMA*. 1999 Aug 25;282(8):771–778.

150. Geiger S, Holdenrieder S, Stieber P, Hamann GF, Bruening R, Ma J, et al. Nucleosomes as a new prognostic marker in early cerebral stroke. *J Neurol*. 2007 May;254(5):617–623.

151. Yip HK, Chang LT, Chang WN, Lu CH, Liou CW, Lan MY, et al. Level and value of circulating endothelial progenitor cells in patients after acute ischemic stroke. *Stroke*. 2008 Jan;39(1):69–74.

152. Brott T, Marler J, Olinger C, Adams H, Tomsick T, Barsan W, et al. Measurements of acute cerebral infarction: lesion size by computed tomography. *Stroke*. 1989;20(7):871–875.

153. Schaechter JD, Moore CI, Connell BD, Rosen BR, Dijkhuizen RM. Structural and functional plasticity in the somatosensory cortex of chronic stroke patients. *Brain*. 2006 Oct;129(Pt 10):2722–2733.

154. Ding G, Jiang Q, Li L, Zhang L, Zhang ZG, Ledbetter KA, et al. Magnetic resonance imaging investigation of axonal remodeling and angiogenesis after embolic stroke in sildenafil-treated rats. *J Cereb Blood Flow Metab*. 2008 Aug;28(8):1440–1448.

155. Marchina S, Zhu LL, Norton A, Zipse L, Wan CY, Schlaug G. Impairment of speech production predicted by lesion load of the left arcuate fasciculus. *Stroke*. 2011 Aug;42(8):2251–2256.

156. Hodics T, Cohen LG, Cramer SC. Functional imaging of intervention effects in stroke motor rehabilitation. *Arch Phys Med Rehabil.* 2006 Dec;87(12 Suppl):36–42.

157. Richards LG, Stewart KC, Woodbury ML, Senesac C, Cauraugh JH. Movement-dependent stroke recovery: a systematic review and meta-analysis of TMS and fMRI evidence. *Neuropsychologia.* 2008 Jan 15;46(1):3–11.

158. Parsons M, Li T, Barber P, Yang Q, Darby D, Desmond P, *et al.* Combined (1)H MR spectroscopy and diffusion-weighted MRI improves the prediction of stroke outcome. *Neurology.* 2000 Aug 22;55(4):498–505.

159. Pendlebury S, Blamire A, Lee M, Styles P, Matthews P. Axonal injury in the internal capsule correlates with motor impairment after stroke. *Stroke.* 1999 May;30(5):956–962.

160. Talelli P, Greenwood RJ, Rothwell JC. Arm function after stroke: neurophysiological correlates and recovery mechanisms assessed by transcranial magnetic stimulation. *Clin Neurophysiol.* 2006 Aug;117(8):1641–1659.

161. Crafton K, Mark A, Cramer S. Improved understanding of cortical injury by incorporating measures of functional anatomy. *Brain.* 2003 Jul;126(Pt 7):1650–1659.

162. Bocti C, Swartz RH, Gao FQ, Sahlas DJ, Behl P, Black SE. A new visual rating scale to assess strategic white matter hyperintensities within cholinergic pathways in dementia. *Stroke.* 2005 Oct;36(10):2126–2131.

163. Hillis AE, Gold L, Kannan V, Cloutman L, Kleinman JT, Newhart M, *et al.* Site of the ischemic penumbra as a predictor of potential for recovery of functions. *Neurology.* 2008 Jul 15;71(3):184–189.

CHAPTER 21

Rehabilitation after stroke

Katharina Stibrant Sunnerhagen

Definition of rehabilitation

The word rehabilitation comes from Latin (re: back/again and habilitas: ability/aptitude) meaning gaining back the capacity to function normally or as close to normally as possible. The aim of rehabilitation is to find an optimal way for a person to return to everyday life and regain reasonable health after an event that led to disability. This implies that something was lost and the aim is to become fit or able again. Having a disability means limitations in doing tasks and/or taking part in some activities. Conventional medical diagnostics form the basis that forecast the prognosis and the content of the rehabilitation intervention. In medicine the person is usually seen as an object and in rehabilitation as a subject.

In order to understand rehabilitation, disability also has to be discussed. How the person is functioning depends on health as well as where and how the person lives in addition to other individual factors. Living with a disability implies that the body is not functioning fully but also that there are limitations in doing some activities or partaking in activities. There is the question of capacity which refers to the ability to do an activity in a barrier-free place. Performance deals with the ability to do a certain task in a real-world setting.

International Classification of Functioning, Disability and Health

The World Health Organization produces international classifications on health so that there is a consensual, meaningful, and useful framework which governments, providers, and consumers can use as a common language. The most commonly known is the International Classification of Disease (ICD) which has a counterpart in the International Classification of Functioning, Disability and Health (ICF) (1). The ICF is a classification of health and health-related domains and was endorsed in May 2001.

The ICF sheds a new light on the terms 'health' and 'disability'. The idea of the ICF is that every person can experience a decrease in health and thereby experience some degree of disability. Disability in this way is not something that only happens to a minority but is a universal experience. The model was developed to assess the consequences of a disorder or a disease for the individual person. The ICF focuses on the person and thereby requires different treatments and interventions depending on that person's goal. In the ICF human functioning and disability are described both as an experience in relation to the health conditions and impairments, and as a result of interaction with the environment (see Figure 21.1).

Body function includes physical as well as mental functions on an organ level. Activity is defined as the execution of a task or an action by an individual. Activity limitations are difficulties in executing activities. Participation is defined as involvement in a life situation and participation restriction is defined as problems an individual may experience while involved in life situations. The contexts are environmental factors and personal factors, which may have an impact on the person. Environmental factors make up the physical, social, and attitudinal environment in which people live and conduct their lives. Personal factors are the particular background of an individual's life and way of living such as gender, age, lifestyle, coping styles, etc.

By shifting the focus from cause to impact it places all health conditions on an equal footing allowing them to be compared using a common metric—the ruler of health and disability. Furthermore, the ICF takes into account the social aspects of disability and does not see disability only as a 'medical' or 'biological' dysfunction. By including contextual factors, in which environmental factors are listed, the ICF allows the impact of the environment on the person's functioning to be recorded.

The rehabilitation process

The rehabilitation process begins when the stroke hits and ends when the person is dead. This viewpoint is that the traditional medical perspective and the rehabilitation perspective are parallel processes, with different impact, however, depending when the crossover occurs. The process is based on the individual's perceived inability, needs, and interests. The process should be goal-oriented and involves complex and coordinated actions; the process should be finite in time but last as long as the need for action exists.

Rehabilitation is in many ways a pedagogical process which aims to alter behaviour (in the person or their family) and much more than just physical training. The stroke rehabilitation process aims to support the person to obtain knowledge and understanding of the stroke and its consequences, to mobilize their own coping strategies, to take responsibility of the life situation, and to become aware of the possibilities considering the resources and limitations in order to reach old and new goals in life. The process is an ongoing procedure where assessment is followed by planning, treatment, and evaluation. After each evaluation, the process starts again if the goal is not yet achieved.

Organization of rehabilitation

Actions that need to be performed within rehabilitation involve medical, physical, social, economical, and vocational interventions all focused on a person with functional limitations. The whole person is affected by the stroke and rehabilitation needs occur and therefore the specific rehabilitation measures are part of a broad strategy.

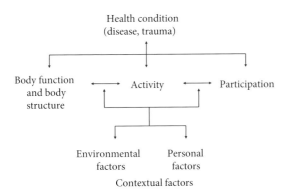

Health condition
(disease, trauma)

Body function
and body
structure   Activity   Participation

Environmental   Personal
factors   factors

Contextual factors

Fig. 21.1 The ICF-model; with 3 domains within Functioning and Disability and 2 domains of Contextual Factors

Rehabilitation solves this problem by working in a team, taking into account both the individual's comprehensive and complex needs and the professional team members' specialist knowledge. The team commonly includes the following members: physicians, nursing staff, occupational therapists, physical therapists, speech and language therapists, psychologists, and social workers. The person's total life situation is taken into consideration in the rehabilitation planning. Individuals have different perceptions of their resources, limitations, wishes, and level of motivation for change. These differences are noted and described by the professional team member with the help of tests, interviews, and accumulated experiences. This means that we as rehabilitation professionals cannot tell what the best is for the person in need of rehabilitation.

Teamwork is highlighted in rehabilitation. Teamwork is an attempt to solve the paradox of the rehabilitation model. How do you address the complex needs that persons in rehabilitation have, with the help of specialized professionals that are trained to assess the reality from a well-defined and narrow perspective? How do we keep the holistic view of the person when we have fragmented fields of knowledge? One way to achieve this is to work in teams. Teamwork that is well functioning has been shown to influence stroke rehabilitation with more efficiency but also with functional improvement in the patients (2, 3). However, to work in a team requires training (3) (Table 21.1).

Goal setting

Rehabilitation aims for behavioural changes and behaviour can be defined as a goal-oriented activity (4). When the patient is taking part in the goal setting, the interventions becomes more patient centred (5). Behavioural changes seem to be easier to achieve if the person wishes to achieve the goal. Behavioural changes are also encouraged by a consistent approach from the team towards the person, helped by team members sharing common goals. Goal setting is in itself a powerful tool to create a rehabilitation plan that includes rehabilitation processes as well as other processes of change (6). The foundation for teamwork is, however, professional assessments. The team's main task is to formulate interdisciplinary goals together with the person in need of rehabilitation in physical, cognitive, psychological, and societal areas. Evaluation of the rehabilitation process should include if the team is setting goals and if these are reached (7).

To formulate a goal in rehabilitation is a demanding and complex task. The team has accumulated knowledge on how to use goal setting and planning techniques that the person in need of rehabilitation is lacking. The questions asked to the person in need of rehabilitation before and during the planning session of the rehabilitation can be perceived as leading, difficult to meet, and constructed. To in part put the responsibility for the process on the person in need of rehabilitation means a change in the care process. The transformation occurs at the change from the medical acute phase into the rehabilitation phase; a transformation from being a more or less passive object in the acute phase to an active subject in the rehabilitation phase. The goal setting requires also that everyone is aware of the difference between wishes and goals. It is important that all are aware that the focus of the planning is on achievable goals and that the team's competence is not sufficient to fulfil wishes. The team thereby admit their limitations and focus the work around what is achievable, taking the limitations into consideration. The goal formulation usually starts by the person in need of rehabilitation with his/her words describing the current situation (8). The professional team members analyse the description and make sure that it includes different life aspects such as the personal situation, family situation, vocational and past time situation, as well as the health situation. After this the main goals are decided by having the person in need of rehabilitation describe what they feel is missing in the different areas. The goal setting can improve if resources and limitations are taken into consideration—this can help in identifying interim goals. The goals have to be relevant and motivational and be of value for the patient. The goals have to express what you want to achieve, not what you are doing. They have to be described in a positive way of what you want to do, not what you want to avoid doing. They have to be concrete and should be expressed in behavioural terms.

Table 21.1 Different teamstructures; advantages and disadvantages

Team	Work structure	Advantages	Disadvantages
Multidisciplinary	Hierarchical structure	Time-efficient team conferences	Not optimal usage of competence
	Parallel assessments and treatments	Clear authority	Difficult for the patient to identify with the goals
	Profession-driven goals	Clear responsibility	Difficult with horizontal communication
	Vertical interaction	Easy adjustment for new members	
Interdisciplinary	Matrix structure	Optimal usage of competence	Time for conferences
	Coordinated assessments and treatments	Synergies	Slow decision process
	Goal by the patient and profession	Quality in decisions	Team education
	Horizontal interaction	Holistic view	Conflicts/responsibilities
		Patient involved	

They have to be clear and understandable and in the way that they are reachable and allow planning. They have to be bold but within reach. Goal fulfilment must be within a reasonable time. The goals have to contain a description of the activity, not the outcome. The goals have to be assessable and be split into interim goals that can be checked during the process.

Rehabilitation interventions in the different domains of the ICF

Body function

Training of motor skills

There are many different approaches of training the motor skills that are affected in patients with stroke. In the early days, the principles from orthopaedic training dominated with a focus on compensatory training of the non-affected side. During the 1950s and 1960s, different methods were developed based on the neurophysiology of the time. In the 1980s, the significance of neuropsychology and motor learning was introduced.

The question is then what treatment to use. A Cochrane review (9) identified 21 randomized controlled studies with more than 900 patients. The aim was to explore if different methods (based on different theories) resulted in different outcome in balance and function in upper and lower extremities. The conclusion was that training with physical therapy was better than no training. No specific therapeutic approach was better than the others for balance control or function in the upper or lower extremity. Training with a combination of approaches resulted in less dependency in activities of daily living (ADL). Another review (10) came to the same conclusion that there are no clear differences in effect of the intervention depending on methodology.

Many persons with paralysis or even paresis after stroke are not able to participate in functional training. The theory is that if there is not enough voluntary activation of muscle to produce functional activity this can be achieved with electro-stimulation. The lack of use of muscles will also lead to changes in the skeletal muscle after stroke because of altered descending neuromuscular drive. The idea is that electro-stimulation given in the correct dose should enhance recovery after stroke more than conventional physical therapy. In a meta-analysis (11) this was investigated and it seems as if the electro-stimulation compared to no training resulted in improved motor performance but compared to physical therapy there were no significant differences. The studies analysed were of different design and varied inclusion time since stroke. There is a need for further research in the area.

Acupuncture has been suggested to improve function after stroke. In different regions of the world, acupuncture is used as an adjunct to training or sometimes as the tool that will make the person better again. Studies have tried to assess the effect of acupuncture on muscle performance, stroke outcome, aphasia, bladder function, etc. There are Cochrane meta-analyses that conclude that there is no clear evidence for effect of acupuncture on body function after stroke (12–14). One reason for lack of evidence going either way is due to a design problem, the difficulties of sham-acupuncture where it is difficult to have an acupuncturist blinded to the treatment. The area is lacking large studies with good design.

Spasticity treatment

Spasticity is a part of the upper motor neuron syndrome. Spasticity is defined as an involuntary, velocity-dependent disorder associated with increased resistance to stretch. Spasticity can present clinically as soft-tissue contracture and/or muscle overactivity (see Figure 21.2). It seems as if symptoms may appear as early as a few days or as late as 18 months after a stroke event. The frequency of spasticity has been reported between 17–46% of stroke survivors depending on sample (15–19). A recent report from a population-based study in Sweden (16) showed that disabling spasticity, defined as spasticity severe enough to warrant some form of intervention, can affect about 4% of stroke survivors 1 year after their initial stroke. Effective treatment of spasticity requires a combined approach, involving physical/occupational therapy, possibly in conjunction with intermittent pharmacological intervention (20). For stroke survivors with focal spasticity, the most commonly used pharmacological treatment is botulinum toxin which decreases the transmission of nerve impulses and thereby reduces spasticity.

Depression

It has been shown from a Norwegian stroke unit that depression and anxiety is present in a higher frequency within the first week after stroke compared to the general population (21). Depression is still common more than a year after rehabilitation as well (22, 23). It is also known that depression is more common (odds ratio (OR) 3.4) even 2 years after stroke than in an age-matched group (24). These results from selected populations were confirmed from the Swedish Riks-Stroke Register where around 12% of the men and 18% of the women acknowledged 'feeling down' at the 1-year follow-up. Medication with antidepressants in the Riks-Stroke group was as expected correlated with acknowledgement of depression in different degrees. However, among those that stated that they were often or always feeling depressed, there was a large variation in whether they received medication or not. Pharmacological intervention has been shown to have a small but significant effect (25). This seems to be an area where there is room for improvement with better awareness of the problem and better follow-up to ensure proper medication and social support.

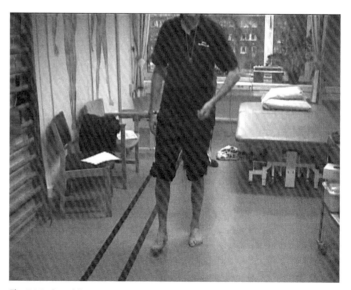

Fig. 21.2 Spasticity.

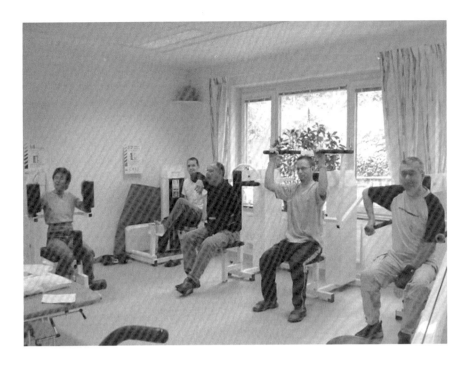

Fig. 21.3 Circuit training.

Activity

Mobility training

A common consequence of the impaired motor function is decreased ability to walk. Many persons after a stroke tell rehabilitation staff that they want to be able to walk again and having enough muscle strength is crucial for this goal. Circuit training in group is a model where exercises and activities which are task specific are performed in an intensive manner (see Figure 21.3). Often the participants complete a series of workstations arranged in a circuit. The focus is on repetitive practice of task-specific training of everyday motor skills. There may also be additional benefits of circuit class therapy related to the peer support and social interaction provided by the group environment. Circuit training has been shown to improve walking distance, walking speed, and there was no increase in level of spasticity (26). A conclusion is that circuit training is safe and effective in improving mobility for people after moderate stroke and may reduce inpatient length of stay.

Walking

Walking is an activity on its own, but also a part of other activities, for example, 'going to the bathroom'. Walking is trained traditionally on the ground together with a therapist. The approaches for walking have been covered in a Cochrane review (9), and it seems that the best way is to have a mixed approach. In the spinal cord there are motor cells that can steer the legs into a gait pattern as can be seen in new-born babies. More steps seem to enhance walking recovery. This background data is the reason for using technical equipment to enhance the number of steps taken. The first efforts dealt with treadmill training with body-weight support (see Figure 21.4). A number of studies were performed and in the beginning they saw diverging results since the control population received 'traditional' physical therapy and this varied a lot. With meta-analysis (27) it was shown that treadmill training with body weight support in the same amount as 'traditional' physical therapy

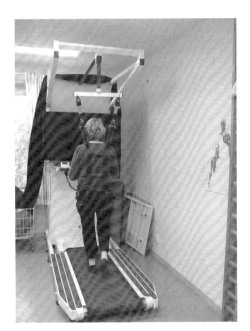

Fig. 21.4 Treadmill training.

did not result in better walking ability. This was probably because there was not much difference in the number of steps taken. A recent meta-analysis (28) has shown that in order to increase walking capacity, the extra time spent in training has to be more than approximately 37 minutes per day. However, treadmill training with body-weight support has been shown to reduce the energy cost of walking (29) and can therefore be an alternative for the person with heart and lung problems.

After a stroke, cardiorespiratory fitness is also often impaired. In a recent Cochrane review (30) 14 trials (651 participants) aiming at improving fitness were included. To walk to improve fitness resulted in improved maximum walking speed, self-selected gait speed and walking capacity. Therefore, cardiorespiratory training should be part of post-stroke rehabilitation programmes for better walking,

Biomechanical gait training

Biomechanical gait training (exoskeletal or foot-platforms) has developed as a result of the ergonomical problems perceived by the therapist in trying to move the paralytic person forwards on the treadmill. Studies have shown the effects of these devices (31) but the best construct is not clear. The studies have usually had a design where the biomechanical training on the treadmill is an add-on to the traditional physical therapy. This of course results in more training time and more steps taken per day and therefore the result of longer walking capacity is not surprising. This longer walking (34 metres or more) is, however, not seen as a clinical meaningful difference (92 metres in walking distance). No effect was seen on walking speed.

Activities of daily living

A meta-analysis (32) was performed where nine studies were included (1258 persons) and the patients were randomized to either training with an occupational therapist or to not receiving occupational therapy. The study subjects were 55–85 years of age, and the proportion of men varied between 19% and 66%. Six of the studies included patients at discharge from the acute unit; one took place on the stroke unit and also included those that were discharged within 2 weeks; one at admittance to the stroke unit; three studies included patients at set intervals after the stroke incidence (within 2 weeks after discharge, 1 month, and within 6 months). One study recruited patients that were not admitted to the hospital for their stroke and one included patients from a nursing home. In spite of this heterogeneous design of studies, the authors were able to draw some conclusions regarding the effect of occupational therapy training. Having training with an occupational therapist resulted in less risk of poor outcome (OR 0–67; confidence interval (CI) 0.51–0.87, p=0.003; number needed to treat 11), as well as increased independence in daily activities (standardized mean difference 0.18; CI 0.04–032, p=0.01).

The generalizability is influenced by the fact that those with communication problems (severe aphasia, severe cognitive problem, or dependent on interpretation) were excluded. The meta-analysis does not give enough information to say what model of occupational therapy intervention should be applied (see Figure 21.5).

Participation

Driving

Being able to drive is key to participation in many Western societies. Driving requires multitasking where input from a complex environment requires fast decisions and motor activities to steer the car in a safe way. It is not unusual that the capacity to drive is altered after a stroke. Often survivors do not realize the difficulties that they might have when driving after a stroke. Some may not know all of the effects of their stroke and may feel that they are to drive. The legal consequences regarding driving after a stroke varies between countries. However, regardless of legal matters, it seems we are all interested in identifying those drivers that should not be driving.

A study from a mobility centre in the UK (33) has shown that important factors affecting outcome were vision (acuity and field),

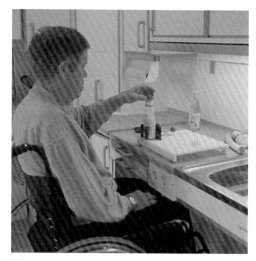

Fig. 21.5 Kitchen.

neuropsychological functions (divided attention), as well as track and/or on-road test (reaction time, anticipation, speed, and positioning). For those who failed during driving test, cognitive impairment was the main problem. Car adaptation, mainly comprising infrared transmitted secondary controls together with automatic transmission, was recommended in 35% of the cases.

A systematic review (34) identified five tests shown to be relevant screening tools of fitness to drive after stroke. These tests assessed executive function, perception, attention and memory, and higher-order planning functions. Some of the tests could also be used to identify unsafe drivers with an accuracy of 80% of more. These were tests were Road Sign Recognition (assesses traffic knowledge and visual comprehension), Compass (examines visuoperceptual and visuospatial abilities, divided attention, mental speed, and executive function), TMT B (evaluates visuomotor tracking, visual scanning, and executive functions).

Work after stroke

According to the Swedish Riks-Stroke Register, about 50% of those who worked prior to the stroke have not returned to work and are not considering this at 1 year post stroke. About one-third are back to the same level as prior to the stroke, 14% at a lower level, and about 6% are still on sick leave but are aiming to return to work. The question then is what factors are influencing return to work? Cognitive impairment at discharge is a hindrance for return to work (35), as is fatigue (36). Positive factors associated with work return are perceived importance of work, not feeling like a burden on others, and support from others for return to work (specifically the closest supervisor) (37).

In vocational rehabilitation the aim is to match the capacity of the person and the demands of the work in order not only to have return to work but also work stability. Factors of importance are to learn labour saving methods including physical/ergonomical and cognitive methods. There is also a need to identify stress factors and find out how these are to be handled in the patient's specific work situation. The general practitioner has an important role in vocational rehabilitation after stroke (38)

The problems after a stroke are varied. Consequently, different interventions and combinations of interventions are required to suit the needs of patients with different problems. There are questions regarding which treatments work best for which patients over the long term, and which models of service represent value for money in the context of life-long care. In future, such questions will need to be set alongside practice-based evidence gathered from large, systematic, longitudinal cohort studies conducted in the context of routine clinical practice.

Environment

Close ones

The need of support from next of kin is quite large. In Sweden, for those who responded 1 year after stroke and were over the age of 75, about one-third stated that they were not dependent on family. In those younger than 75, dependency is less pronounced and slightly more than half are not dependent on family. However, at 2 years post stroke, 70% state that they receive help and support from their partner/close family, 44.8% were partially dependent and 17.2% were totally dependent on their partner/close family. It seems that when the patient has less capacity and low activity level, this result in a strain in the family. A recent study from Hong Kong (39) shows that the families of stroke survivors acknowledge a burden of care. The burden was correlated with anxiety, depression and fatigue in the respondent.

So what can be done to help the family? A meta-analysis (40) has been performed and more than 1000 subjects from eight studies were included. There were no clear results regarding reduction in stress or strain. However, it seems as if structured information and education from a professional will result in reduction in burden and increased well-being in the close family (41).

An enriched environment is of great importance

Current understanding of brain plasticity has altered stroke rehabilitation. A combination of good medical and nursing care with training in an environment that provides confidence, stimulation, and motivation improve outcome (42, 43).

Having stimulation in the environment is important

This can be a garden close to the rehabilitation centre so it is possible to get out and feel the wind and sun (see Figure 21.6). It can also be that there is music on the ward with possibilities to participate in a communal sing-along.

The rehabilitation setting might not function as a learning environment

The learning might be better if the patient is discharged home and the training takes place in a familiar environment. Often the capacity of abstracting is impaired after a stroke and training in another bathroom to stand up from the toilet may lead to results on the ward, but in another environment there is a new situation and most (or all) of the training is 'gone' and there is a need for more rehabilitation.

Personal and environmental factors will influence outcome

The person who has a stroke has a history with comorbidities but also with personal strengths and weakness that need to be taken into consideration. Also the physical environment needs to be considered, such as if the person is living alone or with a partner, in a flat with an elevator from the ground floor to the door, or in an old house with impractical stairs.

Partnership between the patient and the therapist may contribute to patient involvement

A mutual respect between the patient and therapist and an agreement on the need for hard work has an impact on involvement. Getting the patient involved is key to successful rehabilitation.

Organization of rehabilitation

Early supported discharge

A number of studies looking at early supported discharge (ESD) from the stroke unit for certain groups of patients have been performed in different areas of the world. A meta-analysis (44) has been performed and shows that this is safe, economical, and reduces the

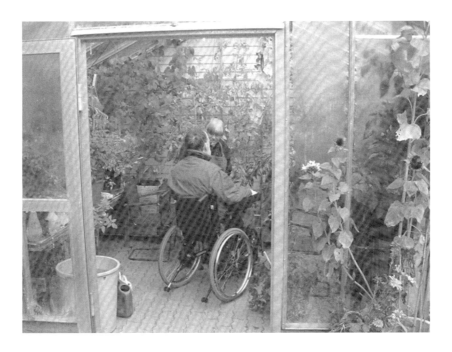

Fig. 21.6 Garden shed.

risk of death and dependency. However, the meta-analysis does not tell how an early supported discharge service should be organized. A recent study (45) where ten early supported discharge trialists participated looked at the key messages from the literature. They also wanted to identify core elements of an ESD service and to describe accessibility to purchasers and service providers. A consensus was reached for some areas regarding the elements of an ESD service. An ESD team should plan and coordinate discharge from hospital and provide rehabilitation and support in the community. There is a key worker, coordinator in the team, and the team should be based in the hospital. Specific eligibility criteria should be followed and these should in part be based on the patient's level of disability, e.g. Barthel Index score between 10 and 17, and the patient should be medically stable. There was no consensus of what the intervention should contain or how long it should be ongoing for. This has been interpreted that the ESD is contextually influenced and that the length of intervention offered by an ESD team should be based on the existence and type of other community-based stroke services operating in the area. There was a consensus reached regarding the multidisciplinary team composition; it should include occupational therapists and physiotherapist, speech and language therapists, physician, nurse and social worker. There was also a recommended case load for 100 patients per year for each profession.

Rehabilitation the first year after discharge

For those that are living at home after stroke there is often an ongoing need of rehabilitation efforts. A meta-analysis (46) has been performed which aimed to assess the effect of physiotherapy, occupational therapy, or multidisciplinary team rehabilitation for persons living at home in the first year after stroke. In these studies there were variations of different organizations of rehabilitation: day-rehabilitation, clinic visits, or training in the home environment. The main efforts have been to improve different task specific behaviours such as walking or dressing. There were 14 studies with more than 1600 patients and the ages varied between 55 and 75 years of age. The conclusion of the meta-analysis is that the rehabilitation efforts given to patients during the first year after stroke who are living at home reduces the risk of death or deterioration in daily living (ADL activities) (OR 0.72; CI 0.57–0.92, p=0.009). The number needed to treat is approximately 13 to avoid that one person deteriorates. The different rehabilitation efforts have a positive effect on the patient's capacity to perform personal and instrumental ADL but the size of the effect remains unclear. We also do not know what type of organization of the rehabilitation is the best and most cost-efficient.

If rehabilitation is efficient after the first year remains unclear. A meta-analysis (47) has been published but only five studies were found and included. Most of the intervention in the studies aimed to diminish functional limitations through problem solving, target-specific, and goal-oriented training to improve personal ADL. The intensity of training varied a lot and only two of the studies had a multidisciplinary team to perform interventions. The outcomes were death or deterioration (more dependent in personal ALD), however, it was not possible to draw any conclusions of whether rehabilitation 1 year after stroke made a difference.

Examples of new techniques/models for rehabilitation

The knowledge of mirror neurons and how they work has influenced rehabilitation (48). These neurons are found in the premotor and parietal cortex and are activated both during activity, but also during observation of actions. This means that the motor system may be activated without overt movement. In rehabilitation, methods are used to activate the mirror neurons and such methods involve action observation, motor imagery, and imitation.

The use of computers

Virtual reality and interactive video gaming are new modalities that can be used in stroke rehabilitation. With virtual reality the patient can get an image of motion of an impaired limb which involves both action observation and motor imagery. The approach in rehabilitation during recent years has been towards environmentally contextual skill training (task-oriented training). Training programmes for enhancing motor skills use patient and goal-tailored exercise schedules and individual feedback on exercise performance. The virtual reality allows the trial of tasks that might be unsafe in the real world (such as crossing the street if you have neglect) (49). Virtual reality can also be goal-oriented and allows for repetitions. Intensive task-specific practice is needed for cortical reorganization as well as for behavioural changes. Virtual reality can offer real-life functional activities to provide ecological validity (see Figure 21.7). Virtual reality tasks have been described as being more interesting, which might lead to higher adherence, then traditional tasks. Games are fun to play and also give feedback on performance. The question is, can this be of use for anything more than amusement? There have been studies assessing the effect of using virtual reality to enhance motor performance. A recent meta-analysis (50) was published with the aim to evaluate the effects of virtual reality and interactive video gaming on motor function after stroke (including both upper and lower extremity). It seems as if the use of virtual reality may be beneficial in improving arm function and ADL function when compared with the same dose of conventional therapy. It is not clear if there is any effect on grip strength or gait speed. Again, it is not clear what characteristics of virtual reality are most important or whether effects are sustained in the longer term. There are few studies on off-the-shelf games and equipment such as Nintendo Wii (see Figure 21.8). More research is needed before these virtual reality and interactive video games can be used as standard treatment.

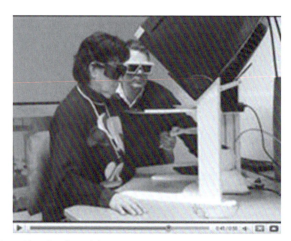

Fig. 21.7 Virtual reality training.

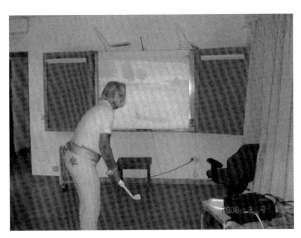

Fig. 21.8 Nintendo golf.

Forced use

Constrained induced motor training is a multifaceted intervention: the restriction to the unaffected limb is accompanied by a certain amount of exercise of the appropriate quality. This is usually limited to participants who have some residual motor power of the paretic arm, the potential for further motor recovery, and with limited pain or spasticity. It seems that for some patients this can be beneficial. However, for disability measured some months after the end of treatment, there was no evidence of persisting benefit. The EXCITE trial (51) showed good results and remaining changes at follow-up. However, the generalizability has to be questioned since the inclusion criteria are so narrow and the average age low in the trials with positive results (below 65 compared to above 70 in most clinical populations).

Music therapy

The use of music to enhance plasticity after stroke has been suggested (52). Different aspects have been tried which includes listening to music and singing in groups. Drums and rhythm has been used as a way of integrating sensory stimulation into training where you can have both the feedback from the drum and the sound of the drum. Bilateral training is advocated by some for upper extremity and in drumming both hands can be used and it becomes obvious to the patient if the sound is different depending on the hand used. Different types of instruments (keyboard) and drum have been used to improve upper extremity function and it seemed to have an effect in a small study of 20 patients (53). Rhythmic auditory stimulation has been used to enhance gait performance after stroke (54) with promising results. However, there are not many well-designed trials regarding the use of music in rehabilitation after stroke. A recent meta-analysis tried to assess the effects of music therapy but there were few studies noted with small numbers of participants (55). It seems as if rhythmic auditory stimulation may be beneficial for improving gait parameters in stroke patients. No other conclusions could be drawn.

References

1. World Health Organization. *International Classification of Functioning, Disability and Health: ICF.* Geneva: WHO; 2001.
2. Schouten LM, Hulscher ME, Akkermans R, van Everdingen JJ, Grol RP, Huijsman R. Factors that influence the stroke care team's effectiveness in reducing the length of hospital stay. *Stroke.* 2008 Sep;39(9):2515–2521.
3. Strasser DC, Falconer JA, Stevens AB, Uomoto JM, Herrin J, Bowen SE, *et al.* Team training and stroke rehabilitation outcomes: a cluster randomized trial. *Arch Phys Med Rehabil.* 2008 Jan;89(1):10–15.
4. Holliday RC, Antoun M, Playford ED. A survey of goal-setting methods used in rehabilitation. *Neurorehabil Neural Repair.* 2005 Sep;19(3):227–231.
5. Holliday RC, Cano S, Freeman JA, Playford ED. Should patients participate in clinical decision making? An optimised balance block design controlled study of goal setting in a rehabilitation unit. *J Neurol Neurosurg Psychiatry.* 2007 Jun;78(6):576–580.
6. Turner-Stokes L. Goal attainment scaling (GAS) in rehabilitation: a practical guide. *Clin Rehabil.* 2009 Apr;23(4):362–370.
7. Ottenbacher KJ, Cusick A. Goal attainment scaling as a method of clinical service evaluation. *Am J Occup Ther.* 1990 Jun;44(6):519–525.
8. Wressle E, Eeg-Olofsson AM, Marcusson J, Henriksson C. Improved client participation in the rehabilitation process using a client-centred goal formulation structure. *J Rehabil Med.* 2002 Jan;34(1):5–11.
9. Pollock A, Baer G, Pomeroy V, Langhorne P. Physiotherapy treatment approaches for the recovery of postural control and lower limb function following stroke. *Cochrane Database Syst Rev.* 2007;1:CD001920.
10. Kollen BJ, Lennon S, Lyons B, Wheatley-Smith L, Scheper M, Buurke JH, *et al.* The effectiveness of the Bobath concept in stroke rehabilitation: what is the evidence? *Stroke.* 2009 Apr;40(4):e89–97.
11. Pomeroy VM, King L, Pollock A, Baily-Hallam A, Langhorne P. Electrostimulation for promoting recovery of movement or functional ability after stroke. *Cochrane Database Syst Rev.* 2006;2:CD003241.
12. Zhang SH, Liu M, Asplund K, Li L. Acupuncture for acute stroke. *Cochrane Database Syst Rev.* 2005;2:CD003317.
13. Wu HM, Tang JL, Lin XP, Lau J, Leung PC, Woo J, *et al.* Acupuncture for stroke rehabilitation. *Cochrane Database Syst Rev.* 2006;3:CD004131.
14. Thomas LH, Cross S, Barrett J, French B, Leathley M, Sutton CJ, *et al.* Treatment of urinary incontinence after stroke in adults. *Cochrane Database Syst Rev.* 2008;1:CD004462.
15. Leathley MJ, Gregson JM, Moore AP, Smith TL, Sharma AK, Watkins CL. Predicting spasticity after stroke in those surviving to 12 months. *Clin Rehabil.* 2004 Jun;18(4):438–443.
16. Lundstrom E, Terent A, Borg J. Prevalence of disabling spasticity 1 year after first-ever stroke. *Eur J Neurol.* 2008 Jun;15(6):533–539.
17. Sommerfeld DK, Eek EU, Svensson AK, Holmqvist LW, von Arbin MH. Spasticity after stroke: its occurrence and association with motor impairments and activity limitations. *Stroke.* 2004 Jan;35(1):134–139.
18. Urban PP, Wolf T, Uebele M, Marx JJ, Vogt T, Stoeter P, *et al.* Occurence and clinical predictors of spasticity after ischemic stroke. *Stroke.* 2010;Sep;41(9):2016–2020.
19. Watkins CL, Leathley MJ, Gregson JM, Moore AP, Smith TL, Sharma AK. Prevalence of spasticity post stroke. *Clin Rehabil.* 2002 Aug;16(5):515–522.
20. Wissel J, Ward AB, Erztgaard P, Bensmail D, Hecht MJ, Lejeune TM, *et al.* European consensus table on the use of botulinum toxin type A in adult spasticity. *J Rehabil Med.* 2009 Jan;41(1):13–25.
21. Fure B, Wyller TB, Engedal K, Thommessen B. Emotional symptoms in acute ischemic stroke. *Int J Geriatr Psychiatry.* 2006 Apr;21(4):382–387.
22. Farner L, Wagle J, Engedal K, Flekkoy KM, Wyller TB, Fure B. Depressive symptoms in stroke patients: a 13 month follow-up study of patients referred to a rehabilitation unit. *J Affect Disord.* 2010;Dec;127(1–3):211–218.
23. Bergersen H, Froslie KF, Stibrant Sunnerhagen K, Schanke AK. Anxiety, depression, and psychological well-being 2 to 5 years poststroke. *J Stroke Cerebrovasc Dis.* 2010;Sep–Oct;19(5):364–369.
24. Linden T, Blomstrand C, Skoog I. Depressive disorders after 20 months in elderly stroke patients: a case-control study. *Stroke.* 2007 Jun;38(6):1860–1863.
25. Hackett ML, Anderson CS, House A, Xia J. Interventions for treating depression after stroke. *Cochrane Database Syst Rev.* 2008;4:CD003437.

26. English C, Hillier SL. Circuit class therapy for improving mobility after stroke. *Cochrane Database Syst Rev*. 2010;7:CD007513.

27. Moseley AM, Stark A, Cameron ID, Pollock A. Treadmill training and body weight support for walking after stroke. *Cochrane Database Syst Rev*. 2005;4:CD002840.

28. Veerbeek JM, Koolstra M, Ket JC, van Wegen EE, Kwakkel G. Effects of augmented exercise therapy on outcome of gait and gait-related activities in the first 6 months after stroke: a meta-analysis. *Stroke*. 2011 Nov;42(11):3311–3315.

29. Danielsson A, Sunnerhagen KS. Oxygen consumption during treadmill walking with and without body weight support in patients with hemiparesis after stroke and in healthy subjects. *Arch Phys Med Rehabil*. 2000;81(7):953–957.

30. Brazzelli M, Saunders DH, Greig CA, Mead GE. Physical fitness training for stroke patients. *Cochrane Database Syst Rev*. 2011;11:CD003316.

31. Mehrholz J, Werner C, Kugler J, Pohl M. Electromechanical-assisted training for walking after stroke. *Cochrane Database Syst Rev*. 2007;4:CD006185.

32. Legg L, Drummond A, Leonardi-Bee J, Gladman JR, Corr S, Donkervoort M, *et al*. Occupational therapy for patients with problems in personal activities of daily living after stroke: systematic review of randomised trials. *BMJ*. 2007 Nov 3;335(7626):922.

33. Ponsford AS, Viitanen M, Lundberg C, Johansson K. Assessment of driving after stroke—a pluridisciplinary task. *Accid Anal Prev*. 2008 Mar;40(2):452–460.

34. Devos H, Akinwuntan AE, Nieuwboer A, Truijen S, Tant M, De Weerdt W. Screening for fitness to drive after stroke: a systematic review and meta-analysis. *Neurology*. 2011 Feb 22;76(8):747–756.

35. Hofgren C, Bjorkdahl A, Esbjornsson E, Stibrant-Sunnerhagen K. Recovery after stroke: cognition, ADL function and return to work. *Acta Neurol Scand*. 2007 Feb;115(2):73–80.

36. Andersen G, Christensen D, Kirkevold M, Johnsen SP. Post-stroke fatigue and return to work: a 2-year follow-up. *Acta Neurol Scand*. 2012;125(4):248–253.

37. Lindstrom B, Roding J, Sundelin G. Positive attitudes and preserved high level of motor performance are important factors for return to work in younger persons after stroke: a national survey. *J Rehabil Med*. 2009 Sep;41(9):714–718.

38. Pollack MR, Disler PB. 2: Rehabilitation of patients after stroke. *Med J Aust*. 2002 Oct 21;177(8):452–456.

39. Tang WK, Lau CG, Mok V, Ungvari GS, Wong KS. Burden of Chinese stroke family caregivers: the Hong Kong experience. *Arch Phys Med Rehabil*. 2011 Sep;92(9):1462–1467.

40. Smith J, Forster A, House A, Knapp P, Wright J, Young J. Information provision for stroke patients and their caregivers. *Cochrane Database Syst Rev*. 2008;2:CD001919.

41. Legg LA, Quinn TJ, Mahmood F, Weir CJ, Tierney J, Stott DJ, *et al*. Non-pharmacological interventions for caregivers of stroke survivors. *Cochrane Database Syst Rev*. 2011;10:CD008179.

42. Teasell R, Bayona NA, Bitensky J. Plasticity and reorganization of the brain post stroke. *Top Stroke Rehabil*. 2005 Summer;12(3):11–26.

43. Johansson BB. Current trends in stroke rehabilitation. A review with focus on brain plasticity. *Acta Neurol Scand*. 2011 Mar;123(3):147–159.

44. Services for reducing duration of hospital care for acute stroke patients. *Cochrane Database Syst Rev*. 2005;2:CD000443.

45. Fisher RJ, Gaynor C, Kerr M, Langhorne P, Anderson C, Bautz-Holter E, *et al*. A consensus on stroke: early supported discharge. *Stroke*. May;42(5):1392–1397.

46. Therapy-based rehabilitation services for stroke patients at home. *Cochrane Database Syst Rev*. 2003;1:CD002925.

47. Aziz NA, Leonardi-Bee J, Phillips M, Gladman JR, Legg L, Walker MF. Therapy-based rehabilitation services for patients living at home more than one year after stroke. *Cochrane Database Syst Rev*. 2008;2:CD005952.

48. Garrison KA, Winstein CJ, Aziz-Zadeh L. The mirror neuron system: a neural substrate for methods in stroke rehabilitation. *Neurorehabil Neural Repair*. 2010 Jun;24(5):404–412.

49. Kim DY, Ku J, Chang WH, Park TH, Lim JY, Han K, *et al*. Assessment of post-stroke extrapersonal neglect using a three-dimensional immersive virtual street crossing program. *Acta Neurol Scand*. 2010 Mar;121(3):171–177.

50. Laver KE, George S, Thomas S, Deutsch JE, Crotty M. Virtual reality for stroke rehabilitation. *Cochrane Database Syst Rev*. 2011;9:CD008349.

51. Wolf SL, Winstein CJ, Miller JP, Taub E, Uswatte G, Morris D, *et al*. Effect of constraint-induced movement therapy on upper extremity function 3 to 9 months after stroke: the EXCITE randomized clinical trial. *JAMA*. 2006 Nov 1;296(17):2095–2104.

52. Altenmuller E, Marco-Pallares J, Munte TF, Schneider S. Neural reorganization underlies improvement in stroke-induced motor dysfunction by music-supported therapy. *Ann N Y Acad Sci*. 2009 Jul;1169:395–405.

53. Schneider S, Schonle PW, Altenmuller E, Munte TF. Using musical instruments to improve motor skill recovery following a stroke. *J Neurol*. 2007 Oct;254(10):1339–1346.

54. Hayden R, Clair AA, Johnson G, Otto D. The effect of rhythmic auditory stimulation (RAS) on physical therapy outcomes for patients in gait training following stroke: a feasibility study. *Int J Neurosci*. 2009;119(12):2183–2195.

55. Bradt J, Magee WL, Dileo C, Wheeler BL, McGilloway E. Music therapy for acquired brain injury. *Cochrane Database Syst Rev*. 2010;7:CD006787.

CHAPTER 22

The long-term management of stroke

Reza Bavarsad Shahripour and Geoffrey A. Donnan

Introduction

In recent years, major advances have been made in stroke management. In acute stroke treatment, the introduction of thrombolytic therapy has been pivotal in improving stroke outcomes; in secondary prevention the use of antiplatelet and other pharmaceutical agents has provided a means to reduce stroke recurrence and, in primary prevention, better control of risk factors has reduced stroke incidence in some countries. However, despite these successes, the burden remains a major global public health problem and the prevalence of self-reported stroke has ranged between 6% to 9% of the general population in most studies (1). Stroke-related problems such as cognitive dysfunction, decreased quality of life (QOL), mood disorders, handicap, and increased long-term mortality persist. Because of the importance of these topics, the World Stroke Organization has developed a checklist to facilitate follow-up of stroke patients. The details of this checklist were presented at the World Stroke Congress in 2012 and included 11 domains such as mobility, incontinence, language, cognition, and mood (2). The checklist is designed to help identify ongoing problems that are experienced by stroke survivors (Table 22.1). In this chapter, we examine commonly experienced sequelae of stroke such as chronic medical complications, mood disturbances, nutritional management, and QOL issues. Importantly, we also discuss the family and their concerns when they are confronted with the reality of long-term stroke management.

Chronic complications after stroke

Several studies have found that medical complications may be the primary cause of hospital-related death in over 50% of stroke patients. There is a bimodal timing, the first peak occurring in the first week, predominantly as a direct consequence of brain damage, and the second peak is several weeks later, mainly because of potentially preventable medical complications such as infection, venous thromboembolism, or cardiac disease (3–5).

The RANTTAS trial showed that serious medical events during hospitalization were associated with a fourfold increase in residual severe disability, independent of stroke severity (97%), and other variables (5, 6). The commonest medical complications have been summarized in Table 22.2 (7–9). It seems that the frequency of complications increases with age of patients and the severity of functional deficits, pre-stroke disability, urinary incontinence, vascular risk factors, markers of poor nutritional status, and length of hospital stay (Table 22.3) (10, 11). Interestingly, it has been reported that complications were

less common in specialized settings such as stroke units (12, 13). This section focuses on discussion about medical complications in the long-term perspective after stroke; some other aspects of complications after stroke are discussed in Chapters 10 and 18.

Specific medical complications

Aspiration pneumonia

A recent meta-analysis has revealed that the incidence of aspiration pneumonia ranges from 51–55% on clinical assessment and from 64–78% when video fluoroscopy is used (5). Dysphagia is associated with a threefold increase in the risk of chest infections, which rises to 11-fold in those with definite aspiration (5). Pneumonia has been reported as the cause of 23% of deaths in the Japanese stroke registry and 31% in the German Stroke Registers Study (12). It seems that two out of three stroke patients who were able to swallow safely on clinical assessment have been shown to have aspiration when assessed by instrumentation (13).

There are several mechanisms that protect the lower airways, ranging from physical processes (voluntary expiration and cough) that clear the airways of the aspirated material to cellular and immunological processes. Absent or weak cough in stroke patients is associated with a higher incidence of aspiration and chest infections (14, 15). This may be related to diaphragmatic involvement on the affected side, disruption of cortico-respiratory neuronal outflow, and decreased expiratory muscle excitation from the affected hemisphere in stroke patients (16). In a mouse model of focal cerebral ischaemia, stroke induced an extensive apoptotic loss of lymphocytes with spontaneous septicaemia and pneumonia, thus suggesting an immune suppression in these animals (17). However, investigators have shown that there is no difference in infection rates at 1 week or 3 months between treated and untreated stroke patients when given antibiotic prophylaxis (18). Unfortunately, there is not enough evidence to support a clear strategy for antibiotic use for prevention and the current policy is to approach by identifying early signs of chest infection and treat aggressively with broad-spectrum antibiotics if any symptoms are present (18–20).

Falling after stroke

In the study by Davenport et al., falling was the most common individual complication and occurred in 22% of patients. Nearly 46% had fallen at least once during their hospitalization and 73% experienced a fall within the first 6 months after stroke (9, 21). In most instances, these falls were benign and only 1–3% of patients who fell suffered a fracture.

Table 22.1 Post-stroke checklist (2)

1. *Secondary prevention* Since your stroke or last assessment, have you received any advice on health-related lifestyle changes or medications for preventing another stroke?	**No**: refer to a primary care physician or stroke neurologist for risk factor assessment and treatment if appropriate **Yes**: observe progress
2. *Activity of daily living* Since your stroke or last assessment, are you finding it more difficult to take care of yourself?	**No**: observe progress **Yes**: do you have difficulty dressing, washing and/or bathing? Do you have difficulty preparing hot drinks and/or meals? Do you have difficulty getting outside?
3. *Mobility* Since your stroke or last assessment, are you finding it more difficult to walk or move safely from bed to chair?	**No**: observe progress **Yes**: are you continuing to receive rehabilitation therapy? If **Yes**, update patient record and review at next assessment If **No**, refer to primary care physician, rehabilitation physician or an appropriate therapist (i.e. OT or PT) for further assessment
4. *Spasticity* Since your stroke or last assessment, do you have increasing stiffness in your arms, hands, and/or legs?	**No**: observe progress **Yes**: is this interfering with activities of daily living, sleep, or causing pain? If **Yes**, refer to a physician with an interest in post-stroke spasticity (i.e. rehabilitation physician or stroke neurologist) for further assessment If **No**, update patient record and review at next assessment
5. *Pain* Since your stroke or last assessment, do you have any new pain?	**No**: observe progress **Yes**: refer to a physician with an interest in post-stroke pain for further assessment and diagnosis
6. *Incontinency* Since your stroke or last assessment, are you having more of a problem controlling your bladder or bowels?	**No**: observe progress **Yes**: refer to healthcare provider with an interest in incontinence
7. *Communication* Since your stroke or last assessment, are you finding it more difficult to communicate with others?	**No**: observe progress **Yes**: refer to specialist speech and language pathologist for further assessment
8. *Mood* Since your stroke or last assessment, do you feel more anxious or depressed?	**No**: observe progress **Yes**: refer to a physician or psychologist with an interest in post-stroke mood changes for further assessment
9. *Cognition* Since your stroke or last assessment, are you finding it more difficult to think, concentrate, or remember things?	**No**: observe progress **Yes**: does this interfere with activity or participation? If **Yes**, refer to a physician or psychologist with an interest in post-stroke cognition for further assessment If **No**, update patient record and review at next assessment
10. *Life after stroke* Since your stroke or last assessment, are you finding things important to you more difficult to carry out (e.g. leisure activities, hobbies, work)?	**No**: observe progress **Yes**: refer to a local stroke support group or a stroke association (i.e. The American Stroke Association or National Stroke Association)
11. *Relationship with family* Since your stroke or last assessment, has your relationship with your family become more difficult or stressed?	**No**: observe progress **Yes**: schedule next primary care visit with patient and family member. If family member is present refer to a local stroke support group

The risk of falls increases with age, severity of stroke deficit, neglect, cognitive impairments, comorbidity, and a tendency to 'push' from the unaffected side (22, 23). The greatest risk of falling in rehabilitation settings is during unsupervised activity, but may be minimized by adapting strategies to prevent falls and good communication with patients to provide a clear understanding of stroke-related impairments. Also managing patients in safe places, trained toileting programmes, and use of some mechanical aids may be of benefit.

Urinary infection

The incidence of urinary infection after stroke ranges from 37–79% and is associated with increased mortality after stroke (7, 24). Many stroke patients suffer from incontinence 2 weeks after stroke, but 15–20% of patients may have persisting problems at 6 months (25). Age, severity of stroke, diabetes, and pre-existing functional comorbidity are risk factors for chronic incontinence after stroke (25). On the other hand, factors associated with increased risk of urinary tract infections include older age, a history of prior stroke, greater stroke severity, use of beta-blockers or antidepressants, and a post-void bladder residual of greater than 150 mL (25).

Incontinence after stroke may be related to stroke-related motor, cognitive, and language impairments or result from bladder hyporeflexia caused by concurrent neuropathy associated with age or diabetes or from concurrent medication. Factors such as stroke-related problems including depression, apathy, confusion, speech difficulties,

Table 22.2 Medical complications reported in stroke patients

Infections	Aspiration pneumonia, chest infections, urinary tract infection, sepsis, cellulitis, *Clostridium difficile* enteritis
Mobility-related problems	Falls, fractures, musculoskeletal pain, oedematous limbs, deep vein thrombosis in calf, thigh, or axilla, pulmonary embolism, loss of skin integrity, breaking skin, pressure ulcers, urinary retention or incontinence, constipation, diarrhoea
Co-morbidity	Angina, myocardial infarction, congestive cardiac failure, atrial or ventricular arrhythmias, cardiac arrest, hypertension, hypotension, poor diabetic control, hypoglycaemia, ischaemic colitis, exacerbation of chronic lung disease, peripheral vascular disease
Others	Non-cardiac pulmonary oedema, gastro-intestinal bleeding, dehydration and electrolyte imbalance, renal impairment, anaemia, malnutrition

dependency on caregiver, and medication history may affect the desire or the ability to communicate voiding needs.

As a rule, treatment begins with behavioural intervention and progresses to medication only if these measures fail, and surgical intervention is only used as a last resort (24). The use of indwelling catheters should be limited to patients with incontinence that cannot be treated by other means, patients with urinary-outlet obstruction, severely impaired patients with skin breakdown in whom frequent bed or clothing changes would be difficult or painful, and patients in whom incontinence interferes with monitoring of fluid and electrolyte balance (24).

Deep vein thrombosis

The incidence of clinically and silent deep vein thrombosis (DVT) may be as high as 45% in acute stroke patients. This rate decreases to 10% or lower in patients in the subacute phase of stroke receiving rehabilitation (24, 26, 27). The incidence of pulmonary embolisms varies between 9% and 15% in patients who have DVT and is lower in those undergoing rehabilitation. DVT and pulmonary embolism have been reported to be associated with a mortality of 1–2% in stroke patients in rehabilitation settings (24). Pulmonary embolism

Table 22.3 Common risk factors for post-stroke complications (8, 10, 13)

Risk factor	Odds ratio (95% CI)
Age	2.4 (1.6–3.8)
Premorbid disability	4.6 (2.7–7.9)
Urinary incontinence	2.7 (1.7–4.3)
Diabetes	8.5 (5.6–13.0)
Hypertension	1.9 (1.1–3.4)
Hypoalbuminaemia	1.8 (1.3–2.6)
Length of stay >30 days	1.7 (1.2–2.5)
Specialist unit management	12.9 (7.7–22.0)
Transfer to acute facilities	0.6 (0.4–0.9)
Elevated admission white blood cell counts	1.9 (1.3–2.8)
Low admission haemoglobin	1.9 (1.3–2.7)
Greater neurological deficit	2.5 (1.4–4.4)
History of cardiac arrhythmia	1.8 (1.2–2.7)

has been implicated as a cause of death in 12–20% of patients after acute stroke and in up to 50% of stroke patients sudden death may be due to pulmonary emboli (28, 29). Clinical symptoms of DVT (pain, swelling, erythema) may be absent in stroke patients with pulmonary emboli. Patients with advanced age, more severe strokes, lower limb plegia, reduced consciousness, obesity, history of a previous DVT, and longer duration of hospital stay have an increased risk for DVT (30). Many reports show that the prevalence of DVT appears higher in patients with haemorrhagic compared with ischaemic strokes, which has partially been attributed to the use of anticoagulant medications in ischaemic stroke patients (31). North American guidelines strongly advise early treatment with anticoagulants, heparin, or other antithrombotic measures to prevent DVT in immobilized stroke patients (32). In contrast, UK guidelines warn again this rule, and recommend the use of aspirin and elastic compression stockings in stroke patients (20). There is very strong evidence in the literature that anticoagulation significantly reduces the incidence of DVT and supports the use of low-molecular-weight heparin over unfractionated heparin, because of its greater clinical efficacy (33).

Oedematous limbs

A recent study in 88 stroke patients on a rehabilitation unit showed that hand swelling was present in 73%, and oedema in 33%, of patients (34). Limb oedema also causes considerable discomfort and concern to stroke survivors, because it may never resolve.

Old age and stroke severity are risk factors for this problem, which also increases the risk of venous thrombosis. The precise aetiology of oedema of the hand of the paralysed arm is not known, but various mechanisms such as complex regional pain syndrome (reflex sympathetic dystrophy), posture, and lack of muscle activity have been suggested.

Interestingly, Geurts et al. found that hand oedema is not due to lymphedema and is associated with increased arterial blood flow, possibly because of autonomic dysregulation (35). Furthermore, there was no specific pharmacological treatment that had any advantage over physical methods for reducing hand oedema (35). Available treatment modalities include elevation of the hand, massage, application of elastic bandages, immersion of the hand in cooled water, and pneumatic compression.

Mood changes and disorders after stroke

Mood disorders have a high frequency in stroke patients. For example, symptoms or signs of depression and anxiety occur at any time after stroke in about 20–60% of patients (36–40). In another published study, after 5 years of patient follow-up 50% had a mood disorder or psychiatric problems (40).

Post-stroke depression and localization

The prevalence of depression in stroke patients is reported to be between 20% and 65% and is dependent on the timing of assessment after stroke (41, 42). Major depression accounts for a minority of cases, with a prevalence of 10–20% in stroke patients while the prevalence of minor depression varies between 5% and 40% (43–45). Post-stroke depression is found to be more frequent in women than men with left hemispheric lesions (46). Patients with left hemisphere lesions may be particularly at risk of developing depression and anxiety after stroke and younger subjects are also at heightened risk (47).

In 'endogenous' depression, stroke patients having computed tomography and magnetic resonance imaging showed a trend toward a reduction in volume of the basal ganglia, hippocampus and amygdala (47–49).

There was also an increase in cortical and subcortical atrophy, white matter hyperintensities, and ventricular enlargement (50, 51). Patients having positron emission tomography (PET) and single-photon emission computed tomography studies showed reduced metabolism with normalization after therapy in the left frontosubcortical and paralimbic circuits, left anterior cingulate, superior temporal and parietal cortex, and caudate (51, 52). The temporal lobes, the connections of hippocampus and amygdale with the neocortex, and the posterior and anterior insular are involved in establishing primary cognitive process (right hemisphere dominance) or social emotions (left hemisphere dominance). The basal ganglia and limbic systems also synchronize mood and motor behaviours (53). Robinson et al. noted the correlation between anterior lesion location and severity of depression (53, 54). During the acute phase, post-stroke depression is associated with left anterior and basal ganglia lesions and after 1–2 years, post-stroke depression is significantly associated with dysfunction of the right hemisphere (55, 56). A past history of mental disorder may also be an important predictor of depression following stroke (57). Several pharmacological treatments have been proposed for patients with post-stroke depression (Table 22.4) (58).

Robinson et al. suggested that major post-stroke depression has a natural course of less than 1 year, while minor depression is often more persistent (59). Tricyclic antidepressants are no longer the treatment of first choice because of concern about the severity and frequency of adverse side effects (60). Serotoninergic neurotransmission also plays an important part in post-stroke pathological crying and citalopram has been found to be an effective and well-tolerated treatment for this condition (60, 61). A recent study comparing combinations of drugs with either noradrenergic effects (desipramine plus mianserin) or noradrenergic and serotonergic effects (imipramine plus mianserin) indicated that drugs with the dual effect may be more effective (61). Some believe that trazodone and lisuride maleate (an ergot derivative and dopamine

Table 22.4 Drugs used in post-stroke depression (67)

Selective serotonin reuptake inhibitors	Sertraline
	Fluoxetine
	Citalopram
	Paroxetine
Psychostimulants	Methylphenidate
	Dextroamphetamine
Tricyclics	Imipramine
	Amitriptyline
	Desipramine
	Amoxapine
MAO inhibitors	Moclobemide
Others	Trazodone
	Maprotiline (tetracyclic)
	Mianserin

D2-agonist) may be good alternative treatments to selective serotonin re-uptake inhibitors (SSRIs) for post-stroke depression (62). It has been reported that improvement of mood disorders with SSRIs may be associated with an enhancement of recovery of neurological function (63, 64). This effect can be quite large (30% recovery), but a close relationship between appropriate early treatment and recovery has not been noted in all studies (65).

Spontaneous remissions may be frequent in the immediate period following stroke in the case of minor depression and after a longer interval (1 or 2 years) in the case of major depression (66). The use of psychostimulant drugs seems an interesting alternative to SSRIs but the interruption of therapy because of adverse drug reactions is not rare. Several reports have found electroconvulsive therapy to be efficacious in isolated cases (67, 68). Cognitive behaviour therapy may be an appropriate treatment and patients with only verbal distress respond better to cognitive therapy alone. Patients with only vegetative symptoms might be best treated with an antidepressant drug, and patients with combined symptoms might require psychological, social, and pharmacological interventions.

Post-stroke mania and psychosis

The incidence of mania in acute stroke is about 1%, but is higher (6–9%) in brain injury (69). This difference is explained by the higher prevalence of lesions involving basotemporal and orbitofrontal cortices in traumatic brain injury patients compared to stroke patients. Most of the case-reported patients had lesions in the non-dominant hemisphere involving the basal medial and frontal area of the temporal lobe, caudate, thalamus, basal ganglia, and ventral pons (69–74). Very few cases of mania have been reported to be a consequence of a left-hemispheric lesion (75). In some patients, hypometabolism involving the right inferior temporal lobe was seen in PET studies. Also, dysfunction of the orbitofrontal and basotemporal cortices has been associated with disinhibited behaviour.

Carbamazepine, lithium, clonidine, valproic acid, and narcoleptics are effective in the treatment of post-stroke mania as they are in primary mania (76). The prevalence of schizophrenia-like symptoms is not an infrequent clinical phenomenon in the acute phases of stroke. Most cases of psychosis have been found with right-hemispheric stroke, especially in the temporo-parieto-occipital junction regions or the thalamus and in patients with pre-existing degenerative disease or cerebral atrophy (77–79). In parieto-temporal-occipital infarcts, patients with psychosis have real hallucinations and sometimes seizures may precede the onset of psychosis (80). Generally, patients have a good response to neuroleptic drugs although anticonvulsant medication can be useful in some treatment-resistant cases.

Anxiety

The incidence of anxiety is probably about 25% in the acute phase, decreasing slightly at 1-year and 3-year follow-up (81, 82). Patients with previous psychiatric disorders are prone to post-stroke anxiety (83). In stroke patients, anxiety is frequently associated with depression (81). There is a correlation between anxiety and left cortical lesions in the case of anxiety with no concurrent depression, and between anxiety and right cortical lesions in the case of anxiodepressive symptoms (82). It is noticed that patients with worries had more anterior lesions, while patients with generalized anxiety disorder had more posterior right-hemispheric lesions (82).

Starkstein et al. showed that post-stroke anxiety may be present in cortical lesions, while patients with combined anxiety and depression may have more subcortical lesions; the volume of the lesion does not correlate with the level of anxiety (84). Benzodiazepines are the most commonly prescribed medications and short-half-life drugs (i.e. lorazepam, oxazepam, and temazepam) are preferable. SSRIs and buspirone can be useful as mood stabilizers.

Suicide

The incidence of suicidal ideation is between 6% in the acute phase and 6–12% in the subsequent 2 years (85). Risk factors for suicide include depression, severe insomnia, chronic illness, organic brain syndrome, younger age, the presence of a sensory deficit, and impaired cognitive functions. In the acute phase, the degree of physical impairment and alcohol abuse seem to be important factors. In the chronic phase, suicidal ideation is an independent sign of major depression and mainly a result of poor social support (86, 87). Patients who are suicidal in the acute phase seem to have lesions with a more anterior location (87). Little has been written about the management of suicide among stroke patients and this is a subject deserving more attention.

Feeding after stroke

The incidence of malnutrition following stroke has been reported to be between 6% and 62%. Some of this variability can likely be attributed to differences in patient characteristics and the timing of assessments among studies (88, 89).

Malnutrition after the first week of stroke is associated with an increased risk of poor outcome at 1 month, a greater incidence of infections and bedsores, and longer lengths of hospital stay. Each decline of 1 g/L in serum albumin at admission was associated with a 1.13-fold increase in mortality at follow-up. Stroke patients consume between 74% and 86% of their energy and protein requirements during the first few weeks following stroke (88, 90–94). Elevations of peripheral plasma catecholamine, cortisol, glucagon, interleukin (IL)-6, IL-1, and acute phase proteins reactant have been demonstrated after stroke and may lead to the decrease of lean body mass (muscle) and fat, which may contribute to the development of malnutrition (95).

Markers used in the assessment of nutrition

Currently, there is no universal consensus on the gold standard for the assessment of nutritional status after stroke. The identification of malnutrition is typically based on the evaluation of a combination of biochemical and anthropometric markers and indicators of skeletal muscle mass and subcutaneous fat store measures. Decline in these indicators may be due to the development of malnutrition, factors secondary to stroke, or a result of atrophy secondary to immobility (96–98). Many of the nutritionally sensitive markers (albumin, pre albumin, transferrin) are affected independently by other acute illnesses, thus sometimes making interpretation difficult (99, 100) (Table 22.5).

Swallowing dysfunction

It is accepted that the presence of dysphagia is itself an indicator of greater stroke severity. Dysphagia is most commonly defined as aspiration detected on video fluoroscopic swallowing study (VFSS) or on fibreoptic endoscopic evaluation of swallowing (FEES). The approach to the treatment of dysphagia is often multidisciplinary, with the team including nurses, speech-language pathologists, dietitians, and occupational therapists) (101, 102). Dysphagia

Table 22.5 Biochemical markers of nutritional status (118)

Measure	Normal reference range	Limitation(s)
Serum albumin	>35 g/L	Large body pool
		Poor specificity to nutritional changes
		Not specific to nutritional status
		Decreased with acute illness
Serum transferrin	2.0–2.60 g/L	Not specific to nutritional status
		Decreased with acute illness
Thyroxin-binding prealbumin	1.6–3.0 g/L	Not specific to nutritional status
		Decreased with acute illness
Retinol-binding protein	0.3–0.8 g/L	Not specific to nutritional status
Total lymphocyte count	2000–3500/mm^3	Poor sensitivity and specificity

diets are individualized according to the degree and site of the oral-pharyngeal impairment.

Enteral feeding

Generally, enteral nutrition as the sole source of nutrient intake is reserved for patients with dysphagia when oral feeding is considered unsafe. The 1-year survival rate of patients with feeding tubes varied between 16% and 70% (101, 102). Aspiration pneumonia is reported in 6–18% of patients with feeding tubes (102).

The data from the Post-Stroke Rehabilitation Outcomes Project provided evidence that tube feeding is an effective intervention (103). A nasogastric (NG) feeding tube is often placed in patients who are expected to return to a full oral diet within 1 month. There is general agreement that permanent feeding access is indicated when a prolonged period of non-oral intake (>1 month) is anticipated (104). There is higher number of treatment failures associated with NG tube feeding while those with percutaneous endoscopic gastrostomy (PEG) may receive a significantly greater proportion of their provided feeds (105–107). Feeding may be provided on a continuous basis, intermittent infusions, or a cyclic method of intermittent infusion or bolus feeding. The latter is a rapid delivery system of feeding into the gastrointestinal tract by syringe or funnel.

Complications of enteral feeding

Complications largely fall into three categories: mechanical, gastrointestinal, and metabolic (108). Mechanical complications are tube blockage, local skin infection at the site of tube insertion, inadvertent insertion in the trachea, nasopharyngeal area erosion, burying of the bumper subcutaneously at the abdominal insertion site, with local pain and swelling (108).

Gastrointestinal complications include haemorrhage, peritonitis, and free air in the abdomen. Metabolic complications in tube-fed populations are often related to fluid balance, electrolyte deficiencies, hyperglycaemia, and dehydration (92, 109).

High-energy (calorie), high-protein diet

Patients with pre-existing malnutrition and those at nutritional risk due to poor intake may benefit from a high-energy, high-protein diet which come in many forms (liquids, bars, and puddings). While some patients may develop malnutrition following stroke, weight gain and obesity are encountered more frequently.

Excess weight is treated by a reduction in total energy intake, while other nutrient requirements remain age-appropriate. In addition, a diet low in fat, particularly saturated and trans fats, is recommended to maximize achievement of the blood lipid targets (110). Although constipation is a common complaint following stroke, this is thought to be due to a variety of factors, including decreased mobility, reduced fluid intake, and medication side effects. Stroke per se is not known to cause constipation but fluid intake of at least 1500 mL should be encouraged (111–113). Exercise and routine schedule for toileting should be encouraged. The risk of dehydration following stroke is a usual concern, particularly in those with dysphagia who are receiving all their nutrition orally (114, 115). The fluid requirement for adults is 20–40 mL/kg of body weight, or 1.0–1.5 mL/kcal of energy expended (116).

Total parenteral nutrition

This kind of nutrition is reserved for stroke patients with a non-functioning gastrointestinal tract, those with a pre-existing stroke medical condition that precludes safe oral or enteral feeding, dysphagic patients who refuse an enteral feeding device, patients with central lines placed for unrelated purposes, or patients with inflammatory bowel disease and when enteral feeding may be contraindicated. Because of the limited use of this feeding modality, there have been no studies about the efficacy of parenteral feeding in post-stroke patients (117).

The FOOD trial

The Feed or Ordinary Diet (FOOD) trials, addressed three clinically relevant questions (92, 109):

1. Does routine oral supplementation decrease the number of patients who have a poor outcome and patients requiring enteral feeding?

2. Do those who receive early feeding have better outcomes than patients whose feeding is delayed?

3. Do patients with PEG tubes have better outcomes than those with NG tubes?

The results of the trial suggest that routine supplementation does not reduce the odds of a poor outcome for all patients (4023 subjects).

The second and third trials, have shown, although not statistically significant, that the odds of death were slightly lower for patients in the early enteral group (95% confidence interval (CI) 1.4–2.7; p=0.5); however, survivors were more likely to be disabled (95% CI 2.3–3.8, p=0.6). In the PEG versus NG tube trial, PEG feeding was associated with a statistically borderline increase in the risk of death or poor outcome (95% CI 0.0–15.5; p=0.05). Interestingly there was no difference between the early tube-feeding and the avoid tube-feeding groups in frequency of recurring stroke, worsening of neurological impairment, or pneumonia, but there were significantly more gastrointestinal haemorrhages in the early group than in the avoid group (92, 118). Most haemorrhages occurred with the PEG or NG tube in place, but a number occurred after the tube was removed and significantly more haemorrhages occurred in the NG group (11%) than in the PEG group (3%) (92,109).

In summary, trials showed no reduction in death or poor outcome with routine oral protein-energy supplementation and NG tube feeding was favoured over PEG as the early route of feeding in dysphasic stroke patients.

Quality of life after stroke

Stroke is the most prevalent disabling disorder requiring neurorehabilitation. It is estimated that approximately 60% of stroke survivors are expected to recover independence, and 75% to walk independently (119). In neurorehabilitation the correct measurement of outcomes is not based on a single factor and the use of less than optimal scales for measuring outcome may cause problems.

QOL has been defined by the World Health Organization Quality of Life (WHOQOL) Group as 'individuals' perceptions of their position in life in the context of the culture and value systems in which they live and in relation to their goals, expectations, standards and concerns (120). The measurement of QOL typically includes physical, functional, psychological, cognitive, and social aspects of life and generally reflects an individual's subjective perception of his/her current function and overall health.

Health-related quality of life (HRQOL) is a self-reported measure consisting of multiple dimensions that includes, but is not limited to, physical, social, and emotional health (121).

Medical advances may prolong life, but it is important to know the nature of that increased life span. Without an assessment of QOL, a treatment may be supposed to be successful despite poor psychosocial functioning or adjustment to impairment. Alternatively, a treatment beneficial to psychosocial status may be rejected because it fails to improve physical function.

Disease-specific quality of life measuring device

Three disease-specific QOL measures have recently been developed for use with patients with stroke. The Stroke Adapted Sickness Impact Profile (SA-SIP30) is a modified version of the 136-item SIPS but it is not as sensitive as the SIP to the decline in QOL reported by the subjects who experienced more severe stroke (122–124). The second scale is version 2.0 of the Stroke Impact Scale (SIS) (125). This self-report measure includes 64 items within eight domains and scales and each domain score has a range of 0–100. SIS domains are sensitive to change as recovery progresses (124). The third and most recently developed stroke specific QOL instrument is the Stroke Specific Quality of Life Measure (SS-QOL). The 12 domains and 49 items included in this measure were initially obtained from interviews with stroke survivors (126). It seems additional research is required to evaluate the sensitivity of generic versus disease-specific QOL measures with stroke survivors and further investigation on the reliability, validity, and sensitivity of the SS-QOL is also necessary with larger numbers of cases (126).

Factors that influence quality of life

Several factors have been identified which contribute to the decreased QOL reported by stroke survivors. Increased age, the severity of motor impairment, lack of social supports, inability to return to work, cognition impairment, the presence of comorbid health problems, and supratentorial site of the lesion, have been correlated with a decreased QOL and should be considered when analysing stroke outcomes (127).

Depression

The presence of depression is highly correlated with and predictive of decreased QOL post stroke. A large percentage of stroke survivors (23–41%) have an acute onset of depression within the first few months of stroke (128–130). Post-stroke depression has been associated with impaired recovery of physical function as well as a decreased QOL and must be mentioned during the rehabilitation process in order to maximize stroke outcomes and improve post-stroke QOL. Moon et al. reported that symptoms of depression in the acute phase of stroke were of importance in predicting low QOL 2 months after stroke (131). Furthermore, Haache et al. and Jönsson et al. found that intervention or treatment targeting mood might improve QOL regardless of physical disability (132, 133).

Aphasia

Since the majority of studies have excluded individuals with significant aphasia, the effect of aphasia on QOL has not been adequately investigated. The few studies that did examine this relationship were inconclusive. Decreased functional independence has been correlated with a decreased QOL in the majority of studies reviewed (134).

Gender

Generally, it is believed that functional prognosis of stroke depends on gender. Some reports demonstrated that there is a connection between gender and cognitive functions of the patient (135). Female patients have been shown to experience more mental disorders, depression, and fatigue, as well as generally lower QOL after stroke compared to male patients. Wyller et al. found that males recorded better results in all questioned areas in their reports (136). Females had worse outcome, not only in motor function, but also in cognitive function and everyday activities (137). Some studies report that female patients with stroke have more dysfunction in daily activity after hospital treatment than male patients (138). In contrast, Wade et al. did not find significant gender differences in the outcome of stroke survivors (138). In a European study female patients were found to have a lower SIS score than men, but it could not be shown significantly (139, 140). This was confirmed in another study in Bosnia and Herzegovina (140, 141). This gender difference in functional outcome can be due to a different approach to their disability. For example, females may show a greater level of insecurity or anxiety and more openly ask for help, while males may present as more self-confident and less willing to ask for help (141).

Side of stroke

There is contradictory data regarding the effect of side of stroke on HRQOL (142). Several investigators have reported HRQOL to be worse in those with right-sided lesions, a finding attributed to neurological disturbances associated with right-sided lesions such as neglect, anosognosia, and spatial disorientation. This may have devastating effects on social functioning and thus on HRQOL (142). One study found that stroke patients with left-brain lesions more likely had communication difficulties secondary to defects of the left hemisphere (143) whereas another found that the side of stroke had little impact on the HRQOL outcomes (144).

Time after stroke

The impact of time since stroke onset on QOL remains controversial. The decrease of QOL over time (6 months to 2 years) in post-stroke survivors has been reported (145). Areas with the most significant decline included self-care needs, personal relationships, handling of life events, home management, and recreation (146). There are some reports of a slight increase in global QOL within the first 1–3 years post stroke (147). A decline in QOL over time may indicate that current strategies to assist patients with community and life re-integration are inadequate and that resources should be directed towards improving this aspect of post-stroke care (147).

Clinical application

These scales are not recommended for setting individual patient goals or monitoring individual patient progress and should not replace existing standardized instruments that examine impairments or functional limitations.

The ideal instrument for measuring QOL post stroke would be a reliable instrument for use by either patients or their proxies would have content validity and it would be responsive to significant patient changes across a wide range of clinical presentations. The potential difference between self-report scores and interview scores should be considered when collecting QOL outcome data as it may bias the data (148). It seems that use of a QOL instrument as one part of an assessment is likely to assist in identifying and targeting all facets of health to provide optimal health outcomes to stroke patients (148).

Stroke and the family

Stroke recovery is the last step that begins with the person's return to community living after acute care or rehabilitation. This stage can last for a lifetime as the stroke survivor and their family learn to live with the effects of the stroke. A family caregiver can be a relative, partner, personal friend, or neighbour who provides assistance to an older person or adult with a chronic or disabling condition. This person forms the core of recovery (149). Roughly 68–74% of stroke survivors are discharged home under the care of family members (149, 150).

Stroke caregivers must suddenly assume the caregiving role after a stroke event, whereas, for example, dementia caregivers typically assume the caregiving role gradually over time (151–154).

The role of family or partner

It is critical that caregivers understand the safety, physical, and emotional requests of the stroke survivor. The partner should participate in education offered to stroke survivors and their families. In addition, a family member could help the patient by exploring employment opportunities, volunteer activities, and by conversation about any concerns about sexual activity. Studies have shown that family caregivers are at risk for depression, psychosocial impairments, and mortality as a result of providing care (155–158).

Preparing a living place

Many stroke survivors can return to their own homes after rehabilitation. The stroke survivor needs a living place that supports continuing recovery or may suggest changes to make it safer. It is often suggested that the stroke survivor go home for a trial visit before discharge from hospital. This will help identify and clarify problems that need to be corrected before the patient returns more permanently. Adjusting to a return to the home or to a new one can be a difficult process.

Impact of stroke on other family members

Family caregivers have a variety of needs and concerns related to stroke care and also experience negative outcomes such as depression, declining health, and other life changes such as social and financial problems. They can reduce these problems by various strategies such as:

◆ Remembering that adjusting to the effects of stroke takes time.

◆ Expecting that knowledge and skills will grow with experience.

◆ Planning for 'breaks' so that you are not together all the time.

◆ Reading about the experiences of other people in similar situations.

◆ Joining or starting a support group for stroke survivors or caregivers.

Caregiver needs and concerns

Information

Having information about stroke is especially important for families because spouses and other family members are commonly the initiators of emergency care for stroke survivors (159–161). It is necessary that health professionals assess the knowledge of stroke warning signs in both patients and caregivers during follow-up visits. It had been reported that only 40% of stroke caregivers recall receiving any information about stroke prevention (162). Additional areas of stroke caregiver informational needs and concerns relate to:

◆ Medication management.

◆ The survivor's condition and treatment plans.

◆ Management of specific symptoms or problems that the survivor may have.

◆ Which health professionals to call for advice.

◆ Where to find books or written materials, support groups, or organizations that can help (160).

Emotions and behaviours

Managing emotional reactions of the stroke survivor are the most stressful aspects for family caregivers (163–167). Studies have documented that approximately one-third of ischaemic stroke survivors suffer from post-stroke depression (168–171). Additional survivor emotions and behaviour that are troublesome for stroke caregivers to manage include: feelings of worthlessness and being a burden on others, moodiness, irritability, anger, loss of temper, negative interpersonal exchanges, emotional dependency, confusion, cognitive difficulty, memory loss, personality changes, inertia waiting for others to do things the survivor can do, lack of participation in social activities, and difficulties in communication (172–175).

Physical care

Stroke caregivers have an important role in assisting the survivor with bathing, toileting, walking, mobility, exercises, meals, managing symptoms and deficits, and medication management (176). Caregivers can suggest such things as using pill boxes for medications, taking the survivor to the mall for exercise, avoiding clutter to prevent falls, taking advantage of resources like Meals on Wheels, following a bladder and bowel regimen, and encouraging the survivor to do as much self-care as possible (160). Health professionals should encourage caregivers to attend therapy sessions with the survivor to learn transfer techniques and how to assist with activities of daily living.

Personal responses to care giving

Caregivers will often share their needs and concerns about the stroke survivors before they will share their own personal needs and concerns (160). Some of this concern is about their own emotions while providing care, shouldering new responsibilities, balancing caregiving with existing responsibilities, asking friends and family members for help, keeping their own social life going, balancing their energy level up, and taking care of their own health (160). The most difficult time for caregivers is during hospitalization and the first few months after the patient is discharged home (162). Hence, there is a need for early caregiver assessment followed by individualized caregiver interventions during these critical time periods following a stroke.

Caregiver outcomes

The caregiving experience is often stressful and can result in negative physical and mental health outcomes for the family caregiver. A comprehensive approach to stroke after care should include comprehensive assessment of caregiver function (177). In fact, some studies have reported higher depression rates in caregivers than in the stroke survivors (178). There is evidence that depression in stroke caregivers worsens the patient's depressive symptoms and predicts poor responses of patients to rehabilitation (155). It has been reported that 54% of the children in patients' families showed at least one behavioural problem or depression between 2 months and 1 year after their parent's discharge (179, 180).

Stroke caregiver intervention research

Jonathan et al. noted in one study that carers in the intervention group had significantly better activity indices, mental health, physical function and general health perception, QOL, satisfaction with understanding of stroke and less depression and anxiety, than those in the control group (176). It seems that caregiver intervention studies that better target the needs and concerns of family caregivers, rather than only the needs of stroke patients, are more useful (176, 181). In addition, combined education with problem-solving strategies is much more effective in improving caregiver knowledge, family functioning, problem-solving strategies, and even patient adjustment than using education alone (182, 183).

References

1. Heuschmann PU, Kolominsky-Rabas PL, Misselwitz B, Hermanek P, Leffmann C, Janzen RW, et al. Predictors of in-hospital mortality and attributable risks of death after ischemic stroke: the German Stroke Registers Study Group. *Arch Intern Med*. 2004;164(16):1761–1768.

2. World Stroke Organization. <http://www.world-stroke.org/index. php>.

3. Dobkin BH. Management of transient ischemic attacks. *Hosp Pract*. 1987;22(3):113–117, 120, 123–124 passim.

4. Dromerick A, Reding M. Medical and neurological complications during inpatient stroke rehabilitation. *Stroke*. 1994;25(2):358–361.

5. Johnston KC, Li JY, Lyden PD, Hanson SK, Feasby TE, Adams RJ, et al. Medical and neurological complications of ischemic stroke: experience from the RANTTAS trial. RANTTAS Investigators. *Stroke*. 1998;29(2):447–453.

6. Kalra L, Yu G, Wilson K, Roots P. Medical complications during stroke rehabilitation. *Stroke*. 1995;26(6):990–994.

7. Roth EJ, Lovell L, Harvey RL, Heinemann AW, Semik P, Diaz S. Incidence of and risk factors for medical complications during stroke rehabilitation. *Stroke*. 2001;32(2):523–529.

8. Siegler EL, Stineman MG, Maislin G. Development of complications during rehabilitation. *Arch Intern Med*. 1994;154(19):2185–2190.

9. Davenport RJ, Dennis MS, Wellwood I, Warlow CP. Complications after acute stroke. *Stroke*. 1996;27(3):415–420.

10. Langhorne P, Stott DJ, Robertson L, MacDonald J, Jones L, McAlpine C, *et al*. Medical complications after stroke: a multicenter study. *Stroke*. 2000;31(6):1223–1229.

11. Evans A, Perez I, Harraf F, Melbourn A, Steadman J, Donaldson N, *et al*. Can differences in management processes explain different outcomes between stroke unit and stroke-team care? *Lancet*. 2001;358(9293):1586–1592.

12. Kimura K, Minematsu K, Kazui S, Yamaguchi T, Japan Multicenter Stroke Investigators C. Mortality and cause of death after hospital discharge in 10,981 patients with ischemic stroke and transient ischemic attack. *Cerebrovasc Dis*. 2005;19(3):171–178.

13. Ramsey D, Smithard D, Kalra L. Silent aspiration: what do we know? *Dysphagia*. 2005;20(3):218–225.

14. Addington WR, Stephens RE, Gilliland KA. Assessing the laryngeal cough reflex and the risk of developing pneumonia after stroke: an interhospital comparison. *Stroke*. 1999;30(6):1203–1207.

15. Smith Hammond CA, Goldstein LB, Zajac DJ, Gray L, Davenport PW, Bolser DC. Assessment of aspiration risk in stroke patients with quantification of voluntary cough. *Neurology*. 2001;56(4):502–506.

16. Urban PP, Morgenstern M, Brause K, Wicht S, Vukurevic G, Kessler S, *et al*. Distribution and course of cortico-respiratory projections for voluntary activation in man. A transcranial magnetic stimulation study in healthy subjects and patients with cerebral ischemia. *J Neurol*. 2002;249(6):735–744.

17. Prass K, Meisel C, Hoflich C, Braun J, Halle E, Wolf T, *et al*. Stroke-induced immunodeficiency promotes spontaneous bacterial infections and is mediated by sympathetic activation reversal by poststroke T helper cell type 1-like immunostimulation. *J Exp Med*. 2003;198(5):725–736.

18. Chamorro A, Horcajada JP, Obach V, Vargas M, Revilla M, Torres F, *et al*. The Early Systemic Prophylaxis of Infection After Stroke study: a randomized clinical trial. *Stroke*. 2005;36(7):1495–1500.

19. Gosney M, Martin MV, Wright AE. The role of selective decontamination of the digestive tract in acute stroke. *Age Ageing*. 2006;35(1):42–47.

20. Party ISW. *National Clinical Guidelines for Stroke* (2nd edn). London: Clinical Effectiveness & Evaluation Unit, Royal College of Physicians; 2004.

21. Forster A, Young J. Incidence and consequences of falls due to stroke: a systematic inquiry. *BMJ*. 1995;311(6997):83–86.

22. Stein J, Viramontes BE, Kerrigan DC. Fall-related injuries in anticoagulated stroke patients during inpatient rehabilitation. *Arch Phys Med Rehabil*. 1995;76(9):840–843.

23. Suzuki T, Sonoda S, Misawa K, Saitoh E, Shimizu Y, Kotake T. Incidence and consequence of falls in inpatient rehabilitation of stroke patients. *Exp Aging Res*. 2005;31(4):457–469.

24. Teasell R, Foley N, Bhogal S, Bagg S, Jutai J. Evidence-based practice and setting basic standards for stroke rehabilitation in Canada. *Top Stroke Rehabil*. 2006;13(3):59–65.

25. Nakayama H, Jorgensen HS, Pedersen PM, Raaschou HO, Olsen TS. Prevalence and risk factors of incontinence after stroke. The Copenhagen Stroke Study. *Stroke*. 1997;28(1):58–62.

26. Zorowitz RD, Smout RJ, Gassaway JA, Horn SD. Prophylaxis for and treatment of deep venous thrombosis after stroke: the Post-Stroke Rehabilitation Outcomes Project (PSROP). *Top Stroke Rehabil*. 2005;12(4):1–10.

27. Wilson RD, Murray PK. Cost-effectiveness of screening for deep vein thrombosis by ultrasound at admission to stroke rehabilitation. *Arch Phys Med Rehabil*. 2005;86(10):1941–1948.

28. Bounds JV, Wiebers DO, Whisnant JP, Okazaki H. Mechanisms and timing of deaths from cerebral infarction. *Stroke*. 1981;12(4):474–477.

29. Wijdicks EF, Scott JP. Pulmonary embolism associated with acute stroke. *Mayo Clin Proc*. 1997;72(4):297–300.

30. Imberti D, Prisco D. Venous thromboembolism prophylaxis in medical patients: future perspectives. *Thrombos Res*. 2005;116(5):365–375.

31. Skaf E, Stein PD, Beemath A, Sanchez J, Bustamante MA, Olson RE. Venous thromboembolism in patients with ischemic and hemorrhagic stroke. *Am J Cardiol*. 2005;96(12):1731–1733.

32. Adams HP, Jr., Adams RJ, Brott T, del Zoppo GJ, Furlan A, Goldstein LB, *et al*. Guidelines for the early management of patients with ischemic stroke: A scientific statement from the Stroke Council of the American Stroke Association. *Stroke*. 2003;34(4):1056–1083.

33. Andre C, de Freitas GR, Fukujima MM. Prevention of deep venous thrombosis and pulmonary embolism following stroke: a systematic review of published articles. *Eur J Neurol*. 2007;14(1):21–32.

34. Boomkamp-Koppen HG, Visser-Meily JM, Post MW, Prevo AJ. Poststroke hand swelling and oedema: prevalence and relationship with impairment and disability. *Clin Rehabil*. 2005;19(5):552–559.

35. Geurts AC, Visschers BA, van Limbeek J, Ribbers GM. Systematic review of aetiology and treatment of post-stroke hand oedema and shoulder-hand syndrome. *Scand J Rehabil Med*. 2000;32(1):4–10.

36. Stroemer RP, Kent TA, Hulsebosch CE. Neocortical neural sprouting, synaptogenesis, and behavioral recovery after neocortical infarction in rats. *Stroke*. 1995;26(11):2135–2144.

37. Kawamata T, Speliotes EK, Finklestein SP. The role of polypeptide growth factors in recovery from stroke. *Adv Neurol*. 1997;73:377–382.

38. Finklestein SP, Caday CG, Kano M, Berlove DJ, Hsu CY, Moskowitz M, *et al*. Growth factor expression after stroke. *Stroke*. 1990;21(11 Suppl):III122–124.

39. Koketsu N, Berlove DJ, Moskowitz MA, Kowall NW, Caday CG, Finklestein SP. Pretreatment with intraventricular basic fibroblast growth factor decreases infarct size following focal cerebral ischemia in rats. *Ann Neurol*. 1994;35(4):451–457.

40. Hackett ML, Anderson CS, Auckland Regional Community Stroke Study G. Frequency, management, and predictors of abnormal mood after stroke: the Auckland Regional Community Stroke (ARCOS) study, 2002 to 2003. *Stroke*. 2006;37(8):2123–2128.

41. Speliotes EK, Caday CG, Do T, Weise J, Kowall NW, Finklestein SP. Increased expression of basic fibroblast growth factor (bFGF) following focal cerebral infarction in the rat. *Brain Res Mol Brain Res*. 1996;39(1–2):31–42.

42. Fedoroff JP, Starkstein SE, Parikh RM, Price TR, Robinson RG. Are depressive symptoms nonspecific in patients with acute stroke? *Am J Psychiatry*. 1991;148(9):1172–1176.

43. Gainotti G, Azzoni A, Gasparini F, Marra C, Razzano C. Relation of lesion location to verbal and nonverbal mood measures in stroke patients. *Stroke*. 1997;28(11):2145–2149.

44. Sutcliffe LM, Lincoln NB. The assessment of depression in aphasic stroke patients: the development of the Stroke Aphasic Depression Questionnaire. *Clin Rehabil*. 1998;12(6):506–513.

45. Ramasubbu R. Denial of illness and depression in stroke. *Stroke*. 1994;25(1):226–227.

46. Ekman P, Friesen WV. Constants across cultures in the face and emotion. *J Pers Soc Psychol*. 1971;17(2):124–129.

47. Starkstein SE, Fedoroff JP, Price TR, Leiguarda R, Robinson RG. Apathy following cerebrovascular lesions. *Stroke*. 1993;24(11):1625–1630.

48. Okada K, Kobayashi S, Yamagata S, Takahashi K, Yamaguchi S. Poststroke apathy and regional cerebral blood flow. *Stroke*. 1997;28(12):2437–2441.

49. Caplan LR, Schmahmann JD, Kase CS, Feldmann E, Baquis G, Greenberg JP, *et al*. Caudate infarcts. *Arch Neurol*. 1990;47(2):133–143.

50. Danel T, Goudemand M, Ghawche F, Godefroy O, Pruvo JP, Vaiva G, *et al*. [Delusional melancholia and multiple lacunar infarcts of the basal ganglia]. *Revue Neurologique*. 1991;147(1):60–62.

51. Degl'Innocenti A, Agren H, Backman L. Executive deficits in major depression. *Acta Psychiatr Scand.* 1998;97(3):182–188.

52. Willeit M, Praschak-Rieder N, Neumeister A, Pirker W, Asenbaum S, Vitouch O, et al. [123I]-beta-CIT SPECT imaging shows reduced brain serotonin transporter availability in drug-free depressed patients with seasonal affective disorder. *Biol Psychiatry.* 2000;47(6):482–489.

53. Chabriat H, Joutel A, Vahedi K, Iba-Zizen MT, Tournier-Lasserve E, Bousser MG. [CADASIS. Cerebral autosomal dominant arteriopathy with subcortical infarcts and leukoencephalopathy]. *Revue Neurologique.* 1997;153(6–7):376–385.

54. Pearlson GD, Robinson RG. Suction lesions of the frontal cerebral cortex in the rat induce asymmetrical behavioral and catecholaminergic responses. *Brain Res.* 1981;218(1–2):233–242.

55. Starkstein SE, Robinson RG, Price TR. Comparison of patients with and without poststroke major depression matched for size and location of lesion. *Arch Gen Psychiatry.* 1988;45(3):247–252.

56. Starkstein SE, Robinson RG, Price TR. Comparison of cortical and subcortical lesions in the production of poststroke mood disorders. *Brain.* 1987;110(Pt 4):1045–1059.

57. Storor DL, Byrne GJ. Pre-morbid personality and depression following stroke. *Int Psychogeriatr.* 2006;18(3):457–469.

58. Carota A, Dieguez S, Bogousslavsky J. [Psychopathology of stroke]. *Psychologie & neuropsychiatrie du vieillissement.* 2005;3(4):235–249.

59. Robinson RG, Price TR. Post-stroke depressive disorders: a follow-up study of 103 patients. *Stroke.* 1982;13(5):635–641.

60. Gustafson Y, Nilsson I, Mattsson M, Astrom M, Bucht G. Epidemiology and treatment of post-stroke depression. *Drugs Aging.* 1995;7(4):298–309.

61. Lauritzen L, Bendsen BB, Vilmar T, Bendsen EB, Lunde M, Bech P. Post-stroke depression: combined treatment with imipramine or desipramine and mianserin. A controlled clinical study. *Psychopharmacology.* 1994;114(1):119–122.

62. Hougaku H, Matsumoto M, Hata R, Handa N, Imaizumi M, Sugitani Y, et al. [Therapeutic effect of lisuride maleate on post-stroke depression]. *Nihon Ronen Igakkai zasshi [Japn J Geriatr].* 1994;31(1):52–59.

63. van de Weg FB, Kuik DJ, Lankhorst GJ. Post-stroke depression and functional outcome: a cohort study investigating the influence of depression on functional recovery from stroke. *Clin Rehabil.* 1999;13(3):268–272.

64. Morris PL, Raphael B, Robinson RG. Clinical depression is associated with impaired recovery from stroke. *Med J Aust.* 1992;157(4):239–242.

65. Robinson RG, Schultz SK, Castillo C, Kopel T, Kosier JT, Newman RM, et al. Nortriptyline versus fluoxetine in the treatment of depression and in short-term recovery after stroke: a placebo-controlled, double-blind study. *Am J Psychiatry.* 2000;157(3):351–359.

66. Parikh RM, Lipsey JR, Robinson RG, Price TR. Two-year longitudinal study of post-stroke mood disorders: dynamic changes in correlates of depression at one and two years. *Stroke.* 1987;18(3):579–584.

67. Murray GB, Shea V, Conn DK. Electroconvulsive therapy for poststroke depression. *J Clin Psychiatry.* 1986;47(5):258–260.

68. Currier MB, Murray GB, Welch CC. Electroconvulsive therapy for post-stroke depressed geriatric patients. *J Neuropsychiatry Clin Neurosci.* 1992;4(2):140–144.

69. Jorge RE, Robinson RG, Starkstein SE, Arndt SV, Forrester AW, Geisler FH. Secondary mania following traumatic brain injury. *Am J Psychiatry.* 1993;150(6):916–921.

70. Starkstein SE, Fedoroff P, Berthier ML, Robinson RG. Manic-depressive and pure manic states after brain lesions. *Biol Psychiatry.* 1991;29(2):149–158.

71. McGilchrist I, Goldstein LH, Jadresic D, Fenwick P. Thalamo-frontal psychosis. *Br J Psychiatry.* 1993;163:113–115.

72. Kulisevsky J, Berthier ML, Pujol J. Hemiballismus and secondary mania following a right thalamic infarction. *Neurology.* 1993;43(7):1422–1424.

73. Bogousslavsky J, Ferrazzini M, Regli F, Assal G, Tanabe H, Delaloye-Bischof A. Manic delirium and frontal-like syndrome with paramedian infarction of the right thalamus. *J Neurol Neurosurg Psychiatry.* 1988;51(1):116–119.

74. Turecki G, Mari Jde J, Del Porto JA. Bipolar disorder following a left basal-ganglia stroke. *Br J Psychiatry.* 1993;163:690.

75. Drake ME, Jr., Pakalnis A, Phillips B. Secondary mania after ventral pontine infarction. *J Neuropsychiatr Clin Neurosci.* 1990;2(3):322–325.

76. Celik Y, Erdogan E, Tuglu C, Utku U. Post-stroke mania in late life due to right temporoparietal infarction. *Psychiatry Clin Neurosci.* 2004;58(4):446–447.

77. Levine DN, Finklestein S. Delayed psychosis after right temporoparietal stroke or trauma: relation to epilepsy. *Neurology.* 1982;32(3):267–273.

78. Price BH, Mesulam M. Psychiatric manifestations of right hemisphere infarctions. *J Nerv Ment Dis.* 1985;173(10):610–614.

79. Pakalnis A, Drake ME, Jr., Kellum JB. Right parieto-occipital lacunar infarction with agitation, hallucinations, and delusions. *Psychosomatics.* 1987;28(2):95–96.

80. Anderson SW, Rizzo M. Hallucinations following occipital lobe damage: the pathological activation of visual representations. *J Clin Exper Neuropsychol.* 1994;16(5):651–663.

81. Schultz SK, Castillo CS, Kosier JT, Robinson RG. Generalized anxiety and depression. Assessment over 2 years after stroke. *Am J Geriatr Psychiatry.* 1997;5(3):229–237.

82. Astrom M. Generalized anxiety disorder in stroke patients. A 3-year longitudinal study. *Stroke.* 1996;27(2):270–275.

83. Astrom M. [Depression after stroke. Antidepressive therapy enhances recovery]. *Lakartidningen.* 1994;91(10):963–966.

84. Starkstein SE, Cohen BS, Fedoroff P, Parikh RM, Price TR, Robinson RG. Relationship between anxiety disorders and depressive disorders in patients with cerebrovascular injury. *Arch Gen Psychiat.* 1990;47(3):246–251.

85. Morrison VL, Johnston M, MacWalter RS, Pollard BS. Improving emotional outcomes following acute stroke: a preliminary evaluation of work-book based intervention. *Scot Med J.* 1998;43(2):52–53.

86. Kishi Y, Kosier JT, Robinson RG. Suicidal plans in patients with acute stroke. *J Nerv Ment Dis.* 1996;184(5):274–280.

87. Kishi Y, Robinson RG, Kosier JT. Suicidal plans in patients with stroke: comparison between acute-onset and delayed-onset suicidal plans. *Int Psychogeriatr.* 1996;8(4):623–634.

88. Davalos A, Ricart W, Gonzalez-Huix F, Soler S, Marrugat J, Molins A, et al. Effect of malnutrition after acute stroke on clinical outcome. *Stroke.* 1996;27(6):1028–1032.

89. Foley NC, Martin RE, Salter KL, Teasell RW. A review of the relationship between dysphagia and malnutrition following stroke. *J Rehabil Med.* 2009;41(9):707–713.

90. Wardlaw JM, Marshall I, Wild J, Dennis MS, Cannon J, Lewis SC. Studies of acute ischemic stroke with proton magnetic resonance spectroscopy: relation between time from onset, neurological deficit, metabolite abnormalities in the infarct, blood flow, and clinical outcome. *Stroke.* 1998;29(8):1618–1624.

91. Collaboration FT. Poor nutritional status on admission predicts poor outcomes after stroke: observational data from the FOOD trial. *Stroke.* 2003;34(6):1450–1456.

92. Dennis MS, Lewis SC, Warlow C, Collaboration FT. Effect of timing and method of enteral tube feeding for dysphagic stroke patients (FOOD): a multicentre randomised controlled trial. *Lancet.* 2005;365(9461):764–772.

93. Aptaker RL, Roth EJ, Reichhardt G, Duerden ME, Levy CE. Serum albumin level as a predictor of geriatric stroke rehabilitation outcome. *Arch Phys Med Rehabil.* 1994;75(1):80–84.

94. Ullegaddi R, Powers HJ, Gariballa SE. Antioxidant supplementation enhances antioxidant capacity and mitigates oxidative damage following acute ischaemic stroke. *Eur J Clin Nutr.* 2005;59(12):1367–1373.

95. Staal-van den Brekel AJ, Dentener MA, Schols AM, Buurman WA, Wouters EF. Increased resting energy expenditure and weight loss are

related to a systemic inflammatory response in lung cancer patients. *J Clin Oncol.* 1995;13(10):2600–2605.

96. Mead GE, Donaldson L, North P, Dennis MS. An informal assessment of nutritional status in acute stroke for use in an international multicentre trial of feeding regimens. *Int J Clin Pract.* 1998;52(5):316–318.

97. Nightingale JM, Walsh N, Bullock ME, Wicks AC. Three simple methods of detecting malnutrition on medical wards. *J R Soc Med.* 1996;89(3):144–148.

98. Deitrick JE, Whedon GD, Shorr E. Effects of immobilization upon various metabolic and physiologic functions of normal men. *Am J Med.* 1948;4(1):3–36.

99. Fleck A. Clinical and nutritional aspects of changes in acute-phase proteins during inflammation. *Proc Nutr Soc.* 1989;48(3):347–354.

100. Akner G, Cederholm T. Treatment of protein-energy malnutrition in chronic nonmalignant disorders. *Am J Clin Nutr.* 2001;74(1):6–24.

101. Yoo SH, Kim JS, Kwon SU, Yun SC, Koh JY, Kang DW. Undernutrition as a predictor of poor clinical outcomes in acute ischemic stroke patients. *Arch Neurol.* 2008;65(1):39–43.

102. Finestone HM, Greene-Finestone LS, Wilson ES, Teasell RW. Malnutrition in stroke patients on the rehabilitation service and at follow-up: prevalence and predictors. *Arch Phys Med Rehabil.* 1995;76(4):310–316.

103. James R, Gines D, Menlove A, Horn SD, Gassaway J, Smout RJ. Nutrition support (tube feeding) as a rehabilitation intervention. *Arch Phys Med Rehabil.* 2005;86(12 Suppl 2):S82–S92.

104. Park RH, Allison MC, Lang J, Spence E, Morris AJ, Danesh BJ, et al. Randomised comparison of percutaneous endoscopic gastrostomy and nasogastric tube feeding in patients with persisting neurological dysphagia. *BMJ.* 1992;304(6839):1406–1409.

105. Hamidon BB, Abdullah SA, Zawawi MF, Sukumar N, Aminuddin A, Raymond AA. A prospective comparison of percutaneous endoscopic gastrostomy and nasogastric tube feeding in patients with acute dysphagic stroke. *Med J Malaysia.* 2006;61(1):59–66.

106. Norton B, Homer-Ward M, Donnelly MT, Long RG, Holmes GK. A randomised prospective comparison of percutaneous endoscopic gastrostomy and nasogastric tube feeding after acute dysphagic stroke. *BMJ.* 1996;312(7022):13–16.

107. Aquilani R, Scocchi M, Boschi F, Viglio S, Iadarola P, Pastoris O, et al. Effect of calorie-protein supplementation on the cognitive recovery of patients with subacute stroke. *Nutr Neurosci.* 2008;11(5):235–240.

108. Lord L, Harrington M. *Enteral Nutrition Implementation and Management* (2nd edn). Silver Springs, MD: American Society for Parenteral and Enteral Nutrition; 2005.

109. Dennis MS, Lewis SC, Warlow C, Collaboration FT. Routine oral nutritional supplementation for stroke patients in hospital (FOOD): a multicentre randomised controlled trial. *Lancet.* 2005;365(9461):755–63.

110. Trumbo P, Schlicker S, Yates AA, Poos M, Food and Nutrition Board of the Institute of Medicine, The National Academies. Dietary reference intakes for energy, carbohydrate, fiber, fat, fatty acids, cholesterol, protein and amino acids. *J Am Diet Assoc.* 2002;102(11):1621–1630.

111. Richmond JP WM. Review of the literature on constipation to enable development of a constipation risk assessment scale. *Clin Effect Nurs.* 2004;8(1):11–25.

112. Finestone HM, Foley NC, Woodbury MG, Greene-Finestone L. Quantifying fluid intake in dysphagic stroke patients: a preliminary comparison of oral and nonoral strategies. *Arch Phys Med Rehabil.* 2001;82(12):1744–1746.

113. Jonnalagadda SS, Thye FW, Robertson JL. Plasma total and lipoprotein cholesterol, liver cholesterol and fecal cholesterol excretion in hamsters fed fiber diets. *J Nutr.* 1993;123(8):1377–1382.

114. Whelan K. Inadequate fluid intakes in dysphagic acute stroke. *Clin Nutr.* 2001;20(5):423–438.

115. Forchielli ML Miller S. *Nutritional Goals and Requirements* (2nd edn). Silver Springs, MD: American Society for Parenteral and Enteral Nutrition; 2005.

116. Garcia ME. Dehydration of the elderly in nursing homes. *Nutr Noteworthy.* 2001;4:1–8.

117. Eskaros S, Ghevariya V, Krishnaiah M, Asarian A, Anand S. Percutaneous endoscopic suturing: an effective treatment for gastrocutaneous fistula. *Gastrointest Endosc.* 2009;70(4):768–771.

118. Buzby GP, Mullen JL, Matthews DC, Hobbs CL, Rosato EF. Prognostic nutritional index in gastrointestinal surgery. *Am J Surg.* 1980;139(1):160–167.

119. Buck D, Jacoby A, Massey A, Ford G. Evaluation of measures used to assess quality of life after stroke. *Stroke.* 2000;31(8):2004–2010.

120. Smith GV, Silver KH, Goldberg AP, Macko RF. "Task-oriented" exercise improves hamstring strength and spastic reflexes in chronic stroke patients. *Stroke.* 1999;30(10):2112–2118.

121. Teixeira-Salmela LF, Olney SJ, Nadeau S, Brouwer B. Muscle strengthening and physical conditioning to reduce impairment and disability in chronic stroke survivors. *Arch Phys Med Rehabil.* 1999;80(10):1211–1218.

122. van der Lee JH, Wagenaar RC, Lankhorst GJ, Vogelaar TW, Deville WL, Bouter LM. Forced use of the upper extremity in chronic stroke patients: results from a single-blind randomized clinical trial. *Stroke.* 1999;30(11):2369–2375.

123. Williams LS. Health-related quality of life outcomes in stroke. *Neuroepidemiology.* 1998;17(3):116–120.

124. Kranciukaite D, Rastenyte D. Measurement of quality of life in stroke patients. *Medicina (Kaunas).* 2006;42(9):709–716.

125. Duncan PW, Wallace D, Lai SM, Johnson D, Embretson S, Laster LJ. The stroke impact scale version 2.0. Evaluation of reliability, validity, and sensitivity to change. *Stroke.* 1999;30(10):2131–2140.

126. Saladin LK, Morrisette DC, Brotherton SS. Making the physical therapy referral. *JAAPA.* 1999;12(2):18–20, 3, 7–32 passim.

127. Sacco RL, Adams R, Albers G, Alberts MJ, Benavente O, Furie K, et al. Guidelines for prevention of stroke in patients with ischemic stroke or transient ischemic attack: a statement for healthcare professionals from the American Heart Association/American Stroke Association Council on Stroke: co-sponsored by the Council on Cardiovascular Radiology and Intervention: the American Academy of Neurology affirms the value of this guideline. *Stroke.* 2006;37(2):577–617.

128. Andersen G, Vestergaard K, Ingemann-Nielsen M, Lauritzen L. Risk factors for post-stroke depression. *Acta Psychiatr Scand.* 1995;92(3):193–198.

129. Astrom M AK. Handicap and quality of life after stroke. In J Bogousslavsky (ed) *Long-Term Effects of Stroke* (pp. 25–50). New York: Marcel Dekker; 2002.

130. Berg A, Psych L, Palomaki H, Lehtihalmes M, Phil L, Lonnqvist J, et al. Poststroke depression – An 18-month follow-up. *Stroke.* 2003;34(1):138–143.

131. Kauhanen ML, Korpelainen JT, Hiltunen P, Brusin E, Mononen H, Maatta R, et al. Poststroke depression correlates with cognitive impairment and neurological deficits. *Stroke.* 1999;30(9):1875–1880.

132. Duncan PW, Wallace D, Lai SM, Johnson D, Embretson S, Laster LJ. The stroke impact scale version 2.0 – Evaluation of reliability, validity, and sensitivity to change. *Stroke.* 1999;30(10):2131–2140.

133. Jonsson AC, Lindgren I, Hallstrom B, Norrving B, Lindgren A. Determinants of quality of life in stroke survivors and their informal caregivers. *Stroke.* 2005;36(4):803–808.

134. Hilari K, Byng S, Lamping DL, Smith SC. Stroke and aphasia quality of life scale-39 (SAQOL-39) – Evaluation of acceptability, reliability, and validity. *Stroke.* 2003;34(8):1944–1950.

135. Zalihic A, Markotic V, Zalihic D, Mabic M. Gender and quality of life after cerebral stroke. *Bosnian J Basic Med.* 2010;10(2):94–99.

136. Gargano JW, Reeves MJ. Sex differences in stroke recovery and stroke-specific quality of life – Results from a statewide stroke registry. *Stroke.* 2007;38(9):2541–2548.

137. Wyller TB, Holmen J, Laake P, Laake K. Correlates of subjective well-being in stroke patients. *Stroke.* 1998;29(2):363–367.

138. Wade DT, Hewer RL, Wood VA. Stroke: influence of patient's sex and side of weakness on outcome. *Arch Phys Med Rehabil.* 1984;65(9):513–516.

139. Gray LJ, Sprigg N, Bath PM, Boysen G, De Deyn PP, Leys D, et al. Sex differences in quality of life in stroke survivors: data from the Tinzaparin in Acute Ischaemic Stroke Trial (TAIST). *Stroke*. 2007;38(11):2960–2964.

140. Zalihic A, Markotic V, Mabic M, Cerni-Obrdalj E, Zalihic D, Pivic G, et al. Differences in quality of life after stroke and myocardial infarction. *Psychiatr Danub*. 2010;22(2):241–248.

141. de Haan RJ, Limburg M, Van der Meulen JH, Jacobs HM, Aaronson NK. Quality of life after stroke. Impact of stroke type and lesion location. *Stroke*. 1995;26(3):402–408.

142. Sturm JW, Donnan GA, Dewey HM, Macdonell RA, Gilligan AK, Srikanth V, et al. Quality of life after stroke: the North East Melbourne Stroke Incidence Study (NEMESIS). *Stroke*. 2004;35(10):2340–2345.

143. Riley JD, Le V, Der-Yeghiaian L, See J, Newton JM, Ward NS, et al. Anatomy of stroke injury predicts gains from therapy. *Stroke*. 2011;42(2):421–426.

144. Hopman WM, Verner J. Quality of life during and after inpatient stroke rehabilitation. *Stroke*. 2003;34(3):801–805.

145. King RB. Quality of life after stroke. *Stroke*. 1996;27(9):1467–1472.

146. Stavem K, Ronning OM. Quality of life 6 months after acute stroke: impact of initial treatment in a stroke unit and general medical wards. *Cerebrovasc Dis*. 2007;23(5–6):417–423.

147. Choi-Kwon S, Choi JM, Kwon SU, Kang DW, Kim JS. Factors that affect the quality of life at 3 years post-stroke. *J Clin Neurol*. 2006;2(1):34–41.

148. Bircher J. Towards a dynamic definition of health and disease. *Med Health Care Philos*. 2005;8(3):335–341.

149. Dewey HM, Thrift AG, Mihalopoulos C, Carter R, Macdonell RA, McNeil JJ, et al. Informal care for stroke survivors: results from the North East Melbourne Stroke Incidence Study (NEMESIS). *Stroke*. 2002;33(4):1028–1033.

150. Dorsey MK, Vaca KJ. The stroke patient and assessment of caregiver needs. *J Vasc Nurs*. 1998;16(3):62–7.

151. Wright LK, Hickey JV, Buckwalter KC, Clipp EC. Human development in the context of aging and chronic illness: the role of attachment in Alzheimer's disease and stroke. *Int J Aging Hum Dev*. 1995;41(2):133–150.

152. Thom T, Haase N, Rosamond W, Howard VJ, Rumsfeld J, Manolio T, et al. Heart disease and stroke statistics—2006 update: a report from the American Heart Association Statistics Committee and Stroke Statistics Subcommittee. *Circulation*. 2006;113(6):e85–151.

153. Kelly-Hayes M, Robertson JT, Broderick JP, Duncan PW, Hershey LA, Roth EJ, et al. The American Heart Association Stroke Outcome Classification. *Stroke*. 1998;29(6):1274–1280.

154. Adams R, Acker J, Alberts M, Andrews L, Atkinson R, Fenelon K, et al. Recommendations for improving the quality of care through stroke centers and systems: an examination of stroke center identification options: multidisciplinary consensus recommendations from the Advisory Working Group on Stroke Center Identification Options of the American Stroke Association. *Stroke*. 2002;33(1):e1–7.

155. Han B, Haley WE. Family caregiving for patients with stroke. Review and analysis. *Stroke*. 1999;30(7):1478–1485.

156. Low JT, Payne S, Roderick P. The impact of stroke on informal carers: a literature review. *Soc Sci Med*. 1999;49(6):711–725.

157. Schulz R, Beach SR. Caregiving as a risk factor for mortality: the Caregiver Health Effects Study. *JAMA* 1999;282(23):2215–2219.

158. Schulz R, Beach SR, Lind B, Martire LM, Zdaniuk B, Hirsch C, et al. Involvement in caregiving and adjustment to death of a spouse: findings from the caregiver health effects study. *JAMA* 2001;285(24):3123–3129.

159. Maze LM, Bakas T. Factors associated with hospital arrival time for stroke patients. *J Neurosci Nurs*. 2004;36(3):136–141.

160. Bakas T, Austin JK, Okonkwo KF, Lewis RR, Chadwick L. Needs, concerns, strategies, and advice of stroke caregivers the first 6 months after discharge. *J Neurosci Nurs*. 2002;34(5):242–251.

161. Hanger HC, Walker G, Paterson LA, McBride S, Sainsbury R. What do patients and their carers want to know about stroke? A two-year follow-up study. *Clin Rehabil*. 1998;12(1):45–52.

162. Visser-Meily A, Post M, Meijer AM, van de Port I, Maas C, Lindeman E. When a parent has a stroke: clinical course and prediction of mood, behavior problems, and health status of their young children. *Stroke*. 2005;36(11):2436–2440.

163. Cameron JI, Cheung AM, Streiner DL, Coyte PC, Stewart DE. Stroke survivors' behavioral and psychologic symptoms are associated with informal caregivers' experiences of depression. *Arch Phys Med Rehabil*. 2006;87(2):177–183.

164. Clark PC, Dunbar SB, Aycock DM, Courtney E, Wolf SL. Caregiver perspectives of memory and behavior changes in stroke survivors. *Rehabil Nurs*. 2006;31(1):26–32.

165. Clark PC, Dunbar SB, Shields CG, Viswanathan B, Aycock DM, Wolf SL. Influence of stroke survivor characteristics and family conflict surrounding recovery on caregivers' mental and physical health. *Nurs Res*. 2004;53(6):406–413.

166. Davis LL, Grant JS. Constructing the reality of recovery: family home care management strategies. *ANS*. 1994;17(2):66–76.

167. Stewart MJ, Doble S, Hart G, Langille L, MacPherson K. Peer visitor support for family caregivers of seniors with stroke. *Can J Nurs Res*. 1998;30(2):87–117.

168. Burvill PW, Johnson GA, Jamrozik KD, Anderson CS, Stewart-Wynne EG, Chakera TM. Prevalence of depression after stroke: the Perth Community Stroke Study. *Br J Psychiatry*. 1995;166(3):320–327.

169. Herrmann N, Black SE, Lawrence J, Szekely C, Szalai JP. The Sunnybrook Stroke Study: a prospective study of depressive symptoms and functional outcome. *Stroke*. 1998;29(3):618–624.

170. Kotila M, Numminen H, Waltimo O, Kaste M. Depression after stroke: results of the FINNSTROKE Study. *Stroke*. 1998;29(2):368–372.

171. Robinson RG, Starr LB, Kubos KL, Price TR. A two-year longitudinal study of post-stroke mood disorders: findings during the initial evaluation. *Stroke*. 1983;14(5):736–741.

172. Pierce LL, Steiner V. What are male caregivers talking about? *Top Stroke Rehabil*. 2004;11(2):77–83.

173. Williams LS, Brizendine EJ, Plue L, Bakas T, Tu W, Hendrie H, et al. Performance of the PHQ-9 as a screening tool for depression after stroke. *Stroke*. 2005;36(3):635–638.

174. Anderson CS, Linto J, Stewart-Wynne EG. A population-based assessment of the impact and burden of caregiving for long-term stroke survivors. *Stroke*. 1995;26(5):843–849.

175. Anderson C, Rubenach S, Mhurchu CN, Clark M, Spencer C, Winsor A. Home or hospital for stroke rehabilitation? results of a randomized controlled trial : I: health outcomes at 6 months. *Stroke*. 2000;31(5):1024–1031.

176. Grov EK, Fossa SD, Tonnessen A, Dahl AA. The caregiver reaction assessment: psychometrics, and temporal stability in primary caregivers of Norwegian cancer patients in late palliative phase. *Psycho-oncol*. 2006;15(6):517–527.

177. Anderson C, Mhurchu CN, Rubenach S, Clark M, Spencer C, Winsor A. Home or hospital for stroke Rehabilitation? Results of a randomized controlled trial : II: cost minimization analysis at 6 months. *Stroke*. 2000;31(5):1032–1037.

178. Berg A, Palomaki H, Lonnqvist J, Lehtihalmes M, Kaste M. Depression among caregivers of stroke survivors. *Stroke*. 2005;36(3):639–643.

179. Lackey NR, Gates MF. Adults' recollections of their experiences as young caregivers of family members with chronic physical illnesses. *J Adv Nurs*. 2001;34(3):320–328.

180. King RB, Semik PE. Stroke caregiving: difficult times, resource use, and needs during the first 2 years. *J Gerontol Nurs*. 2006;32(4):37–44.

181. Visser-Meily A, van Heugten C, Post M, Schepers V, Lindeman E. Intervention studies for caregivers of stroke survivors: a critical review. *Patient Educ Couns*. 2005;56(3):257–267.

182. Evans RL, Matlock AL, Bishop DS, Stranahan S, Pederson C. Family intervention after stroke: does counseling or education help? *Stroke*. 1988;19(10):1243–1249.

183. van den Heuvel ET, de Witte LP, Nooyen-Haazen I, Sanderman R, Meyboom-de Jong B. Short-term effects of a group support program and an individual support program for caregivers of stroke patients. *Patient Educ Couns*. 2000;40(2):109–120.

CHAPTER 23

Primary prevention of stroke

Anna M. Cervantes-Arslanian and Sudha Seshadri

Introduction

Stroke follows cardiovascular disease as the leading cause of death worldwide, the two together being responsible for 17.1 million deaths each year (1). In the United States (US) and United Kingdom (UK), stroke ranks third among leading causes of death (behind cardiac disease and cancers in the US and behind cardiac disease and lower respiratory infections in the UK) (2, 3). Cardiovascular and cerebrovascular disease are often thought to be diseases of high-income nations, yet nearly 85% of all stroke deaths occur in low- to middle-income nations (4, 5). In many low–middle-income nations, with large populations, e.g. China, stroke has now become the leading cause of death (6). This contrasts with trends in the US, where stroke death rates fell by 34.3% over the last decade (9).

Declining stroke mortality in the US and most high-income nations, is largely attributable to improvements in the control of hypertension. An analysis of 50 years of data from the Framingham Heart Study (FHS), a largely Caucasian population in Massachusetts, showed a decline in the age-adjusted incidence of stroke across three consecutive epochs 1950–1977, 1978–1989, and 1990–2004. The age-adjusted incidences of first stroke per 1000 person-years in each of the three periods were 7.6, 6.2, and 5.3 in men and 6.2, 5.8, and 5.1 in women, respectively (Table 23.1) (7, 8).

Over the past 40 years in high-income countries, the age-adjusted stroke incidence has decreased by 42% from 163 per 100,000 in 1970–1979 to 94 per 100,000 in 2000–2008 (p=0.0004). However over the same time period, the incidence increased by over 100% in low- to middle-income countries that are going through a demographic transition, from 52 per 100,000 to 117 per 100,000 (p <0.0001) (9). The risk of stroke is now higher in low- to middle-income countries than in high-income countries.

A review of 56 population based studies examined stroke incidence in 18 high-income countries and 20 low- to middle-income countries, as defined by the World Bank, found that lower- to middle-income countries had higher first ever stroke incidence and early case-specific mortality rates compared to higher-income countries (Figure 23.1) (9). When macro socioeconomic status (SES) was more precisely defined as per capita GDP adjusted for purchasing power parity (PPP-aGDP) or total healthcare expenditures per capita at purchasing power parity (PPP-aTHE), it was again shown that poorer SES was associated with higher incident stroke risk, higher stroke mortality, a greater proportion of ICH among all strokes, and a younger age at first stroke (9). In a 22-nation study, countries with lower SES tended to invest less in health expenditures on both an absolute and relative basis. Wealthy countries tended to spend a higher proportion of their economic resources on healthcare (10). The problem is compounded by the fact that the prevalence of vascular risk factors is higher in nations with less economic resources available to dedicate to prevention and treatment of stroke (11).

Data also suggest that within nations, both on an individual basis and at a population level, SES is inversely associated with risk of stroke. Even in countries with high investment in healthcare resources, individuals within the nation who have a lower SES have a higher risk of stroke (11). The higher prevalence of vascular risk factors in populations of lower SES partly, but not entirely, explains this risk (12). Further, even within a single country, different races and ethnic groups have consistently demonstrated differences in the rates of cardiovascular risk factors and stroke. In the US, the age-adjusted incidence of all stroke types is greater in black people and Hispanics than in white people (191 per 100,000, 149 per 100,000 and 88 per 100,000, respectively). Mortality rates are also higher in minority groups compared to white populations (13). Data from the Greater Cincinnati/Northern Kentucky Stroke Study (GCNKSS) show that in black people, the incidence of stroke has not decreased since the 1990s, in contrast to the decrease described earlier for white people in the FHS and that observed among white people in Rochester, Minnesota (14).

Stroke is the leading cause of disability in the developed world with a quarter of all survivors left permanently disabled. Stroke survivors report a poor quality of life, and their families are often devastated emotionally and financially as the lifetime costs of stroke per individual are estimated at $140,000 (USD). The economic burden of this disease at a national level is substantial, with an estimated $73.7 billion in direct and indirect costs in the US (15).

Therefore, the primary prevention of stroke will have a great impact on populations worldwide; this involves both the identification of modifiable risk factors and the identification of non-modifiable risk factors and risk markers that can be used to identify and more intensively follow individuals at high risk. The identification of risk factors is the first step towards developing an effective public health and public education strategy for the primary prevention of stroke and the primordial prevention of risk factors predisposing to stroke.

Non-modifiable risk factors

Across all races, ethnicities, and geographic regions, age is the strongest determinant of stroke risk. Other non-modifiable markers of increased stroke risk include male sex, family history, low birth weight, and black or Hispanic ethnicity (13, 14, 16–19). These risk factors are addressed in detail in Chapter 2.

Table 23.1 Annual age-adjusted incidence of clinical stroke and atherothrombotic brain infarction

	Men				Women			
	1950–1977	1978–1989	1990–2004	P for Trend	1950–1977	1978–1989	1990–2004	P for Trend
Total person-years	30,348	19,779	24,065		41,332	27,189	29,991	
Clinical stroke No. of cases	168	134	148		181	191	208	
Age-adjusted annual incidence per 1000 person-years	7.6	6.2	5.3		6.2	5.8	5.1	
Relative risk (95% CI)	1.00	0.86 (0.68–1.08)	0.75 (0.59–0.95)	.02	1.00	0.85 (0.68–1.05)	0.76 (0.61–0.94)	.01
Atherothrombotic brain infarction No. of cases	111	80	95		113	111	119	
Age-adjusted annual incidence per 1000 person-years	4.9	3.7	3.6		3.7	3.4	2.9	
Relative risk (95% CI)	1.00	0.80 (6.50–1.07)	0.76 (0.59–1.02)	.07	1.00	0.79 (0.59–1.04)	0.69	.01

CI: confidence interval. Table modified from Carandang R, Seshadri S, Beiser A, Kelly- Hayes M, Kase CS, Kannel WB, *et al*. Trends in incidence, lifetime risk, severity, and 30-day mortality of stroke over the past 50 years. *JAMA*. 2006 ; 296 (24): 2939–2946.

Potentially modifiable risk factors

A simple risk prediction algorithm that predicts a stroke-free individual's risk of developing a stroke in the next 10 years based on their current levels of various modifiable risk factors, has been proposed. This was based on FHS data but has been validated in various other population and clinical samples and illustrates the substantial impact of common, modifiable risk factors (Table 23.2) (20).

Hypertension

Hypertension is the single most powerful modifiable risk factor in all geographic and ethnic groups and for all stroke subtypes. Elevations in systolic blood pressure, diastolic blood pressure, or both values are associated with an increased risk of stroke. In addition, it has been shown that increased variability of blood pressure itself is an independent risk factor for stroke (21). Though various groups including

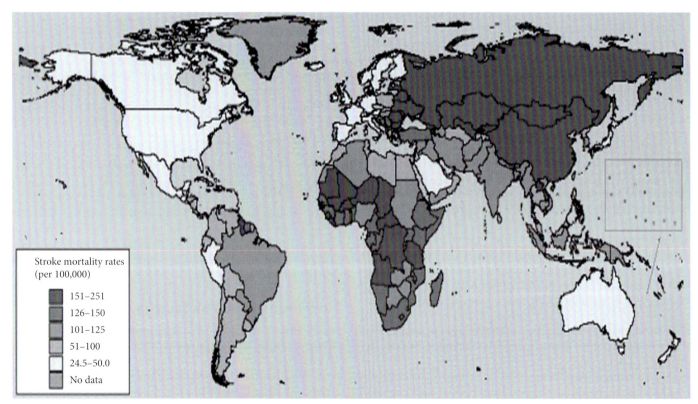

Fig. 23.1 Age-adjusted and sex-adjusted stroke mortality rates. Rates and highest in eastern Europe, north Asia, central Africa and the south Pacific.

Table 23.2 Probability or stroke within 10 years for men aged 55–84 years and free of previous stroke: Framingham study

Risk factor	Points										
	0	1	2	3	4	5	6	7	8	9	10
Age (yr)	54–56	57–59	60–62	63–65	66–68	69–71	72–74	75–77	78–80	81–83	84–86
SBP (min Hg)	95–105	106–116	117–126	127–137	138–148	149–159	100–170	171–181	182–191	192–202	203–213
Hyp Rx	No		Yes								
DM	No		Yes								
Cigs	No			Yes							
CVD	No			Yes							
AF	No				Yes						
LVH	No						Yes				

Points	10-yr probability	Points	10-yr probability	Points	10-yr probability
1	2.6%	11	11.2%	21	41.7%
2	3.0%	12	12.9%	22	46.6%
3	3.5%	13	14.8%	23	51.8%
4	4.0%	14	17.0%	24	57.3%
5	4.7%	15	19.5%	25	62.8%
6	5.4%	16	22.4%	26	68.4%
7	6.3%	17	25.5%	27	73.8%
8	73%	18	29.0%	28	79.0%
9	8.4%	19	32.9%	29	83.7%
10	9.7%	20	37.1%	30	87.9%

AF: history of atrial fibrillation; CHD; history of myocardial infarction angina pectoris, or coronary insufficiency; Cigs; smokes cigarettes; CVD: history of intermittent claudication or congestive heart failure; DM; history of diabetes mellitus; Hyp Rx; under antihypertensive therapy; LVH: left ventricular hypertrophy on electrocardiogram; SBP; systolic blood pressure. Table modified from Wolf PA, D'Agostino RB, Belanger AJ, Kannel WB. Probability of stroke: a risk profile from the Framingham Study. *Stroke*. 1991; 22 (3): 312–318.

the Seventh Joint National Committee (JNC-7) target specific blood pressure goals, it is important to recognize that the risks associated with elevations in blood pressure increase continuously with increasing blood pressures, beginning even within the non-hypertensive range (22). Stratification of the FHS original cohort by JNC-7 criteria demonstrated that compared to men with normal (<120/80 mmHg) blood pressure, those with pre-hypertension (120–140/80–90 mmHg) had a 40% higher lifetime risk of stroke and those with stage 1 or 2 hypertension (>140/90 mmHg) had twice the lifetime risk of stroke. For women, compared to those with normal blood pressure, those with pre-hypertension had a 25% higher lifetime risk of stroke and those with stage 1 or 2 hypertension had a 76% higher lifetime risk of stroke (Figure 23.2) (7). Furthermore, data collected from 1 million adults in prospective studies show that the risk of death due to cardiovascular disease and stroke doubles for each increment of 20 mmHg systolic or 10 mmHg diastolic above 115/75 mmHg (22, 23).

In addition to severity of elevated blood pressure, the duration of the hypertensive state also contributes to stroke risk. Elevated blood pressure during midlife increases the risk of stroke later in life such that at age 60, after adjusting for systolic blood pressure, diabetes and smoking status at baseline, the blood pressure during the preceding decade (age 50–59 years increased the relative risk of stroke by 1.92 (95% confidence interval (CI) 1.39–2.66) per standard deviation (SD) increment in men and 1.68 (95% CI 1.25–2.25) per SD increment in women; level of blood pressure when the

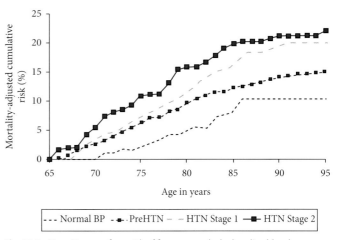

Fig. 23.2 Men, 65 years of age: risk of first-ever stroke by baseline blood pressure (BP); LTR of all-stroke within four BP categories defined using systolic (SBP) and diastolic blood pressure (DBP); subjects categorized using higher of two values: (i) normal BP: SBP <120 and DBP <80 mmHg; (ii) pre-hypertension (PreHTN): 120≤SBP<140 or 80≤DBP<90; (3) stage 1 hypertension (HTN stage 1): 140 ≤SBP<160 or 90≤DBP<100; (4) stage 2 hypertension (HTN stage 2) SBP ≥160 or DBP ≥100. Figure modified from Seshadri S, Beiser A, Kelly-Hayes M, Kase CS, Au R, Kannel WB, *et al*. Th e lifetime risk of stroke: estimates from the Framingham Study. *Stroke*. 2006; 37 (2): 345–350.

same person had been 40–49 years old increased risk by 48% (95% CI 1.07–2.07) in women and 54% (95% CI 0.96–2.45) in men (24).

Numerous studies have shown that treatment of elevated blood pressure reduces the risk of stroke (25). A meta-analysis of 23 clinical trials involving various classes of antihypertensive medications showed that any drug treatment reduced the relative risk (RR) of stroke (RR 0.69; 95% CI 0.61–0.76) compared to no treatment (26). Multiple studies have tried to determine if one particular class of antihypertensive medications is more effective than another. A Cochrane review in 2009 showed all antihypertensives reduce the risk of stroke with thiazide diuretics to have a RR of 0.62 (95% CI 0.57–0.71), beta-blockers a RR 0.83 (95% CI 0.72–0.97), angiotensin-converting enzyme (ACE) inhibitors a RR 0.65 (95% CI 0.52–0.82), and calcium channel blockers a RR 0.58 (95% CI 0.41–0.84) (27). Overall, the impact of anti-hypertensive medications in preventing stroke is proportional to the degree to which the blood pressure is controlled (28). However, for a given reduction in blood pressure, drug class-specific effects on stroke risk exist. This may be partly explained by differences in the extent to which a drug class decreases blood pressure variability, with calcium channel blockers being the most efficacious and beta-blockers the least (29, 30). Several studies, including the Hypertension in the Very Elderly Trial (HYVET) (31), Systolic Hypertension in the Elderly Program (SHEP) (32), and European Working Party on Hypertension in the Elderly (EWPHE) (33) trials have shown that reduction of blood pressure even in the elderly (>80 years old) is not only tolerable but beneficial in reducing the risk of stroke.

To reduce the risk of stroke, the American Heart Association and American Stroke Association (AHA/ASA) Guidelines for primary prevention of stroke (34), endorse using the JNC-7 guideline (23) recommendations for a goal of <140/90 mmHg for individuals without other cardiovascular risk factors, and <130/80 mm Hg for individuals with diabetes mellitus or chronic kidney disease. They suggest that all individuals should be counselled on lifestyle modifications and for those at a higher risk, pharmacological treatment of blood pressure should be employed.

The specific choice of antihypertensive agent may be tailored to an individual patient's characteristics or comorbidities. Diabetics with hypertension are at an even higher risk of stroke than non-diabetics and should be managed aggressively. Certain classes of antihypertensives, such as ACE inhibitors, may reduce stroke risk via additional mechanisms independent of direct effects on blood pressure. ACE inhibitors combined with diuretic agents are currently the recommended combination for secondary prevention of stroke, though it is not clear if this is also the best combination for primary prevention (35).

Dyslipidaemia

The relationship between lipid levels and stroke suggests that elevated serum total cholesterol, elevated low-density lipoprotein (LDL) levels, and lower high-density lipoprotein (HDL) levels are associated with an increased risk of stroke. Many large trials including the Multiple Risk Factor Intervention Trial (MRFIT) (36), Asia Pacific Cohort Studies Collaboration (APCSC) (37), and Women's Health Study (WHS) (38), have found that higher total cholesterol levels are associated with an increased risk of stroke. However, several other studies including the ARIC (39), the Physician's Health Study (PHS) (40), and the FHS, found weak or inconsistent associations between total cholesterol level and stroke incidence. Most studies have shown that higher levels of HDL are protective

against risk of stroke (41). Despite the inconsistencies seen in the relationship between lipid level and risk of stroke, there is a consistent reduction of stroke risk with the use of statins. In a large meta-analysis of more than 90,000 patients statin use reduced the risk of incident stroke by approximately 21% (95% CI 15–27%) (42). In several secondary prevention studies, statins appear to have pleiotropic effects lowering the risk of stroke independent of their impact on LDL levels. Though statins may be of particular effectiveness in reducing stroke risk among persons with coronary artery disease (CAD), the Anglo-Scandinavian Cardiac Outcomes Trial—Lipid Lowering Arm (ASCOT-LLA) provided evidence that statins were effective for primary prevention of stroke even in individuals without CAD. In patients with hypertension but normal or low cholesterol, treatment with atorvastatin 10 mg was associated with a reduced risk of stroke with a hazard ratio (HR) of 0.73 (95% CI 0.56–0.96, P=0.024) (43).

Several studies have found an association between low cholesterol, in particular LDL levels and an increased risk of haemorrhagic stroke. In a pooled analysis of data from prospective cohorts, an inverse association was seen between LDL levels and intracerebral haemorrhage (ICH) with a RR of 0.52 (95% CI 0.31–0.88, P=0.0085) when comparing the top quartile (158.8–504.6 mg/dL) to the lower three quartiles (4–158.8 mg/dL) (44). However, a recent retrospective cohort study found no association between statin use and ICH (HR 0.87; 95% CI 0.65–1.17) (45).

To reduce the risk of stroke, the National Cholesterol Education Program Adult Treatment Panel III (NCEP-ATP III) recommends checking lipid profiles at least once every 5 years in individuals above the age of 20 and targeting LDL levels based on the presence of other cardiovascular risk factors and the estimated over-all 10-year risk of any cardiovascular event (46). First-line therapy should also include counselling on lifestyle modifications, including diet and physical activity. Statins are the first-line pharmacological treatment for elevated LDL, and have demonstrated benefit in primary and secondary prevention of stroke. This is discussed in detail later in this chapter. Fibrates and nicotinic acid may be considered for elevated triglycerides and low HDL, though it has not been established if such treatment will prevent stroke (34).

Diabetes mellitus

Worldwide an estimated 171 million people above the age of 20 had diabetes in 2000. Projections conservatively estimate that the prevalence of diabetes will rise from 2.8% to 4.4% by 2030 (47). The burden of disease is relatively higher in the US, Central America, and Oceania where over 10% of the population is estimated to have diabetes. American Indian and Polynesian populations have a higher prevalence of diabetes, likely reflecting a combination of genetic and SES factors. Diabetic patients have an independently increased risk of stroke (from 1.8- to 6-fold) even after adjusting for the fact that they are also more likely to have hypertension and hypercholesterolemia (34). In addition to the usual stroke risk factors, two important risk factors among diabetics are impaired glucose tolerance and microalbuminuria. However, although impaired glucose tolerance increases the risk of stroke, tight glycaemic control has not been shown to decrease the risk of incident stroke. In the CARDS (Collaborative Atorvastatin Diabetes) trial, the presence of microalbuminuria, measured as an albumin:creatinine ratio (ACR) of higher than 2.5, doubled the risk of stroke (48, 49).

Strategies to reduce the risk of stroke in diabetics are focused on decreasing the risk of co-morbidities. Reducing blood pressure in diabetics is the main strategy to reduce stroke risk; the AHA/ASA recommends that diabetics lower blood pressure to less than 130/80 mmHg. Oftentimes, two drug therapies are needed to reach this goal and ACE inhibitors, angiotensin receptor blockers (ARBs), thiazide diuretics, beta-blockers, and calcium channel blockers have all been shown to reduce stroke risk in diabetics (23). Most studies have also shown that using statins reduces stroke risk in diabetics. A meta-analysis of 14 randomized trials of statins, involving more than 18,600 subjects, demonstrated a 21% reduction in stroke risk among diabetics who were also on statins compared to diabetics who were not on statins (OR 0.79; 95% CI 0.67–0.93). This parallels the reduction in stroke risk observed in persons without diabetes (50). The CARDS study showed that in diabetics with at least one other risk factor for stroke (smoking, hypertension, retinopathy, albuminuria) and LDL levels below 160 mg/dL, statin treatment reduced the risk of stroke by 48% (95% CI 11–69%) (51). The benefits of aspirin use for primary prevention of stroke in diabetics remains unclear, however the AHA/ASA opines that it may be reasonable to use, especially if the diabetic patient is at high risk of cardiovascular disease (34).

Cigarette smoking

Cigarette smoking has declined in many parts of the world, but remains a major contributor to the risk of cardiovascular disease and stroke, being associated with 12–14% of all stroke deaths (52). There is a graded dose–response relationship between exposure to cigarette smoke and stroke risk (53). Both active and passive exposure to cigarette smoke have been associated with increased risks of ischaemic stroke and subarachnoid haemorrhage, and may also be a risk factor for intracerebral haemorrhage (54, 55). Smoking has been shown to increase systolic blood pressure and heart rate, and to decrease arterial distensibility (34, 56). Smoking may accelerate atherosclerosis via endothelial damage, increased levels of circulating inflammatory markers, and greater platelet aggregability (57). There is also a synergistic effect between smoking and oral contraceptive use in increasing the risk of stroke (58).

All patients should be counselled about the dangers of cigarette smoke to themselves and those around them and encouraged to quit smoking. The US Preventive Services Task Force recommends a combination of counselling and medications (such as replacement nicotine, bupropion therapy) for maximal effectiveness (59). The risk of stroke declines following smoking cessation. In the FHS, a risk reduction of 60% was seen in smokers who quit smoking and the risk of smoking may return to the level of non-smokers within 5 years (55).

Atrial fibrillation

Atrial fibrillation (AF) is the most common arrhythmia in the elderly. An estimated 2.3 million people in the US and 4.5 million in the European Union have chronic or paroxysmal atrial fibrillation, a number that is likely to increase dramatically as the population ages (60). AF results in stasis within the left atrium or left atrial appendage allowing for clot formation and is the most common cause for cardioembolic stroke. Both chronic AF and paroxysmal AF confer an increased risk of stroke (61). Approximately 10% of strokes in all age groups are attributable to AF. The risk of stroke attributed to AF increases with age such that in the FHS study, among individuals in the 80–89 year age group, 36.2% of strokes were attributable to AF (62).

The AHA/ASA recommends that all individuals older than 65 years old be screened for AF via pulse assessment followed by electrocardiography for those with an irregular pulse (63). The CHADS$_2$ score is commonly used to stratify an individual's risk of stroke with AF and to guide treatment recommendations (64). Several other stratification schemes exist and are quite similar, most taking into account age and presence of other vascular risk factors such as congestive heart failure, hypertension, diabetes, and prior thromboembolic events including transient ischaemic attacks or strokes. For most patients, (risk >2.5–7% per year) warfarin is the treatment of choice, with an INR goal between 2.0 and 3.0 (65). For those persons with non-valvular AF and a very low risk of stroke (~1%/year), the Stroke Prevention in Atrial Fibrillation III (SPAF III) trial has shown that daily aspirin alone (75–325 mg) may be considered (66).

Anticoagulation therapy is not without its own risks. In clinical trials, 1.0–1.5% of patients with monitored therapeutic international normalized ratio (INR) had major haemorrhages annually. Studies have shown that only half of all warfarin users have INR values in the appropriate range. The emergence of anticoagulation clinics has helped to decrease patients' risk of complications from sub- and supra-therapeutic INRs (67). Treatment of hypertension is dually important in AF patients, both for lowering risk of ischaemic stroke and for reducing likelihood of anticoagulation associated intracerebral haemorrhage (68).

New medications, including the factor Xa inhibitors and direct thrombin inhibitors offer alternatives to warfarin (69–71). In the Randomized Evaluation of Long-term Anticoagulation therapy (RE-LY) trial, dabigatran, the first Food and Drug Administration-approved factor Xa inhibitor, was shown to reduce the risks of stroke and systemic embolism to the same extent as warfarin with equivalent or reduced risk of major haemorrhage (69). Apixaban, an oral direct thrombin inhibitor, was shown to be superior to warfarin in preventing strokes with lower risks of bleeding and death (70). Another new thrombin inhibitor, rivaroxaban, was shown to be equivalent to warfarin in reduction of stroke and bleeding risk (71). These new medications will likely become very popular since they do not require therapeutic anticoagulation monitoring. However there are currently no available agents for reversal of anticoagulation effect in the event of catastrophic bleeding and these newer anticoagulants cannot be safely used in patients with renal dysfunction.

Alcohol

An intriguing relationship exists between alcohol consumption and stroke risk. High alcohol consumption has been associated with a linear increase in risk of haemorrhagic stroke (72). However, for ischaemic stroke, the association appears J-shaped. Low to moderate consumption of alcohol, in particular red wine, has been associated with a lower risk of ischaemic stroke compared to those who do not drink alcohol at all. High consumption of alcohol is associated with an increased risk for ischaemic stroke (73, 74). No trials have demonstrated that reducing alcohol intake modifies an individual's ischaemic or haemorrhagic stroke risk. Given the myriad detrimental health effects attributable to alcohol overuse and abuse, the overall recommendation from the stroke community is for non-drinkers to continue avoidance of alcohol and for low to moderate consumption by those who already drink.

Sickle cell

Sickle cell disease (SCD) is an autosomal recessive condition causing a mutation within the haemoglobin B chain. This disease is an important cause of stroke within the paediatric population, particularly amongst African Americans, with stroke subtypes varying with age. Stroke is most common in homozygous SCD, with lower risks in those who carry both the sickle and β-thalassemia traits and minimal elevations of risk in heterozygote carriers of the SC mutation. In early childhood (ages 2–9), and over the age of 30 years, ischaemic stroke is more common, with a risk close to 1% per year. In early adulthood (ages 20–30), haemorrhagic stroke is more common (75). Primary prevention in SCD is based on identification of children at higher risk via transcranial Doppler ultrasound and treatment of these children with exchange transfusions. The Stroke Prevention Trial in Sickle Cell Anemia (STOP) demonstrated the benefit of transfusion in primary prevention of stroke in SCD (76). Children between the ages of 2 and 16 with SCD should undergo routine surveillance every 6–12 months via transcranial Doppler (TCD) ultrasound of the internal carotid and middle cerebral arteries. Elevated middle cerebral artery velocities (>170 cm/sec) are associated with an increased risk of stroke with risks exceeding 10% per year at greater than 200 cm/sec. Therefore, at middle cerebral artery velocities greater than 170 cm/sec, chronic transfusion therapy (simple or exchange, packed red blood cells) is advised with target reduction of sickle cell haemoglobin to less than 30% (77). Once initiated, there is currently no definitive data on when transfusions may be safely discontinued. In the STOP II follow-up study a high rate of reversion to abnormal blood-flow velocities on TCD and an increased risk of stroke was observed in patients who had discontinued transfusions (78). There may be significant adverse effects of chronic transfusions including iron overload and transfusion related infection, so alternative therapies need to be developed. Other strategies including the use of hydroxyurea are under investigation but have shown mixed results (79, 80).

Postmenopausal hormonal therapy

Observational studies had suggested that postmenopausal hormonal replacement therapy (HRT) might reduce the risk of cardiovascular disease including stroke. This led to the Women's Health Initiative (WHI), which was a large (>160,000 women) randomized controlled trial testing the use of conjugated oestrogens plus progestin against placebo. The trial was stopped early since interim data analysis showed significant adverse effects (81). Over an average follow-up period of 5.2 years, the risk of ischaemic stroke was increased in persons on HRT (HR 1.55; 95% CI 1.19–2.01), but there was no difference in the risk of haemorrhagic stroke (HR 0.64; 95% CI 0.35–1.18) (82). Both the WHI and the Nurses' Health Study (NHS) found that the increased risk of stroke was independent of age at initiation of HRT (83). Other medications used for the prevention of osteoporosis such as tibolone have also been associated with an increased risk of stroke (84). Raloxifene, a selective oestrogen receptor modulator (SERM), has been associated with an increased risk of fatal stroke (85).

Hormone replacement therapies should not be used for primary prevention of stroke in postmenopausal women. The use of SERMs and tibolone, though proven to be beneficial for prevention of breast cancer and osteoporosis, should be used with caution in persons at a high risk of stroke.

Oral contraceptives

Historically oral contraceptives (OC) were considered a risk factor for stroke. Today, it appears the overall risk of stroke with use of low-dose OC is low (58, 86). This change most likely stems from the use of lower doses of oestrogens and progestin, in combination with prescribing recommendations limiting use to healthy young women without cardiovascular disease. Data from the UK suggest that the incidence of stroke in all young women is 3.56 per 100,000 per year and that the OR for those using OC compared to others is 2.3 (95% CI 1.15–4.59) (87). More recent Danish studies show an even lower absolute risk of thrombotic stroke with OC (RR averaging 1.60–1.97; 95% CI 1.37–2.66, depending upon the dose of ethinyl oestradiol and type of progestin), however higher risks were seen with transdermal contraceptive patches and vaginal rings (3.15 and 2.49). Implantation of a progestin only intrauterine device did not increase stroke risk (86). The risk of stroke associated with the use of hormonal contraceptives is lower than the risk associated with a pregnancy (22 per 100,000 per year) (88).

The risk of stroke associated with hormonal contraceptives use is higher amongst some categories of women (smokers, those with hypertension, obesity, or hypercholesterolemia) and their use should probably be avoided in these groups (89).

Elevated homocysteine

Debate continues as to the significance of elevated circulating homocysteine levels within the adult population (90). Many observational studies including the FHS, have related mild to moderate elevations in circulating homocysteine levels to the risk of incident stroke (91). However, clinical trials of homocysteine lowering treatments (vitamins folate and B$_{12}$), in the Vitamin Intervention for Stroke Prevention trial (VISP) and the more recent Vitamins to Prevent Stroke recurrence (VITATOPS) trials have shown little benefit (92, 93).

At this time routine screening for hyperhomocysteinaemia is not indicated unless particular conditions (such as a family history of hyperhomocysteinaemia or current use of drugs interfering with folate metabolism) exist. The AHA/ASA suggests that the use of B-complex vitamins may be considered for ischaemic stroke prevention. By eating fortified grains, leafy green vegetables, fruits, legumes, limited quantities of meats, poultry, and fish, most patients will fulfil dietary recommendations for folate consumption and avoid hyperhomocystenaemia.

Sleep disordered breathing/ obstructive sleep apnoea

Sleep disordered breathing, specifically, obstructive sleep apnoea (OSA) is associated with several conditions, including hypertension (94), abdominal obesity, and atrial fibrillation (95), that predispose to stroke and other cardiovascular events. Evidence is growing that OSA itself is also an independent risk factor for stroke. In a cohort of 1022 consecutive stroke- and myocardial infarction (MI)-free persons referred to the Yale Center for Sleep Medicine, the presence of OSA (defined as a polysomnogram documented obstructive apnoea-hypopnea index (OAHI) ≥5) doubled the combined risk of stroke or death due to any cause, even after adjustment for traditional cardiovascular risk factors (HR 1.97; 95% CI 1.12–3.4) (96). The Sleep Heart Health Study followed 5422 middle-aged and older community-based cohort participants for an average of 8.7 years and observed a graded increase in risk of incident stroke among men; each one point increase in the OAHI was associated with a 6% (95% CI 2–10%) increase in stroke risk and men in the highest quartile (a OAHI ≥19) had thrice the risk of men in the lowest quartile (OAHI ≤4); HR 2.86 (95% CI 1.1–7.4). There was however a threshold effect among women such that only women with severe OAHI (>25) appeared to have an increased risk of stroke (97). The Vitoria Sleep Project found that among both elderly men and women, aged 70–100 years, severe OSA hypopnea (OAHI >30) increased the risk of ischaemic stroke (98).

Treatment of OSA via continuous positive airway pressure (CPAP) has been shown to decrease blood pressure and cardiovascular risk but has not been shown to specifically decrease the risk of stroke (99) (100). Sleep disordered breathing could lead to stroke through multiple mechanisms including intermittent hypoxemia triggering sympathetic surges, reductions in cerebral blood flow, arrhythmias, altered endothelial function, acceleration of atherosclerosis, and impaired cerebral vaso-regulation. Given the association between sleep disordered breathing and cardiovascular disease including stroke, routine screening for OSA is prudent and polysomnograms should be performed when indicated. CPAP or bi-level positive airway pressure (BiPAP) devices should be employed for sleep apnoea as their use has been shown to be successful in reducing the prevalence of drug resistant hypertension in OSA (101).

Obesity

The prevalence of overweight and obesity has been increasing worldwide. In the US, 66.3% of adults are considered either overweight or obese (body mass index (BMI) >25). Ethnic minorities are disproportionately affected compared to white people, with 45% of black people, 36% of Hispanics, and 30% of white people considered overweight or obese (102). A high correlation exists between BMI and waist circumference (a measure of central obesity and a proxy for abdominal fat or visceral adiposity). Increased abdominal fat is a strong predictor of stroke risk, though it is not clear whether the increased risk is mediated by the effect of central obesity on other stroke risk factors, in particular hypertension (103). Weight reduction has been consistently shown to decrease both systolic and diastolic blood pressure (104). Other stroke risk factors such as sleep disordered breathing, poor nutrition, and lower levels of physical activity are also associated with obesity and may mediate the increased risk observed in obese persons.

Nutrition

A wide range of studies have found that certain dietary habits have an impact on stroke risk. High consumption of sodium-containing foods and low potassium intake has both been associated with an increased stroke risk (105). A recent meta-analysis found a strong association between low fruit and vegetable intake and an increased risk of stroke (106). Since the relationship between sodium intake and elevated blood pressure is direct and progressive, low-sodium

diets, such as the DASH diet, are recommended and have been shown to be effective in reducing blood pressure (107). The Mediterranean diet is rich in whole grains, monounsaturated fats, and fish, with lower consumption of red meat, refined grains, and sugars than is the norm in the typical Western diet. In the NHS, women who more closely adhered to a Mediterranean diet were found to have a lower risk of stroke and CHD (108). This was similarly demonstrated in both men and women in the Northern Manhattan Study (NOMAS) where increased consumption of a Mediterranean diet was associated with decreased risk of ischaemic stroke, MI, and all cause vascular death (109). In the Health Professional Follow-up Study (HPFS), men who ate fish as little as once per month had a decreased risk of ischaemic stroke (110).

Exercise

Increased physical activity has been shown to decrease the risk of ischaemic stroke in both women and men. In the NHS increasing physical activity in women was inversely associated with risk of ischaemic stroke with a dose–response effect so that across quintiles of increasing physical activity the relative risks (RRs) were 1.00, 0.87, 0.83, 0.76, and 0.52; P for trend=0.003, respectively (111). In the NOMAS and FHS cohorts, a dose–response effect was not seen, but when compared to sedentary men, those participating in physical activity of moderate to heavy intensity had decreased relative risk of stroke (112, 113). This may be mediated through reductions in the prevalence and levels of other cardiovascular risk factors such as blood pressure, diabetes, and obesity. Physically active adults have a 25–30% lower risk of stroke or death than the most inactive group (114). The 2008 US Department of Health and Human Services Physical Activity Guidelines for Americans recommends at least 150 minutes of moderate intensity aerobic activity per week for all adults (115).

Exercise is also an important component of the 'low-risk lifestyle'. In a prospective cohort study involving the participants of the Health Professionals Follow-up Study and the NHS, the combination of modest exercise (30 minutes per day or more) when combined with avoidance of smoking, a BMI lower than 25 kg/m², modest alcohol consumption, and consumption of a healthy diet was associated with a reduced risk of ischaemic stroke. Women and men with all five low-risk factors had relative risks of 0.21 (95% CI 0.12–0.36) and 0.31 (95% CI 0.19–0.53) respectively, for total stroke compared with women or men who had none of these factors (116).

Metabolic syndrome

The metabolic syndrome (Met S) refers to a cluster of potentially modifiable subclinical and clinical conditions that when present together appear to increase an individual's risk of vascular disease including stroke. The NCEP-ATP III criteria for diagnosis of Met S require that at least three of the following criteria be present: (i) abdominal obesity (waist circumference >102 cm or 40 inches for men and >88 cm or 35 inches for women), (ii) hypertriglyceridemia (TG >150 mg/dL), (iii) low HDL (HDL <40 mg/dL in men and <50 mg/dL in women), (iv) elevated blood pressure (>130/85 mm Hg), and (v) glucose intolerance (fasting glucose >110 mg/dL) (46). Other groups have established similar criteria that differ only in the cut-offs for waist circumference. Worldwide the prevalence of the Met S is increasing. Among middle–high-income nations, the prevalence varies between 14% in Danish women to 45% in Turkish women (117). Individual components of the Met S may contribute to stroke risk as described in other sections and each should be treated appropriately. Amongst stroke patients of all ethnic groups, ages, and both sexes, Met S is prevalent amongst the majority (118). However, it remains uncertain whether the Met S is an independent risk factor for stroke with a synergistic interaction between the individual components or simply represents the sum effect of independent, albeit interrelated stroke risk factors. In the FHS, the Met S was present in 24% of men and 20% of women, which is similar to the prevalence reported in the US nationwide. In a study of 2097 stroke-free Framingham Offspring participants (aged 50–81 years) it was observed that a combination of both diabetes and the Met S was associated with a relative risk of stroke of 3.28 (95% CI 1.82–5.92), while each component alone had a lower but still elevated relative risk of stroke (Met S alone RR 2.10, 95% CI 1.37–3.22; diabetes alone RR 2.47, 95% CI, 1.31–4.65) (119). Other studies including ARIC and NOMAS as well as of a large cohort in Finland have demonstrated an increased risk of stroke in men and women, white people and black people with the Met S (120–122). Given the higher prevalence of metabolic syndrome compared with diabetes it has been estimated that the population attributable risk of Met S may be as high as 30%. Thus, components of the Met S represent a significant target for public health interventions to reduce stroke (119).

The biological mechanisms linking the metabolic syndrome to stroke risk are likely related to insulin resistance, the key feature of the metabolic syndrome. Randomized secondary prevention studies using oral hypoglycaemic agents to reduce insulin resistance in persons with the metabolic syndrome are currently underway (123).

Chronic kidney disease

Chronic kidney disease (CKD) is a marker of exposure to vascular risk factors such as hypertension and diabetes. It also results in an increased prevalence of stroke risk factors such as AF and hyperhomocysteinaemia (124). In the ARIC study, a reduced estimated glomerular filtration rate (eGFR) was associated with a greatly increased risk of stroke, but only in the presence of anaemia (HR 5.4; 95% CI 2.04–14.41) (125). A recent meta-analysis of data from 33 prospective cohort studies and clinical trials assessed the risk of incident stroke among 284,672 persons in whom eGFR estimates were available. The data showed that risk of incident stroke was increased in persons with an eGFR less than 60 mL/min/1.73 m^2 (RR 1.43; 95% CI 1.31–1.57, P <0.001) but not amongst those with an eGFR of 60–90 mL/min/1.73 m^2 (RR 1.07; 95% CI 0.98–1.17, P=0.15). After adjusting for other known cardiovascular risk factors the risk of stroke was reduced (RR 1.45; 95% CI 1.26–1.68) but remained higher than in persons with a normal eGFR suggesting that CKD was an independent risk factor for stroke. Further, a dose–response relationship was observed with persons at an eGFR of <40 mL/min/1.73 m^2 being at greater risk than those with an eGFR in the 40–60 mL/min/1.73 m^2 range (126).

Both haemodialysis and peritoneal dialysis are associated with an increased risk of stroke that may be five to ten times higher than in the general population (127–130). Persons on dialysis also have higher stroke mortality, partly attributable to the higher proportion of haemorrhagic strokes in these patients (131). Among patients on dialysis, stroke risk is higher in persons with diabetic nephropathy or hypertensive nephrosclerosis likely due to pre-existent atherosclerosis. Patients with diabetic nephropathy or hypertensive

nephrosclerosis also tend to have strokes earlier after initiation of dialysis whereas strokes occur later in persons on haemodialysis due to primary glomerulonephritis (132). Recipients of renal transplants, though off haemodialysis, still harbour an increased risk of stroke compared to those without CKD (133). In a retrospective study of 400 renal transplant recipients, 8% suffered from a stroke within 10 years post transplantation. As with patients still on dialysis, intracerebral haemorrhage was more prevalent in the renal transplant population, and not surprisingly all those who suffered strokes, ischaemic or haemorrhagic, had hypertension. As with other CKD patients, those patients with renal transplant secondary to diabetic nephropathy were at higher risk (133, 134).

Inflammation and infection

Inflammation appears to promote atherogenesis via initiation, growth, and progression, as well as destabilization of atherosclerotic plaques leading to clinical thrombotic events (135). Over the past decade several serum markers of inflammation have been identified with high sensitivity C-reactive protein (hs-CRP) drawing the most attention. Data from several studies including the FHS have shown that in men and women, an elevation of hs-CRP levels even within the normal range results in an increased risk of stroke and TIA (136). Patients with rheumatoid arthritis (RA) have a higher risk of stroke than patients with osteoarthritis (OA) (137).

Several chronic infections (*Chlamydia pneumoniae*, *Helicobacter pylori*, periodontitis, chronic bronchitis, herpes viruses, hepatitis C virus, HIV, and most recently human papillomavirus) have been associated with increased stroke risk in some but not all studies (138–143). Whether the observed association is causal remains uncertain (144). The microbe with the most extensive research link to atherosclerosis is *C. pneumoniae*. It is a Gram-negative intracellular bacterium, which is present worldwide. Serological evidence of *C. pneumoniae* has been associated with MI and numerous studies have demonstrated the presence of the organism within atherosclerotic plaques but not in normal vessel walls (145, 146).

Randomized trials of antibiotic treatment of *C. pneumoniae* with azithromycin to prevent vascular events in patients with chronic infection have not demonstrated a reduction in risk of cardiovascular events (147). It seems unlikely that any specific infectious agent is responsible for provoking all atherosclerotic cardiovascular events, however there may exist an aggregate 'infectious burden' resulting in an increased risk of atherosclerosis and vascular disease (148). Acute infection has consistently been shown to transiently increase the risk of stroke. Influenza has been associated with an increased risk of cardiovascular death (149). Unlike treatment of chronic infection, treatment of influenza with antivirals and prevention of influenza via vaccination have both been shown to decrease the risk of stroke and all-cause mortality (150, 151).

Pharmacological agents for primary prevention in otherwise healthy adults

Aspirin

Aspirin is the mainstay of secondary stroke prevention. Meta-analyses have shown that over a range of doses, aspirin decreases the relative risk of recurrent stroke by 15% (152). However, the data regarding the use of aspirin for primary prevention of stroke in otherwise healthy adults are less clear. In the PHS,

325 mg of aspirin taken every other day was shown to have a clear benefit in preventing MI but did not prevent ischaemic strokes. Moreover, the use of aspirin was associated with a small increase in haemorrhagic strokes (153). In a meta-analysis of five studies in men aspirin reduced the risk of MI by 32% (odds ratio (OR) 0.68; 95% CI 0.54–0.86, P=0.001) but did not alter the risk of ischaemic stroke (OR 1.00; 95% CI 0.72–1.41, P=0.98) although it increased the risk of haemorrhagic stroke (OR 1.69; 95% CI 1.04–2.73, P=0.03) (154). Curiously, the WHS found the opposite; aspirin therapy (100 mg, every other day) was associated with a reduction in risk of ischaemic strokes (RR 0.76; 95% CI 0.69–0.93, P=0.009) but not a significant reduction in risk of MI (155). The risk of haemorrhagic stroke was not significantly increased (RR 1.24; 95% CI 0.82–1.87, P=0.31). Older women and those with other cardiovascular risk factors appeared to derive greater benefit from aspirin. The reason for the differences observed in men and women is not currently understood. Current AHA Guidelines recommend aspirin 75 mg daily for those patients with a Framingham 10-year risk score of any cardiovascular event of 10% or higher (156). Given the more recent findings that daily aspirin use also reduces risk of cancer, the combined beneficial impact appears to further tilt the risk-benefit ratio in favour of prophylactic aspirin use (157).

Statins

Given the overwhelming evidence supporting the beneficial impact of statins on secondary prevention of stroke, current research focuses on identifying groups in which statins may have a role in primary prevention. In the Justification for the Use of Statins in Prevention: an Intervention Trial Evaluating Rosuvastatin (JUPITER) 17,802 apparently healthy persons with normal LDL (defined as <130 mg/dL) but elevated hs-CRP (≥2.0 mg/L) were randomized to receive either rosuvastatin 20 mg daily or placebo. The trial was stopped at a mean follow-up of 1.9 years due to strong evidence that those on statin treatment benefited from a reduction in the incidence of major cardiovascular events including stroke (HR 0.52; 95% CI 0.34–0.79, P=0.002), and reduction in all-cause mortality (HR 0.80; 95% CI 0.67–0.97, P=0.02). This benefit was observed even in low-risk groups such as persons with LDL lower than 100 mg/dL and those with only elevated C-reactive protein but no other risk factors (158). As discussed in the 'Dyslipidaemia' section, the ASCOT-LLA trial also showed a benefit from atorvastatin use in hypertensive persons with normal or low cholesterol levels reducing stroke risk by 27% (43). Whether statins might reduce stroke risk in persons without any identifiable stroke risk factor is unknown.

Calculating individual stroke risk and global risk of cardiovascular disease

A number of stroke risk-assessment tools have been developed which integrate the most prevalent and high-impact risk factors into a simple clinical tool. The FHS developed a model that uses age, systolic blood pressure, diabetes mellitus, cigarette smoking, prior cardiovascular disease, AF, left ventricular hypertrophy on electrocardiogram, and the use of antihypertensive medication to determine a 10-year risk of stroke (25). This risk assessment tool has been endorsed and is used in treatment guidelines by the AHA/ASA, the British cardiovascular societies, and the European cardiovascular societies (34, 159, 160). Since the risk of stroke does not

occur in isolation from the risks of other cardiovascular events, a global cardiovascular risk score had been described. Two models have been developed for use in a primary care setting both of which estimate a 'heart age/vascular age.' The first model is based on components of all the traditional risk factors including laboratory values and the second model requires only data that may easily be obtained in an office setting. From the general risk score, individual risks of coronary heart disease, stroke, congestive heart failure, and peripheral vascular disease may also be determined (161).

Public health strategies for stroke prevention

Most strokes are a result of chronic disease caused by accumulation of risk factors. In this sense, stroke has a long latency period before becoming symptomatic. Thus most strokes are 'preventable.' In general, the earlier an intervention to prevent atherosclerotic disease is initiated, the greater its efficacy in preventing strokes.

We can determine the relative impact of the various causes of 'preventable' strokes by estimating a population-attributable risk (PAR) fraction for each risk factor; this depends on both the prevalence of the specific risk factor and the relative risk associated with it. Thus correcting a common risk factor such as a modest elevation in blood pressure would have a greater impact than addressing a relatively rarer risk factor such as SCD. PAR has been described as the reduction in disease incidence that would be observed if a given risk factor could be eliminated in the population (162).

Public health strategies to prevent stroke can be categorized into two main approaches, the 'mass' strategy and the 'high-risk' strategy (162, 163). The mass approach focuses on health education and a government commitment via legislative and economic measures to encourage healthy lifestyles. A 'prevention paradox' exists however, whereby a prevention that has a large benefit at a community level may not benefit an individual patient to the same degree (164). The high-risk approach focuses on identifying individual patients at high risk, through the use of risk-assessment profiles such as the Framingham risk score (see earlier) followed by targeted risk factor reduction in such individuals (164). On a community level, this approach is less effective and may fail to prevent most events that occur in the larger subset of the population that has mild elevation in risk factors levels below the threshold that would trigger clinical action (19). The most successful approach to the primary prevention of stroke will require the simultaneous use of both individual and community-based approaches.

Community-based interventions

In the HPFS and NHS, a low-risk lifestyle was defined as non-smoking, with a normal BMI (<25 kg/m^2), exercise for at least 30 minutes each day, modest consumption of alcohol, and eating a healthy diet rated in the upper 40% of all diets evaluated in the study sample. In these studies, women with a low-risk lifestyle had an almost 80% lower risk of stroke while men had an almost 70% lower risk compared to those without any of the low-risk lifestyle factors (165).

The AHA Guide for Improving Cardiovascular Health at the Community Level (166) and the UK's National Institute for Health and Clinical Excellence (NICE) guidelines (167) focus on decreasing population level CVD via community level education about vascular disease and its risk factors. The specific goals include lowering the salt, saturated fat and trans-fat contents of foods at a nationwide level via public education and economic incentives. Another goal is to increase average levels of physical activity via improved access to parks, community activity centres, and physical education programmes in schools. Policy changes are encouraged to reduce overall cigarette smoking and to reduce smoking initiation by adolescents and young adults; specific methods proposed include education, graphic risk warnings on cigarette cartons, increasing tariffs on cigarettes, and restrictions on advertising. Long-term community-based interventions can also improve smoking cessation rates. In the North Karelia region of Finland, a community-based intervention resulted in a complete smoking abstinence rate of 0.3% in the targeted group, compared with an average of 0.1% in other areas (p <0.001) (168).

In 2011, the Department of Health and Human Services together with the AHA announced the 'Million Hearts' initiative to prevent 1 million heart attacks and strokes within the next 5 years. This campaign ties together both an individualized high risk and a mass intervention approach. One goal will be based on attention to each individual's 'ABCs' for heart disease and stroke prevention: appropriate Aspirin use, Blood pressure control, Cholesterol control, and Smoking cessation. The second goal seeks to expand community programmes for reducing tobacco use and second-hand smoke exposure, reducing blood pressure, and improving nutrition (169, 170).

Commonality of risk factors and the international agenda for stroke prevention

The United Nations (UN) has acknowledged that the burden of non-communicable disease (NCD) is increasing. Today two-thirds of all deaths are attributed to NCD with four-fifths of these deaths occurring in low- and middle-income countries (171). Stroke prevention is an integral part of this overall goal of preventing non-communicable diseases since stroke shares risk factors with coronary heart disease, diabetes, peripheral vascular disease, and many types of cancer. The INTERSTROKE study looked at 22 countries worldwide, with 86% being low- to middle-income countries, to assess stroke risk factors across geographic regions and national income levels. Their findings suggest that ten risk factors are associated with 88.1% (99% CI 82.3–92.2) of the PAR for all strokes. These ten risk factors are hypertension, current smoking, waist-to-hip ratio, poor diet, lack of regular physical activity, diabetes, high alcohol intake, psychosocial factors including stress and depression, AF and other cardiac causes, and the ratio of apolipoproteins B to A1 (172). Of these, the most important remains controls of elevated blood pressures; in the INTERSTROKE study, hypertension had a PAR of 34.6% (99% CI 30.4–39.1) (172). Other studies have found that in low- to middle-income countries up to 54% of stroke mortality is attributable to elevated blood pressure (5). The common set of risk factors with the highest PARs worldwide have been targeted by the UN and the World Health Organization (WHO) as priority interventions that are most likely to rapidly reduce the burden of NCD. These 'Best-buys' have been deemed cost-effective in almost all countries; they again include targeting tobacco use, consumption of dietary salt, obesity and poor nutrition, physical inactivity, harmful alcohol use, and more specific cardiovascular risk reduction interventions targeted towards individuals at high risk of cardiovascular disease (171, 173, 174) (Table 23.3).

Table 23.3 'Best buy' interventions

Risk factor/disease	Interventions
Tobacco use	Tax increases
	Smoke-free indoor workplaces and public places
	Health information and warnings
	Bans on tobacco advertising, promotion and sponsorship
Harmful alcohol use	Tax increases
	Restricted access to retailed alcohol
	Bans on alcohol advertising
Unhealthy diet and physical inactivity	Reduced salt intake in food
	Replacement of trans fat with polyunsaturated fat
	Public awareness through mass media on diet and physical activity
Cardiovascular disease (CVD) and diabetes	Counselling and multi-drug therapy for people with a high risk of developing heart attacks and strokes (including those with established CVD)
	Treatment of heart attacks with aspirin
Cancer	Hepatitis B immunization to prevent liver cancer (already scaled up)
	Screening and treatment of pre-cancerous lesions to prevent cervical cancer

Conclusion

Stroke is a major cause of disability and death worldwide with several known risk factors. Efforts should be made at the individual level to identify high-risk individuals but this should be combined with approaches aimed at primordial prevention, that is preventing the development of key modifiable risk factors for cardiovascular and cerebrovascular disease. Prevention and management of hypertension, hyperlipidaemia, diabetes mellitus, obesity, cigarette smoking, and AF would substantially reduce the burden of stroke. Today these risk factors are no longer exclusive to the affluent, but are commonly found in the lower–middle-income populations throughout the world. Prevention of stroke alongside other NCDs strives to reduce the economic burden of managing chronic expensive medical conditions and reduce the cost of long-term disability that frequently accompanies cerebrovascular events.

References

1. Partridge EE, Mayer-Davis EJ, Sacco RL, Balch AJ. Creating a 21st century global health agenda: the General Assembly of the United Nations High Level Meeting on Non-Communicable Diseases. *Circulation*. 2011;123(25):3012–3014.
2. Jiaquan X, Kochanek KD, Murphy SL, Tejada-Vera B, Division of Vital Statistics. Deaths: final data for 2007.*NVSS*. 2007;58:19.
3. World Health Organization. *Global Health Repository Data. Mortality Country Fact Sheet 2006: United Kingdom*. <http://www.who.int/whosis/mort/profiles/mort_euro_gbr_unitedkingdom.pdf> (accessed 30 September 2011).
4. World Health Organization. *Chronic disease and Health Promotion. Stroke Surveillance*. <http://www.who.int/chp/steps/stroke/en/index.html> (accessed 30 September 2011).
5. Strong K, Mathers C, Bonita R. Preventing stroke: saving lives around the world. *Lancet Neurol*. 2007;6(2):182–187.

6. Lozano R, Naghavi M, Foreman K, Lim S, Shibuya K, Aboyans V, *et al.* Global and regional mortality from 235 causes of death for 20 age groups in 1990 and 2010: a systematic analysis for the Global Burden of Disease Study 2010. *Lancet.* 2012;380(9859):2095–2128.

7. Seshadri S, Beiser A, Kelly-Hayes M, Kase CS, Au R, Kannel WB, *et al.* The lifetime risk of stroke: estimates from the Framingham Study. *Stroke.* 2006;37(2):345–350.

8. Carandang R, Seshadri S, Beiser A, Kelly-Hayes M, Kase CS, Kannel WB, *et al.* Trends in incidence, lifetime risk, severity, and 30-day mortality of stroke over the past 50 years. *JAMA.* 2006;296(24):2939–2946.

9. Feigin VL, Lawes CM, Bennett DA, Barker-Collo SL, Parag V. Worldwide stroke incidence and early case fatality reported in 56 population-based studies: a systematic review. *Lancet Neurol.* 2009;8(4):355–369.

10. Sposato LA, Saposnik G. Gross domestic product and health expenditure associated with incidence, 30-day fatality, and age at stroke onset: a systematic review. *Stroke.* 2012;43(1):170–177.

11. Kurth T, Berger K. The socioeconomic stroke puzzle. *Stroke.* 2007;38(1):4–5.

12. Kuper H, Adami HO, Theorell T, Weiderpass E. The socioeconomic gradient in the incidence of stroke: a prospective study in middle-aged women in Sweden. *Stroke.* 2007;38(1):27–33.

13. Sacco RL, Boden-Albala B, Gan R, Chen X, Kargman DE, Shea S, *et al.* Stroke incidence among white, black, and Hispanic residents of an urban community: the Northern Manhattan Stroke Study. *Am J Epidemiol.* 1998;147(3):259–268.

14. Kissela B, Broderick J, Woo D, Kothari R, Miller R, Khoury J, *et al.* Greater Cincinnati/Northern Kentucky Stroke Study: volume of first-ever ischemic stroke among blacks in a population-based study. *Stroke.* 2001;32(6):1285–1290.

15. Roger VL, Go AS, Lloyd-Jones DM, Adams RJ, Berry JD, Brown TM, *et al.* Heart disease and stroke statistics—2011 update: a report from the American Heart Association. *Circulation.* 2011;123(4):e18–e209.

16. Kiely DK, Wolf PA, Cupples LA, Beiser AS, Myers RH. Familial aggregation of stroke. The Framingham Study. *Stroke.* 1993;24(9):1366–1371.

17. Petrea RE, Beiser AS, Seshadri S, Kelly-Hayes M, Kase CS, Wolf PA. Gender differences in stroke incidence and poststroke disability in the Framingham heart study. *Stroke.* 2009;40(4):1032–1037.

18. Seshadri S, Beiser A, Pikula A, Himali JJ, Kelly-Hayes M, Debette S, *et al.* Parental occurrence of stroke and risk of stroke in their children: the Framingham study. *Circulation.* 2010;121(11):1304–1312.

19. Wolf PA. Cerebrovascular risk. In Izzo JL, Black HR (eds) *Hypertension Primer: The Essentials of High Blood Pressure* (3rd edn, pp. 239–242). Philadelphia, PA: Lippincott, Williams & Williams; 2003.

20. Wolf PA, D'Agostino RB, Belanger AJ, Kannel WB. Probability of stroke: a risk profile from the Framingham Study. *Stroke.* 1991;22(3):312–318.

21. Rothwell PM, Howard SC, Dolan E, O'Brien E, Dobson JE, Dahlof B, *et al.* Prognostic significance of visit-to-visit variability, maximum systolic blood pressure, and episodic hypertension. *Lancet.* 2010;375(9718):895–905.

22. Lewington S, Clarke R, Qizilbash N, Peto R, Collins R. Age-specific relevance of usual blood pressure to vascular mortality: a meta-analysis of individual data for one million adults in 61 prospective studies. *Lancet.* 2002;1:1903–1913.

23. Chobanian AV, Bakris GL, Black HR, Cushman WC, Green LA, Izzo JL, Jr, *et al.* The Seventh Report of the Joint National Committee on Prevention, Detection, Evaluation, and Treatment of High Blood Pressure: the JNC 7 report. *JAMA.* 2003;289(19):2560–2572.

24. Seshadri S, Wolf PA, Beiser A, Vasan RS, Wilson PW, Kase CS, *et al.* Elevated midlife blood pressure increases stroke risk in elderly persons: the Framingham Study. *Arch Intern Med.* 2001;161(19):2343–2350.

25. D'Agostino RB, Wolf PA, Belanger AJ, Kannel WB. Stroke risk profile: adjustment for antihypertensive medication. The Framingham Study. *Stroke.* 1994;25(1):40–43.

26. Psaty BM, Lumley T, Furberg CD, Schellenbaum G, Pahor M, Alderman MH, *et al.* Health outcomes associated with various antihypertensive therapies used as first-line agents: a network meta-analysis. *JAMA.* 2003;289(19):2534–2544.

27. Wright JM, Musini VM. First-line drugs for hypertension. *Cochrane Database Syst Rev.* 2009;3:CD001841.

28. Major outcomes in high-risk hypertensive patients randomized to angiotensin-converting enzyme inhibitor or calcium channel blocker vs diuretic: The Antihypertensive and Lipid-Lowering Treatment to Prevent Heart Attack Trial (ALLHAT). *JAMA.* 2002;288(23):2981–2997.

29. Webb AJ, Fischer U, Mehta Z, Rothwell PM. Effects of antihypertensive-drug class on interindividual variation in blood pressure and risk of stroke: a systematic review and meta-analysis. *Lancet.* 2010;375(9718):906–915.

30. Webb AJ, Fischer U, Rothwell PM. Effects of beta-blocker selectivity on blood pressure variability and stroke: a systematic review. *Neurology.* 2011;77(8):731–737.

31. Beckett NS, Peters R, Fletcher AE, Staessen JA, Liu L, Dumitrascu D, *et al.* Treatment of hypertension in patients 80 years of age or older. *N Engl J Med.* 2008;358(18):1887–1898.

32. Prevention of stroke by antihypertensive drug treatment in older persons with isolated systolic hypertension. Final results of the Systolic Hypertension in the Elderly Program (SHEP). SHEP Cooperative Research Group. *JAMA.* 1991;265(24):3255–3264.

33. Amery A, Birkenhager W, Brixko P, Bulpitt C, Clement D, Deruyttere M, *et al.* Mortality and morbidity results from the European Working Party on High Blood Pressure in the Elderly trial. *Lancet.* 1985;1(8442):1349–1354.

34. Goldstein LB, Bushnell CD, Adams RJ, Appel LJ, Braun LT, Chaturvedi S, *et al.* Guidelines for the primary prevention of stroke: a guideline for healthcare professionals from the American Heart Association/ American Stroke Association. *Stroke.* 2011;42(2):517–584.

35. Randomised trial of a perindopril-based blood-pressure-lowering regimen among 6105 individuals with previous stroke or transient ischaemic attack. *Lancet.* 2001;358(9287):1033–1041.

36. Iso H, Jacobs DR Jr, Wentworth D, Neaton JD, Cohen JD. Serum cholesterol levels and six year mortality from stroke in 350,977 men screened for the multiple risk factor interventional trial. *N Engl J Med.* 1989.

37. Zhang X, Patel A, Horibe H, Wu Z, Barzi F, Rodgers A, *et al.* Cholesterol, coronary heart disease, and stroke in the Asia Pacific region. *Int J Epidemiol.* 2003;32(4):563–572.

38. Kurth T, Everett BM, Buring JE, Kase CS, Ridker PM, Gaziano JM. Lipid levels and the risk of ischemic stroke in women. *Neurology.* 2007;68(8):556–562.

39. Shahar E, Chambless LE, Rosamond WD, Boland LL, Ballantyne CM, McGovern PG, *et al.* Plasma lipid profile and incident ischemic stroke: the Atherosclerosis Risk in Communities (ARIC) study. *Stroke.* 2003;34(3):623–631.

40. Bowman TS, Sesso HD, Ma J, Kurth T, Kase CS, Stampfer MJ, *et al.* Cholesterol and the risk of ischemic stroke. *Stroke.* 2003;34(12):2930–2934.

41. Sanossian N, Saver JL, Navab M, Ovbiagele B. High-density lipoprotein cholesterol: an emerging target for stroke treatment. *Stroke.* 2007;38(3):1104–1109.

42. Amarenco P, Labreuche J, Lavallee P, Touboul PJ. Statins in stroke prevention and carotid atherosclerosis: systematic review and up-to-date meta-analysis. *Stroke.* 2004;35(12):2902–2909.

43. Sever P, Dahlof B, Poulter N, Wedel H, Beevers G, Caulfield M, *et al.* Prevention of coronary and stroke events with atorvastatin in hypertensive patients who have average or lower-than-average cholesterol concentrations, in the Anglo-Scandinavian Cardiac Outcomes Trial? Lipid Lowering Arm (ASCOT-LLA): a multicentre randomised controlled trial. *Lancet.* 2003;361(9364):1149–1158.

44. Sturgeon JD, Folsom AR, Longstreth WT, Jr, Shahar E, Rosamond WD, Cushman M. Risk factors for intracerebral hemorrhage in a pooled prospective study. *Stroke.* 2007;38(10):2718–2725.

45. Hackam DG, Austin PC, Huang A, Juurlink DN, Mamdani MM, Paterson JM, et al. Statins and intracerebral hemorrhage: a retrospective cohort study. *Arch Neurol*. 2011.

46. Executive Summary of The Third Report of The National Cholesterol Education Program (NCEP) Expert Panel on Detection, Evaluation, And Treatment of High Blood Cholesterol In Adults (Adult Treatment Panel III). *JAMA*. 2001;285(19):2486–2497.

47. Wild S, Roglic G, Green A, Sicree R, King H. Global prevalence of diabetes: estimates for the year 2000 and projections for 2030. *Diabet Care*. 2004;27(5):1047–1053.

48. Effect of intensive blood-glucose control with metformin on complications in overweight patients with type 2 diabetes (UKPDS 34). *Lancet*. 1998;352(9131):854–865.

49. Duckworth W, Abraira C, Moritz T, Reda D, Emanuele N, Reaven PD, et al. Glucose control and vascular complications in veterans with type 2 diabetes. *N Engl J Med*. 2009;360(2):129–139.

50. Kearney PM, Blackwell L, Collins R, Keech A, Simes J, Peto R, et al. Efficacy of cholesterol-lowering therapy in 18,686 people with diabetes in 14 randomised trials of statins: a meta-analysis. *Lancet*. 2008;371(9607):117–125.

51. Colhoun HM, Betteridge DJ, Durrington PN, Hitman GA, Neil HA, Livingstone SJ, et al. Primary prevention of cardiovascular disease with atorvastatin in type 2 diabetes in the Collaborative Atorvastatin Diabetes Study (CARDS): multicentre randomised placebo-controlled trial. *Lancet*. 2004;364(9435):685–696.

52. Thun MJ, Apicella LF, Henley SJ. Smoking vs other risk factors as the cause of smoking-attributable deaths: confounding in the courtroom. *JAMA*. 2000;284(6):706–712.

53. Shinton R, Beevers G. Meta-analysis of relation between cigarette smoking and stroke. *BMJ*. 1989;298(6676):789–794.

54. Moritsugu KP. The 2006 Report of the Surgeon General: the health consequences of involuntary exposure to tobacco smoke. *Am J Prev Med*. 2007;32(6):542–543.

55. Wolf PA, D'Agostino RB, Kannel WB, Bonita R, Belanger AJ. Cigarette smoking as a risk factor for stroke. The Framingham Study. *JAMA*. 1988;259(7):1025–1029.

56. Nakamura K, Barzi F, Lam TH, Huxley R, Feigin VL, Ueshima H, et al. Cigarette smoking, systolic blood pressure, and cardiovascular diseases in the Asia-Pacific region. *Stroke*. 2008;39(6):1694–1702.

57. Howard G, Wagenknecht LE, Burke GL, Diez-Roux A, Evans GW, McGovern P, et al. Cigarette smoking and progression of atherosclerosis: The Atherosclerosis Risk in Communities (ARIC) Study. *JAMA*. 1998;279(2):119–124.

58. Ischaemic stroke and combined oral contraceptives: results of an international, multicentre, case-control study. WHO Collaborative Study of Cardiovascular Disease and Steroid Hormone Contraception. *Lancet*. 1996;348(9026):498–505.

59. U.S. Preventive Services Task Force. Counseling and Interventions to Prevent Tobacco Use and Tobacco-Caused Disease in Adults and Pregnant Women: U.S. Preventive Services Task Force Reaffirmation Recommendation Statement. *Ann Intern Med*. 2009;150(8):551–555.

60. Fuster V, Ryden LE, Cannom DS, Crijns HJ, Curtis AB, Ellenbogen KA, et al. ACC/AHA/ESC 2006 Guidelines for the Management of Patients with Atrial Fibrillation: a report of the American College of Cardiology/American Heart Association Task Force on Practice Guidelines and the European Society of Cardiology Committee for Practice Guidelines (Writing Committee to Revise the 2001 Guidelines for the Management of Patients With Atrial Fibrillation): developed in collaboration with the European Heart Rhythm Association and the Heart Rhythm Society. *Circulation*. 2006;114(7):e257–354.

61. Marini C, De Santis F, Sacco S, Russo T, Olivieri L, Totaro R, et al. Contribution of atrial fibrillation to incidence and outcome of ischemic stroke: results from a population-based study. *Stroke*. 2005;36(6):1115–1119.

62. Wolf PA, Abbott RD, Kannel WB. Atrial fibrillation: a major contributor to stroke in the elderly. The Framingham Study. *Arch Intern Med*. 1987;147(9):1561–1564.

63. Fitzmaurice DA, Hobbs FD, Jowett S, Mant J, Murray ET, Holder R, et al. Screening versus routine practice in detection of atrial fibrillation in patients aged 65 or over: cluster randomised controlled trial. *BMJ*. 2007;335(7616):383.

64. Gage BF, Waterman AD, Shannon W, Boechler M, Rich MW, Radford MJ. Validation of clinical classification schemes for predicting stroke: results from the National Registry of Atrial Fibrillation. *JAMA*. 2001;285(22):2864–2870.

65. Hart RG, Pearce LA, Aguilar MI. Meta-analysis: antithrombotic therapy to prevent stroke in patients who have nonvalvular atrial fibrillation. *Ann Intern Med*. 2007;146(12):857–867.

66. Patients with nonvalvular atrial fibrillation at low risk of stroke during treatment with aspirin: Stroke Prevention in Atrial Fibrillation III Study. The SPAF III Writing Committee for the Stroke Prevention in Atrial Fibrillation Investigators. *JAMA*. 1998;279(16):1273–1277.

67. Singer DE, Albers GW, Dalen JE, Go AS, Halperin JL, Manning WJ. Antithrombotic therapy in atrial fibrillation: the Seventh ACCP Conference on Antithrombotic and Thrombolytic Therapy. *Chest*. 2004;126(3 Suppl):429S–56S.

68. Hart RG, Tonarelli SB, Pearce LA. Avoiding central nervous system bleeding during antithrombotic therapy: recent data and ideas. *Stroke*. 2005;36(7):1588–1593.

69. Connolly SJ, Ezekowitz MD, Yusuf S, Eikelboom J, Oldgren J, Parekh A, et al. Dabigatran versus warfarin in patients with atrial fibrillation. *N Engl J Med*. 2009;361(12):1139–1151.

70. Granger CB, Alexander JH, McMurray JJ, Lopes RD, Hylek EM, Hanna M, et al. Apixaban versus warfarin in patients with atrial fibrillation. *N Engl J Med*. 2011;365(11):981–992.

71. Patel MR, Mahaffey KW, Garg J, Pan G, Singer DE, Hacke W, et al. Rivaroxaban versus warfarin in nonvalvular atrial fibrillation. *N Engl J Med*. 2011;365(10):883–891.

72. Donahue RP, Abbott RD, Reed DM, Yano K. Alcohol and hemorrhagic stroke. The Honolulu Heart Program. *JAMA*. 1986;255(17):2311–2314.

73. Sacco RL, Elkind M, Boden-Albala B, Lin IF, Kargman DE, Hauser WA, et al. The protective effect of moderate alcohol consumption on ischemic stroke. *JAMA*. 1999;281(1):53–60.

74. Berger K, Ajani UA, Kase CS, Gaziano JM, Buring JE, Glynn RJ, et al. Light-to-moderate alcohol consumption and risk of stroke among U.S. male physicians. *N Engl J Med*. 1999;341(21):1557–1564.

75. Ohene-Frempong K, Weiner SJ, Sleeper LA, Miller ST, Embury S, Moohr JW, et al. Cerebrovascular accidents in sickle cell disease: rates and risk factors. *Blood*. 1998;91(1):288–294.

76. Adams RJ, McKie VC, Hsu L, Files B, Vichinsky E, Pegelow C, et al. Prevention of a first stroke by transfusions in children with sickle cell anemia and abnormal results on transcranial Doppler ultrasonography. *N Engl J Med*. 1998;339(1):5–11.

77. Adams RJ. Stroke prevention and treatment in sickle cell disease. *Arch Neurol*. 2001;58(4):565–568.

78. Adams RJ, Brambilla D. Discontinuing prophylactic transfusions used to prevent stroke in sickle cell disease. *N Engl J Med*. 2005;353(26):2769–2778.

79. Zimmerman SA, Schultz WH, Burgett S, Mortier NA, Ware RE. Hydroxyurea therapy lowers transcranial Doppler flow velocities in children with sickle cell anemia. *Blood*. 2007;110(3):1043–1047.

80. National Heart, Lung, and Blood Institute (NHLBI) press release, 6 April 2010. <http://public.nhlbi.nih.gov/newsroom/home/GetPressRelease.aspx?id=2709> (accessed 11 October 2010)>.

81. Rossouw JE, Anderson GL, Prentice RL, LaCroix AZ, Kooperberg C, Stefanick ML, et al. Risks and benefits of estrogen plus progestin in healthy postmenopausal women: principal results From the Women's Health Initiative randomized controlled trial. *JAMA*. 2002;288(3):321–333.

82. Hendrix SL, Wassertheil-Smoller S, Johnson KC, Howard BV, Kooperberg C, Rossouw JE, et al. Effects of conjugated equine estrogen on stroke in the Women's Health Initiative. *Circulation.* 2006;113(20):2425–2434.

83. Grodstein F, Manson JE, Stampfer MJ, Rexrode K. Postmenopausal hormone therapy and stroke: role of time since menopause and age at initiation of hormone therapy. *Arch Intern Med.* 2008;168(8):861–866.

84. Cummings SR, Ettinger B, Delmas PD, Kenemans P, Stathopoulos V, Verweij P, et al. The effects of tibolone in older postmenopausal women. *N Engl J Med.* 2008;359(7):697–708.

85. Mosca L, Grady D, Barrett-Connor E, Collins P, Wenger N, Abramson BL, et al. Effect of raloxifene on stroke and venous thromboembolism according to subgroups in postmenopausal women at increased risk of coronary heart disease. *Stroke.* 2009;40(1):147–155.

86. Lidegaard O, Lokkegaard E, Jensen A, Skovlund CW, Keiding N. Thrombotic stroke and myocardial infarction with hormonal contraception. *N Engl J Med.* 2012;366(24):2257–2266.

87. Nightingale AL, Farmer RD. Ischemic stroke in young women: a nested case-control study using the UK General Practice Research Database. *Stroke.* 2004;35(7):1574–1578.

88. Kuklina EV, Tong X, Bansil P, George MG, Callaghan WM. Trends in pregnancy hospitalizations that included a stroke in the United States from 1994 to 2007: reasons for concern? *Stroke.* 2011;42(9):2564–2570.

89. Kemmeren JM. Risk of Arterial Thrombosis in Relation to Oral Contraceptives (RATIO) Study: Oral Contraceptives and the Risk of Ischemic Stroke. *Stroke.* 2002;33(5):1202–1208.

90. Mudd SH, Skovby F, Levy HL, Pettigrew KD, Wilcken B, Pyeritz RE, et al. The natural history of homocystinuria due to cystathionine beta-synthase deficiency. *Am J Hum Genet.* 1985;37(1):1–31.

91. Bostom AG, Rosenberg IH, Silbershatz H, Jacques PF, Selhub J, D'Agostino RB, et al. Nonfasting plasma total homocysteine levels and stroke incidence in elderly persons: the Framingham Study. *Ann Intern Med.* 1999;131(5):352–355.

92. Ebbing M, Bleie O, Ueland PM, Nordrehaug JE, Nilsen DW, Vollset SE, et al. Mortality and cardiovascular events in patients treated with homocysteine-lowering B vitamins after coronary angiography: a randomized controlled trial. *JAMA.* 2008;300(7):795–804.

93. B vitamins in patients with recent transient ischaemic attack or stroke in the VITAmins TO Prevent Stroke (VITATOPS) trial: a randomised, double-blind, parallel, placebo-controlled trial. *Lancet Neurol.* 2010;9(9):855–865.

94. Nieto FJ, Young TB, Lind BK, Shahar E, Samet JM, Redline S, et al. Association of sleep-disordered breathing, sleep apnea, and hypertension in a large community-based study. Sleep Heart Health Study. *JAMA.* 2000;283(14):1829–1836.

95. Gami AS, Pressman G, Caples SM, Kanagala R, Gard JJ, Davison DE, et al. Association of atrial fibrillation and obstructive sleep apnea. *Circulation.* 2004;110(4):364–367.

96. Yaggi HK, Concato J, Kernan WN, Lichtman JH, Brass LM, Mohsenin V. Obstructive sleep apnea as a risk factor for stroke and death. *N Engl J Med.* 2005;353(19):2034–2041.

97. Redline S, Yenokyan G, Gottlieb DJ, Shahar E, O'Connor GT, Resnick HE, et al. Obstructive sleep apnea-hypopnea and incident stroke: the sleep heart health study. *Am J Respir Crit Care Med.* 2010;182(2):269–277.

98. Munoz R, Duran-Cantolla J, Martinez-Vila E, Gallego J, Rubio R, Aizpuru F, et al. Severe sleep apnea and risk of ischemic stroke in the elderly. *Stroke.* 2006;37(9):2317–2321.

99. Pepperell JC, Ramdassingh-Dow S, Crosthwaite N, Mullins R, Jenkinson C, Stradling JR, et al. Ambulatory blood pressure after therapeutic and subtherapeutic nasal continuous positive airway pressure for obstructive sleep apnoea: a randomised parallel trial. *Lancet.* 2002;359(9302):204–210.

100. Buchner NJ, Sanner BM, Borgel J, Rump LC. Continuous positive airway pressure treatment of mild to moderate obstructive sleep

101. apnea reduces cardiovascular risk. *Am J Respir Crit Care Med.* 2007;176(12):1274–1280.

101. Lozano L, Tovar JL, Sampol G, Romero O, Jurado MJ, Segarra A, et al. Continuous positive airway pressure treatment in sleep apnea patients with resistant hypertension: a randomized, controlled trial. *J Hypertens.* 2010;28(10):2161–2168.

102. Ogden CL, Carroll MD, Curtin LR, McDowell MA, Tabak CJ, Flegal KM. Prevalence of overweight and obesity in the United States, 1999-2004. *JAMA.* 2006;295(13):1549–1555.

103. Suk SH, Sacco RL, Boden-Albala B, Cheun JF, Pittman JG, Elkind MS, et al. Abdominal obesity and risk of ischemic stroke: the Northern Manhattan Stroke Study. *Stroke.* 2003;34(7):1586–1592.

104. Neter JE, Stam BE, Kok FJ, Grobbee DE, Geleijnse JM. Influence of weight reduction on blood pressure: a meta-analysis of randomized controlled trials. *Hypertension.* 2003;42(5):878–884.

105. Appel LJ, Brands MW, Daniels SR, Karanja N, Elmer PJ, Sacks FM. Dietary approaches to prevent and treat hypertension: a scientific statement from the American Heart Association. *Hypertension.* 2006;47(2):296–308.

106. He FJ, Nowson CA, MacGregor GA. Fruit and vegetable consumption and stroke: meta-analysis of cohort studies. *Lancet.* 2006;367(9507):320–326.

107. Sacks FM, Svetkey LP, Vollmer WM, Appel LJ, Bray GA, Harsha D, et al. Effects on blood pressure of reduced dietary sodium and the Dietary Approaches to Stop Hypertension (DASH) diet. DASH-Sodium Collaborative Research Group. *N Engl J Med.* 2001;344(1):3–10.

108. Fung TT, Rexrode KM, Mantzoros CS, Manson JE, Willett WC, Hu FB. Mediterranean diet and incidence of and mortality from coronary heart disease and stroke in women. *Circulation.* 2009;119(8):1093–1100.

109. Gardener H, Wright CB, Gu Y, Demmer RT, Boden-Albala B, Elkind MS, et al. Mediterranean-style diet and risk of ischemic stroke, myocardial infarction, and vascular death: the Northern Manhattan Study. *Am J Clin Nutr.* 2011;94(6):1458–1464.

110. He K, Rimm EB, Merchant A, Rosner BA, Stampfer MJ, Willett WC, et al. Fish consumption and risk of stroke in men. *JAMA.* 2002;288(24):3130–3136.

111. Hu FB, Stampfer MJ, Colditz GA, Ascherio A, Rexrode KM, Willett WC, et al. Physical activity and risk of stroke in women. *JAMA.* 2000;283(22):2961–2967.

112. Kiely DK, Wolf PA, Cupples LA, Beiser AS, Kannel WB. Physical activity and stroke risk: the Framingham Study. *Am J Epidemiol.* 1994;140(7):608–620.

113. Willey JZ, Moon YP, Paik MC, Boden-Albala B, Sacco RL, Elkind MS. Physical activity and risk of ischemic stroke in the Northern Manhattan Study. *Neurology.* 2009;73(21):1774–1779.

114. Lee CD, Folsom AR, Blair SN. Physical activity and stroke risk: a meta-analysis. *Stroke.* 2003;34(10):2475–2481.

115. Services UDoHaH. *Physical Activity Guidelines Advisory Committee Report, 2008.* <http://www.health.gov/paguidelines/> (accessed 14 October 2011).

116. Chiuve SE, Rexrode KM, Spiegelman D, Logroscino G, Manson JE, Rimm EB. Primary prevention of stroke by healthy lifestyle. *Circulation.* 2008;118(9):947–954.

117. Cornier MA, Dabelea D, Hernandez TL, Lindstrom RC, Steig AJ, Stob NR, et al. The metabolic syndrome. *Endocrine Rev.* 2008;29(7):777–822.

118. Ninomiya JK, L'Italien G, Criqui MH, Whyte JL, Gamst A, Chen RS. Association of the metabolic syndrome with history of myocardial infarction and stroke in the Third National Health and Nutrition Examination Survey. *Circulation.* 2004;109(1):42–46.

119. Najarian RM, Sullivan LM, Kannel WB, Wilson PW, D'Agostino RB, Wolf PA. Metabolic syndrome compared with type 2 diabetes mellitus as a risk factor for stroke: the Framingham Offspring Study. *Arch Intern Med.* 2006;166(1):106–111.

120. Ballantyne CM, Hoogeveen RC, McNeill AM, Heiss G, Schmidt MI, Duncan BB, et al. Metabolic syndrome risk for cardiovascular disease

and diabetes in the ARIC study. *Int J Obes (Lond)*. 2008;32(Suppl 2):S21–S24.

121. Rundek T, White H, Boden-Albala B, Jin Z, Elkind MS, Sacco RL. The metabolic syndrome and subclinical carotid atherosclerosis: the Northern Manhattan Study. *J Cardiometabol Syndr*. 2007;2(1):24–29.

122. Wang J, Ruotsalainen S, Moilanen L, Lepisto P, Laakso M, Kuusisto J. The metabolic syndrome predicts incident stroke: a 14-year follow-up study in elderly people in Finland. *Stroke*. 2008;39(4):1078–1083.

123. Insulin Resistance Intervention after Stroke Trial. <http://www.iristrial. org/> (accessed 15 October 2011).

124. Fabbian F, Catalano C, Lambertini D, Tarroni G, Bordin V, Squerzanti R, *et al.* Clinical characteristics associated to atrial fibrillation in chronic hemodialysis patients. *Clin Nephrol*. 2000;54(3):234–239.

125. Abramson JL, Jurkovitz CT, Vaccarino V, Weintraub WS, McClellan W. Chronic kidney disease, anemia, and incident stroke in a middle-aged, community-based population: the ARIC Study. *Kidney Int*. 2003;64(2):610–615.

126. Lee M, Saver JL, Chang KH, Liao HW, Chang SC, Ovbiagele B. Low glomerular filtration rate and risk of stroke: meta-analysis. *BMJ*. 2010;341:c4249.

127. Cheung AK, Sarnak MJ, Yan G, Dwyer JT, Heyka RJ, Rocco MV, *et al.* Atherosclerotic cardiovascular disease risks in chronic hemodialysis patients. *Kidney Int*. 2000;58(1):353–362.

128. Kawamura M, Fijimoto S, Hisanaga S, Yamamoto Y, Eto T. Incidence, outcome, and risk factors of cerebrovascular events in patients undergoing maintenance hemodialysis. *Am J Kidney Dis*.1998;31(6):991–996.

129. Seliger SL, Gillen DL, Longstreth WT, Jr, Kestenbaum B, Stehman-Breen CO. Elevated risk of stroke among patients with end-stage renal disease. *Kidney Int*. 2003;64(2):603–609.

130. Sozio SM, Armstrong PA, Coresh J, Jaar BG, Fink NE, Plantinga LC, *et al.* Cerebrovascular disease incidence, characteristics, and outcomes in patients initiating dialysis: the choices for healthy outcomes in caring for ESRD (CHOICE) study. *Am J Kidney Dis*. 2009;54(3):468–477.

131. Power A, Chan K, Singh SK, Taube D, Duncan N. Appraising stroke risk in maintenance hemodialysis patients: a large single-center cohort study. *Am J Kidney Dis*. 2012;59(2):249–257.

132. van der Sande FM, Hermans MM, Leunissen KM, Kooman JP. Noncardiac consequences of hypertension in hemodialysis patients. *Semin Dial*. 2004;17(4):304–306.

133. Abedini S, Holme I, Fellstrom B, Jardine A, Cole E, Maes B, *et al.* Cerebrovascular events in renal transplant recipients. *Transplantation*. 2009;87(1):112–117.

134. Oliveras A, Roquer J, Puig JM, Rodriguez A, Mir M, Orfila MA, *et al.* Stroke in renal transplant recipients: epidemiology, predictive risk factors and outcome. *Clin Transplant*. 2003;17(1):1–8.

135. Libby P, Ridker PM, Hansson GK. Inflammation in atherosclerosis: from pathophysiology to practice. *J Am Coll Cardiol*. 2009;54(23):2129–2138.

136. Rost NS, Wolf PA, Kase CS, Kelly-Hayes M, Silbershatz H, Massaro JM, *et al.* Plasma concentration of C-reactive protein and risk of ischemic stroke and transient ischemic attack: the Framingham study. *Stroke*. 2001;32(11):2575–2579.

137. Wolfe F, Freundlich B, Straus WL. Increase in cardiovascular and cerebrovascular disease prevalence in rheumatoid arthritis. *J Rheumatol*. 2003;30:36–40.

138. Cole JW, Pinto AN, Hebel JR, Buchholz DW, Earley CJ, Johnson CJ, *et al.* Acquired immunodeficiency syndrome and the risk of stroke. *Stroke*. 2004;35(1):51–56.

139. Danesh J. Coronary heart disease, Helicobacter pylori, dental disease, Chlamydia pneumoniae, and cytomegalovirus: meta-analyses of prospective studies. *Am Heart J*. 1999;138(5 Pt 2):S434–S437.

140. Grau AJ, Buggle F, Ziegler C, Schwarz W, Meuser J, Tasman AJ, *et al.* Association between acute cerebrovascular ischemia and chronic and recurrent infection. *Stroke*. 1997;28(9):1724–1729.

141. Kuo HK, Fujise K. Human papillomavirus and cardiovascular disease among US women in the National Health and Nutrition Examination Survey, 2003 to 2006. *J Am Coll Cardiol*. 2011;58:2001–2006.

142. Lee MH, Yang HI, Wang CH, Jen CL, Yeh SH, Liu CJ, *et al.* Hepatitis C virus infection and increased risk of cerebrovascular disease. *Stroke*. 2010;41(12):2894–2900.

143. Markus HS, Mendall MA. Helicobacter pylori infection: a risk factor for ischaemic cerebrovascular disease and carotid atheroma. *J Neurol Neurosurg Psychiatry*. 1998;64(1):104–107.

144. Lindsberg PJ, Grau AJ. Inflammation and infections as risk factors for ischemic stroke. *Stroke*. 2003;34(10):2518–2532.

145. Grayston JT. Background and current knowledge of Chlamydia pneumoniae and atherosclerosis. *J Infect Dis*. 2000;181 Suppl 3:S402–S410.

146. Saikku P, Leinonen M, Mattila K, Ekman MR, Nieminen MS, Makela PH, *et al.* Serological evidence of an association of a novel Chlamydia, TWAR, with chronic coronary heart disease and acute myocardial infarction. *Lancet*. 1988;2(8618):983–986.

147. Grayston JT, Kronmal RA, Jackson LA, Parisi AF, Muhlestein JB, Cohen JD, *et al.* Azithromycin for the secondary prevention of coronary events. *N Engl J Med*. 2005;352(16):1637–1645.

148. Elkind MS. Infectious burden: a new risk factor and treatment target for atherosclerosis. *Infect Disord Drug Targets*. 2010;10(2):84–90.

149. Warren-Gash C, Smeeth L, Hayward AC. Influenza as a trigger for acute myocardial infarction or death from cardiovascular disease: a systematic review. *Lancet Infect Dis*. 2009;9(10):601–610.

150. Madjid M, Curkendall S, Blumentals WA. The influence of oseltamivir treatment on the risk of stroke after influenza infection. *Cardiology*. 2009;113(2):98–107.

151. Nichol KL, Nordin J, Mullooly J, Lask R, Fillbrandt K, Iwane M. Influenza vaccination and reduction in hospitalizations for cardiac disease and stroke among the elderly. *N Engl J Med*. 2003;348(14):1322–1332.

152. Johnson ES, Lanes SF, Wentworth CE, 3rd, Satterfield MH, Abebe BL, Dicker LW. A metaregression analysis of the dose-response effect of aspirin on stroke. *Arch Intern Med*. 1999;159(11):1248–1253.

153. Final report on the aspirin component of the ongoing Physicians' Health Study. Steering Committee of the Physicians' Health Study Research Group. *N Engl J Med*. 1989;321(3):129–135.

154. Berger JS, Roncaglioni MC, Avanzini F, Pangrazzi I, Tognoni G, Brown DL. Aspirin for the primary prevention of cardiovascular events in women and men: a sex-specific meta-analysis of randomized controlled trials. *JAMA*. 2006;295(3):306–313.

155. Ridker PM, Cook NR, Lee IM, Gordon D, Gaziano JM, Manson JE, *et al.* A randomized trial of low-dose aspirin in the primary prevention of cardiovascular disease in women. *N Engl J Med*. 2005;352(13):1293–1304.

156. Pearson TA, Blair SN, Daniels SR, Eckel RH, Fair JM, Fortmann SP, *et al.* AHA Guidelines for Primary Prevention of Cardiovascular Disease and Stroke: 2002 Update: Consensus Panel Guide to Comprehensive Risk Reduction for Adult Patients Without Coronary or Other Atherosclerotic Vascular Diseases. American Heart Association Science Advisory and Coordinating Committee. *Circulation*. 2002;106(3):388–391.

157. Rothwell PM, Price JF, Fowkes FG, Zanchetti A, Roncaglioni MC, Tognoni G, *et al.* Short-term effects of daily aspirin on cancer incidence, mortality, and non-vascular death: analysis of the time course of risks and benefits in 51 randomised controlled trials. *Lancet*. 2012;379(9826):1602–1612.

158. Ridker PM, Danielson E, Fonseca FA, Genest J, Gotto AM, Jr, Kastelein JJ, *et al.* Rosuvastatin to prevent vascular events in men and women with elevated C-reactive protein. *N Engl J Med*. 2008;359(21):2195–2207.

159. Joint British recommendations on prevention of coronary heart disease in clinical practice: summary. British Cardiac Society, British Hyperlipidaemia Association, British Hypertension Society, British Diabetic Association. *BMJ*. 2000;320(7236):705–708.

160. De Backer G, Ambrosioni E, Borch-Johnsen K, Brotons C, Cifkova R, Dallongeville J, et al. European guidelines on cardiovascular disease prevention in clinical practice. Third Joint Task Force of European and Other Societies on Cardiovascular Disease Prevention in Clinical Practice. Eur Heart J. 2003;24(17):1601–1610.

161. D'Agostino RB, Sr., Vasan RS, Pencina MJ, Wolf PA, Cobain M, Massaro JM, et al. General cardiovascular risk profile for use in primary care: the Framingham Heart Study. Circulation. 2008;117(6):743–753.

162. Rose G. Strategy of prevention: lessons from cardiovascular disease. BMJ (Clin Res Ed). 1981;282(6279):1847–1851.

163. Gorelick PB. Stroke prevention. An opportunity for efficient utilization of health care resources during the coming decade. Stroke. 1994;25(1):220–224.

164. Gorelick PB. Stroke prevention. Arch Neurol. 1995;52(4):347–355.

165. Chiuve SE, Rexrode KM, Spiegelman D, Logroscino G, Manson JE, Rimm EB. Primary prevention of stroke by healthy lifestyle. Circulation. 2008;118(9):947–954.

166. Pearson TA. American Heart Association Guide for Improving Cardiovascular Health at the Community Level: A Statement for Public Health Practitioners, Healthcare Providers, and Health Policy Makers From the American Heart Association Expert Panel on Population and Prevention Science. Circulation. 2003;107(4):645–651.

167. National Institute for Health and Clinical Excellence. NICE Public Health Guidance 25:Prevention of Cardiovascular Disease at Population Level. <http://www.nice.org.uk/guidance/PH25> (accessed 19 October 2011).

168. Korhonen T, Urjanheimo EL, Mannonen P, Korhonen HJ, Uutela A, Puska P. Quit and Win campaigns as a long-term anti-smoking intervention in North Karelia and other parts of Finland. Tob Control. 1999;8(2):175–181.

169. Tomaselli GF, Harty MB, Horton K, Schoeberl M. The American Heart Association and the Million Hearts Initiative: a presidential advisory from the American Heart Association. Circulation. 2011;124(16):1795–1799.

170. Frieden TR, Berwick DM. The "Million Hearts" initiative—preventing heart attacks and strokes. N Engl J Med. 2011;365(13):e27.

171. Beaglehole R, Bonita R, Horton R, Adams C, Alleyne G, Asaria P, et al. Priority actions for the non-communicable disease crisis. Lancet. 2011;377(9775):1438–1447.

172. O'Donnell MJ, Xavier D, Liu L, Zhang H, Chin SL, Rao-Melacini P, et al. Risk factors for ischaemic and intracerebral haemorrhagic stroke in 22 countries (the INTERSTROKE study): a case-control study. Lancet. 2010;376(9735):112–123.

173. World Health Organization. Global Atlas on Cardiovascular Disease Prevention and Control. Geneva: World Health Organization; 2011.

174. Bloom D. From Burden to "Best Buys":Reducing the Economic Impact of Non-Communicable Diseases in Low- and Middle-Income Countries. World Health Organization, World Economic Forum, and the Harvard School of Public Health; 2011 <http://www.weforum.org/EconomicsOfNCD> (accessed 1 February 2013).

175. Johnston SC, Mendis S, Mathers CD. Global variation in stroke burden and mortality: estimates from monitoring, surveillance, and modelling. Lancet Neurol. 2009;8(4):345–354.

CHAPTER 24

Organized stroke care: Germany and Canada

Silke Wiedmann, Peter U. Heuschmann, and Michael D. Hill

Introduction

Organization of stroke services varies across different countries due to variations in healthcare systems, financing, facilities, and involvement of the government. We compare the organization of stroke services in one European (Germany) and one Northern American country (Canada) as paradigms of stroke organization. Evidence has shaped the care of stroke patients over the last two decades but care is still very much influenced by political and financial considerations. Stroke unit care remains an excellent example of the evidence-to-care gap; we know how patients should be cared for but many patients do not receive such care for a multiplicity of reasons. We try to highlight these factors in contrasting the two health systems.

Background

Stroke rates

Based on recent estimates from population-based stroke registers about 196,000 incident strokes and 66,000 recurrent strokes occur each year in Germany (total German population in 2008) (1). The rate of stroke occurrence is estimated at 174 per 100,000 population in Erlangen, Germany (2). Stroke is the third leading cause of death with about 63,000 documented deaths in 2008 according to routine statistics (1). About 50% of all incident strokes occur in women, mean age at first onset is between 72 and 75 years (3, 4). About 5% of patients who have suffered from a first stroke are not being admitted to hospital (3, 4). Stroke is a major contributor to healthcare costs in Germany with approximately 7 billion EUR direct costs per year (estimated for 2004 for first ischaemic strokes) (5).

Stroke rates and deaths are similar in Canada. Stroke occurs at 120–175 persons per 100,000 population and is the fourth leading cause of death, and the most important cause of adult-onset neurological disability (6, 7). The costs are similarly large with estimated direct costs of 3 billion CDN$ annually (8, 9).

Globally, stroke is the second leading cause of death with widely varying access to stroke services and stroke mortality (10). Costs are high (11). Variation in stroke services with economic resources of a given region or country is paramount (12, 13).

Components of stroke unit care

Organized stroke care is an intuitive approach to management of the complex problem of hospitalized stroke patients. Randomized trials of stroke unit care, summarized by Langhorne et al. have broadly included both stroke units that focused on acute management and stroke units focused on rehabilitation (14, 15). Stroke patients admitted to a general medical ward and subsequently transferred to a subacute care and rehabilitation unit fare better than those who remain on a general medical ward. Stroke patients admitted directly to an acute stroke unit similarly fare better than those admitted to a general medical ward. Conceptually, it is clear that grouping patients in a single, geographic ward and providing care with a multidisciplinary team of healthcare professionals results in better outcomes. But what are the components of such care?

Broadly, organized stroke care can be categorized into: (i) pre-hospital care, (ii) hyper-acute care in the first 48 hours, (iii) subacute care, and (iv) rehabilitation and prevention-focused care. Pre-hospital and emergency management of stroke requires tremendous logistical organization to be able to safely and effectively provide acute thrombolysis for ischaemic stroke. Similar logistical concerns arise for the management of transient ischaemic attack (TIA) and minor stroke to be able to provide urgent investigation and preventive treatments, including carotid revascularization within 2 weeks of the ictus. In the subacute phase, a multidisciplinary team of physicians (stroke physician, neurosurgeon, physiatrist), nurses, therapists (occupational, physical, speech language), and social workers is needed to prevent medical complications, investigate the stroke cause, manage relevant preventive measures, begin mobilization and rehabilitation, and manage the transition to rehabilitation services and then back to the community. The relative degree to which each of these components contributes to reductions in mortality and morbidity and improvements in quality of life are poorly defined. However, it is abundantly clear that all of these factors are important in achieving the best possible outcome after stroke (14, 15). Globally, the availability of each of these components of care is highly variable.

The structure of the healthcare system

The German health system is based on a model of social insurance. About 90% of the population has statutory health insurance, which provides a standardized level of coverage. Dependent on income, insurance is funded by a combination of employee contributions and employer contributions. The remaining part of the population is privately insured, where contribution is depends upon health status instead of income level. The different sectors of the healthcare system (e.g. ambulant practices, hospitals, rehabilitation) have separate reimbursement structures. Due to these separations within the German healthcare system, acute care and rehabilitation after stroke are for the most part offered in separate settings. Since 2004 diagnosis-related groups adapted to the German healthcare system (G-DRG) were implemented for reimbursement of acute care hospitals. Specific OPS (German Procedure Classification) were published allowing reimbursement of hospitals for early rehabilitation of stroke patients (2004), stroke unit treatment (2006), and neurological telemedicine consultation of stroke patients (2011) (16) Dependent on the patient's age, employment, and the cause of the disease, different providers (health insurance, pension insurance, accident insurance) cover rehabilitation costs (17).

The Canadian health system is based within each province and primarily paid for from general taxation revenues at the provincial level. Thus, each provincial government functions as the single insurer for all hospital care and physician care. Federally, the Canada Health Act (18) mandates equality of access across the ten provinces and three territories, in exchange for a federal funding contribution (~20% of costs) indirectly through transfer of federal tax dollars to the provinces. In practice, this means that any citizen's hospital and physician costs are entirely covered by the provincial insurance system. Stroke care is no exception; any hospital stay, procedures and inpatient rehabilitation are paid from general universal provincial insurance scheme. An advantage of this system is that cost savings achieved at the front end from thrombolysis or stroke unit care will be realized in the reduced utilization in rehabilitation and long-term care. Therefore, it is facile to show how the changes at one end of the continuum of care will both benefit the patient and the financial bottom line. Not all aspects of care are equally well insured; these include long-term care, some types of outpatient rehabilitation, drug costs, dental and eye care. For an acute condition, such as stroke, the system provides exemplary acute care. But, for long-term care issues such as long-term therapy and other types of outpatient therapy, private insurance is needed and available.

Pre-hospital services

In Germany, it is estimated that about 60–70% of all acute strokes were admitted by emergency medical services, about 25–30% were self-admission, and about 5% were in-hospital strokes or admitted by other ways. Based on figures from regional stroke registers currently about 30% of all stroke and TIA patients reach the hospital in the first 3 hours after onset of symptoms (1). The percentage of patients admitted during the first 3 hours remained relatively constant during recent years in many regions in Germany, as has been exemplary shown by the quality register 'Northwest Germany' (Table 24.1) (1).

One reason for long time intervals between onset of symptoms and acute hospital admission are delays in emergency calls of patients or carers (19). In addition, patients admitted via ambulance have significantly shorter onset to admission times compared to patients coming by private cars or via a clinic office (20). For improving pre-hospital stroke services, a number of regional initiatives using telemedicine services were initiated recently. The 'stroke angle' project, for example, transfers basic patient data from the ambulance to the stroke unit by telemedicine linage leading to a

Table 24.1 Time trends in time interval from onset of stroke to hospital admission in the stroke register Northwest Germany from 2007 to 2009[a]

Time interval from onset to admission, %	2007	2008	2009
<3 hours	29	30	32
3–<6 hours	20	21	19
6–<24 hours	21	21	21
≥24 hours	19	18	18
Unknown onset of symptoms	11	10	10

[a] Data from 74 hospitals with continuous documentation, n=115,705.
Modified according to (1).

halving of door-to-computed tomography (CT) time (21). Other initiatives are currently under the way aim to improve early diagnosis and treatment in the ambulance, by integrating a mobile CT unit in an ambulance (22). While stroke is a well-recognized emergency in the medical community, the general public in Germany is often unaware of stroke symptoms and the urgency for immediate treatment (23). Several stroke awareness campaigns aiming to improve public awareness of stroke signs and symptoms as well as correct action knowledge in case of stroke have been performed on regional or national levels in Germany with varying degrees of success. One of the regional campaigns using information brochures for the general population at high risk reported for example shortening of admission time in women only (24).

Similar data are not available nationally in Canada. However, from selected stroke centres, the estimates are similar. Stroke is equally well recognized in the medical community but the public are far less aware of stroke symptoms and what to do about them. In surveys in Ontario (the most populace province) some 50% of the general public can name one symptoms of stroke. This improved to 72% after a public information campaign but then regressed after the campaign ended (25, 26).

Ambulance services are well organized in most large metropolitan areas to recognize and transport stroke victims to regional stroke centres. Increasingly, stroke care is becoming centralized with designated comprehensive stroke centres and designated primary stroke centres. Ambulance services have pre-planned bypass rules to the nearest stroke centre. Approximately, 90% of the Canadian population lives within a 1-hour ambulance drive of a CT scanner (27). However, because of the vast distances in Canada, persons living in rural or remote areas simply will not have access to the same type of emergency care. Telemedicine as a solution to the geography is increasingly well developed in Ontario (28) and Alberta and less so in other provinces. Telemedicine services are underdeveloped.

Acute care

Stroke unit concept in Germany

The first stroke units in Europe were established in Scandinavian hospitals in the 1980s followed by other countries such as the UK (29, 30). Based on these experiences, stroke units in Germany were established from 1996 onwards including evidence-based management of stroke patients on organized stroke units exclusively treating stroke patients by a stroke-specialized multi-professional team (31). Compared to the Scandinavian and British concept, stroke units in Germany have focused at the beginning especially on stroke treatment and management in the hyperacute phase including early admission, multimodal monitoring of vital functions, rapid diagnosis, and early initiation of secondary prevention. One reason for this model is that acute care including early rehabilitation and early mobilization is separated from subsequent rehabilitation and aftercare in Germany. Future stroke unit concepts in Germany propose to integrate and to continue subsequent rehabilitation treatment in the acute care setting (32). The advantage of such a comprehensive stroke unit concept would be the better care of patients after the monitoring phase by a common stroke unit team and the avoidance of problems arising by missing interfaces when patients are admitted from stroke units to general wards or to rehabilitation facilities (32).

Stroke unit care in Canada

The first established stroke in Canada was the MacLachlan Stroke Unit at Sunnybrook Hospital in Toronto in 1975 (33). The unit made seminal observations about cardiac arrhythmias in the setting of acute stroke. Unfortunately, funding for the unit was not continued and other priorities at the hospital led it to be disbanded in the late 1980s. Like Germany, few other stroke units existed in Canada until the late 1990s. An integrated stroke unit concept evolved in Hamilton at McMaster University and continues to date. Patients are cared for acutely with integrated rehabilitation and as they progress are moved to inpatient rehabilitation beds on the same unit. The unit has a small gym and rooms for occupational therapy and speech language assessment on the ward. A similar acute style stroke unit was established in Halifax (34) and in Calgary (35, 36) around the same time and both continue to this day. Acute stroke treatment units have been or are being developed in other major teaching hospitals (Vancouver General Hospital, Toronto Western Hospital and others).

However, most patients with stroke in Canada are still cared for on general medical wards or on a general neurology ward. Most stroke patients are not primarily cared for by a neurologist as the most responsible physician. Apart from two centres, Neurology continues to be structurally organized as a Division of Medicine in most hospitals leading to the treatment of stroke on general medical wards.

There are active plans in many centres to change this. It is well recognized by the medical establishment that stroke units save lives, disability, and are most likely extremely cost-effective. Their lack in many large hospitals in this country is due among other reasons, until now, to a dearth of stroke neurologists as champions and to the structure of stroke care falling under general medicine. A major initiative is currently underway in British Columbia to develop stroke units in all major hospitals in that province. Many other major hospitals are in various stages of planning the development of acute stroke units.

Stroke unit certification

To ensure quality of structures and processes required for appropriate care of acute stroke patients a quality seal for stroke units was implemented in Germany in 1996. Depending on equipment and expertise, stroke units are divided into local stroke units and regional stroke units according to this model. Regional stroke units provide all therapeutic and diagnostic facilities for stroke diagnosis, treatment, and management also including, for example,

interventional neuroradiology and neurosurgery. According to the current criteria of the German Stroke Society (DSG) and the German Stroke Foundation (SDSH) 190 stroke units were certified in Germany in 2011; the proportion between local and regional stroke units is approximately 1:1 (1). The majority of certified Stroke Units in Germany is allocated at Departments of Neurology (1). It is estimated that up to 60% of acute stroke patients are currently being treated on a certified stroke unit bed. The number of hyperacute stroke unit beds on certified stroke units was in 2008 on average 5.7 (mean) with a range of 4–14 (1). The average length of stay on a hyperacute stroke unit was 3 days in 2008 (1).

Through the efforts of the Canadian Stroke Strategy, a new stroke centre certification process was launched by Accreditation Canada in 2010 (37). Several levels of certification are available at all levels of stroke care from acute through rehabilitation and secondary prevention. This certification recognizes achievement on excellence in care on multiple indicators. The Calgary Stroke Unit is the only unit to have achieved a full certification in comprehensive stroke care. Nationally, the process of stroke centre certification is only just beginning. Provincially, stroke centre designation has more to do with funding and routing of acutely sick patients and location of stroke clinics. To date, provincial designation has not been tied to performance.

Telestroke networks in rural areas

Stroke units are usually established in large hospitals in urban areas. To improve management of stroke patients in rural areas with restricted access to hospitals providing acute stroke unit services, several telemedical stroke networks between community hospitals and specialized stroke centres were established in different regions of Germany, for example, in Bavaria (STENO (38), TEMPiS (39), TESS (40)), or Eastern Saxony (SOS-NET (41)). Core elements of telemedical stroke networks in community hospitals include: providing telemedical support for treatment of defined stroke patients by specialized stroke centres, establishing dedicated stroke wards, training of members of staff, and establishing a multidisciplinary stroke team (42). The evaluation of the TEMPiS network has shown that patients treated in a telemedical network had a reduced probability of poor outcome at 3 months (death, institutionalization, or disability) compared to usual stroke care (odds ratio 0.62; 95% confidence interval 0.52–0.74) with effects sustaining over 30 months (43, 44). Based on these results, in 2011 a specific OPS was published nationwide allowing the community hospitals to get reimbursed for this specific procedure (16).

Telestroke resources in Canada have been reviewed and are developing rapidly (45). The most extensive system is located in Ontario, where a distributed system is available servicing multiple rural hospitals. The system has been shown to be comparable to in-person care and has resulted in improved emergency access to acute stroke expertise (46). A similar system has been developed in Alberta (47). These telemedicine systems are also being used for stroke prevention clinic style appointments and consultation for stroke rehabilitation.

Initiative for monitoring quality of acute care

German national and regional audits

Since 1994, regional quality assurance programmes documenting quality of acute stroke care have been established in Germany

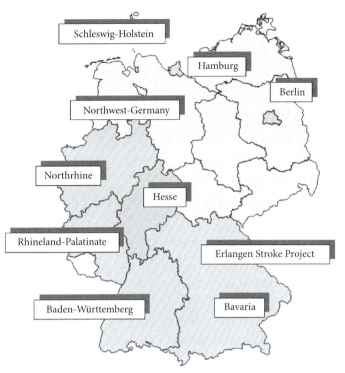

Fig. 24.1 The German Stroke Register Study Group (as at 31 December 2010).

Table 24.2 Examples of quality indicators of acute stroke care and corresponding target values where applicable in Germany

Quality indicator	Target value (%)
Antithrombotic therapy—antiplatelet medication within 48 h after stroke onset	95
Antithrombotic therapy—antiplatelet medication at discharge	95
Antithrombotic therapy—anticoagulation at discharge in patients with atrial fibrillation	80
Brain imaging in stroke suspicious patients	95
Vascular imaging in patients with ischaemic stroke or TIA	90
Screening of patients for swallowing disorders	90
Early rehabilitation—physiotherapy/occupational therapy	90
Early rehabilitation—speech therapy	80
Early mobilization	90
Stroke education of patients and relatives	90
Early brain imaging within 1 h of admission in patients admitted within 2 h after stroke onset	90
Percentage of eligible patients receiving intravenous thrombolytic therapy	60
Seven day in-hospital case-fatality for ischaemic stroke patients	–
Hospital-acquired pneumonia rate for ischaemic stroke patients	–

(Figure 24.1) (48). These regional registers cooperate in the German Stroke Registers Study Group (ADSR), which was founded in 1999 as a voluntary association of the regional registers to ensure standardization of data collection (49). According to the criteria of the German Stroke Society and the German Stroke Foundation, participation in one of the regional registers of the ADSR is mandatory for all certified stroke units; in several other regions it is also mandatory for all hospitals treating stroke patients to document quality of acute stroke care in a standardized way. Defined processes and treatment outcomes are benchmarked on the basis of quality indicators in defined time intervals between participating hospitals. Data from all regional registers participating in the ADSR are regularly pooled and analysed to address questions related to patient care on a national level. Since the beginning of the quality assurance programmes the number of documented patients as well as the number of participating hospitals is steadily increasing: currently 210,000 patients are documented within the ADSR in more than 500 hospitals across Germany (2009).

Quality indicators

Standardized quality indicators for measuring and comparing quality of acute stroke care between German hospitals have been developed in an evidence-based multidisciplinary process between 2003 and 2006 (50). Since 2007 the regional stroke registers in the ADSR agreed to document quality of stroke care using these standards. Based on these quality indicators, performance of an individual hospital is benchmarked against all participating hospitals on a regional level at least once a year. Quality indicators are updated every 2–3 years. Since 2010 quality targets for the quality indicators have also also defined and implemented (Table 24.2).

Currently, quality indicators are focusing on process and outcome measures during the acute treatment phase of stroke patients

in a hospital-based setting. Measures of quality of long-term stroke care of individual stroke patients or of inpatient or outpatient rehabilitation after discharge from acute care hospital are currently hampered by the separation of acute care, rehabilitation, and aftercare settings in the German healthcare system. Moreover, the use of patient reported outcome measures (PROMs) such as health-related quality of life to measure effectiveness of stroke care from the patient perspective on a large-scale population basis is limited to regional activities, although this might offer potential to improve the quality and results of health services (51).

tPA treatment as example for quality of acute care in Germany

Administration of tPA (tissue plasminogen activator) is an approved treatment for patients with ischaemic stroke that received approval in Germany in August 2000. The proportion of patients being thrombolysed is high, with about 7–10% of all ischaemic stroke patients documented in the regional registers of the ADSR receiving tPA in 2008 (1). The proportion of patients treated with tPA is increasing over time, e.g. from 8.5% in 2007, to 9.6% in 2008, and to 12.1% in 2009 in the Stroke Register 'Northwest Germany' (Table 24.3) (1).

Canadian Best Practice Guidelines and the Canadian Stroke Audit

The Canadian Stroke Strategy spearheaded the development of the Canadian Best Practice guidelines; along with these guidelines, a set of quality indicators was published to encourage the measurement and benchmarking of stroke care (52, 53). These quality indicators have been presented in full and in an abridged core set of indicators

Table 24.3 Canadian core clinical indicators for quality stroke care

	Canadian stroke strategy core system indicators 2010
1	Proportion of the population aware of two or more signs of stroke
2	The proportion of patients in the population that has any identified risk factors for stroke including: hypertension, obesity, smoking history, low physical activity, hyperlipidaemia, diabetes, atrial fibrillation, and carotid artery disease
3	The emergency department admission volumes for patients with ischaemic stroke, intracerebral haemorrhagic stroke, subarachnoid haemorrhage, and TIA. The hospital inpatient admission volumes for patients with ischaemic stroke, intracerebral haemorrhagic stroke, subarachnoid haemorrhage, and TIA
4	Total acute inpatient hospital length of stay (active LOS + ALC = total) Total inpatient rehabilitation hospital length of stay (active LOS + days waiting-service interruptions = total)
5	Stroke death rates for 7-day in-hospital stroke fatality; 30 day all-cause mortality; 1-year all-cause mortality, for patients with ischaemic stroke, intracerebral haemorrhagic stroke, subarachnoid haemorrhage, and transient ischaemic attack
6	Proportion of acute stroke and TIA patients that are discharged alive that are then readmitted to hospital with a new stroke or TIA diagnosis within 90 days of index acute care discharge
	Canadian stroke strategy core clinical indicators 2010
7	Proportion of acute ischaemic stroke patients who arrive at hospital within 3.5 hours of stroke symptom onset
8	Proportion of all ischaemic stroke patients who receive acute thrombolytic therapy
9	Proportion of all thrombolysed ischaemic stroke patients who receive acute thrombolytic therapy within 1 hour of hospital arrival
10	The proportion of all acute stroke patients who are managed on a designated, geographically defined, integrated, acute, and/or rehabilitation stroke unit at any point during hospitalization Median total time spent on a stroke unit for each patient during inpatient stay
11	Proportion of stroke patients who receive a brain CT/MRI within 24 hours of hospital arrival
12	Proportion of patients with documentation of an initial dysphagia screening during admission to emergency department or acute inpatient care or inpatient rehabilitation
13	Proportion of acute ischaemic stroke and TIA patients who receive acute antiplatelet therapy within the first 48 hours of hospital arrival
14	Proportion of stroke patients with a rehabilitation assessment within 48 hours of hospital admission for acute ischaemic stroke and within 5 days of admission for haemorrhagic stroke
15	Proportion of acute ischaemic stroke patients discharged on antithrombotic therapy unless contraindicated
16	Proportion of acute ischaemic stroke patients with atrial fibrillation who are treated with anti-coagulant therapy unless contraindicated
17	Proportion of patients with TIA who are investigated and discharged from the emergency department who are referred to organized secondary stroke prevention services Percentage of patients referred to organized secondary stroke prevention services who are seen within 72 hours
18	Wait time from ischaemic stroke or TIA symptom onset to carotid revascularization
19	Distribution of discharge locations (dispositions) for acute stroke patients from acute inpatient care to: home (with and without services), inpatient rehabilitation (general or specialized), long-term care, and to palliative care (each stratified by stroke type and severity)
20	Wait times for inpatient stroke rehabilitation services from stroke onset to rehabilitation admission Wait times for outpatient stroke rehabilitation services from stroke onset to outpatient rehabilitation admission
21	Distribution of discharge locations (dispositions) from inpatient rehabilitation to: home (with and without services), acute care (for acute medical issues or as repatriation to home community), and to long term care (each stratified by stroke type and severity)

Adapted from reference (54).

for most programmes. They were designed to be practical and provide defined measurement tools along with the indicators (54).

These indicators have been assessed in the Canadian Stroke Audit, a national chart audit of the care of 10,000 stroke patients. This audit was conducted with oversampling of rural and smaller regions in an attempt to provide a national level picture of the quality of stroke care. Results have been presented as a white paper (9). Key findings from this audit include:

1. Two-thirds of patients with an ischaemic stroke do not arrive at the hospital in time to potentially receive thrombolytic treatment

2. Only 40% of patients arriving within 3.5 hours from stroke onset received a brain CT or MR scan within 60 minutes.

3. The median door-to-needle time for thrombolytic treatment was 72 minutes.

4. Less than 1% of patients who live in rural settings are benefitting from telestroke services.

5. Less than a quarter (23%) of patients are treated in a formal stroke unit.

6. Less than half of stroke victims have a documented swallowing assessment on the hospital record.

These findings make for sober reading considering the gross domestic product of Canada and highlight the large evidence-to-practice gap that remains in stroke care, even in developed countries. There is dramatic room for improvement.

Stroke rehabilitation

Stroke rehabilitation is offered in Germany as inpatient as well as outpatient neurological rehabilitation. The majority of patients receive inpatient rehabilitation after acute stroke in dedicated neurological rehabilitation hospitals separated from acute care facilities. Approximately 25% of stroke patients are currently transferred to an inpatient rehabilitation hospital immediately after discharge from acute care hospital (Table 24.4) (1). About half of the patients showing a relevant functional deficit at discharge receive inpatient rehabilitation in the 3 months following acute treatment (55).

Organization of rehabilitation is characterized by different insurance systems and institutions, depending on the severity of the clinical deficit and working status. In *neurological* rehabilitation patients are categorized to one of the stages from B to D according to their functional independence and activity limitations (57, 58). Rehabilitation in a *stage B* institution includes unconscious stroke patients or patients with disturbed level of consciousness who are, for example, in need of intensive care; the main objective of this stage is to increase the patient's capability of active participation in rehabilitation efforts. Stage B rehabilitation units are mostly located at specialized rehabilitation facilities, but could be also attached to acute hospitals. S*tage C* patients are of clear consciousness and are able to actively cooperate in the rehabilitation process, although they are still dependent on support in several activities of daily living (defined by Barthel Index 30–65). Overall objective in this stage is to reach independence in daily activities. Patients in *stage D* are already largely independent from the assistance of others and able to take active part in further rehabilitation (defined by Barthel Index 70–100). Phase D rehabilitation can be funded either by the health insurance or the German Pension Scheme, depending on the vocational status of the patient (59). These stages of medical rehabilitation can be followed by rehabilitation of stage E (social and professional rehabilitation) and stage F (activating long-term care) (57, 58).

Stroke is also a major indication for geriatric rehabilitation. Patients aged 70 years and older suffering comorbid conditions might also benefit from a geriatric rehabilitation, which combines continuous medical surveillance and therapy with rehabilitation and nursing care (60). Geriatric rehabilitation is provided both in inpatient and day clinic settings. Phase D rehabilitation funded by the German Pension Scheme is supervised by a quality assurance system which is mainly based on structure and process indicators (amount of therapy), patient interviews, and assessment of discharge letter quality (61).

Regional initiatives are currently under the way for monitoring quality of stroke rehabilitation after hospital discharge using evidence-based performance measures specifically designed for inpatient and outpatient facilities in a more general approach (62).

From the Canadian Stroke Audit, we found that there are similar gaps in stroke rehabilitation. Patients with moderate to severe stroke may benefit most from rehabilitation in a specialized inpatient facility. However, only 37% of all moderate to severe stroke cases are discharged to a rehabilitation facility. In general, there is a lack of reliable information on the quality of inpatient and outpatient rehabilitation. Mandatory reporting is beginning in Canada but the data are not comprehensive, even within provinces. The Canadian Stroke Strategy has spearheaded efforts to get organized, begin collecting better data with the ultimate aim of improving management.

In Calgary, we have begun routine monitoring of rehabilitation effectiveness using simple tools. Measuring the AlphaFIM at entry to the rehabilitation stream and at exit has demonstrated that reproducible gains can be made with routine and regular therapy. However, even in the controlled hospital setting, we are not achieving common agreed upon standards, such as 3 hours of hands-on therapy per day. Much more needs to be done to improve the intensity and availability of therapy.

Long-term follow-up programmes

Limited data on care and outcome of stroke patients after discharge from acute care or rehabilitation hospital are currently available in Germany. Due to the separation of acute care, rehabilitation, and stroke aftercare in the German healthcare system, data on long-term care of stroke are available mainly from stroke registers, regional initiatives to follow up stroke patients or health services research projects (1). Data from the stroke register 'Northwest-Germany', for example, showed, that 3 months after stroke or TIA about 68% of patients were living independently at home, about 22% were dependent at home, and about 6% were living in a nursing home (55). Long-term follow-up of a subgroup of these patients showed that about 22.5% of stroke patients had applied for any nursing care during an average of 3.6 years after stroke (63). After the age of 40 the risk of dependency on nursing care 1 year after stroke increases by 13% with every additional year of life as has been shown by secondary data analysis of statutory health insurance data (64).

Long-term secondary prevention measures are mainly supervised by general practitioners or outpatient specialists. Three months after stroke, 66–85% of patients with stroke or TIA received secondary prevention medication as recommended on discharge from the acute hospital (55); adherence to antihypertensive treatment was 85%, for antiplatelets 75%, for oral hypoglycaemic drugs 67%, for anticoagulation therapy 72%, and for lipid-lowering agents 75% (55).

There are similar gaps in knowledge about the long-term prognosis and outcome of stroke patients in Canada. There are not enough stroke physicians to supervise long-term secondary prevention

Table 24.4 Stroke patient discharges from acute care

Discharge destination if discharged alive	Total	Disability at discharge[a]		
		Severe	Moderate	Mild
Home	57	10	21	73
Institutionalized	7	27	14	2
Other ward	5	8	7	4
External acute hospital	4	10	6	3
Inpatient rehabilitation	26	45	52	18
Unknown	**1**	**1**	**1**	**1**

[a] Calculated based on the 3-item-Barthel Index (BI) according to (56) and categorized into severe (BI 0–25), moderate (BI 30–65), and mild disability (BI 70–100).

Modified according to (1).

and these roles are similarly supervised by family physicians. The long-term adherence to secondary prevention medications among the stroke population is unknown.

Carer support

In Germany, there are currently no official nationwide programmes established (e.g. contact points) for providing advice to carers of stroke patients over the different treatment phases. However, there are several regional self-help groups or regional stroke offices for stroke patients and their carers. In addition, for certified stroke units a standardized consultation of patients or care givers is mandatory by the in-hospital acute social service. To assure post-acute quality of care of stroke patients a discharge management by the social service is in principle foreseen in most federal states. The German Stroke Foundation is offering structured information about different aspects of the disease for stroke patients and carers, is doing press and media work to raise awareness for stroke, its symptoms, and risk factors, and is offering seminars and meetings for the qualification of volunteers. Optional carer training is also offered by statutory health insurance companies for specific conditions, for example, for the care of ventilated patients. In Canada, the situation is very similar. Long term carer support is dominated by volunteer groups, not-for-profit groups and self-organized patient groups. Support from the Heart & Stroke Foundation of Canada, a national charitable organization which supports stroke research, stroke awareness and prevention, exists varying by province.

Summary and perspective

Germany and Canada are both developed, wealthy nations where stroke care ought to be optimal. Many advances have been made in the last couple of decades, following the proven evidence. However, stroke care is dominated by the vast chasm of the evidence-to-practice gap. Many patients are simply not getting the kind of care, which we know is possible and needed. Further, application is simple and to a large extent depends upon the establishment and measurement of standards. This is a major reason why simple advances in stroke care can be so remarkably cost-effective (8).

In contrast, stroke is an emerging and grave problem in the developing countries. Changes in lifestyle, the more widespread prevalence of smoking in Asia, Africa and Middle East mean that stroke is a major global problem. In contrast to stroke falling to the fourth leading cause of death in North America, globally stroke has risen to the second leading cause of death (10). Hypertension is the relevant risk factor and it remains poorly treated worldwide. Stroke care is even more haphazard globally. Neurologically disabling conditions require hands-on care, which in turn requires resources and a social safety net. Where this net does not exist, the burden falls to families.

As stroke occurs, organized stroke care will be needed and there is great scope for improvement in such care in both the developed and developing world.

Acknowledgements

MDH was funded by grants from the Heart & Stroke Foundation of Alberta/NWT/Nunavut and by Alberta Innovates Health Solutions. PUH received in the recent years research support from the European Union, the Federal Ministry of Education and Research (BMBF) in Germany, the German Stroke Foundation, and the Charité–Universitätsmedizin Berlin. SW received research support by the Federal Ministry of Education and Research (BMBF) of Germany by the Comprehensive Heart Failure Centre, University Hospital Würzburg.

References

1. Heuschmann PU, Busse O, Wagner M, Endres M, Villringer A, Rother J, et al. Frequency and care of stroke in Germany. *Aktuelle Neurologie.* 2010;37(7):333–340.
2. Kolominsky-Rabas PL, Sarti C, Heuschmann PU, Graf C, Siemonsen S, Neundoerfer B, et al. A prospective community-based study of stroke in Germany—the Erlangen Stroke Project (ESPro): incidence and case fatality at 1, 3, and 12 months. *Stroke.* 1998;29(12):2501–2506.
3. Palm F, Urbanek C, Rose S, Buggle F, Bode B, Hennerici MG, et al. Stroke Incidence and Survival in Ludwigshafen am Rhein, Germany: the Ludwigshafen Stroke Study (LuSSt). *Stroke.* 2010;41(9):1865–1870.
4. Kolominsky-Rabas PL, Sarti C, Heuschmann PU, Graf C, Siemonsen S, Neundoerfer B, et al. A prospective community-based study of stroke in Germany—the Erlangen Stroke Project (ESPro): incidence and case fatality at 1, 3, and 12 months. *Stroke.* 1998;29(12):2501–2506.
5. Kolominsky-Rabas PL, Heuschmann PU, Marschall D, Emmert M, Baltzer N, Neundorfer B, et al. Lifetime cost of ischemic stroke in Germany: results and national projections from a population-based stroke registry: the Erlangen Stroke Project. *Stroke.* 2006;37(5):1179–1183.
6. Canada PHAo. *Tracking Heart Disease and Stroke in Canada.* Report. Ottawa: Canada PHAo; 2011.
7. Field TS, Green TL, Roy K, Pedersen J, Hill MD. Trends in hospital admission for stroke in Calgary. *Can J Neurol Sci.* 2004;31(3):387–393.
8. Krueger H, Lindsay P, Cote R, Kapral MK, Kaczorowski J, Hill MD. Cost avoidance associated with optimal stroke care in Canada. *Stroke.* 2012;43(8):2198–2206.
9. Lindsay P, Cote R, Hill MD, Kapral MK, Kaczorowski J, Korner-Bitensky N, et al. *The Quality of Stroke Care in Canada.* Ottawa: Canadian Stroke Network; 2011.
10. Kim AS, Johnston SC. Global variation in the relative burden of stroke and ischemic heart disease. *Circulation.* 2011;124(3):314–323.
11. Meretoja A, Kaste M, Roine RO, Juntunen M, Linna M, Hillbom M, et al. Direct costs of patients with stroke can be continuously monitored on a national level: performance, effectiveness, and Costs of Treatment episodes in Stroke (PERFECT Stroke) Database in Finland. *Stroke.* 2011;42(7):2007–2012.
12. Johnston SC, Mendis S, Mathers CD. Global variation in stroke burden and mortality: estimates from monitoring, surveillance, and modelling. *Lancet Neurol.* 2009;8(4):345–354.
13. Sposato LA, Saposnik G. Gross domestic product and health expenditure associated with incidence, 30-day fatality, and age at stroke onset: a systematic review. *Stroke.* 2012;43(1):170–177.
14. How do stroke units improve patient outcomes? A collaborative systematic review of the randomized trials. Stroke Unit Trialists' Collaboration. *Stroke.* 1997;28(11):2139–2144.
15. Collaborative systematic review of the randomised trials of organised inpatient (stroke unit) care after stroke. Stroke Unit Trialists' Collaboration. *BMJ.* 1997;314(7088):1151–1159.
16. Kidwell CS, Saver JL, Mattiello J, Starkman S, Vinuela F, Duckwiler G, et al. Diffusion-perfusion MRI characterization of post-recanalization hyperperfusion in humans. *Neurology.* 2001;57(11):2015–2021.
17. Lyden P, Brott T, Tilley B, Welch KM, Mascha EJ, Levine S, et al. Improved reliability of the NIH Stroke Scale using video training. NINDS TPA Stroke Study Group. *Stroke.* 1994;25(11):2220–2226.
18. *Canada Health Act.* Ottawa: Government of Canada; 1985.
19. Röther J, Gerloff C, Heuschmann P. Optimierte Schlaganfallversorgung durch protokollgestützte Therapie. *Der Notarzt.* 2011;27:216–218.

20. Rossnagel K, Jungehulsing GJ, Nolte CH, Muller-Nordhorn J, Roll S, Wegscheider K, et al. Out-of-hospital delays in patients with acute stroke. Ann Emerg Med. 2004;44(5):476–483.

21. Ziegler V, Rashid A, Müller-Gorchs M, Kippnich U, Hiermann E, Kögerl C, et al. Einsatz mobiler Computing-Systeme in der präklinischen Schlaganfallversorgung. Anaesthesist. 2008;57(7):677–685.

22. Walter S, Kostpopoulos P, Haass A, Helwig S, Keller I, Licina T, et al. Bringing the hospital to the patient: first treatment of stroke patients at the emergency site. PLoS One. 2010;5(10):e13758.

23. Kraywinkel K, Heidrich J, Heuschmann PU, Wagner M, Berger K. Stroke risk perception among participants of a stroke awareness campaign. BMC Public Health. 2007;7:39.

24. Muller-Nordhorn J, Wegscheider K, Nolte CH, Jungehulsing GJ, Rossnagel K, Reich A, et al. Population-based intervention to reduce prehospital delays in patients with cerebrovascular events. Arch Intern Med. 2009;169(16):1484–1490.

25. Hodgson C, Lindsay P, Rubini F. Can mass media influence emergency department visits for stroke? Stroke. 2007;38(7):2115–2122.

26. Canada HaSF. Environics Omnibus Stroke Survey Results Report. Ottawa: Heart and Stroke Foundation Canada; 2009.

27. Scott PA, Temovsky CJ, Lawrence K, Gudaitis E, Lowell MJ. Analysis of Canadian population with potential geographic access to intravenous thrombolysis for acute ischemic stroke. Stroke. 1998;29(11):2304–2310.

28. Ontario Telestroke Network website. <http://otn.ca/en/programs/telestroke> (accessed 2 March 2013).

29. Kalra L. The influence of stroke unit rehabilitation on functional recovery from stroke. Stroke. 1994;25(4):821–825.

30. Strand T, Asplund K, Eriksson S, Hagg E, Lithner F, Wester PO. A non-intensive stroke unit reduces functional disability and the need for long-term hospitalization. Stroke. 1985;16(1):29–34.

31. Busse O. Stroke units and stroke services in Germany. Cerebrovasc Dis. 2003;15(Suppl 1):8–10.

32. Ringelstein EB, Muller-Jensen A, Nabavi DG, Grotemeyer KH, Busse O. [Comprehensive stroke unit].Nervenarzt. 2011;82(6):778–784.

33. Norris JW, Hachinski VC. Intensive care management of stroke patients. Stroke. 1976;7(6):573–577.

34. Phillips SJ, Eskes GA, Gubitz GJ. Description and evaluation of an acute stroke unit. Cmaj. 2002;167(6):655–660.

35. Hill MD. Stroke units in Canada. CMAJ. 2002;167(6):649–650.

36. Zhu HF, Newcommon NN, Cooper ME, Green TL, Seal B, Klein G, et al. Impact of a stroke unit on length of hospital stay and in-hospital case fatality. Stroke. 2009;40(1):18–23.

37. Accreditation Canada—Stroke Services Distinction. 2012. <http://www.accreditation.ca/accreditation-programs/distinction/stroke-services/> (accessed 3 March 2013).

38. Handschu R, Littmann R, Reulbach U, Gaul C, Heckmann JG, Neundorfer B, et al. Telemedicine in emergency evaluation of acute stroke: interrater agreement in remote video examination with a novel multimedia system. Stroke. 2003;34(12):2842–2846.

39. Audebert HJ, Kukla C, Clarmann von Claranau S, Kuhn J, Vatankhah B, Schenkel J, et al. Telemedicine for safe and extended use of thrombolysis in stroke: the Telemedic Pilot Project for Integrative Stroke Care (TEMPiS) in Bavaria. Stroke. 2005;36(2):287–291.

40. Wiborg A, Widder B. Teleneurology to improve stroke care in rural areas: The Telemedicine in Stroke in Swabia (TESS) Project. Stroke. 2003;34(12):2951–2956.

41. Gahn G, Becker U, Goldhagen T, Eulitz M, Dreischer T, Schiller S, et al. Schlaganfall-Ostsachsen-Netzwerk (SOS-NET): Aufbau einer flächendeckenden Schlaganfallversorgung auf Basis eines unabhängigen Qualitätsmanagement-Systems. Akt Neurol. 2008;35:P558.

42. Audebert HJ, Wimmer ML, Hahn R, Schenkel J, Bogdahn U, Horn M, et al. Can telemedicine contribute to fulfill WHO Helsingborg Declaration of specialized stroke care? Cerebrovasc Dis. 2005;20(5):362–369.

43. Audebert HJ, Schenkel J, Heuschmann PU, Bogdahn U, Haberl RL. Effects of the implementation of a telemedical stroke network: the Telemedic Pilot Project for Integrative Stroke Care (TEMPiS) in Bavaria, Germany. Lancet Neurol. 2006;5(9):742–748.

44. Audebert HJ, Schultes K, Tietz V, Heuschmann PU, Bogdahn U, Haberl RL, et al. Long-term effects of specialized stroke care with telemedicine support in community hospitals on behalf of the Telemedical Project for Integrative Stroke Care (TEMPiS). Stroke. 2009;40(3):902–908.

45. Deshpande A, Khoja S, McKibbon A, Rizo C, Jadad AR. Telehealth for Acute Stroke Management (Telestroke): Systematic Review and Environmental Scan. Ottawa: Canadian Agency for Drugs and Technologies in Health; 2008.

46. Waite K, Silver F, Jaigobin C, Black S, Lee L, Murray B, et al. Telestroke: a multi-site, emergency-based telemedicine service in Ontario. J Telemed Telecare. 2006;12(3):141–145.

47. Khan K, Shuaib A, Whittaker T, Saqqur M, Jeerakathil T, Butcher K, et al. Telestroke in Northern Alberta: a two year experience with remote hospitals. Can J Neurol Sci. 2010;37(6):808–813.

48. Heuschmann PU, Berger K. International experience in stroke registries: German Stroke Registers Study Group. Am J Prev Med. 2006;31(6 Suppl 2):S238–S239.

49. Heuschmann P, Hermanek P, Elsner S, Walter G, Kolominsky-Rabas P, Streuf R, et al. Hintergründe und Ergebnisse der Datenpoolung der ADSR von 2000 bis 2005. Nervenheilkunde. 2009;28(3):108–113.

50. Heuschmann PU, Biegler MK, Busse O, Elsner S, Grau A, Hasenbein U, et al. Development and implementation of evidence-based indicators for measuring quality of acute stroke care: the Quality Indicator Board of the German Stroke Registers Study Group (ADSR). Stroke. 2006;37(10):2573–2578.

51. Cella D, Yount S, Rothrock N, Gershon R, Cook K, Reeve B, et al. The Patient-Reported Outcomes Measurement Information System (PROMIS): progress of an NIH Roadmap cooperative group during its first two years. Med Care. 2007;45(5 Suppl 1):S3–S11.

52. Lindsay MP, Bayley M, Hellings C, Hill MD, Woodbury E, Phillips S. Canadian Best Practice Recommendations for Stroke Care (Updated 2008). CMAJ. 2008;179(12 (suppl)):E1–E93.

53. Lindsay MP, Kapral MK, Gladstone D, Holloway R, Tu JV, Laupacis A, et al. The Canadian Stroke Quality of Care Study: establishing indicators for optimal acute stroke care. Cmaj. 2005;172(3):363–365.

54. Group CIaEW. Canadian Stroke Strategy Core Performance Indicator Update 2010. June 2010. <http://www.strokebestpractices.ca/wp-content/uploads/2012/07/Stroke_Core_ENG.pdf> (accessed 3 March 2013).

55. Schneider K, Heise M, Heuschmann P, Berger K. Situation of life and care in patients with a stroke. Nervenheilkunde. 2009;28(3):114–118.

56. Ellul J, Watkins C, Barer D. Estimating total Barthel scores from just three items: the European Stroke Database 'minimum dataset' for assessing functional status at discharge from hospital. Age Ageing. 1998;27(2):115–122.

57. Bundesarbeitsgemeinschaft für Rehabilitation. Schriftenreihe der Bundesarbeitsgemeinschaft für Rehabilitation (eds). Rehabilitation. Bf. Arbeitshilfe für die Rehabilitation von Schlaganfallpatienten (Vol. 4). Frankfurt: BAR; 1998.

58. Bundesarbeitsgemeinschaft für Rehabilitation (eds). Empfehlungen zur Neurologischen Rehabilitation von Patienten mit schweren und schwersten Hirnschädigungen in den Phasen B und C. Frankfurt: BAR; 1995.

59. Schupp W. Externe Qualitätssicherungsprogramme der gesetzlichen Sozialversicherungen für die neurologische Rehabilitation-Übersicht der Vorgehensweisen und erste Ergebnisse. Neurol Rehabil. 2006;12(3):113–127.

60. Borchelt M, Pientka L, Wrobel N. Abgrenzungskriterien der Geriatrie. 2004. <http://wwwdggg-onlinede/pdf/abgrenzungskriterien_geriatrie v13pdf>.

61. Schupp W. [Current aspects of neurologic and neurosurgical rehabilitation in ambulatory medicine]. Z Arztl Fortbild (Jena). 1996;90(6):501–509.

62. Grube MM, Dohle C, Djouchadar D, Rech P, Bienek K, Dietz-Fricke U, *et al.* Evidence-based quality indicators for stroke rehabilitation. *Stroke.* 2012;43(1):142–146.

63. Diederichs C, Muhlenbruch K, Lincke HO, Heuschmann PU, Ritter MA, Berger K. Predictors of dependency on nursing care after stroke: results from the Dortmund and Munster stroke registry. *Dtsch Arztebl Int.* 2011;108(36):592–599.

64. van den Bussche H, Berger K, Kemper C, Barzel A, Glaeske G, Koller D. Incidence, relapse, nursing care dependency and mortality of stroke in Germany. A secondary analysis of statutory insurance claims data. *Aktuelle Neurologie.* 2010;37(3):131–135.

Index

Note: page numbers in *italics* refer to figures and tables.

'3H' syndrome 86
ABCD² score *81*
'ABCs' for heart disease and stroke prevention
    264
abducens nerve palsy
    after subarachnoid haemorrhage 68, 74
    Gasperini syndrome 89
absolute risk, definition *9*
abulia 88
acidosis 114
acoustic radiations, arterial supply 19
ACTIVE-A trial 167
ACTIVE-W trial 167
activities of daily living, rehabilitation 238, 240
activity-based therapies 226, *237–8*
acupuncture 236
acute myocardial infarction, stroke prevention
    169
Acute Stroke Accurate Prediction model *187*
ADDTC criteria, diagnosis of vascular dementia
    217
age
    as a prognostic marker 186, *187*
    relationship to stroke risk 5, 6, *9–10*
        silent cerebral infarcts *197*
AGES-Reykjavik Study, prevalence of cerebral
    microbleeds 199
agraphia, associated lesions 86, 88
airway management *109*
alcohol consumption
    'best buy' interventions *264*
    recommendations 263
    relationship to stroke risk 259
    as a risk factor 13, 14, 15
        for subarachnoid haemorrhage 62
alexia, associated lesions 86, 88
alteplase (recombinant tissue plasminogen
    activator) 124
ATLANTIS trial 125–6
    see also thrombolysis
Alternate Healthy Eating Index (AHEI) 14
Alzheimer disease
    association with post-stroke dementia 220
    cerebral microbleeds 199
amaurosis fugax 80
    differential diagnoses *82*
aminocaproic acid 140, *144*
amitriptyline, in neuropathic pain *213*
amnesia 217
    associated lesions 87, 88
    in subcortical vascular dementia 219
amygdaloid nucleus, arterial supply 27

amyloidosis *see* cerebral amyloid angiopathy
anaemia
    after subarachnoid haemorrhage 147
    causes *156*
analgesia *109*
aneurysms
    arteriovenous malformations 55
    associated disorders 158
    causes 63
    imaging *71–2, 73*, 103
    intracerebral haemorrhage *73, 74*
    location according to pattern of SAH *70*
    middle cerebral artery *64*
    mycotic 66
    prevalence 61
    repair 142–3, 144
    risk factors for 62–3
    risk of rupture 63
    see also subarachnoid haemorrhage
angiogenesis 225
angiography
    after intracerebral haemorrhage 57
    ulcerative plaques *36*
    see also computed tomography angiography;
        digital subtraction angiography;
        magnetic resonance angiography
anosognosia
    associated lesions 85, 86, 88
    recovery factors 188–9
anterior cerebellar vein *32, 33*
anterior cerebral artery (ACA) *27*
    leptomeningeal branches 27
    perforating branches *22, 24*
anterior cerebral artery infarcts 88
    clinical features 88
anterior choroidal artery (AChA) *27–8, 27, 29*
    perforating branches 19, *22–3*
    territory *21*
anterior choroidal artery infarcts 86–7
anterior commissure, arterial supply 19, 24, 26
anterior communicating artery (ACoA) *27*
    perforating branches 19, *22*
anterior inferior cerebellar artery (AICA)
    27–8, 29
    territory *20, 21*
anterior inferior cerebellar artery infarcts 91
anterior opercular syndrome 86
anterior parietal artery infarcts 86
anterior spinal artery *27–8*
    territory *20*
anteromedian medullary vein *32*
anteromedian pontine vein *32*

antibiotics
    in pneumonia 204
    prophylactic 204
    in urinary tract infections 203
anticoagulation
    after intracerebral haemorrhage 117, 132
    after ischaemic stroke 127–8
    in atrial fibrillation 259
    as cause of subarachnoid haemorrhage 67
    DVT prophylaxis and treatment 116–17,
        205, 245
    implications of cerebral microbleeds 200
    novel anticoagulants, stroke prevention in
        NVAF *167, 168*
    patients with dementia 221
    reversal 57, 131–2
    secondary prevention
        comparison with antiplatelet therapy
            163, *165*
        patients with intracranial stenosis 177
        patients with left ventricular thrombus 169
        patients with mechanical heart valves 169
    stroke risk 14
antidepressants 211–12, 236, 246
antiepileptic drugs 213
    after subarachnoid haemorrhage 142
    in mania and psychosis 246
antifibrinolytic therapy 140, *144*
antihypertensive medication, impact on stroke
    risk 257–8
anti-neutrophilic cytoplasmic antibodies
    (ANCA) 160
antiphospholipid antibodies, stroke risk 12
antiplatelet medication
    after ischaemic stroke 127
    cerebral microbleeds 200
    in rarer causes of stroke 162
    secondary prevention 163–6
        in atrial fibrillation 167
        comparison with warfarin *165*
        patients with intracranial stenosis 177–8
        patients with left ventricular thrombus 169
        patients with mechanical heart valves 169
    stroke risk 14
    see also aspirin
Anton syndrome 88
anxiety 246–7
aorta, as source of embolisms 13, 37
aphasia
    associated lesions 85, 86–7, 88
    cardioembolic strokes 91
    impact on quality of life 249

associated lesions (*Cont.*)
　recovery factors 189
　transient ischaemic attack 80
apixaban
　in atrial fibrillation *167*, 168, 259
　risk of intracerebral haemorrhage 132, *167*
APOE gene variations 10
apraxia, associated lesions 85, 86, 88
area under the curve (AUC), prognostic
　　studies 186
Argyll Robertson pupils 156
ARIC study 262
ARISTOTLE trial *167*, 168
arrhythmias 119, 148, 206–8
　congestive heart failure 208
　see also atrial fibrillation
arterial anatomy 19
　of brainstem *20–1*, 27–8
　of cerebellum *20–1*, 24, 29
　of cerebral hemispheres 19, *22–3*, 24–7
　of midbrain *21*, 29
　of pons *20–1*, 28–9
　variations 29
arterial diseases, stroke risk 13
arterial imaging 99–101, *100*
　see also angiography
arterial tortuosity syndrome *154*
arteriolosclerosis, intracerebral
　　haemorrhage 54
arteriopathies
　non-atherosclerotic inflammatory *155*, 160
　non-atherosclerotic non-inflammatory *155*,
　　159–60
arteriovenous malformations (AVMs) 54–5
　associated disorders 158
　imaging 103
　subarachnoid haemorrhage 63–4, *65*
arteritis 44
artery-to-artery embolism 35–7
　imaging *36*
　posterior cerebral artery infarcts 88
　Takayasu disease 44
ASCO classification system 46–7
ASCOT-LLA trial 258, 263
aspiration pneumonia *204*, 243
aspiration risk 127
　reduction 110, 115
aspirin
　DVT prophylaxis 116
　primary prevention 262–3
　　in atrial fibrillation 259
　　in diabetes 259
　in rarer causes of stroke 162
　secondary prevention 163, *164*, 165
　　in atrial fibrillation 167
　　patients with intracranial stenosis 177–8
　　patients with left ventricular
　　　thrombus 169
　　patients with mechanical heart valves 169
　　prevention of early recurrence 165–6
　see also antiplatelet medication
asthma, associated disorders 153
ataxia
　associated lesions 86, 87, 89, 90–1
　recovery factors 189
atenolol, in secondary prevention *171*
atheromatous branch occlusion (BAD) 41
atherosclerosis 35
　intracranial 37–40
　plaque destabilization 35–6

atorvastatin, in secondary prevention 174
atrial fibrillation (AF) 206
　detection 166
　Holter monitoring 207–8
　ECG *207*
　embolic infarction 43
　　posterior cerebral artery occlusion *42*
　primary prevention of stroke 259
　relationship to genetic variations 10
　secondary prevention of stroke 167–9
　stroke risk 11, 166
atrial septal aneurysms 170
atrial septal defects 11
atrophy of infarcts 96
attack rate, definition *2*
Austrian Stroke Prevention Study, prevalence of
　　cerebral microbleeds 199
AVERROES trial *167*, 168
awareness campaigns 271

Babinski–Nageotte syndrome 90
bacteriuria 203
BAD (atheromatous branch occlusion) 41
Balint syndrome 86
barbiturates, reduction of intracranial
　　pressure 134
Barthel Index (BI) score, prognostic
　　significance 187
basal vein *31*, 32, *32*
basilar artery 27–8, *27*, *29*
　as source of embolisms 37
　territory *20*, *21*
basilar artery occlusion, clinical features 90
beading of cerebral arteries
　associated disorders 158
　reversible cerebral vasoconstriction
　　syndrome 161
Behçet disease *155*, 156, 157, 158, 160
　epidemiology 153
Benedikt syndrome 89
benign idiopathic subarachnoid haemorrhage
　　(benign perimesencephalic
　　haemorrhage) 63, *64*
benzodiazepines 247
beta-carotene supplementation 179
Binswanger disease 219
biomarkers 229
biomechanical gait training 238
birth weight, relationship to stroke risk 9
bladder training 209
bladder ultrasound scanning 209
blood pressure
　relationship to stroke risk 170, 256–8
　target levels 258, 259
　see also hypertension
blood pressure management 173
　acute stroke 111–*12*
　　pharmacological agents *113*
　after intracerebral haemorrhage 130–1
　in diabetes 258–9
　secondary prevention 170–3
　subarachnoid haemorrhage 140, *144*
blood pressure variability, stroke risk 172
body temperature management *109*, 112,
　　114, 132
Boston criteria for cerebral amyloid angiopathy
　　53–4
botulinum toxin, spasticity treatment 236
brain biopsy 159
brain injury minimization 106

brain oedema
　management 117–19, 128
　pathophysiology 117
　see also intracranial hypertension
brain organization, influence on recovery 228
brain repair
　clinical trials 228–9
　definition 225
　principles of 227–8
　promotion of 225–7
brainstem
　arterial supply *20–1*, 27–8
　venous drainage *32*
brainstem infarcts, clinical features 89–90
brain stimulation therapies 226–7
branch occlusion 38, *39*, *40*
breathing, monitoring and management *109*
bridging therapy 126–7
Broca's aphasia 85, 86
bronchopneumonia 203–4
buspirone 247
B vitamin supplements 179, 260

CADASIL (cerebral autosomal dominant
　　arteriopathy with subcortical infarcts and
　　leucoencephalopathy) 10, 44, *154*, 159, 219
　cerebral microbleeds 199
calcium blockers, in vasospastic disorders 162
Canada
　carer support 276
　healthcare system 271
　long-term follow-up 275–6
　pre-hospital services 271
　quality of care 273–5
　rehabilitation 275
　stroke rates 270
　stroke units 272
　telestroke networks 272
Canadian Core Clinical Indicators for Quality
　　Stroke Care *274*
Canadian Stroke Audit 274
cancer-associated stroke 44, *45*
candesartan, in secondary prevention *171*
cannabis use, stroke risk 14
CAPRIE trial 163, *164*
CARASIL (cerebral autosomal recessive
　　arteriopathy with subcortical infarcts
　　and leucoencephalopathy) 10, *154*
　epidemiology 153
carbamazepine 213
cardiac complications 206, *207*
　arrhythmias 206–8
　heart failure 208
　ischaemic heart disease 208
cardiac control *110*
cardiac function monitoring 119
cardiac imaging 101
cardioembolic strokes 41–3
　causes *43*
　　atrial fibrillation 43
　　infective endocarditis 43–4
　　patent foramen ovale 44
　clinical patterns 91–2
　imaging 102
　posterior cerebral artery infarcts 88
　secondary prevention 166–70, *171*
cardiomyopathy
　after subarachnoid haemorrhage 72–3
　　management *144*
　stroke prevention 169

cardiorespiratory training 237–8
Cardiovascular Health Study, prevalence of silent cerebral infarcts 196
CARDS (Collaborative Atorvastatin Diabetes) trial 258, 259
caregivers
    impact of stroke 249–50
    information provision 250
    involvement in rehabilitation 239
    support of 276
CARESS trial 165
Carney syndrome *154*
carotid angioplasty and stenting (CAS) 176–7
carotid arterial disease, stroke risk 13
carotid Doppler ultrasound 99, *101*, 102, 104
carotid endarterectomy (CEA) 174–5
carotid TIA, suggestive symptoms *80*
case–control studies, definition *2*
case-fatality, definition *2*
catheterization 245
caudate nucleus, arterial supply 19, 24
Causative Classification System (CCS) 46–7
CAVATAS trial 176
cavernomas (cerebral cavernous malformations) 55–6
cavernous haemangioma, imaging *103*
cavernous sinus 30, 31, *31*
    malformations 64, 66
cavitation, silent cerebral infarcts 195
CCM genes 56
central sulcus artery territory infarcts 86
central venous pressure 141
centrum ovale, arterial supply 29
cerebellar infarcts, clinical patterns 90–1
cerebellar intracranial haemorrhage, surgical treatment 135–6
cerebellar oedema 117
    decompressive surgery 118–19
    management 128
cerebellum
    arterial supply *20–1*, 29
        variations 29
    venous drainage *32–3*
cerebral abscesses, diffusion MRI 96
cerebral amyloid angiopathy (CAA) 53–4, *95*, *154*
    cerebral microbleeds 199
    convexal subarachnoid haemorrhage 63
    distinction from TIA 82
    imaging 216
cerebral blood flow (CBF) 98
    regulation 111
cerebral blood volume (CBV) 97
cerebral hemispheres
    anatomical structures *22–3*, 25–6
    arterial supply 19, *22–3*, 24, *26–7*, 27
        variations 29
    arterial territories *26*
cerebral infarction *see* ischaemic stroke
cerebral microbleeds (CMB) 54, *196*, 199–200, *220*
    definitions and terminology 194
    discovery 194
    role in cognitive impairment 220
cerebral microinfarcts 195
cerebral perfusion pressure management 133
    after subarachnoid haemorrhage 140–1, *143*
cerebral salt wasting syndrome 147
cerebral sinus thrombosis, hemicraniectomy 135

cerebral venous thrombosis (CVT) 56, 66, 161
    risk factors 15
cerebroretinal vasculopathy *154*
cerebrospinal fluid examination *see* lumbar puncture
cervical artery dissection (CEAD) 64, *66*, 159
CHA$_2$DS$_2$VASc score *12*, 43, *44*
CHADS$_2$ score 11, 43, *44*
Chagas disease
    epidemiology 153
    as risk factor for stroke 13
CHANCE trial 166
CHARISMA trial *164*, 165
Cheyne–Stokes breathing 110
CHHIPS (Controlling Hypertension and Hypotension Immediately Post-Stroke) trial 112
Chlamydia pneumoniae, associated stroke risk 262
cholesterol levels
    as a risk factor 12, 14, 173–4, 258
        for subarachnoid haemorrhage 62
    secondary prevention of stroke 173–4
cholinesterase inhibitors 221
chronic kidney disease, stroke risk 262
Churg–Strauss syndrome 153, 160
Cincinnati prognostic score *190*
cingulate gyrus, arterial supply 19
circle of Willis *27*
circuit training *237*
circulation management *109*
citalopram 211, 246
citicoline 127
CLAIR trial 165
classification of stroke 45–7, 91
Claude's syndrome 89
clevidipine, in hypertension *113*
clinical features
    anterior cerebral artery infarcts 88
    brainstem infarcts 89–90
    cardioembolic strokes 91–2
    cerebellar infarcts 90–1
    combined hemispherical infarcts 88–9
    intracerebral haemorrhage 52
    lacunar syndromes 91
    middle cerebral artery infarcts 85–6
    OCSP classification 91
    posterior cerebral artery infarcts 87–8
    rarer causes of stroke 154–5
    striatocapsular infarcts 86–7
    subarachnoid haemorrhage 67–9
    transient ischaemic attack 79–81
clipping of aneurysms 142–3
clopidogrel
    secondary prevention 163, *164*, 165
        in atrial fibrillation 167
        prevention of early recurrence 165–6
    see also antiplatelet medication
CLOSURE-1 trial 169, *170*, *171*
coagulation disorders 44, *156*, 161
    cancer-associated *45*
    laboratory investigations 158
    stroke risk 12
coagulation factors, assessment of 58
coagulation tests, in DOAC therapy 132
cocaine abuse 66–7
    as a risk factor 14
cognitive impairment
    association with cerebral microbleeds 199
    association with silent cerebral infarcts 197–8
    contributing factors 220, *221*

organic delirium 210–11
prognostic significance 216
treatment 211–12
vascular
    clinical patterns 217
    diagnosis 216–17
    epidemiology, after stroke 215
    epidemiology, patients without clinical evidence of stroke 216
cognitive therapies 227, 246
cohort studies, case-fatality *2*
coil embolization 143
COL4A1 gene variations 10
collateral circulation 37
collicular artery *27–8*, 29
    territory *21*
colour agnosia 88
combined hemispherical infarcts, clinical features 88–9
community-based risk reduction 263–4
complications 243, *245*
    acute *108*
        prevention and treatment 107–8
    anxiety 246–7
    aspiration pneumonia 243
    cardiac 206, *207*
        arrhythmias 206–8
        heart failure 208
        ischaemic heart disease 208
    constipation 209–10
    depression 211–12, 245–6
    emotionalism 212–13
    of enteral feeding 247
    falls 208–9, 243–4
    incontinence 244–5
    infections 203–4
    lower urinary tract symptoms 209
    mania and psychosis 246
    oedematous limbs 245
    organic delirium 210–11
    pain 213
    post-stroke fatigue 213
    pressure ulcers 209
    risk factors for *108*, *245*
    seizures 213
    of subarachnoid haemorrhage 72–5
    suicidal ideation 247
    urinary tract infections 244–5
    venous thromboembolism 205–6, 245
    see also cognitive impairment; dementia
compression stockings 116, 132, 205
COMPRESS trial *166*
computed tomography (CT) 102-3, 104
    after intracerebral haemorrhage 57, 102–3
    after TIA and ischaemic stroke 94–6, *95*, 98–9
    Fisher grading scale *141*
        modified *142*
    in subarachnoid haemorrhage *70*
        MDCTA 71–2
    venography (CTV) 101, 102
    computed tomography angiography (CTA) *100*, 101, 102-3, 104
computers, use in rehabilitation 240–1
conduction aphasia 86, 88
confusional state
    associated lesions 86, 88
    transient ischaemic attack 81
congestive heart failure (CHF) 208
conivaptan 147

connective tissue disorders 63, *154*, 155, 156, 157, 160
consciousness alteration
basilar artery occlusion 90
cardioembolic infarcts 91
  cerebellar infarcts 91
  intracerebral haemorrhage 52
  mesencebral infarcts 89
  middle cerebral artery infarcts 85
  pontine infarcts 89
  subarachnoid haemorrhage 68
  transient ischaemic attack 81
constipation 209–*10*, 248
constraint-induced therapy 226, 241
convexal subarachnoid haemorrhage 63
  diagnosis, non-contrast CT 94
  distinction from TIA 82
Copenhagen Stroke Study 189
corpus callosum, arterial supply 19, 27
cortical cerebral veins *31*, 32
cortical vascular dementia 218
corticosteroids
  prevention of hyponatraemia 147
  in vasculitides 162
COSSACS (Continue or Stop Post-Stroke Antihypertensives Collaborative Study) 112
COSS trial 175, 177, *178*
costs of stroke 255
cranial nerve palsies
abducens nerve palsy 68, 74, 89
facial nerve palsy 89, 90, 91
  Gasperini syndrome 89
glossopharyngeal nerve palsy 90, 91
oculomotor nerve palsy 68, *69*, 74, 89
  after subarachnoid haemorrhage 68, *69*, 74
trigeminal nerve deficits 90, 91
vagus nerve palsy 90, 91
vestibulocochlear nerve palsies 91
CREST trial *176*, 177
cryptogenic stroke 45
c-statistic, prognostic studies 186

dabigatran
  associated intracerebral haemorrhage 132
  in atrial fibrillation *167*, 168, 259
  risk of intracerebral haemorrhage *167*
  secondary prevention, patients with mechanical heart valves 169
D-dimer 205
DECIMAL (decompressive craniectomy in malignant middle cerebral artery infarcts) trial 128
decompressive surgery 118–19, 128, 135–6
  after subarachnoid haemorrhage 140
  indications 89
  in rarer causes of stroke 162
deconvolution 97–8
deep vein thrombosis (DVT) 205–6, 245
  diagnosis 116
  prophylaxis 116–17, 132–3, *144*
  risk factors 115–16
  treatment *116*, 117
dehydration avoidance 248
Dejerine's syndrome 90
delayed cerebral ischaemia (DCI) 145
  after subarachnoid haemorrhage 74, *75*
  management 146
  monitoring for 145–6
  prevention 146

delirium, organic 210–11
dementia
  association with stroke 215
  diagnosis 216–17
  epidemiology
    after stroke 215
    patients without clinical evidence of stroke 216
  prognostic significance 216
depression 236, 245–6
  association with silent cerebral infarcts 197
  Geriatric Depression Scale *212*
  impact on quality of life 249
  incidence 211
  symptoms and diagnosis 211
  vascular dementia 217
deserpine, in secondary prevention *171*
DESTINY (decompressive surgery for the treatment of malignant infarction of the middle cerebral artery) trial 128
diabetes mellitus
  hyperglycaemia 114
  primary prevention of stroke 258–9
  secondary prevention of stroke 178, *179*
  stroke risk 12, 14
diagnosis 35
intracranial haemorrhage 52, 57–8
  rarer causes of stroke *154*
    history-taking 153–5
    imaging 157–8
    laboratory investigations 158
    physical examination 155–7
    subarachnoid haemorrhage 67–9
      imaging 70–2
      lumbar puncture 71
    TIA and ischaemic stroke
      diffusion MRI *96*–7
      non-contrast CT 94–6, *95*
diaschisis 225
Dide–Botcazo syndrome 88
diet 247–8
  'best buy' interventions *264*
  recommendations 263–4
  relationship to stroke risk 14, 261
diffusion MRI 83, 85, *96*–7, 103
  after transient ischaemic attack 98
  of embolic stroke *36*, 37
  reversibility of lesions 97
digital subtraction angiography (DSA) 101, 158
  in subarachnoid haemorrhage 71, *72*
digoxin loading *207*
diplopia 90
  subarachnoid haemorrhage 68
  transient ischaemic attack 80
dipyridamole, secondary prevention 163
direct oral anticoagulants, associated intracerebral haemorrhage 132
disability 234
disability-adjusted life years (DALYs) 1
  definition *2*
discharge from hospital
  destinations *275*
  preparations for 249
dissections 44
  cervical artery 64, *66*, 159
dizziness
  subarachnoid haemorrhage 68
  transient ischaemic attack 81
dobutamine 146
dolichoectasia, associated disorders 158

'do not resuscitate' (DNR) orders
  after intracerebral haemorrhage 53
  impact on prognostic studies 190–1
Doppler ultrasound imaging 99–100, 158
  DVT diagnosis 205, *206*
driving 238
drug abuse
  as cause of subarachnoid haemorrhage 66–7
  epidemiology 153
  skin changes 156
  stroke mechanisms 161
  stroke risk 13–14
DSM-IV criteria, diagnosis of vascular dementia *216*
dural arteriovenous fistulas 64, *65*
dural venous sinuses 30–31,
Dutch TIA trial *171*, 198
dysarthria
  associated lesions 86, 89, 90–1, 92
  transient ischaemic attack 80–1
dysexecutive syndrome 217, 219
dyslipidaemia, as a risk factor 258
dysphagia 247
associated lesions 86, 89
  evaluation and management 115
  recovery factors 189
  transient ischaemic attack 80
dysphagia screening 204–*5*
dysphonia 89

early death
  combined hemispherical infarcts 88–9
  pseudotumoural cerebellar infarcts 91
  subarachnoid haemorrhage 74
early ischaemic changes 94, *95*
early recurrence, prevention 106
  aspirin and clopidogrel 165–6
early supported discharge (ESD) 239–40
ECASS trials 125–6
echocardiography 101, 102
ECST trial 175
Ehlers–Danlos syndrome 10, *154*, 157
  intracranial aneurysms 63
EKOS micro-infusion system 126
electrocardiography (ECG) 119, 206–8
electro-stimulation therapy 236
embolisms
  artery-to-artery 35–7
  basilar artery 90
  cardiac 41–4
  as cause of lacunar infarcts 41
  as cause of subarachnoid haemorrhage 66
emotionalism 212–13
  vascular dementia 217
'empty delta' sign *102*
enalaprilat, in hypertension *113*
endovascular cooling 127
enteral feeding 115, 247
  FOOD trials 248
epidemiology 1
  age-adjusted incidence rates *5*
  definitions of common terms *2*
  incidence
    age-adjusted rates *256*
    geographical variation *256*
    in Germany and Canada 270
    relationship to socioeconomic status 255
  of intracerebral haemorrhage 51
  population-based studies 1–2

population differences in stroke subtype frequencies 7
rarer causes of stroke 153
stroke burden
    gender and ethnic differences 4–7
    high-income countries 2–4
    low- to middle-income countries 4
epilepsy
    associations with intracerebral haemorrhage 57
    focal, distinction from TIA 82
epistaxis, associated disorders 153
EPITHET trial 125
eprosartan, in secondary prevention 172
erythema 155
escitalopram, promotion of brain repair 226
esmolol, in hypertension 113
ESPIRIT trial 163, 164, 165
ESPS-2 trial 163, 164
Essen ICH score 190
Essen prognostic model 186, 187
ethnic differences in stroke risk 4–6, 10, 14
    rarer causes of stroke 153
    subarachnoid haemorrhage 61
EVA-3S trial 176, 177
EXCITE trial 226, 241
exercise
    recommendations 263
    relationship to stroke risk 14, 261
        subarachnoid haemorrhage 62
    in secondary prevention 179
experience-dependence, brain repair 227
external ventricular drainage (EVD) 136, 140, 144
extracranial atherosclerosis, arterial occlusion 37
extracranial–intracranial (EC–IC) bypass 175
    EC–IC Bypass trial 177, 178
eyes, physical examination 156–7

Fabry disease 10, 153, 154, 155, 157, 159
    treatment 162
facial nerve palsy
    basilar artery occlusion 90
    cerebellar infarcts 91
    Gasperini syndrome 89
    medullary infarcts 90
facial vein 31
fainting, and TIA 81
falls 208–9, 243–4
familial hemiplegic migraine 154
familial intracranial aneurysms syndrome 62
familial risk factors 10
    for intracerebral haemorrhage 57
family
    impact of stroke 249–50
    involvement in rehabilitation 239
    see also caregivers
family history, rarer causes of stroke 154
FASTER trial 166
FAST trial 131
fatigue 213
fenoldopam, in management of high blood pressure 113
fever see hyperthermia
FEVER trial 171
fibromuscular dysplasia (FMD) 63, 159–60
Field Administration of Stroke Therapy–Magnesium Phase III (FAST-MAG) trial 127
fingers, physical examination 157

Fisher grading scale 69, 70, 139, 141
    modified 142
FLAIR (fluid-attenuated inversion recovery) imaging
    perfusion imaging 97–8
    principles of 97
FLAME study 226
fluid intake 248
fluid status assessment 141–2
fluoxetine, promotion of brain repair 226
focal epilepsy, distinction from TIA 82
focal subarachnoid haemorrhage (focal superficial siderosis) see convexal subarachnoid haemorrhage
'fogging' 96
Foix–Chavany–Marie syndrome 86
folic acid supplements 179
follow-up 275–6
follow-up checklist 243, 244
FOOD (Feed or Ordinary Diet) trials 248
foramen coecum artery 28
    territory 20, 21
fornix, arterial supply 19
fosphenytoin 142
Framingham Heart Study
    prevalence of cerebral microbleeds 199
    prevalence of silent cerebral infarcts 196
Framingham risk prediction algorithm 257
fresh frozen plasma (FFP), reversal of anticoagulation 131–2
frontal syndrome 86
functional score 190

gait-based therapies 226, 238
Gasperini syndrome 89
gastric protection 144
gemfibrozil, in primary prevention 174
gender differences in outcome 249
gender differences in stroke risk 6–7, 9, 15, 256
    subarachnoid haemorrhage 61
genetic risk factors 10, 154, 159
    CCM genes 56
    for subarachnoid haemorrhage 62
genetic testing 158
geniculate bodies, arterial supply 19, 27
Geriatric Depression Scale 212
German Stroke Registers Study Group (ADSR) 273
Germany
    carer support 276
    healthcare system 270–1
    long-term follow-up 275
    pre-hospital services 271
    quality of care 272–3
    rehabilitation 275
    stroke rates 270
    stroke units 271–2
    telestroke networks 272
Gerstmann syndrome 86
GESICA study 178
Get With The Guidelines programme, mortality prediction 188
GIST-UK trial 132
Glasgow Coma Score (GCS) 139, 140
    after intracerebral haemorrhage 53
Global Agenda for Stroke vii
Global Burden of Disease Project 4
global cerebral ischaemia, after subarachnoid haemorrhage 74
globus pallidus, arterial supply 19, 24

glossopharyngeal nerve palsy
    cerebellar infarcts 91
    medullary infarcts 90
glycaemic control 110, 114–15, 132
    after subarachnoid haemorrhage 144, 147
    in secondary prevention 178, 179
glycerol therapy 128
goal setting 235–6
gradient echo (GRE), GRE susceptibility vessel sign (GRE SVS) 42–3
great cerebral vein (of Galen) 31
grey-white differentiation, loss of 94, 95
growth factors, therapeutic use 225–6
growth inhibitor blockade 226

haematological disorders 156, 161
haematoma evacuation, in supratentorial ICH 134–5
haematoma expansion 51–2
haemodilution 110
haemodynamic failure 41
haemodynamic infarction/TIA 38–40, 41
haemoglobin levels, relationship to outcome 109, 111
haemorrhagic infarcts
    causes 158
    see also intracerebral haemorrhage; subarachnoid haemorrhage
haemorrhagic transformation 56–7
    cardioembolic strokes 42, 90–1
    imaging 94–5
    risk from intravenous thrombolysis 125
    risk prediction 99
haemostatic therapy 131
haloperidol, in organic delirium 211
HAMLET (hemicraniectomy after middle cerebral artery infarction with life-threatening oedema) trial 128
HANAC (hereditary angiopathy, nephropathy, aneurysm, and muscle cramps) 10, 154
hands, physical examination 157
hazard ratio, definition 9
HDAC9 gene variations 10
headache
    basilar artery occlusion 90
    cerebellar infarcts 91
    intracerebral haemorrhage 52
    medullary infarcts 90
    posterior cerebral artery infarcts 87
    rarer causes of stroke 154–5
    subarachnoid haemorrhage 67
    thunderclap headache 56, 66, 67, 161
head position 109, 118
    after subarachnoid haemorrhage 144
health-related quality of life (HRQOL) 248
hearing loss, associated disorders 153
heart conditions, as risk factor for stroke 11–12, 13
heart failure 208
Helsinki Young Stroke Study, prevalence of silent cerebral infarcts 198
hemianopia
associated lesions 85, 86, 87, 88
recovery factors 188
hemicraniectomy 118, 128, 135
hemifacial spasms, pontine infarcts 89
heminaesthesia, medullary infarcts 90
hemiparesis, associated lesions 85, 86, 87, 88, 89, 90, 91
hemiplegia–hemianopia syndrome 88

hemisensory loss, associated lesions 85, 86, 87
heparin
    after intracerebral haemorrhage 117
    after ischaemic stroke 127–8
    DVT prophylaxis 116
        after subarachnoid haemorrhage *144*
    reversal of effect 131
hepatic dysfunction, after subarachnoid
        haemorrhage 73
hereditary haemorrhagic telangiectasia 153, *154*
HERNS (hereditary endotheliopathy, retinopathy,
        nephropathy, and strokes) 10, *154*
hiccups, associated lesions 90, 91
high-energy, high-protein diet 247–8
high-risk approach to prevention 263
hippocampal artery 27
history-taking
    intracerebral haemorrhage 57
    rarer causes of stroke 153–4
HMG-CoA reductase inhibitors *see* statins
Holter monitoring 166, 207–8
homocystinuria 10, 12, *154*, 159, 260
    B vitamin supplements 179
homonymous hemianopia, transient ischaemic
        attack 80
HOPE trial *171*
hormone replacement therapy as risk factor
        14, 260
    for subarachnoid haemorrhage 62
Horner syndrome 156
    associated lesions 90, 91
HPS study 174
HSCSG trial *171*
HTRA gene variations 10
human immunodeficiency virus (HIV),
        epidemiology 153
Hunt–Hess grading system 68, *69*, 139, *140*
hydralazine *113*
hydration *110*
hydrocephalus
    after subarachnoid haemorrhage 140, *144*
        acute *73*
        subacute or chronic 74–5
    prevention of 136
hydrochlorothiazide, in secondary prevention
        171
hyperbaric oxygen therapy 111
hyperdense artery sign 94, *95*
hyperglycaemia 132
    after subarachnoid haemorrhage 147
    effect on outcome 114
    management 115
hypernatraemia, after subarachnoid
        haemorrhage 146
hypertension
    arteriolosclerosis 54
    intracerebral haemorrhage *55*
    management
        in acute stroke 111–*12*, *113*, 130–1
        after subarachnoid haemorrhage 140, *144*
        secondary prevention 170–*3*
    relationship to outcome 111–12
    as a risk factor 11, 14–15, 53, 170, 256–8
        for silent cerebral infarcts 197
        for subarachnoid haemorrhage 62
    see also intracranial hypertension
hyperthermia
    infections 203
    management *109*, 112, 114, 132
        after subarachnoid haemorrhage *144*, 147

hypertonic saline, osmotherapy 118, 133, 141
hyperventilation, effect on intracranial pressure
        118, 134
hyperviscosity states *156*, 161
hypokalaemia 146
hypomagnesaemia 146
hyponatraemia 73, 146–7
    management *144*
hypoperfusion 38–40
    moyamoya disease 44
    Takayasu disease 44
hypothalamus, arterial supply 19, 26
hypothermia 132
    neuroprotection 114, 127
hypoxia
    causes 109
        low haemoglobin 109
        sleep-disordered breathing 109–10
    hyperbaric oxygen therapy 111
    oxygen therapy 108–9

ICD-10 criteria, diagnosis of vascular dementia
        217
ICH score *53*, *190*
ICSS trial *176*, 177
ICTUS (International Citicoline Trial on acUte
        Stroke) 127
imaging 157–8
    arterial 99–101, *100*
    cardiac 101
    cerebral microbleeds 199
    in dementia 216
    after intracerebral haemorrhage 57–8
    in pneumonia *204*
    of silent cerebral infarcts *195*–6
    after subarachnoid haemorrhage 70–1
    after transient ischaemic attack 83
    venous 101
    of venous thromboembolism *205*
    see also angiography; computed tomography;
        magnetic resonance imaging
immobilization, associated disorders 153
IMPACT 24 trial 127
impaired glucose tolerance, stroke risk 258
incidence
    age-adjusted rates *5*, *6*, *256*
    definition *2*
    geographical variation *256*
    in Germany and Canada 270
    high-income countries 2–4
    relationship to socioeconomic status 255
    of subarachnoid haemorrhage 61
incidence studies 1–2
    gold standards *3*
    STEP-wise approach to surveillance *3*
incontinence 244–5
indapamide, in secondary prevention 170, *171*
infections
    frequencies and causes 203–4
    as risk factor for stroke 13, 262
infective endocarditis
    diagnosis 58
    septic emboli 43–4
inferior anastomotic vein (of Labbé) 32
inferior cerebellar peduncle vein *32*
inferior petrosal sinus *30*, 31, *31*
inferior sagittal sinus *30*, *31*
inferior vena cava filters 116–17
inferior vermian vein 33
inferolateral (thalamogeniculate) infarcts 87

inferolateral thalamic arteries *see*
        thalamogeniculate arteries
inflammation
    after intracerebral haemorrhage 51
    stroke risk 262
influenza, associated stroke risk 262
infratentorial intracranial haemorrhage, clinical
        features 52
in situ thrombotic occlusion 37–8
    branch occlusion 38
insula, arterial supply 29
insulin treatment 115
    after subarachnoid haemorrhage 147
INTERACT trial 130–1
intercaverous sinus *30*
interdisciplinary approach *235*
intermittent pneumatic compression, DVT
        prophylaxis 116
internal capsule, arterial supply 19, 24
internal carotid artery (ICA) 27
    atherosclerosis 35
    perforating branches 19, *22*
    as source of embolisms 35–6, 37
internal cerebral vein *31*
internal jugular vein *31*
International Classification of Functioning,
        Disability and Health (ICF) 234, *235*
international normalized ratio (INR) 57
    reduction of 131–2
    therapeutic level maintenance 167
International Stroke Trial 3 (IST-3) 125
interpeduncular fossa artery 28
    territory *21*
interpeduncular veins *32*
INTERSTROKE study 264
Interventional Management of Stroke Part 3
        (IMS III) trial 126–7
intra-arterial thrombolysis (IAT) 126
    bridging therapy 126–7
    patient selection 99
intracerebral haemorrhage (ICH)
    aetiological workup
        history 57
        laboratory investigations 58
        radiology 57–8
    causes 53, *54*
        aneurysm rupture 73, *74*
        cerebral amyloid angiopathy 53–4
        cerebral microbleeds 54
        cerebral venous thrombosis 56
        hypertension 54, *55*
        intracranial vascular malformations 54–6
        reversible cerebral vasoconstriction
            syndrome 56
    definition and terminology 51
    diagnosis 52
        distinction from ischaemia, use of non-
            contrast CT 94
        distinction from TIA 82
    DVT prophylaxis 117
    epidemiology 2–3, 51
        proportional frequency in selected
            populations *7*
    imaging 94, 102–3, *104*
    management
        anticoagulation resumption 132
        anticoagulation reversal 131–2
        of blood pressure 130–1
        of body temperature 132
        glycaemic control 132

haemostatic therapy 131
mechanical ventilation 130
neuromonitoring 133
pulmonary embolism and deep vein
thrombosis prevention 132–3
of raised intracranial pressure 133–4
recommendations for surgical or
conservative treatment 135
seizure control 132
surgical procedures 134–6
mortality 3
pathophysiology 51–2
prognosis 189–91
prognostic scales 53
risk factors 14
oral anticoagulation 167–8
risk factors for complications 108
secondary prevention, blood pressure
lowering 172–3
volume categories 51
see also haemorrhagic transformation
intracranial atherosclerosis
arterial occlusion 37–40
secondary prevention 177–8
intracranial hypertension 133
after subarachnoid haemorrhage 73, 74–5,
140–1, 143
management 117–19, 118, 128, 133–4,
140–1, 143
pathophysiology 117
intracranial pressure monitoring 133
intracranial vascular malformations (IVMs)
arteriovenous malformations 54–5
cerebral cavernous malformations 55–6
intravenous fluid management, after
subarachnoid haemorrhage 141–2, 144
intravenous thrombolysis (IVT) 124
bridging therapy 126–7
efficacy 124–5
indications and contraindications 124
safety 125–6
intraventricular haemorrhage, external
ventricular drainage 136
intubation
after intracerebral haemorrhage 130
prognostic studies 189
involuntary movements, associated lesions 87,
89, 90
iris, disorders of 157
ISAT (International Subarachnoid
Haemorrhage Aneurysm Trial) 143
ischaemic heart disease 208
ischaemic stroke 85
clinical patterns
anterior cerebral artery infarcts 88
brainstem infarcts 89–90
cerebellar infarcts 90–1
combined hemispherical infarcts 88–9
middle cerebral artery infarcts 85–6
posterior cerebral artery infarcts 87–8
striatocapsular infarcts 86–7
differential diagnosis 94
epidemiology
incidence 2–4
proportional frequency in selected
populations 7
imaging 98–9, 103–4
diffusion MRI 96–7
non-contrast CT 94–6, 95, 96
management

antiplatelet therapy 127
blood pressure reduction, current
guidelines 173
of brain oedema and raised intracranial
pressure 128
bridging therapy 126–7
early anticoagulation 127–8
intra-arterial thrombolysis 126
intravenous thrombolysis 124–6
neuroprotection 127
thrombectomy 126
mortality 3
OCSP classification 91
pathophysiology 35
artery-to-artery embolism 35–7
cardiac embolism 41–4
hypoperfusion 38–40
large artery disease 35
non-atherosclerotic causes 155
in situ thrombotic occlusion 37–40
small artery disease 40–1
uncommon causes or mechanisms 44
prognosis
mortality prediction 188
recovery prediction 186–8
risk factors
lifestyle factors 13–14
non-modifiable factors 9–13
risk factors for complications 108
iScore model 187
mortality prediction 188

joints, physical examination 157
J-ROCKET AF trial 167, 168
JUPITER trial 263

Kawasaki disease 156, 160
epidemiology 153
KCNN3 gene 10

labetalol, in hypertension 113
laboratory investigations 158
after intracerebral haemorrhage 58
lactate, CSF levels 158
lacunar anterior circulation infarcts (LACI) 91
lacunar infarcts 38, 39, 196
in diabetes 12
hyperglycaemia 114
pontine 89
role of hypoperfusion 39–40
small artery disease 40–1
SPS3 trial 171, 172
vascular dementia 219–20
lacunar syndromes 86, 91
lamina terminalis, arterial supply 19
lamotrigine
in neuropathic pain 213
for seizures 213
large artery disease (LAD) 35
imaging 102
L-arginine, in MELAS 162
lateral medullary vein 32
lateral mesencephalic vein 32
lateral pontine artery, territory 21
lateral sinus 30–1, 31
lateropulsion, cerebellar infarcts 90, 91
LEAPS trial 226, 227
left atrial occlusion, secondary prevention
168–9
left ventricular thrombus, stroke prevention 169

lens, disorders of 157
lenticulostriate arteries 24, 26
leptomeningeal arteries 19, 27
variations 29
leucoencephalopathy
role in cognitive impairment 220
stroke risk 11
vascular dementia 219
levodopa, promotion of brain repair 226
lifestyle, risk factors for stroke 13–14
lifestyle modification 178–9
community-based interventions 263–4
low-risk lifestyle 263
Lindegaard index 146
lipid levels, as a risk factor 12, 14, 173–4, 258
lipohyalinosis, lacunar infarcts 38, 40–1
Lisch spots 157
lisuride maleate 246
locked-in syndrome 89, 90
Loeys–Dietz syndrome 154
low-density lipoprotein (LDL) reduction
intracerebral haemorrhage risk 258
role in stroke prevention 174
lower urinary tract symptoms (LUTS) 209
low-molecular-weight heparin (LMWH)
DVT prophylaxis 116, 132, 205, 245
after subarachnoid haemorrhage 144
reversal of effect 131
lumbar drains 140
lumbar puncture 158
serial 140
in subarachnoid haemorrhage 71
lupus anticoagulant, stroke risk 12

magnesium
after subarachnoid haemorrhage 146
neuroprotection 127
magnetic resonance angiography (MRA) 100,
101, 102
in subarachnoid haemorrhage 72, 73
magnetic resonance imaging (MRI) 103, 104,
157–8
after intracerebral haemorrhage 57, 103
after ischaemic stroke 85
after transient ischaemic attack 83
cerebral microbleeds 199
in dementia 216
fates of small vessel disease-related lesions
195
in subarachnoid haemorrhage 70–1
venography (MRV) 101, 102
see also diffusion MRI; FLAIR imaging
malignant MCA infarct 88–9
management 118, 128
risk prediction 117
malnutrition 247
mamillary body, arterial supply 26
management
of intracerebral haemorrhage, medical
therapies 130–4
multidisciplinary approach 106, 119–20
nutrition 247–8
promotion of brain repair 225–7
of rarer causes of stroke 161–2
see also decompressive surgery; supportive
care; thrombectomy; thrombolysis
mania 246
mannitol, osmotherapy 118, 128, 133
Marfan syndrome 10, 154, 155, 157
intracranial aneurysms 63

mass approach to prevention 263
MATCH trial *164*, 165, 166
mean transit time (MTT) 98
mechanical heart valves, secondary prevention of stroke 169
median callosal artery 19
Mediterranean diet 261
medulla, arterial supply *20*, 28, 29
medullary infarcts 89–90
MELT (Middle Cerebral Artery Embolism Local Fibrinolytic Intervention Trial) 126
memantine 221
memory defects 217
    associated lesions 87, 88
    in subcortical vascular dementia 219
meningeal spaces, anatomy *62*
meningeal symptoms, subarachnoid haemorrhage 68
menopause, changes in stroke risk 9
mental status examination 216
Merci Retriever 126
mesencephalic infarcts 89
mesencephalic vein 33
metabolic disorders *157*, 161
metabolic syndrome 261–2
methylclothiazide, in secondary prevention *171*
metoprolol, in hypertension *113*
microalbuminuria, stroke risk 258
microbleeds *see* cerebral microbleeds
microscopic polyangiitis 160
midbrain, arterial supply *21*, 29
middle cerebral artery (MCA) *27*
    aneurysm of 63–4
    leptomeningeal branches 27
    perforating branches 24, 26
        variations 29
middle cerebral artery infarcts *37–8*, *85*, *218*
    brain oedema 117
    clinical patterns 85–6
    DWI studies 37
migraine
    distinction from TIA 82
    stroke risk 12–13, 160–1
migraine-associated infarcts 88
'Million Hearts' initiative 264
Mills–Guillain syndrome 90
Mini Mental Status Examination (MMSE) 216
mirror neurons 240
mirtazapine 211
miscarriage, associated disorders 153
MISTIE trial 135
mitochondrial encephalopathy, lactic acidosis, and stroke-like episodes (MELAS) 10, 158, 159, 161
    treatment 162
mobility training 237
modality-specific endpoints 228
Montreal Cognitive Assessment (MoCA) 216
mood changes
    vascular dementia 217
    see also depression
mortality 1
    definition *2*
    high-income countries 3
mortality prediction
    after intracerebral haemorrhage 189–91
    after ischaemic stroke 188
MOSES trial 172
motor deficits, associated lesions 85–7, 88, 89, 90

motor recovery, prognostic factors 188
motor skills training 236
mouth, physical examination 156
moyamoya disease 44, *154*, 160
    epidemiology 153
    subarachnoid haemorrhage 66
    treatment 162
multidetector CT angiography 71–2
multidisciplinary approach 106, 119–20
    in rehabilitation *235*
Multi MERCI (Multi Mechanical Embolus Removal in Cerebral Ischaemia) trial 126
multiple infarcts, causes 158
muscle biopsy 159
music therapy 241
mutism, anterior cerebral artery infarcts 88
mycotic aneurysms 66
myocardial infarction 208
myocytolysis 119

nails, physical examination 157
NASCET trial 175
National Institute of Neurological Disorders and Stroke (NINDS), Recombinant Tissue Plasminogen Activator Study 124, 125
National Institutes of Health Stroke Scale (NIHSS) 53
    prognostic significance 186, 187
        mortality prediction 188
nausea
    associated lesions 90
    subarachnoid haemorrhage 68
neck stiffness, subarachnoid haemorrhage 68
neglect
    associated lesions 85, 86–7, 88, 91
    recovery factors 188–9
NEST trials 127
net reclassification improvement (NRI) 186
neurocysticercosis 153
neuroendocrine effects of SAH 72–3
neurofibromatosis type 1 *154*
    intracranial aneurysms 63
neurogenic pulmonary oedema 147–8
neurogenic stress cardiomyopathy 72–3, 147–8, 208
    management *144*
neuromonitoring 133
neuropathic pain *213*
neuroprotection 127
    hypothermia 114
nicardipine, in hypertension *113*, 131
NICE-SUGAR trial 132
nicotinic acid, in stroke prevention 174
nimodipine
    neuroprotection 146
    in vasospastic disorders 162
NINDS–AIREN criteria, diagnosis of vascular dementia *217*
nitrendipine, in secondary prevention 172
nitroglycerine, in hypertension *113*
N-methyl-D-aspartate (NMDA) receptor blockade 127
NOMAS (Northern Manhattan Study) 261
non-valvular atrial fibrillation (NVAF)
    as cause of stroke 166
    detection 166
    secondary prevention of stroke 167–9
    see also atrial fibrillation
NOTCH3 gene variations 10, 159, 219

nutrition *110*, 115, 247–8
    after subarachnoid haemorrhage *144*
    risk factors for stroke 261
nutritional status, biochemical markers *247*
nystagmus, associated lesions 90, 91

obesity 261
    as a risk factor 14
obstructive sleep apnoea 13, 260–1
occipital sinus *30*
occipital vein *31*
occupational therapy 238
oculomotor disturbance
    associated lesions 87, 89, 90
    after subarachnoid haemorrhage 68, *69*, 74
odds ratio, definition *9*
oedema 245
    formation after intracerebral haemorrhage 51
oestrogen therapy as a risk factor 14, 15
    for subarachnoid haemorrhage 62
ophthalmic vein *31*
ophthalmological symptoms, in subarachnoid haemorrhage 68
optic chiasm, arterial supply 26
optic radiations, arterial supply 19
optic tract, arterial supply 26
optocerebral syndrome 88
oral contraceptives as a risk factor 14, 15, 260
    for subarachnoid haemorrhage 62
organic delirium 210–11
organized stroke care 270
    acute care 271–2
    carer support 276
    long-term follow-up 275–6
    monitoring quality 272–5
    pre-hospital services 271
    rehabilitation 275
    telestroke networks 272
oscillopsia 90
osmotherapy 118, 133
osteogenic protein-1 227
outcome
    gender differences 6–7
    population-based studies 1–2
oxcarbamazepine 213
Oxfordshire Community Stroke Project (OCSP), stroke subtyping classification 91
Oxford Vascular Study 9, 79, 81
oxygen therapy 108–9, 110
    hyperbaric oxygen therapy 111
    in pneumonia 204
    after subarachnoid haemorrhage *144*

pain 213
palatal myoclonus, pontine infarcts 89
paramedian thalamic arteries (thalamoperforating arteries) 19, 26
paramedian thalamic infarcts 87
paraterminal gyrus, arterial supply 19
parietal MCA branch territory infarcts 86
parkinsonian symptoms, anterior cerebral artery infarcts 88
paroxysmal atrial fibrillation 43
partial anterior circulation infarct (PACI) 91
passive smoking, stroke risk 13
patent foramen ovale (PFO) 11–12, 13, 44
    secondary prevention of stroke 169–*70*, *171*
pathophysiology
    of intracerebral haemorrhage 51–2
    of ischaemic stroke and TIA 35

artery-to-artery embolism 35–7
cardiac embolism 41–4
hypoperfusion 38–40
large artery disease 35
in situ thrombotic occlusion 37–8
small artery disease 40–1
uncommon causes or mechanisms 44
PATS trial *171*
PC Trial 169, *170*, *171*
pelvic muscle training 209
penumbra 39
brain injury minimization 106
fate of, influencing factors *107*
Penumbra System 126
Percheron artery 87
percutaneous endoscopic gastrostomy (PEG) 115, 247
FOOD trials 248
perforating arteries 19, 24, 26
occlusion of 38, *39*
variations 29
perfusion imaging 97–8
perfusion thresholds 98
pericallosal artery 27
perindopril, in secondary prevention 170, *171*
periodontitis, as risk factor for stroke 13
perivascular spaces, distinction from silent cerebral infarcts 195, *196*
PFO-ASA study 169, 170
phenprocoumon, reversal of effect 131–2
phenylephrine, in delayed cerebral ischaemia 146
phenylpropanolamine abuse 66–7
phenytoin 142
phlebography 205, *206*
physical activity *see* exercise
physical examination, signs of rarer causes of stroke 155–7
pial arteries (leptomeningeal arteries) 19, 27
variations 29
pial middle cerebral artery infarcts, clinical features 85
pineal vein 33
pioglitazone, in secondary prevention 178
pituitary apoplexy 66
PITX gene 10
pneumonia 110, 203–4
aspiration pneumonia 243
POINT trial *166*
polyarteritis nodosa 160
polycystic kidney disease, intracranial aneurysms 63
pons, arterial supply 20–1, 28, 28–9, 29, *30*
pontine infarcts 89, *90*
'popcorn' appearance, caverous haemangioma *103*
population attributable risk (PAR) 9
definition *2*, 9
population-based studies 1–2
gold standards *3*
in high-income countries 2–4
in low- to middle-income studies 4
STEP-wise approach to surveillance *3*
positive end-expiratory pressure (PEEP) levels 130
positron emission tomography (PET), in dementia 216
possible TIA, symptoms *80–1*
postcentral sulcus artery territory infarcts 86
posterior cerebral artery (PCA) 27–8, *27*, 29
embolic occlusion *42*

leptomeningeal branches 27
perforating branches 19
territory *21*
posterior cerebral artery infarcts *88*
clinical features 87–8
posterior choroidal arteries (PChA) 19, 26–7
posterior choroidal artery infarcts 87
posterior circulation infarcts (POCI) 91
posterior communicating artery (PCoA) *27*
perforating branches 19, *22*, 26
posterior fossa TIA, hypoperfusion *40*
posterior fossa veins 32–3
posterior inferior cerebellar artery (PICA) 27–8, 29
territory 20
variations 29
posterior inferior cerebellar artery infarcts *91*
cerebellar oedema 117
posterior parietal artery territory infarcts 86
posterior spinal artery 27
territory 20
posteromedial choroidal artery 28, 29
territory *21*
posteromedian medullary vein *32*
post-stroke dementia (PSD) 215
epidemiology 215
prognostic significance 216
post-stroke fatigue 213
precentral artery territory infarcts 86
pregabalin, in neuropathic pain *213*
pre-hospital services 271
premamillary artery 19, 26
pressure reactivity index 141
pressure ulcers 209
prevalence
definition *2*
of subarachnoid haemorrhage 61
prevention
antiplatelet medication 163–6
in patients with silent cerebral infarcts 198–9
public health strategies 7
see also primary prevention; secondary prevention
prevention paradox 263
primary angiitis of the central nervous system (PACNS) 160
primary prevention
alcohol consumption 259
atrial fibrillation management 259
'best buy' interventions *264*
blood pressure management 256–8
in chronic kidney disease 262
community-based interventions 263–4
diabetes management 258–9
dietary modification 261
dyslipidaemia management 258
exercise 261
in homocystinuria 260
and hormone replacement therapy 260
in inflammatory conditions and infections 262
in metabolic syndrome 261–2
in obstructive sleep apnoea 260–1
and oral contraceptives 260
pharmacological agents
aspirin 262–3
statins 263
public health strategies 263
in sickle cell disease 260
smoking cessation 259
weight reduction 261

PROACT II (Prolyse in Acute Cerebral Thromboembolism II) study 126
PROactive study 178
probable TIA, symptoms *80*
PRoFESS trial 163, *164*, *171*, 172
prognosis, influence of post-stroke dementia 216
prognostic scales, intracerebral haemorrhage 53
prognostic studies 185–6
intracerebral haemorrhage 189–91
ischaemic stroke
mortality prediction 188
recovery prediction 186–8
recovery of specific neurological deficits 188–9
of silent cerebral infarcts 197–8, *198*
PROGRESS trial 11, 170, *171*, 172, 173, 199
prosopagnosia 88
protamine sulphate 131
PROTECT-AF trial 168–9
prothrombin complex concentrate (PCC), reversal of anticoagulation 131–2
pseudotumoural cerebellar infarcts 91
pseudoxanthoma elasticum 10, *154*
intracranial aneurysms 63
skin changes 156
psychosis 246
psychostimulants 246
pterygoid plexus *31*
public health, preventive strategies 7, 263
pulmonary embolism (PE) 116, 205–6, 245
prevention 132–3
pulmonary oedema
after subarachnoid haemorrhage 73
neurogenic 147–8
pulvinar, arterial supply 26, 27
pupillary disorders, basilar artery occlusion 90
putamen, arterial supply 24

quality indicators *273*, *274*
quality of care, Germany and Canada 272–5
quality of life (QOL) 248
influencing factors 248–9

raised intracranial pressure *see* intracranial hypertension
ramipril, in secondary prevention 171
randomized clinical trials (RCTs), definition 2
RANTTAS trial 243
rarer causes of stroke 157
demographic features 153
diagnosis, genetic testing 158
family history 154
genetic disorders *154*, 159
haematological disorders *156*, 161
medical history 153–4
metabolic disorders *157*, 161
monogenic disorders *154*
non-atherosclerotic inflammatory arteriopathies *155*, 160
non-atherosclerotic non-inflammatory arteriopathies *155*, 159–60
physical examination 155–7
specific diagnostic tests *154*
symptoms at admission 154–5
treatment 161–2
vasospastic disorders *156*, 160–1
RE-ALIGN trial 169
rebleeding 52
after subarachnoid haemorrhage 74
risk after endovascular therapy 143
risk factors 139–40

recanalization
    after cardioembolic infarcts 42
    see also thrombectomy; thrombolysis
recombinant activated factor VII (rFVIIa)
        therapy 131
recombinant tissue plasminogen activator
        (rtPA) 124, 225
    see also thrombolysis
recovery
    spontaneous 225
    see also brain repair
recovery period, duration 187–8
recovery prediction
    ischaemic stroke 186–7
    specific neurological deficits 188–9
recreational drug use 57, 58
rectus gyrus, arterial supply 24
recurrence, prognostic studies 185
rehabilitation
    definition 234
    environmental factors 239
    family involvement 239, 249
    in Germany and Canada 275
    goal setting 235–6
    new techniques/models 240–1
    organization 234–5
        early supported discharge 239–40
        first year after discharge 240
    patient–therapist relationship 239
rehabilitation interventions
    activity 237–8
    body function 236
    participation in society 238–9
rehabilitation process 234
relative risk, definition 9
RE-LY trial 167, 168, 259
renal disease, stroke risk 13
renal transplant recipients, stroke risk 262
reperfusion injury, prevention 127
RESPECT trial 169, 171
restorative therapies 225–7
retina, disorders of 157
retro-olivary vein 32
reversible cerebral vasoconstriction syndrome
        (RCVS) 14, 56, 161
rheumatoid arthritis 154, 157, 160
rhythmic auditory stimulation 241
risk assessment tools 263
risk factors 1, 4, 9
    for cerebral microbleeds 199
    for cerebral venous thrombosis 15
    $CHADS_2/CHA_2DS_2VASc$ scores 12, 43, 44
    chronic kidney disease 262
    for complications 108
    definitions of common terms 9
    gender and ethnic differences 4–7
    homocystinuria 260
    inflammation and infections 262
    interaction 14
    for intracerebral haemorrhage 14, 53
    for ischaemic stroke
        lifestyle factors 13–14
        non-modifiable factors 9–13
    modifiable
        alcohol consumption 259
        atrial fibrillation 259
        cigarette smoking 259
        diabetes mellitus 258–9
        diet 261
        dyslipidaemia 258

exercise 261
        hormone replacement therapy 260
        hypertension 256–8
        metabolic syndrome 261–2
        obesity 261
        obstructive sleep apnoea 260–1
        oral contraceptives 260
    non-modifiable 255
    for post-stroke complications 245
    for post-stroke dementia 215
    sickle cell disease 260
    for silent cerebral infarcts 197, 198
    for subarachnoid haemorrhage 14–15, 62–3
risk prediction algorithm 257
rivaroxaban
    in atrial fibrillation 167, 168, 259
    risk of intracerebral haemorrhage 132, 167
robot-assisted therapy 226
ROCKET-AF trial 167, 168
rolandic artery territory infarcts 86
Rome criteria for constipation 210
rosiglitazone 178
Roth's spots 157
Rotterdam Scan Study
    prevalence of cerebral microbleeds 199
    prevalence of silent cerebral infarcts 196

sagittal sinus thrombosis 102
salt intake, relationship to stroke risk 14
SAMMPRIS trial 165, 177, 178
SCAST (Scandinavian Candesartan Acute
        Stroke Trial) 112
sclera, disorders of 157
SCOPE trial 171
secondary prevention
    antiplatelet medication 163–6
    blood pressure management 170–3
    of cardioembolic stroke 166–70, 171
    carotid surgery and stenting 174–7
    cholesterol levels 173–4
    intracranial atherosclerosis 177–8
    lifestyle modification 178–9
    patients with dementia 221
    in patients with silent cerebral infarcts 198–9
    prevention of early recurrence 106
sedation 109
seizures 213
    after intracerebral haemorrhage 52, 132
    after subarachnoid haemorrhage 68, 74, 142
    focal, distinction from TIA 82
    management 110, 132, 142
    prophylaxis 144
selective serotonin reuptake inhibitors
        (SSRIs) 246
    in anxiety 247
sensory loss
    associated lesions 85–6, 87, 88, 90, 91
    recovery factors 189
sentinel headache 67
SENTIS trial 127
septal nuclei, arterial supply 19
septic emboli 57
septum pellucidum, arterial supply 19
severity of impairment, prognostic significance
        186, 187, 188
sickle cell disease 10, 154, 159, 161
    as cause of subarachnoid haemorrhage 66
    epidemiology 153
    primary prevention of stroke 260
    treatment 162

side of stroke, relationship to quality of life 249
SIFAP study, prevalence of silent cerebral
        infarcts 198
sigmoid sinus 30–1
silent cerebral infarcts (SCIs)
    definitions and terminology 194
    diagnostic issues 194–5
    discovery 194
    occurrence after stroke 198
    in patients without prior TIA and stroke
        effects and prognostic implication 197–8
        imaging characteristics 196
        management 198
        prevalence 196, 197
        risk factors 197
    in patients with symptomatic cerebral
        ischaemia 198
    prognostic significance 197, 198
    stroke risk 11
simvastatin, in secondary prevention 174
single-nucleotide polymorphisms (SNPs) 10
SITS-MOST (Safe Implementation of
        Thrombolysis in Stroke-MOnitoring
        STudy) 125
Six Simple Variables prognostic model 186, 187
skin, physical examination 155–6
skin biopsy 158–9
skin care 209
sleep-disordered breathing (SDB) 109–10, 260–1
Sleep Heart Health Study 261
small artery disease (SAD) 40–1
SMART Study, prevalence of silent cerebral
        infarcts 196
smoking
    'best buy' interventions 264
    community-based interventions 264
    as a risk factor 13, 14–15, 259
        for subarachnoid haemorrhage 62
smoking cessation 178
Sneddon syndrome 154, 155, 156
socioeconomic factors in stroke risk 4, 14, 255
sodium nitroprusside, in hypertension 113
Solitaire flow restoration device 126
SPACE trial 176, 177
SPAF III (Stroke Prevention in Atrial
        Fibrillation III) trial 259
SPARCL trial 174
spasticity, treatment 236
sphenoparietal sinus 30, 31
spinal arteriovenous malformations 64
SPIRIT trial 165
splenial artery 27
spontaneous intracerebral haemorrhage 51
'spot' sign 57, 103
SPS3 (Secondary Prevention of Small
        Subcortical Strokes) trial 164, 165,
        171, 172
SSS- TOAST (Stop Stroke Study Trial of Org
        10172) classification 46–7
statins
    after subarachnoid haemorrhage 146
    risk reduction 174, 258, 263
        in diabetes 259
status epilepticus 213
stem cell therapies 226
stents 126
    carotid artery 176–7
    for intracranial stenosis 177, 178
STEP-wise approach to surveillance 3
sterotactic haematoma removal 135

STICH (Surgical Trial in Intracerebral Haemorrhage) 134–5
STOP (Stroke Prevention Trial in Sickle Cell Anaemia) 260
straight sinus 30, 31
strategic infarct vascular dementia 218
stress, as risk factor 14
striatocapsular infarcts 87
    clinical features 86–7
string-of-beads appearance 159
Stroke Adapted Sickness Impact Profile (SA-SIP30) 248
stroke burden
    high-income countries 2–4
    low- to middle-income countries 4
stroke centres, effectiveness 119–20
stroke data bank score 190
Stroke Impact Scale (SIS) 248
Stroke Specific Quality of Life Measure (SS-QOL) 248
stroke subtypes, population differences 7
stroke syndromes 10
stroke units
    certification 272
    in Germany and Canada 271–2
subarachnoid haemorrhage (SAH)
    aneurysm repair 142–3, 144
    causes 63
        arteriovenous malformations 55
        benign idiopathic SAH 63
        convexal SAH 63, 94, 95
        diagnosis of 71–2, 73
        intracranial aneurysms 63
        rare medical causes 66–7
    clinical features
        headache 67
        neurological examination 68–9
        presentation 67–8
    clinical scores 139, 140
    complications 147
        acute 72–4
        delayed cerebral ischaemia 145–6
        electrolyte disturbances 146–7
        secondary 74–5
    definition 61
    diagnosis
        differentiation from ischaemia 94
        imaging 70–1
        lumbar puncture 71
    epidemiology 61–2
        incidence in high-income countries 2–3
        proportional frequency in selected populations 7
    gender differences in risk 9
    management 140, 144–5
        of intracranial hypertension 140–1, 143
        new therapies 148
        of seizures 142
        of volume status 141–2
    mortality 3
    prognosis 139
    risk factors 14–15, 62–3
subarachnoid space 62
subcallosal gyrus, arterial supply 19, 24
subclavian steal syndrome 44
subcortical infarcts see lacunar infarcts
subcortical vascular dementia 219–20
subdural haematoma
    after subarachnoid haemorrhage 73

differentiation from ischaemia 94
differentiation from TIA 82
subdural space 62
subhyaloidal haemorrhages (Terson syndrome) 68, 69
suboccipital craniectomy 118–19
suicidal ideation 247
superficial middle cerebral artery infarcts, clinical features 85
superior anastomotic vein (of Trolard) 32
superior cerebellar artery (SCA) 27–8, 29
    territory 21
superior cerebellar artery infarcts, clinical features 90–1
superior petrosal sinus 30, 31, 31
superior petrosal vein (of Dandy) 32, 33
superior sagittal sinus 30, 31
supportive care
    blood pressure management 111–12
        pharmacological agents 113
    body temperature management 112, 114
    brain oedema management 117–19
    cardiac function monitoring 119
    DVT and PE prevention and treatment 115–17
    dysphagia evaluation and nutrition 115
    general issues 109
    glycaemic control 114–15
    goals 106–8
    maintenance of tissue oxygenation 108–11
    specific issues 110
supratentorial intracranial haemorrhage
    clinical features 52
    haematoma evacuation 134–5
    hemicraniectomy 118, 128, 135
susceptibility-weighted MRI 103
swallowing dysfunction see dysphagia
sylvian 'dot' sign 94, 95
syndrome of inappropriate antidiuretic hormone secretion (HSIADH) 73, 146–7;
systemic lupus erythematosus (SLE) 154, 155, 156, 157, 160
    treatment 162

T2-weighted MRI see FLAIR imaging
Takayasu disease 44, 160
    epidemiology 153
Takotsubo cardiomyopathy syndrome (transient cardiac ballooning syndrome) 72–3, 119, 208
    management 144
tamoxifen, as risk factor 14
TARDIS trial 166
teamwork, rehabilitation 235
telestroke networks 272
telmisartan, in secondary prevention 171, 172
temporal artery biopsy 159
temporal evolution
    of haematomas 103
    of ischaemic lesions 95–6
temporal MCA territory infarcts 86
Terson syndrome 68, 69
TEST trial 171
thalamic infarcts 87, 218
thalamogeniculate arteries (inferolateral thalamic arteries) 26
thalamoperforating arteries (paramedian thalamic arteries) 19, 26
thalamus, arterial supply 19, 26, 27, 29

thalassaemia, epidemiology 153
THAM (tris-hydroxy-methyl-aminomethan, tromethamine) 133–4
therapeutic windows 106, 107, 227
    for intravenous thrombolysis 125
thiazides, in secondary prevention 170, 171
three-tube test, subarachnoid haemorrhage 71
thrombectomy 126
    in rarer causes of stroke 161
thromboembolism
    prophylaxis 116–17, 132
    see also deep vein thrombosis; pulmonary embolism
thrombolysis 225
    bridging therapy 126–7
    impact on stroke subtype presentation 85
    implications of cerebral microbleeds 199–200
    intra-arterial 126
    intravenous 124
        efficacy 124–5
        indications and contraindications 124
        safety 125–6
    intraventricular 136
    patient selection
        blood pressure 112
        imaging 99
    patients with dementia 221
    in rarer causes of stroke 161
    therapeutic window 107
    use in Germany 273
thrombophilias 115–16
    history-taking 153
thunderclap headache 67, 154
    cerebral venous thrombosis 66
    reversible cerebral vasoconstriction syndrome 56, 161
time-of-flight (TOF) MRA 101, 102
time since stroke, relationship to quality of life 249
time to peak (TTP), perfusion imaging 97, 98
time trends, in subarachnoid haemorrhage 62
'tissue clock', FLAIR imaging 97
TOAST (Trial of Org 10172 in Acute Stroke Treatment) classification 45–7, 46, 153
top of the basilar syndrome
    basilar artery occlusion 90
    cardioembolic strokes 91
    cerebellar infarcts 90
torcular herophilii 30, 31
total anterior circulation infarcts (TACI) 91
total parenteral nutrition 248
tranexamic acid 140
transcranial Doppler ultrasound 99, 101, 102
    diagnosis of vasospasm 143–6
transcranial duplex sonography (TDS), after intracerebral haemorrhage 58
transient cardiac ballooning syndrome (Takotsubo cardiomyopathy syndrome) 72–3, 119, 144, 208
transient global amnesia (TGA), distinction from TIA 82
transient ischaemic attack (TIA)
    definition 79
    diagnosis 83
        imaging 80, 94–7, 98
        inter-observer agreement 81
    differential diagnoses 81–2, 94
    pathophysiology 35
        artery-to-artery embolism 35–7
        cardiac embolism 41–4

transient ischaemic attack (TIA) (*Cont.*)
    hypoperfusion 38–*40*
    large artery disease 35
    small artery disease 40–1
    uncommon causes or mechanisms 44
  prognostic studies 185
  stroke risk 11
    predictors of early stroke (ABCD² score) 81
  symptoms
    clinical features 79–81, *80*
    duration 79
transoesophageal echocardiography (TOE)
    see echocardiography
transthoracic echocardiography (TTE)
    see echocardiography
transverse sinus 30, 31
trauma, associated disorders 153–4
traumatic subarachnoid haemorrhage 70
trazodone 246
treadmill training *237*
Treating to New Targets trial 174
tremor, associated lesions 87, 88, 90
Trevo receiver 126
TREX mutations 10, *154*
tricyclic antidepressants 246
trigeminal nerve deficits
    cerebellar infarcts 91
    medullary infarcts 90
triglyceride levels, relationship to stroke risk 14
triple H therapy 146
tromethamine (THAM) 133–4
troponin levels 119, 147–8, 208
tuberothalamic infarcts 87
tumours, differentiation from ischaemia 94, *96*

ultrasound examination
    of bladder 209
    see also Doppler ultrasound imaging
uncus, arterial supply 27
urinary control *110*
urinary tract infections 203, 244–5

vagus nerve palsy
    cerebellar infarcts 91
    medullary infarcts 90
VA-HIT trial 174
valproic acid 213
VASCT trial 175
vascular dementia (VaD) 215, *216–17*
    in absence of detectable stroke lesions 216
    clinical patterns 217
    diagnosis 216–17

epidemiology
    after stroke 215
    patients without clinical evidence of
      stroke 216
  management 221
  multifactorial origin 220–*1*
  subtypes 218–20
vasculitides 44, *155*, 160
    as cause of subarachnoid haemorrhage 66, *67*
    treatment 162
vasospasm 74, *143*, *156*, 160–1
    management 146, 162
    monitoring for 143–6
    prevention 146
VECTORS trial 226
venous circulation 30, *31*
    cortical cerebral veins 32
    deep cerebral veins 31–2
    dural venous sinuses 30–31
    posterior fossa veins *32–3*
venous imaging 101, 102
venous sinus thrombosis
    hemicraniectomy 135
    imaging *102*
venous thromboembolism 115–17, 205–6, 245
    see also deep vein thrombosis; pulmonary
      embolism
ventilatory support *109*, 130
ventricular ectopic beats 207
ventricular tachycardia 207
ventriculostomy 128
vermis, arterial supply 29
vertebral artery 27–8
    dissection 66
    dural arteriovenous fistula 65
    as source of embolisms 37
    territory *20*
vertebral artery occlusion, clinical features 90
vertebrobasilar TIA, suggestive symptoms *80*, 81
vertigo
    associated lesions 86, 89, 90, 91
      transient ischaemic attack 80
vestibular signs, medullary infarcts 90
vestibulocochlear nerve palsies 91
video games, use in rehabilitation 240–1
Virchow's postulate 115
virtual reality training 240–1
visual agnosia 88
visual field defects
    associated lesions 86, 87, 88, 89
    cardioembolic infarcts 91
    rarer causes 156–7

recovery factors 188
transient ischaemic attack 80
vitamin supplements
    in primary prevention 260
    in secondary prevention 179
VITATOPS trial 179
Vitoria Sleep Project 261
vocational rehabilitation 238–9
vomiting
    associated lesions 90, 91
    intracerebral haemorrhage 52
    subarachnoid haemorrhage 68

walking ability
    recovery factors 189
    rehabilitation 237–8
Wallenberg's syndrome 90, 91
    cardioembolic strokes 91
WARCEF trial 169
warfarin
    in atrial fibrillation 259
    DVT treatment 117
    implications of cerebral microbleeds 200
    reversal of effect 131–2
    risk of intracerebral haemorrhage 167–8
    secondary prevention
      comparison with antiplatelet therapy
        163, *165*
      patients with intracranial stenosis 177
      patients with left ventricular
        thrombus 169
      patients with mechanical heart
        valves 169
WARSS trial *165*
WASID trial *165*, 177, *178*
WATCHMAN device 168–9
WATCH trial 169
Wegener's granulomatosis 160
weight reduction 248, 261
Wernicke's aphasia 86
    cardioembolic strokes 91
white matter disease *see* leucoencephalopathy
white matter hyperintensity *195*, *196*
    effects and prognostic implication 197–8
within-subject treatment effects 228–9
work, return to 238–9
World Federation of Neurological Surgeons
    (WFNS) grading system 68, *69*, 139, *140*

xanthochromia, CSF 71

ZHFX3 gene 10

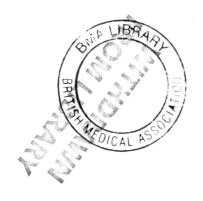